TEXTBOOK OF IMMUNOLOGY

An Introduction to Immunochemistry and Immunobiology

TEXTBOOK OF IMMUNOLOGY

An Introduction to Immunochemistry and Immunobiology

James T. Barrett, Ph.D.

Professor of Microbiology
University of Missouri School of Medicine
Columbia, Missouri

FIFTH EDITION

With 198 illustrations

The C. V. Mosby Company

St. Louis • Washington, D.C. • Toronto   1988

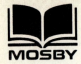

MOSBY

A TRADITION OF PUBLISHING EXCELLENCE

Editor: Stephanie Bircher
Assistant Editor: Anne Gunter
Project Manager: Teri Merchant
Manuscript Editor: EDP
Production Editor: Suzanne C. Glazer
Design: Susan E. Lane

Cover photo: © Frieder Michler–Peter Arnold, Inc.

FIFTH EDITION

The C. V. Mosby Company
11830 Westline Industrial Drive, St. Louis, Missouri 63146

Library of Congress Cataloging-in-Publication Data

Barrett, James T., 1927-
   Textbook of immunology.

   Includes bibliographies and index.
   1. Immunology.   I. Title.   [DNLM: 1. Immunity.
2. Immunochemistry.   3. Serology.   QW 504 B274t]
QR181.B28   1987   616.07'9   87-21987
ISBN 0-8016-0530-X

C/VH/VH   9 8 7 6 5 4 3 2 1   02/B/247

To
my former students

They who are not in the habit of conducting experiments
may not be aware of the coincidence of circumstances necessary
for their being managed so as to prove perfectly decisive;
nor how often men engaged in professional pursuits are liable
to interruptions which disappoint them almost at the instant
of their being accomplished: however, I feel no room for hesitation. . . .

Edward Jenner, 1798

Preface

Before writing this, I reread the preface to the first edition of this text. That preface was written in 1969, and the book was published in 1970. At that time, I stated that immunology was experiencing a rebirth, not only because of developments within its own science, but also through the application of its methodology into other subjects. Inevitably, these other sciences—biochemistry and genetics to mention two—were also influencing the thinking of immunologists. Thus I claimed that teachers and students of immunology needed more breadth of information and instruction than ever before. Toward that goal, this text was designed to present immunology in its broadest sense, simultaneously incorporating data from other biologic and chemical sciences. This goal has been retained in subsequent editions, including the present.

In 1970 there were only a handful of journals dealing with immunology. Today, it is claimed that there are more than 50 journals with the word *immunology,* or other derivations of its Latin origin, in their title. Scores of other journals occasionally publish articles on immunologic subjects. The American Association of Immunologists claims over 4000 members. Some of these immunologists are trying to repair immunodeficiencies, and others, in their attempts to suppress the rejection of a transplant, are creating an immunodepressed state. While some use hormones to stimulate immunoreactive cells and enhance immunity, others are trying to suppress these same cells in order to relieve an autoimmune disease. These examples indicate the extremes within which present-day immunologists work and emphasize the breadth of understanding immunologists need for a successful application of their talents. This breadth of understanding, in addition to adequate education in other sciences, commences with a strong general education in immunology itself. Toward this purpose, this fifth edition of *Textbook of Immunology* does not (nor should any general text) omit a description of allergy in order to emphasize the genetics of the immunoglobulins, nor does it devote chapter after chapter to cellular immunology, thereby forcing a discussion of serology or immunity to so few pages that it approaches an apology. Yes, the goal here remains the same—to provide a well-balanced discussion from the broad view needed by students in their first course in immunology. I believe this goal is perhaps even more worthy in this age of specialization than it was earlier. In an age of specialization, it is easy to be ignorant of subjects that border on your own specialty unless the early stages of your education are sufficient to prevent this.

I find it amusing that virtually every preface ends with an apology and a statement of gratitude. The apology is included for those inevitable errors that are the responsibility of the author. The thank you recognizes colleagues, artists, secretaries, students, the publisher, and others who have helped in the preparation of the work. I can find no honest way to avoid the former and little to strengthen the importance of the latter, but it is true this text would not be possible without the truly excellent assistance of Karen Ehlert, Arlene Dethloff, Barbro Barrett, and many enthusiasts of the C.V. Mosby Company.

The generosity of Eugene Garfield and ISI Press to permit the use of Citation Classics from Current Contents, Life Sciences, **25**(20):20, 1982; **25**(46): 14, 1982; **26**(15):26, 1983; **27**(27):20, 1984; **27**(27): 21, 1984; and, **28**(3):19, 1985 is especially appreciated.

James T. Barrett

Preface to the first edition

In its most recent growth, immunology has expanded from its origins in the medical sciences to permeate all of biology. The recognition by biologists of immunologic methods as important and sensitive research weapons has been responsible in a large measure for this rebirth of immunology. At the same time the utilization of modern biochemical knowledge and technology has given immunologists a new insight into their own science. These developments have presented additional problems to both students and teachers of immunology. On the one hand, undergraduate students who have had little opportunity to master complex chemical and biologic problems are drawn early to immunology as an exciting and "new" science. On the other hand, students who might have been content to continue in their chosen specialty now see a need to include immunology in their curriculum. The teacher is thus presented with a more varied audience than ever before. A partial solution to this dilemma is a textbook of immunology that will be equally useful to undergraduate and graduate students. This does not necessarily mean that the interests of students in the health sciences have been ignored, as is pointed out below.

To meet the demands of a broad audience the contents of this book have been tailored in several ways. First, the book is intended as a general textbook of immunology—one that overemphasizes neither immunochemistry nor immunobiology. Consequently complementary sections on the chemistry of the immunoglobulins and immunochemistry are balanced by sections on the phylogeny of the immune response and cellular aspects of the immunoglobulin response. A similar balance has been attempted in other sections. For example, the chapters on immunity and hypersensitivity, subjects of considerable interest to students in the medical and paramedical sciences, have been developed from the viewpoint that the fundamentals of these topics are essential to all students of immunology. Second, the references have been limited and chosen to emphasize reviews and specialty books. Several excellent immunologic review series are now available. These provide extended discussions of various items and lengthy bibliographies. In this way a broad base of additional readings has been provided without the necessity of a voluminous and, all too soon, outdated bibliography in this volume. Only a few students have the time for extensive outside reading during their course work in any case. Third, a brief appendix, which summarizes the highlights of macromolecular biochemistry, is included for those who are as yet uninitiated or need a quick refresher on the subject. Fourth, a genuine effort has been made to use a concise and intelligible writing style.

Introspection is an unreliable witness to the origin of ideas, and this is no more evident that in authorship. Many of the concepts incorporated here were derived from my past professors, current colleagues, and perhaps, most vitally, interested students. To this legion, I give a salute of gratitude, with the hope that my efforts have in some small measure been worthy of them. Of those persons whom I wish to name, that of my wife, Barbro, must come first, both for her many hours of silent support and her active participation as an artist. To those wonderful girls at the typewriters, especially Anne, Carol, Linda, and Vera, I give my thanks for a job well done.

J.T.B.

ix

Contents

FOUNDATION OF IMMUNOLOGY

The history of immunology

≡ GLOSSARY

antitoxin An antibody (or antiserum) prepared in response to a toxin or toxoid.

attenuation Weakening the virulence of a pathogenic organism while retaining its viability.

immunity Condition of being resistant to an infection.

Within the last decades immunology has emerged as an individual science, and, like all modern sciences, it draws from and contributes to many other closely related biologic and chemical sciences, including microbiology, biochemistry, genetics, medicine, zoology, and pathology. The recent outburst of advances in immunology has followed very closely and in some instances has been responsible for notable progress in these other sciences. Virtually the entire history of immunology has been recorded in the past 100 years; even if we calculate the origin of immunology from the time of the introduction of smallpox vaccination into the western world, immunology has existed for only about 150 years. During that time the development of immunology and the sciences on which it has depended has been gradual and uneven. Consequently it is only within the past century that the growth of subdisciplines within the area of immunology has become apparent.

The first of the subdivisions of immunology to emerge was *immunity*. In its infancy immunology was devoted almost exclusively to the prevention of infectious diseases by vaccination and immunization. In the 1880s immunology and immunity were synonymous, but this is no longer true. Even though considerable effort still is being directed toward the improvement of old vaccines and toward the improvement of immunizing techniques, new topics such as synthetic vaccines, genetically engineered vaccines, and new adjuvants and the fantastic recent advances in cell-mediated immunity have magnified immunity as a distinct discipline within the broader subject of immunology.

Serology also could be thought of as a subdivision of immunity, but it is such a vast subject that it deserves an equal status. Like immunity, serology has obvious practical implications for human and veterinary medicine, but as a diagnostic rather than a preventive aid. Today's serologists seek not only to discover new specific serologic tests for disease, such as those employing fluorescent, electron microscopy or enzyme-labeled antibodies, but also to improve existing serologic techniques, analyze the behavior of serum complement, and purify and improve antigen and antiserum preparations.

A third subdivision of immunology emerged with the others at the turn of the twentieth century. It attempted to view immunologic phenomena primarily as macromolecular phenomena, as expressions of complex chemical reactions between antigens and haptens with immunoglobulins and complement. In the beginning this new area of *immunochemistry* was almost totally dominated by Landsteiner and his studies with haptens. Gradually, as biochemical and biophysical procedures became more sophisticated, macromolecular antigens, antibodies, and complement became subjects of truer chemical investigation. Already vast rewards have been harvested, including a knowledge of the chemical basis of antigenic determinants, the structure and chemistry—including the nucleotide and amino acid sequence—of immunoglobulins, the chemistry of complement, the means by which the components of the complement system influence chemotaxis and anaphylaxis, and the chemistry of immunosuppression.

In contrast to immunochemistry, a fourth area, perhaps poorly described as *immunobiology* but certainly based on broad biologic principles, has evolved. Many aspects of immunobiology are primarily immunologically oriented; theories of antibody formation, development of allergies and hypersensitivities, immunologic tolerance, and the origin of autoimmune disease are examples, but these and subjects such as the genetics of the immune response, the cellular biology of immunology, and transplantation and tumor immunity all have obvious ramifications into other biologic sciences.

These four subdivisions *(immunity, serology, immunochemistry,* and *immunobiology)* encompass the field of immunology as it exists today. The dividing lines between these areas of immunology are all but invisible and in fact make subdivision rather artificial. Consideration of these four entities as individual units is intended only as an organizational convenience. After all, if a scientist is studying the chemistry of the transplantation antigens involved in serologic tests for tissue rejection, it is clear that scientist is working in all four of the subdisciplines of immunology. Indeed several immunologists have made important contributions of nearly equal importance in two or more areas of immunology, although these contributions have been categorized somewhat arbitrarily in the following pages. The Nobel Prize in Physiology and Medicine has been awarded to several of these scientists whose discoveries were of paramount importance to science as a whole (Table 1-1).

IMMUNITY

The first exciting area of study for immunologists and the foundation for the whole of immunology was that of immunity to infectious diseases. Many unrecorded observers must have noted that the contraction of and recovery from certain diseases resulted in

TABLE 1-1

Nobel prize winners in immunology and closely related subjects

1901	Emil von Behring	Antiserum therapy
1905	Robert Koch	Tuberculosis research
1908	Paul Ehrlich	Theories of immunity
	Elie Metchnikoff	Phagocytosis
1912	Alexis Carrell	Organ grafting
1913	Charles Richet	Anaphylaxis
1919	Jules Bordet	Complement and theories of immunity
1930	Karl Landsteiner	Human blood groups
1951	Max Theiler	Yellow fever vaccine
1957	Daniel Bovet	Antihistamine research
1960	Macfarlane Burnet and Peter Medawar	Immunologic tolerance
1972	Rodney R. Porter and Gerald M. Edelman	Structure of immunoglobulins
1977	Rosalyn Yalow	Radioimmunoassay
1980	Baruj Benacerraf, Jean Dausset, and George Snell	Immunogenetics and histocompatibility
1984	Cesar Milstein, Georges Köhler, and Nils Jerne	Hybridoma technology and contributions to theoretical immunology
1987	Susumu Tonegawa	Immunoglobulin genetics

a permanent resistance to recurrence of the same illness. Despite such knowledge among the lay population, it was not until the early eighteenth century that the purposeful contraction of a disease with the intent of creating immunity came under study. The disease was smallpox.

Although ancient Chinese and Arabic writings recorded the deliberate transmission of smallpox to healthy persons by inhalation of powdered smallpox crusts from diseased persons, immunization against smallpox was not practiced in the western world until 1721. Even so, this followed by several years correspondence to the Royal Society by physicians traveling to China and Turkey that the custom was widespread there. Credit is given to Lady Mary Wortley Montagu, wife of the British Ambassador to Turkey, for introducing variolization to England and Europe. Shortly after her arrival in Turkey in 1717 Lady Montagu wrote to a friend in England*:

> The small-pox, so fatal, and so general amongst us, is here entirely harmless. . . . People send to one another to know if any of their family has a mind to have the small-pox: they make parties for this purpose, and when they are met (commonly 15 or 16 together), the old woman comes with a nutshell of the matter of the best sort of small-pox, and asks what vein you please to have opened. She immediately rips open that you offer her, with a large needle (which gives you no more pain than a common scratch) and puts into the vein, as much matter as can lie upon the head of her needle. . . . There is no example of anyone that had died in it: and you may believe I am well satisfied of the safety of this experiment, since I intend to try it on my dear little son. I am patriot enough to take pains to bring this useful invention into fashion in England.

Lady Montagu was faithful to this proclamation and had her son inoculated in March of 1718. Three years later her daughter became the first person to be so immunized in England.

Despite the favorable claims for variolization (smallpox was then known as variola), it was not without hazard. The disease did not always take the mild course seen in the donor, and occasional infec-

*From Dixon, C.W.: Smallpox, London, 1962, J. & A. Churchill, Ltd.

tions of other types such as leprosy or syphilis were transmitted. Still the risk was less than that from acquiring "wild smallpox," which was extremely disfiguring, if not fatal. Variolization became widespread in England and in the American colonies and by the middle of the eighteenth century was common in central Europe.

Shortly after this time a more scientific and far safer approach to smallpox immunization was developed by Edward Jenner, a country physician in England (Fig. 1-1). Jenner (1749-1823), a vicar's son, was born in May 1749. By the time he was 13 years old he exhibited an intense interest in nature and was apprenticed to a physician. He was later a student in London but returned to his hometown to practice medicine; he also pursued interests in zoology, music, and poetry.

Jenner's observations on cowpox and smallpox spanned a quarter of a century before he performed his famous experiment. He became impressed, first

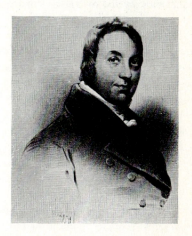

FIG. 1-1
Edward Jenner (1749-1823). From his objective observations that milkmaids who contracted cowpox were thereafter resistant to smallpox, Jenner transformed rumor into a scientific procedure that saved millions of lives. Jenner's announcement in 1798 of a new method of vaccination was at first rebuked, but since it was based on sound scientific fact, it was soon accepted as the great immunologic discovery that it truly was. (From Smith, A.L.: Principles of microbiology, ed. 6, St. Louis, 1969, The C.V. Mosby Co.)

by rumor and later by his own observations, that persons who acquired cowpox were thereafter protected against smallpox. Cowpox is a mild viral pox of cattle that is easily transmitted to herders and dairy workers.

Jenner's experiments with cowpox and smallpox are said to have begun on May 14, 1796, when he transferred matter from a cowpox lesion on the hand of Sarah Nelmes to the arm of a lad named James Phipps. Nearly 6 weeks later he subjected young Master Phipps to an inoculation of pus taken directly from a smallpox pustule. No infection followed. By 1798 Jenner had published a booklet on the nature of cowpox and how it prevented variola. After an initial few years of resistance and neglect, jennerian vaccination became accepted. Today there is some dispute about whether Jenner's vaccine virus was cowpox or some other virus. The present vaccine virus is not identical to cowpox. Jennerian vaccination has eliminated smallpox as a human disease, according to a declaration made by the World Health Organization in 1979.

That for almost a century no further advances in immunity followed Jenner's discovery is not really surprising, since the infectious agents were just then being described, and it was still uncertain which organisms caused a specific disease. Pure culture techniques were just being developed, and many uncertainties surrounded the sparse understanding of microorganisms. In addition, smallpox was a very exceptional case—it is one of the few diseases that is entirely preventable by recovery from another closely related illness. Cross-immunity of this sort now can be explained in exact chemical terms, but its discovery 190 years ago, and in its most absolute form, must have been confusing.

The next great discoveries in immunity were made by Louis Pasteur (1822-1895), a French chemist turned biologist, who by accident hit on two different methods of reducing the virulence of pathogenic microbes (Fig. 1-2). Pasteur found that aged cultures of the chicken cholera bacillus would not cause disease in chickens. Subsequent injections of young cultures, which ordinarily killed normal chickens, had no effect on the birds previously inoculated with the impotent culture. Aged cultures of the chicken cholera organisms thus became the first attenuated vaccine.

Pasteur noted that a similar type of protection against anthrax resulted when sheep were inoculated with cultures of *Bacillus anthracis* that had been cultivated at 42° C. At their usual growth temperature of 37° C these organisms are fully pathogenic for sheep, but this virulence is lost on cultivation at the higher temperature. However, animals first inoculated with the 42° C culture were immune to subsequent inoculations with the 37° C culture. Attenuation (virulence reduction) of a pathogen by these or

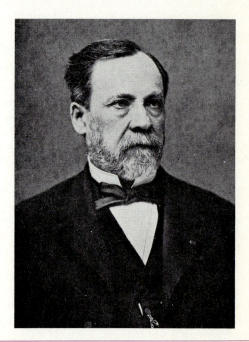

FIG. 1-2

Louis Pasteur (1822-1895). The genius of Pasteur, first evidenced by his discovery that polarization of light could be related to the structure of crystals, carried him to the solution of many problems: the spoilage of beers and wines, with the accompanying pasteurization process; the discovery of anaerobic bacteria, virus vaccines, and attenuation of virulence; and studies of spontaneous generation. His studies in immunology have rightly earned him the position as father of the science. (From Carpenter, P.L.: Microbiology, ed. 2, Philadelphia, 1967, W.B. Saunders Co.)

other means such as radiation or genetic selection has been the key to the development of vaccines against tuberculosis, yellow fever, poliomyelitis, rabies, measles, mumps, and other infectious diseases. Incidentally, Pasteur coined the term *vaccination* for these immunization procedures in honor of Jenner's initial discoveries with cowpox (Latin *vacca,* cow). In its present usage vaccination generally refers to immunization with cellular vaccines.

Pasteur's most famous immunization was that developed against rabies (Fig. 1-3). The causative agent had not yet been identified as a virus when Pasteur found he could perpetuate the disease in dogs or rabbits by injecting spinal-cord extracts from rabid animals into normal animals. Extracts prepared from infected cords that had been dried for several days at room temperature were less infectious than those not dried, and infected cords that were dried

for longer periods were not infectious at all. Pasteur correctly deduced, in parallel with his earlier studies with fowl cholera and anthrax, that injections of the inactive cord extract and then the weakened extracts with a progression toward more potent virus-containing extracts would protect his animals against otherwise fully active rabies virus.

The first human test occurred on July 6, 1885. A young boy named Joseph Meister had been bitten severely, some 14 times, just 2 days before. After much persuasion from the boy's parents Pasteur initiated his treatment of 12 injections, gradually increasing the potency of the virus-cord extract over a 2-week period. Despite Pasteur's many fears, the boy survived the rabid dog bites and the active virus present in the final injections of the series.

A few weeks later Pasteur presented his report on rabies prevention to the Academy of Sciences.

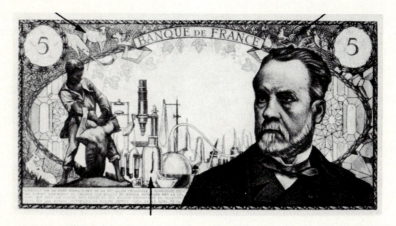

FIG. 1-3

French 5-franc notes illustrate many of Pasteur's scientific accomplishments in a true art form. Upper left and upper right arrows point to sheep and chickens that commemorate development of attenuated vaccines for anthrax and chicken cholera. Lower arrow indicates rabid rabbit spinal cord in a drying jar first used to treat Joseph Meister, the young boy shown battling a rabid dog. Rabbits in lower left corner possibly portray Pasteur's entry into bacterial warfare and his deliberate infection of rabbits who were burrowing into a friend's wine cellar and dislodging the masonry with disastrous results. Crystals at left and right center illustrate relationships of crystal structure to optic rotation. Grape clusters refer to Pasteur's study of diseases of wine and discovery of pasteurization, and swan-necked flask near Pasteur's portrait is a reminder of his disputation of the theory of spontaneous generation. Flagellated bacilli surrounding the number 5 in each upper corner of note refer to his discovery of anaerobic life. The reverse side of the bill is also beautiful and illustrates fungi, mulberry, and grapes with the portrait of Pasteur.

Within a year the Pasteur treatment was applied to 350 persons without one fatality. Pasteur's fame quickly spread around the world. Pasteur Institutes, first in Paris and then in other major European cities, were constructed with funds contributed for vaccine production and research. Many young physicians and scientists begged to come and study under Pasteur in Paris. The Pasteur Institutes quickly assumed a dominant role in the battle to control infectious diseases.

Pasteur died in 1895 after a lifetime of scientific accomplishment, first in chemistry and then in biochemistry, microbiology, immunology, and medicine. The impact of this one man on science can hardly be envisioned. Born the son of a humble tanner in 1822, he first had an interest in art and later in chemistry. It is written that he was not an exceptional scholar even as a college student, but his keen observations, his willingness to test hypotheses experimentally, and his courage in the face of the unknown have rightfully earned him the title "father of immunology."

Pasteur's remains are housed at the Pasteur Institute in Paris. By a strange twist of fate, Joseph Meister became the gatekeeper there. In 1940, 55 years after being immunized with rabies vaccine, he took his own life. German military forces had requested his keys to Pasteur's crypt, and, rather than surrender them to what he thought would be plunder and dishonor, he committed suicide.

At about the time of Pasteur's discoveries and shortly thereafter there emerged a strong conviction that immunity was totally dependent on certain body cells. These cells were described by the Russian zoologist Elie Metchnikoff (1845-1916) and were called phagocytic (cell-eating) cells (Fig. 1-4).

Metchnikoff was a brilliant student of zoology at the University of Kharkov. He studied in Germany before obtaining his doctorate at St. Petersburg and becoming a docent (assistant professor) at the University of Odessa. In one of his periods of depression that followed the death of his wife in 1873, Metchnikoff made an unsuccessful attempt on his life by taking an overdose of morphine. After his recovery he returned to work but disliked certain changes in the university. A few years later (in

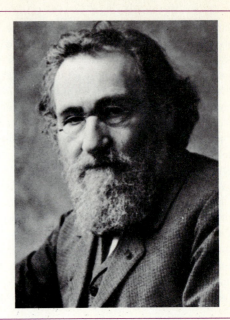

FIG. 1-4

Elie Metchnikoff (1845-1916). The electrifying and persistent personality of Metchnikoff allowed him to convert his discoveries of phagocytosis into a doctrine that gained many disciples from his coterie of students. His doctrine of cellular immunity eventually was united with the doctrine of humoral immunity approximately 10 years before his death. (From Dubos, R., and Hirsch, J.: Bacterial and mycotic infections of man, ed. 4, Philadelphia, 1965, J.B. Lippincott Co.)

1881) he was again so despondent that he attempted suicide, this time by self-inoculation with the organisms that cause relapsing fever.

Although Metchnikoff became seriously ill, it was not his fate to die. Within a year he resigned from the university and took his second wife and her orphaned brothers and sisters to Italy. While his family was away at a circus, he began to study the motile cells that he could see microscopically in transparent starfish larvae. He thought that these cells might be protective in a digestive way, much like the cells that gather at points of infection near splinters in human skin; he stuck some rose thorns into the larvae. The next day the thorns were surrounded by these ameboid cells.

Shortly thereafter he returned to Russia, and while studying the water flea *(Daphnia)* he observed that phagocytic cells could ingest and destroy yeasts *(Monospora bicuspidata)* that were pathogenic to the flea. Metchnikoff published a paper on these studies in 1884. Metchnikoff spent the rest of his life studying the phenomenon of phagocytosis in higher animals. In 1908 he shared a Nobel Prize with Ehrlich for his early contributions to immunity.

Those who supported the theory of phagocytosis as the prime source of immunity were not long without antagonists. George Nuttall, an American bacteriologist working in Goettingen, Germany, found in 1888 that defibrinated blood was bactericidal in itself. He suggested that, although phagocytosis also occurred, the phagocytic white blood cells merely removed the bacteria killed by some heat-labile, serum substance. Other investigators, including Emil von Behring, began to study the bactericidal quality of blood for several different pathogenic microbes. Pfeiffer published a report of his studies of the cholera bacillus in 1894 that clearly showed that peritoneal fluids and immune serum would lyse the cholera vibrio (Pfeiffer's phenomenon).

Perhaps the greatest support for the humoral theory arose from the studies of Behring (1854-1917), who stated in 1890 that immunity to diphtheria or tetanus was dependent on the capacity of blood to inactivate diphtheria or tetanus exotoxin. It was easily proved that this antitoxic activity resided in the cell-free portion of the blood. In 1901 Behring became the first Nobel laureate in Physiology and Medicine for his work with antiserum therapy (Fig. 1-5).

Behring led a life unlike that of Metchnikoff. Behring was born into a poor family. He nearly passed up medical school in favor of free university training in theology but was able to enter the army medical school in Berlin. As a military physician, he apparently had a rather unrestrained bachelorhood, but he was professionally able and worked diligently. He was transferred in 1889 to Robert Koch's laboratories in Berlin and moved later (in 1891) with Koch into the Institute for Infectious Diseases. After his successes with antitoxin therapy were proved in human beings, Behring achieved tremendous fame. After all, diphtheria and tetanus were the great kill-

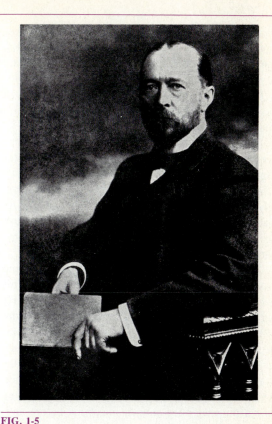

FIG. 1-5

Emil von Behring (1854-1917). Behring's discoveries of antitoxin and the principles of antiserum therapy placed him strongly on the side of those favoring humoral substances as the cause of immunity. He established one of the first corporations to produce immunobiologic products. (From Parish, H.J.: A history of immunization, Edinburgh, 1965, E. & S. Livingstone, Ltd.)

ers of that day. Koch, jealous of Behring and his discoveries, forced a transfer of Behring's appointment from the Institute into the university system, but Behring was a poor teacher and soon resigned. His fame continued to grow, however, and he was honored first by being brought into the nobility and then by being awarded the Nobel Prize. Later he created the Behring Werke, which still exists today, for manufacturing biologic products.

By 1903 it had become apparent to Almroth Wright (1861-1947), an English physician and later teacher of Sir Alexander Fleming (the discoverer of penicillin), that neither the cellular theory nor the

humoral theory was wrong and that both were correct. In 1903, with Stewart Douglass, he published
convincing evidence that serum substances, which
he termed *opsonins,* functioned by aiding phagocytosis of bacteria. By this simple discovery he resolved
the differences between the humoralists and the cel-
lularists.

During these same years a man named Paul Ehrlich was making unique contributions to immunology, contributions that were both original and correl-
ative in nature. Ehrlich (1854-1915) attended several
schools, eventually earning his doctorate in 1878. As
a student he was noted for his intense love of histology and staining. One of his earliest scientific contributions was the discovery of mast cells.

An addicted cigar smoker, note taker, and memo
writer, Ehrlich had considerable disregard for his
personal appearance and that of his laboratory. He
was an original thinker and is honored as the founder
of chemotherapy. Prior to his work with chemotherapeutics, especially during the years 1890 to 1896 after recovering from tuberculosis, he worked at the
famous Institute for Infectious Diseases in Berlin,
where he studied immunity. He discovered that there
was a time lag after antigen injections before antibody was formed. Ehrlich also discovered the anamnestic or booster response and standardized antitoxins and toxins. He found that immunity could be
transferred from mother to offspring. His theory of
antibody formation, the side chain hypothesis, paved
the way for the theories of Burnet and later Jerne
that contributed to their winning Nobel Prizes. Ehrlich renamed complement (from Bordet's alexin),
developed the concept of horror autotoxicus, and
made many other contributions to immunology. For
these he shared the Nobel Prize in 1908 with Metchnikoff (Fig. 1-6).

After Ehrlich it was approximately 25 years before anyone made another truly major contribution to
immunity. Gaston Ramon, a Frenchman, observed
in 1923 that toxins could be converted to toxoids
with formaldehyde. The toxoids retained essentially
all the antigenic activity of the toxin without its nox-
ious effects. Toxoids, much more stable than toxins,
were quickly used to replace the toxin-antitoxin mixtures then used in immunization. Ramon also devel-

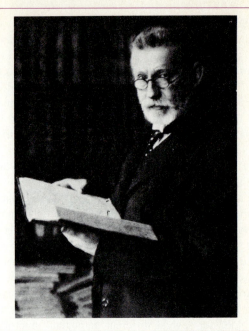

FIG. 1-6

Paul Ehrlich (1854-1915). An exact contemporary of
Metchnikoff but of much different background and personality, Ehrlich has been described as the greatest scientific
worker in medicine prior to World War II. He was a his-
tologist, hematologist, chemotherapist, bacteriologist,
physician, and immunologist. (From Burdon, K., and Williams, R.P.: Microbiology, ed. 6, New York, 1968, Macmillan, Inc.)

oped his own form of the precipitation test, which he
based on antibody dilution. Ramon's test is a truer
measure of antitoxin than the animal protection tests
developed by Ehrlich.

The final landmark to be considered in this res-
ume of historically important contributions to immunity (Table 1-2) is the discovery of interferon. Interferons are substances excreted by cells harboring an
intracellular parasite. The interferons enter adjacent
cells and protect them against the inducing and other
antigenically unrelated intracellular parasites. The
antigenic nonspecificity of interferons is an important difference between interferons and antibodies.
The original interferon was discovered by Isaacs and
Lindenmann in 1957; Isaacs continued his studies of
interferons until his death in 1967.

TABLE 1-2

Historical landmarks in immunity

1721	Lady Mary Wortley Montagu	Smallpox immunization
1798	Edward Jenner	Smallpox immunization
1880	Louis Pasteur	Age attenuation of vaccines
1881	Louis Pasteur	Heat attenuation of vaccines
1884	Elie Metchnikoff	Discovery of phagocytosis
1885	Louis Pasteur	Rabies vaccination
1888	George Nuttall	Bactericidal property of blood
1890	Emil von Behring	Antitoxin therapy
1897	Paul Ehrlich	Studies in immunity
1903	Almroth Wright and Stewart Douglass	Role of serum in phagocytosis
1923	Gaston Ramon	Toxoid immunization
1957	Alick Isaacs and Jean Lindenmann	Interferons

TABLE 1-3

Historical landmarks in serology

1896	Max Grüber and Herbert Durham	Agglutination test
1896	G. Fernand Widal	Agglutination test for typhoid fever
1897	Rudolf Kraus	Precipitation test
1898	Jules Bordet	Complement
1901	Jules Bordet and Octave Gengou	Demonstrate complement fixation
1906	August von Wassermann	Complement-fixation test for syphilis
1942	Albert Coons	Fluorescent antibody
1945	R.R.A. Coombs	Antiglobulin tests
1946-1948	Örjan Ouchterlony, Jacques Oudin, and Stephen Elek	Gel diffusion tests
1953	Pierre Grabar and Curtis Williams	Immunoelectrophoresis
1959-1960	Solomon Berson and Rosalyn Yalow	Radioimmunoassay

SEROLOGY

Closely associated with the history of vaccines and immunizing preparations was the development of a dichotomy between those who believed immunity depended on cellular constituents of the body and those who believed in acellular serum components (serology) as the basis of immunity. Metchnikoff's contribution already has been described; later discoveries are listed in Table 1-3.

The first serologic reaction described was bacterial agglutination. The agglutination reaction, or the clumping of bacteria by specific antisera, was described by Max Grüber and Herbert Durham in 1896. They showed that the cholera vibrio was agglutinated by cholera antiserum, and the typhoid bacillus was agglutinated by antityphoid serum, but not vice versa. Immediately after publication of their paper and in the same year G. Fernand Widal described the agglutination test as a diagnostic aid for typhoid fever and bacterial agglutination soon became known as the Widal test. By the use of red blood cells as the antigen the test has been extended to hemagglutination, which is important in blood grouping and blood transfusion.

The second serologic test to be described, the precipitation test was, like the agglutination test, discovered in Austria; Rudolf Kraus discovered that bacterial culture filtrates or glass-ground extracts of bacteria were precipitable by bacterial antisera. He also determined the serologic specificity of the reaction between plague, typhoid, and cholera bacilli. The various modifications of the precipitin test have allowed its application in diagnostic microbiology and medicine.

The discovery that serologic precipitation tests could be performed in gels was announced during 1946 to 1948 by Örjan Ouchterlony, Stephen Elek, and Jacques Oudin in three separate laboratories in Sweden, the United States, and France, respectively. These immunodiffusion tests differed in their physical design but were based on the observation that antigens and antisera could diffuse from reservoirs placed in agar through that agar until they met in concentrations adequate for precipitation. The fact that the Ouchterlony test is very simple to prepare and to interpret and that it has a somewhat more general application accounts for its greater popularity today.

The first modification of the gel immunodiffusion test was immunoelectrophoresis, developed by Pierre Grabar and Curtis Williams in 1953. In this procedure an electrophoretic separation of antigens in a mixture of antigens precedes the immunodiffusion portion of the test, which is conducted essentially as in the Ouchterlony tests. The antigens are displaced and segregate themselves according to their ionic properties, thus facilitating the enumeration and identification of the precipitates that form.

Another useful modification of immunodiffusion referred to as *radial* or *quantitative immunodiffusion* was first described by Feinberg in 1957; however, the test is known as the Mancini test, since it was most extensively studied by Mancini. In this technique antigen diffuses radially from a well placed in an antibody-containing gel. The zone of precipitate that forms is an accurate measure of the quantity of antigen added. Other important variants of the immunodiffusion method such as crossed immunoelectrophoresis, counterimmunoelectrophoresis, and the Laurell, or rocket, technique are discussed in Chapter 12.

One of the major early contributions to the field of serology was made by Jules Bordet (1870-1961), a Belgian who completed his medical studies by the age of 22 and entered the Pasteur Institute under Metchnikoff in Paris. Within 3 years of his graduation he published his paper on alexin (later renamed complement by Ehrlich), a normal serum substance that was heat labile and strongly bactericidal when antibody was present.

Bordet also found that complement did not increase in quantity during immunization. He made several contributions to medical bacteriology. He returned to Belgium as director of the Pasteur Institute in Brussels. At the Free University he resumed research in immunology, studying the mechanism of in vitro serologic reactions and conglutination.

Productive as he was, Bordet is most remembered for his discovery of complement, which allowed Au-

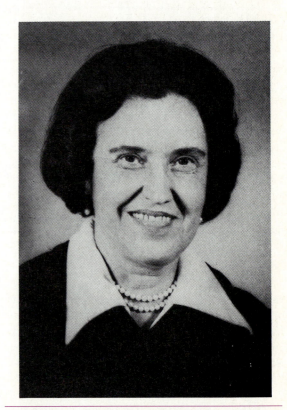

FIG. 1-7

Rosalyn Yalow, the first woman to receive a Nobel Prize in Physiology and Medicine (in 1977) for her research in immunology. With Solomon Berson she developed the first radioimmunoassays.

gust von Wassermann to develop his famous test for syphilis. Of course the great advantage of the complement-fixation test is not in its single application to the serodiagnosis of syphilis but in its wide applicability to many diseases. The Nobel Committee recognized this and awarded the Prize to Bordet in 1919.

The covalent bonding of fluorescein isocyanate or isothiocyanate to antibody molecules provided a remarkably useful histochemical reagent for locating antigen in tissue preparations. This technique, developed by Albert Coons in 1942, required the use of ultraviolet microscopy but was immediately accepted as a technique superior to the use of azo-labeled antigens for the same purpose. Later development of the indirect procedure, or immunologic sandwich technique, extended the method and increased its sensitivity.

The radioimmunoassay procedures in such widespread use today for detecting nanogram or even picogram quantities of antigens and haptens rely on methods founded by Rosalyn Yalow and Solomon Berson in the years immediately after 1956 (Fig. 1-7). Yalow and Berson's use of radioactive tracers to detect insulin (the antigen) and antiinsulin greatly extended the sensitivity of serologic tests, which are also noted for their high specificity. The methods originally designed for insulin now have been applied to the detection and quantitation of a myriad of antigens and haptens, including human growth hormone, lactogenic hormone, corticosteroids, several different antibiotics, many enzymes, tumor antigens, and viruses.

This remarkable advance also signaled the development of other labeled antigen (or antibody) tests, most notably enzyme immunoassays. For her contributions Yalow was awarded the Nobel Prize in Physiology and Medicine in 1977, which she shared with two others who did research on a separate although related subject. Yalow is the first woman to receive this coveted award for studies in immunology.

IMMUNOCHEMISTRY

Svante August Arrhenius was the first to use the term *immunochemistry,* in 1903; he published a monograph bearing that title in 1907. Other books emphasizing the chemistry of immunity and immunology were published by Wells in 1929, Karl Landsteiner in 1936, Marrack in 1934, and Kabat and Mayer in 1948; immunochemistry has long been accepted as a subdivision of immunology (Table 1-4).

The first major contribution to immunology with a distinctive chemical imprint resulted from the study of haptens. The word *hapten* was coined by the famous Landsteiner (1868-1943) in 1921 to refer to small chemical groups that could be attached to already existing antigens that would add specificity to the antigen. Earlier (in 1906) Obermayer and Pick had discovered that mild nitration or iodination would alter the serologic specificity of a protein; unlike Landsteiner, they did not learn that low-molecular weight—nitrated or iodinated—compounds alone

TABLE 1-4

Historical landmarks in immunochemistry

1906	F. Obermayer and E. Pick	Altered protein antigens
1907	S. Arrhenius	Monograph on immunochemistry
1917	Karl Landsteiner	Haptens
1929	Michael Heidelberger	Quantitative chemical serology
1934	J. Marrack	Antigen-antibody reaction
1938	Elvin Kabat and Arne Tiselius	Antibodies as globulins
1958	Rodney R. Porter	Structure of immunoglobulins
1959	Gerald M. Edelman	Structure of immunoglobulins
1966-1968	K. Ishizaka, H. Bennich, and S.G.O. Johansson	Studies with IgE

could react with antibodies to the chemically modified antigen.

Landsteiner pursued the subject of chemically modified antigens and haptens for over 25 years, from his initial studies in 1917 until his death in 1943. Of his 167 publications, 95 can easily be cited as relating to haptens, conjugated antigens, and serologic specificity. Many of the remaining papers were devoted to blood grouping and blood-group specificity (not included in the 95), and these, too, often were oriented toward antigen specificity. It was his work with blood groups that led to his Nobel Prize award in 1930 (Fig. 1-8).

During the 1920s and 1930s chemistry was the basis for new insight into serologic reactions, as exemplified by the studies of Michael Heidelberger with Avery and Goebel in their chemical descriptions of pneumococcal polysaccharide antigens. Later, with Kendall, Heidelberger devised the quantitative precipitin technique. The impact of this work

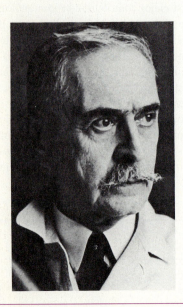

FIG. 1-8
Karl Landsteiner (1868-1943). This physician left the practice of medicine and yet made one of the most significant contributions to that science in the last 80 years: his discovery of the human ABO blood groups. (From Dubos, R., and Hirsch, J.: Bacterial and mycotic infections of man, ed. 4, Philadelphia, 1965, J.B. Lippincott Co.)

was so great that immunochemists ever since have expressed the quantity of antibody in terms of milligrams of protein per milliliter in preference to the often meaningless quotation of antibody titer. The initial studies with quantitative precipitation were possible largely through the availability of the nitrogen-free pneumococcal polysaccharide antigen that Heidelberger had earlier helped to prepare.

Once Heidelberger and Kendall had established that analytical chemical techniques could be applied to the precipitation reaction, chemical procedures were applied to other serologic reactions. Elvin Kabat, one of Heidelberger's students, applied quantitative techniques to the agglutination reaction. While doing postgraduate research in Sweden, Kabat conclusively proved that antibodies are in the γ-globulin fraction of serum, a fact he determined by the use of the analytical ultracentrifuge that had just been developed in Sweden. Since that time (1939) Kabat has been especially concerned with the immunochemistry of the human blood group antigens.

Also in the 1930s Marrack, an Englishman, made an important contribution of a more theoretic sort to immunochemistry. In 1934 he proposed a new model for antigen-antibody reactions based on the multivalence (multiple combining sites) of each. With a combination of their specific reactive groups a latticework of alternating antigen and antibody molecules could be created.

This concept of lattice formation is fundamentally an extension of some of Bordet's ideas on serologic reactions, but Marrack emphasized the genuine attractiveness of antigen and antibody for each other based on the special chemistry of each. Marrack's lattice hypothesis may be considered as proved today and has been very useful in explaining serologic reactions, not only with multivalent reactants but also with haptens and monovalent antibodies.

In 1972 two immunochemists, Rodney R. Porter and Gerald M. Edelman (Figs. 1-9 and 1-10) were recognized by the Nobel Committee for their outstanding contributions toward determining the structure of immunoglobulins. Both men worked on the same immunoglobulin, the one now known as IgG, but each used slightly different methods. Porter used an enzyme method to cleave the antibody molecule into three parts, two that were identical and contained the antibody activity, and a third portion by which the antibody molecule attaches itself to cells. Edelman disrupted the normal structure of immunoglobulins by strong disulfide reagents in high-molarity urea. Under these conditions the molecule was fragmented into two types of polypeptide chains, one of which (L-chain) was approximately half the size and weight of the other (H-chain). Within 3 years of these discoveries it was possible to synthesize this information into a single structure for IgG. This is the four-peptide structure, which is similar for all five known immunoglobulins.

It is quite probable that the discovery of IgE by K. Ishizaka and his co-workers and by H. Bennich and S.G.O. Johansson in the years 1966 to 1968 also should be considered a landmark discovery in immunology. The fact that a unique immunoglobulinlike factor in serum was responsible or closely associated with various forms of allergic disease was known from the studies of Prausnitz and Küstner in 1921. A quarter of a century later these allergies were related to the activity of a new immunoglobulin, IgE, which, unlike the ordinary antibodies, is essentially destructive in behavior rather than protective.

IMMUNOBIOLOGY

Since immunology is fundamentally a biologic science, every facet of it could be considered under an umbrella called immunobiology. Obviously the use of the word *immunobiology* here, as a subdivision of immunology, is intended for those segments of immunology that have not yet achieved the status (at least from a historical point of view) of immunity, serology, and immunochemistry. When items

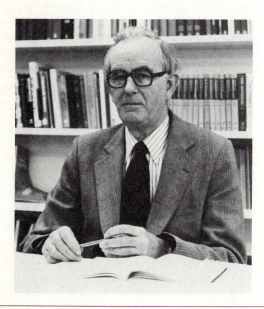

FIG. 1-9
Rodney R. Porter (1917-1985) of Oxford University shared the Nobel Prize in Physiology and Medicine with Gerald M. Edelman. It is interesting that their fundamental studies in the chemistry of immunoglobulins should win an award in medicine, underscoring the dependence of advances in medicine on chemistry and immunology.

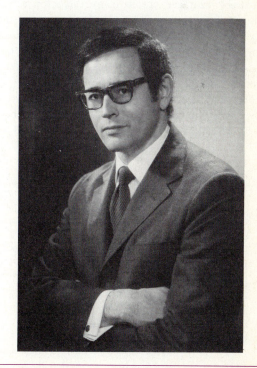

FIG. 1-10
Gerald M. Edelman of Rockefeller University was only 43 years of age when he shared the Nobel Prize with Rodney R. Porter in 1972. The discoveries for which the Nobel Prize was awarded were made by Edelman in the middle 1960s. (Photograph by Fabian Bachrach.)

such as allergy and hypersensitivity, theories of antibody formation, autoimmune disease, tissue transplantation, tumor immunology, immunologic tolerance, red blood cell grouping, and erythroblastosis fetalis are discussed under a single heading, the ramifications of immunology into the medical sciences become very apparent (Table 1-5).

The concept that disease could be caused by antibodies was a complete antithesis to the pioneer work of Behring, Ehrlich, Bordet, and the many others who had conclusively demonstrated that antibodies and serum substances were protective. Today there is no longer room for speculation; the whole subject of allergy and hypersensitivity is replete with documented examples of antibody-associated illnesses. Antibodies to foreign serum proteins, to plant pollens, to animal danders, and even to self-antigens are associated with and are in many cases the actual cause of a disease condition. Antibodies are not the only initiators of immune disease; there is a form of immune illness that is cell dependent rather than humoral. This latter class, the delayed-hypersensitivity reaction, was the first to be described.

The discovery of delayed hypersensitivity was a direct outgrowth of Robert Koch's studies of tuberculosis. Koch (1843-1910) noted that laboratory guinea pigs are highly susceptible to tuberculosis and that inoculating these animals with tubercle bacilli will kill them in 4 to 8 weeks. If such tuberculous guinea pigs are given a second subcutaneous injection of more tubercle bacilli, they are able to mobilize defenses that tend to wall off the new inoculum. The second injection site becomes reddened, tissue death follows, and the dead tissue and tuberculosis germs are sloughed off, leaving an ulcer that will heal. This is the Koch phenomenon. Although the record is somewhat incomplete and confused, Koch apparently thought that dead tubercle bacilli or growth products of these organisms, called tuberculin, could be injected into persons who already had tuberculosis and that a curative effect would be obtained. The idea was apparently that these injections would cause the tubercle bacilli, wherever they were located, to be sloughed, as in the Koch phenomenon in tuberculous guinea pigs. However, this reaction did not occur.

Injections of tuberculin into the skin of tuberculous individuals caused a gradual reddening at the injection site, followed by induration. This process peaked about 48 to 72 hours after the injection and did not occur in nontuberculous persons. This delayed hypersensitivity skin test is an example of an

---

TABLE 1-5

Historical landmarks in immunobiology

1890	Robert Koch	Delayed hypersensitivity
1901	Karl Landsteiner	Human blood groups
1902	Charles Richet and Paul Portier	Anaphylaxis
1905	Clemens von Pirquet	Serum sickness
1908	Paul Ehrlich	Theories of antibody formation and other studies
1921	Carl Prausnitz and Heinz Küstner	Reagin discovery
1930	Felix Haurowitz and others	Template theories of antibody formation
1940	Karl Landsteiner and Alexander Wiener	Discovery of Rh antigens
1942	Karl Landsteiner and Merrill Chase	Cellular transfer of delayed hypersensitivity
1944-1960	Macfarlane Burnet and Peter Medawar	Immunologic tolerance
1956	Ernest Witebsky	Autoimmunity studies
1960	Baruj Benacerraf, Jean Dausset, and George Snell	Immunogenetics and histocompatibility
1984	Cesar Milstein, Georges Köhler, and Nils Jerne	Hybridoma technology and contributions to theoretical immunology

allergy of infection. Skin tests of this type are employed in epidemiologic studies of several infectious diseases, of which tuberculosis is a prime example. Similar delayed hypersensitivity tests are employed to determine drug hypersensitivity.

Koch made many contributions to medical bacteriology; it is unfortunate that his efforts to cure and to immunize against tuberculosis failed. He has many scientific credits, among which are proof of the life cycle of anthrax bacillus and its causative role in the disease, improvement in staining procedures, identification of the tubercle bacillus, Koch's postulates, Koch's phenomenon, tuberculin, and discovery of the cholera bacillus.

As a youngster, Koch was active and keenly interested in nature. His family, although poor, mustered sufficient funds to send him through medical school. He practiced medicine in Berlin, Hamburg, and several small villages. Koch's extensive research was done in his own humble laboratories until 1880, when he received an appointment in the Imperial Health Office in recognition of his studies with anthrax. Later at the University Institute Pfeiffer, Behring, Ehrlich, and other noted immunologists were his students. In 1891 Koch became the first director of the research Institute for Infectious Diseases. In 1905 he was awarded the Nobel Prize in Physiology and Medicine for his research in tuberculosis (Fig. 1-11).

The next important mark in the history of immunobiology is the description of anaphylaxis by the French scientists Paul Portier and Charles Richet (1850–1935) in 1902. In 1913 Richet received the Nobel Prize for these studies. This work began in the French Mediterranean, where the sea anemone and the Portuguese man-of-war populations were dense. Both of these animals have fairly potent toxins. While trying to immunize dogs against the sea anemone toxin, Portier and Richet found that small sublethal quantities injected into a previously immunized dog could throw the dog into extensive convulsions and collapse, terminating in death. They suggested the term *anaphylaxis* (meaning without or against protection). This was the first unequivocal demonstration that antibodies could be detrimental to one's health. The evidence had a tremendous impact on the practice of medicine; this was the era of antiserum therapy, and injections of antiserum were par-

ticularly likely to initiate anaphylaxis. The replacement of antiserum therapy with antibiotic therapy has not alleviated the dangers of anaphylaxis, which is all too often the result of antibiotic treatment.

At the beginning of the twentieth century several researchers, including Ehrlich and Otto in Germany and Smith in the United States, were studying serum sickness, a kind of protracted anaphylaxis resulting from injections of large quantities of antitoxin. Serum sickness was a gentler form of anaphylaxis than that described by Richet; although seldom fatal, it was quite common. Schick and Clemens von Pirquet subsequently summarized much of the available information on serum sickness, which they published in the form of a monograph in 1905. Because of this publication, they are generally, although erroneously, cited as the discoverers of serum sickness; the discovery probably should be credited to Smith. Even so, von Pirquet formulated many novel ideas about allergy, many of which are still valid today.

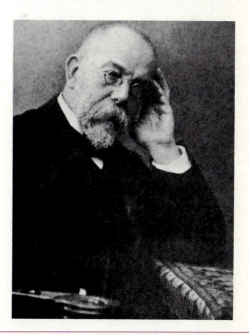

FIG. 1-11
Robert Koch (1843-1910). Although Koch is probably most famous as a bacteriologist, his discovery of delayed hypersensitivity always has been considered a hallmark in immunology. (From Burdon, K., and Williams, R.P.: Microbiology, ed. 6, New York, 1968, Macmillan, Inc.)

The Prausnitz-Küstner test is not widely used today, but few would dispute the importance of this test or the importance of the contributions that Carl Prausnitz and Heinz Küstner made to the study of allergy. In 1921 they published their data on reagin, a serum antibody-like substance apparently associated with food allergies, hay fever, asthma, hives, and other allergic conditions. Until the 1960s nearly all the information we had about reagin came from the work of Prausnitz and Küstner and from experimentation with the Prausnitz-Küstner test. The chemical nature of reagin is now accepted as being identical to that of IgE.

Landsteiner was awarded the Nobel Prize in 1930 for his description in 1901 of the major human blood groups, the ABO system. Practically every student of biology is cognizant of the pivotal role this theory played in clarifying the problems in blood transfusion reactions and in solving them by the proper matching of blood. Eventually the solution to many tissue transplantation problems became based on antigenic typing of cells. After all, blood transfusions are a special form of transplantation.

Landsteiner teamed with Wiener in 1940 for another important contribution to immunohematology, the discovery of the Rh antigen system common to humans and to the rhesus monkey (for which the antigen was named). This discovery, amplified by Wiener, Levine, and others, provided the basis for a scientific understanding of certain transfusion reactions and erythroblastosis fetalis.

Beyond his contributions to blood group immunology and to the nature of antigenic determinants, Landsteiner also made with Merrill Chase in 1942 the discovery that a class of allergies known as the delayed hypersensitivities could be transferred from the allergic animal to a normal recipient with lymph node cells (lymphocytes). This was the initial step in unraveling the cellular and molecular basis of important phenomena such as contact dermatitis and certain other drug allergies, the tuberculin reaction and certain other allergies of infection, some aspects of transplantation immunology, and, of course, much of the cellular basis of other immunologic conditions.

Much of the original work on organ-specific antigens was initiated by Witebsky and his students, although the discovery of tissue-specific antigens dates back to Uhlenhuth's work in 1903. A fuller comprehension of these antigens is necessary before tissue transplantations can be successful on a routine basis. Closely associated with this is the role of tissue antigens in autoimmune diseases. Witebsky established four criteria for proof of an autoimmune disease: (1) the autoimmune response must be regularly associated with the disease; (2) the disease must be replicable in laboratory animals; (3) pathologic changes in the human and experimental condition should parallel each other; and (4) transfer of the autoimmune illness should result from the transfer of serum or lymphoid cells from the diseased individual to a normal recipient. In 1956 examination of Hashimoto's thyroiditis in humans and rabbits by Witebsky confirmed that it was an autoimmune disease; this opened a new era of medicine.

The development of the modern theories of antibody formation is largely the result of the hypotheses and scientific investigations of Haurowitz and Macfarlane Burnet (Fig. 1-12). In 1930 Haurowitz formulated the template theory of antibody formation, which suggested that antigen was retained by the antibody-forming cells and served as a template or mold about which antibody was synthesized. In this way antibody and antigen (the lock and key described by Ehrlich) have a physical compatibility that permits their later specific combination in serologic reactions. The template theory is an example of an instructive mechanism for antibody synthesis.

Burnet's ideas about antibody formation evolved gradually, until in 1959 he conceived of the clonal selection theory, the essence of which is that cells are already endowed with the genetic ability to make a certain antibody, and the antigen, through combination with its specific cell, causes that cell to proliferate and hence result in observable antibody formation. The two theories have obvious irreconcilable differences, but the differences do not detract from their usefulness in stimulating immunologic opinion and experimentation.

An attractive portion of the clonal selection theory is its application to specific immunologic tolerance, the failure to make antibody to a normally antigenic

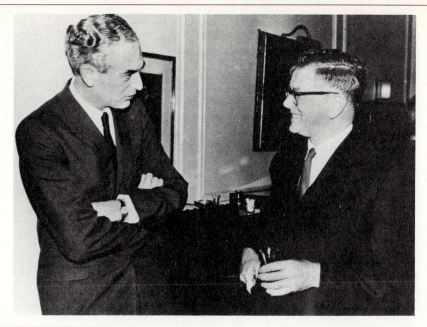

FIG. 1-12

Peter Medawar *(left)* and Macfarlane Burnet (1899-1985). This photograph of the Nobel Prize winners in Physiology and Medicine was taken about the time of their award in 1960 for developing the concept of immunologic tolerance. (From Burnet, F.M.: Changing patterns, St. Kilda, Australia, 1969, William Heinemann, Ltd.)

material because of a previous exposure to the antigen. Burnet suggested that self-recognition occurs in neonatal life by contact of antibody-forming cells with new antigens as the fetus first forms them. The result in utero is a functional shutdown of such a cell, so that one does not make antibodies to his own antigens. Peter Medawar tested this hypothesis with neonatal exposure to non-self-antigens and measured the results the theory predicted, that is, that the animal, when grown to adulthood, will not respond to the antigen. For their contributions to immunology Burnet and Medawar shared the 1960 Nobel Prize (Fig. 1-12).

The 1980 Nobel Prize in Physiology and Medicine was shared by three scientists for their collective yet separate studies of immunogenetics and histocompatibility. George Snell, a geneticist, joined the staff at the Bar Harbor Laboratories in Maine in 1935 and devoted his life to the development of con-

genic mouse strains, that is, mice that differ at only a single gene locus (Fig. 1-13). From this effort, and in conjunction with Peter Gorer, he determined that genes controlled the synthesis of antigen II (later named H-2 for histocompatibility) and the success or failure of grafts between mice that were otherwise identical. Hence a genetic basis for the study of transplantation immunology and histocompatibility in experimental animal species was created.

Meanwhile Jean Dausset found that human patients who had received multiple blood transfusions usually produced antibodies to white blood cells of the donor. These antibodies reacted with antigens on the surface of the donor's leukocytes (human leukocyte antigens, or HLA) or with the same antigen on the leukocytes of other persons. The generation of an immune response to HLA soon was related to graft failure, parallel to the studies found with the H-2 system in mice.

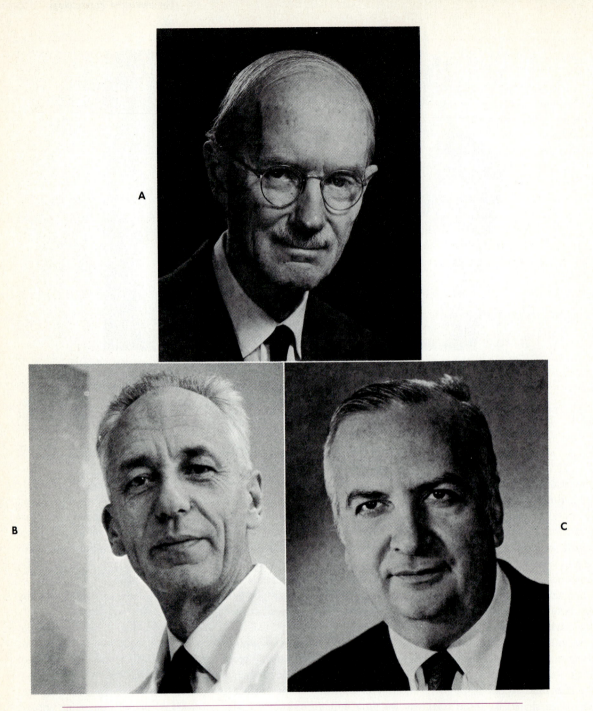

FIG. 1-13
Three recent immunologists to receive the Nobel Prize in Physiology and Medicine are George Snell (**A**), Jean Dausset (**B**), and Baruj Benacerraf (**C**). Separately these three conducted research on the transplantation antigens and the ability of an animal to develop an immune response. These characteristics were determined to be regulated by structural genes on the same chromosome.

Baruj Benacerraf began his progress toward the Nobel Prize by studying synthetic polypeptides as simplified models of more complex antigens. When he found that some guinea pigs made antibodies to a specific synthetic antigen and others failed to respond to the antigen, he theorized the presence of immune-response genes in the responders that were not present in the nonresponders. Further studies localized the immune-response gene on the same chromosome that controlled the synthesis of the histocompatibility antigens. McDevitt also had shown that this condition existed in mice. Thus the genes that regulate the synthesis of the transplantation antigens accompany the genes that regulate the immune response.

In the mid-1970s research conducted primarily at Cambridge University in England by Milstein and Köhler (Fig. 1-14) led to the description of immunoglobulin-synthesizing hybridomas. A myeloma cell—a neoplastic cell that normally secretes antibody and grows well in culture—is fused with a second cell to form the hybrid. In the experiment as it is now conducted, a nonsecreting myeloma cell is used as one parent. The second cell is a lymph node or spleen cell from an animal recently immunized with some antigen of special interest. The two cells are incubated together under conditions that allow their cell membranes to fuse, producing a binuclear hybrid. The hybrid usually discards some chromosomes after the fusion. The hybrid cells then are placed in a medium containing compounds that prevent the growth of the parent myeloma cell and spleen cell. Only the hybrid cells will grow in this medium. The growing cells are screened to determine if they have retained the spleen cell gene for antibody formation, that is, they are examined for their ability to synthesize antibody. Clones of active cells are then perpetuated in culture. Such cells will produce a monomolecular antibody that is specific for a single site of the antigen. Such monoclonal antibodies have application in studies of immunoglobulin chemistry and synthesis, antigen analysis, immunoassay, immunogenetics, and other areas. For the discovery and development of hybridoma technology Köhler and Milstein received the Nobel Prize in Physiology and Medicine in 1984.

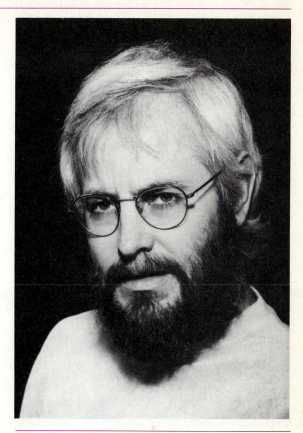

FIG. 1-14

Georges Köhler, currently Director of the Max-Planck Institute for Immunobiology in Freiburg, Germany, shared a 1984 Nobel Prize with Cesar Milstein for studies of hybridoma technology conducted at Cambridge England.

Nils Jerne (Fig. 1-15) also shared the 1984 Nobel Prize. In contrast to the highly technical hybridoma procedure advanced by Köhler and Milstein, Jerne's contributions were often theoretic or speculative, though subject to experimental proof. For example, Jerne modernized the selective theory of antibody formation first conceived by Ehrlich and later modified by Burnet. This theory stated that an animal had a preexisting capability to synthesize antibodies before antigen exposure. Jerne's plaque-forming cell assay, developed in association with Nordin, conclusively demonstrated the existence of this phenomenon.

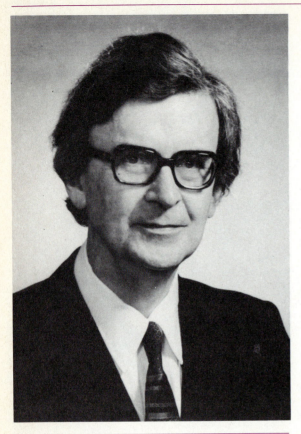

FIG. 1-15

Nils K. Jerne, a prolific theorist, as well as experimenter, received the Nobel Prize in 1984. Cited for this award was his application of the plaque forming cell assay, the identification of antibody forming cells, as proof of a genetic capacity to produce antibodies prior to exposure to antigen. His formulation of the idiotypic network as a method to downgrade the antibody response was a second major contribution.

Jerne also first conceptualized immune regulation through an idiotypic network. He predicted that an antibody molecule, each of which contains a unique immunogenic region termed an *idiotypic marker,* would stimulate the formation of a second antibody that would react with this marker. Since the second antibody would also contain an idiotypic marker, a third antibody would be induced. This sequence would continue ad nauseam and result in a downgrading of the antibody response since each antibody would react with and tend to neutralize the immediately previous antibody in the network. Again Jerne's prediction was substantiated by experimentation.

Jerne contributed to other aspects of immunology as diverse as the affinity of antibody molecules for antigen, for which he proposed the term *avidity,* and antigen-recognition sites on lymphocytes.

The 1987 Nobel Prize in Medicine and Physiology was awarded to the Japanese American Susumu Tonegawa for two important discoveries based on his analysis of immunoglobulin genes. Tonegawa used the knowledge then available about the amino acid sequence of immunoglobulins to synthesize "artificial genes" that represented a copy of the natural genes that determined specific sequences. These artificial genes were in reality only small portions of the total gene and are more accurately described as copy or cDNA. Tonegawa found that his cDNA for the portion of the immunoglobulin that had a variable amino acid sequence (from one specimen to another) would bind to a different region of the chromosome than the cDNA for the constant sequence of the immunoglobulin. This conclusion, based on the study of DNA from fetal tissues, clearly indicated that more than one gene was involved in the synthesis of a single peptide. Thus the dogma of one gene–one protein, for so many years a basic tenet in genetics, was destroyed. Surprisingly, this same type of analysis performed on adult tissues proved that the variable (V) and constant (C) genes were now situated adjacent to each other on the chromosome. This unexpected mobility and realignment of immunoglobulin genes was also a novel discovery. A companion to these discoveries was the observation that the antibody-forming cell has several V genes, one of which is chosen and then linked to the solitary C gene to provide the specificity that the antibody needs for a certain antigen. Obviously other V genes would be chosen during the response to a different antigen. Tonegawa's discovery of a multigene–one protein relationship and the movement of genes with an accompanying elimination of the unrequired DNA has importance in many areas of biology outside immunology (see also p. 70).

REFERENCES

Baxby, D.: Jenner's smallpox vaccine, Exeter, N.H., 1981, Heinemann Educational Books, Inc.

Benacerraf, B.: Role of MHC gene products in immune regulation, Science **212:**1229, 1981.

Brock, T.: Milestones in microbiology, Englewood Cliffs, N.J., 1961, Prentice-Hall, Inc.

Bulloch, W.: The history of bacteriology, London, 1938, Oxford University Press.

Burnet, F.M.: Changing patterns, New York, 1969, American Elsevier Publishers, Inc.

Cope, Z.: Almroth Wright, founder of modern vaccine therapy, London, 1966, Thomas Nelson & Sons, Ltd.

Dausset, J.: The major histocompatibility complex in man, Science **213:**1469, 1981.

Dixon, C.W.: Smallpox, London, 1962, J. & A. Churchill, Ltd.

Dubos, R.J.: Louis Pasteur, free lance of science, Boston, 1950, Little, Brown & Co.

Edelman, G.M.: Antibody structure and molecular immunology, Science **180:**830, 1973.

Jerne, N.K.: The generative grammar of the immune system, Science **229:**1057, 1985.

Köhler, G.: Derivation and diversification of monoclonal antibodies, Science **233:**1281, 1986.

Lechevalier, H.A., and Solotorovsky, M.: Three centuries of microbiology, New York, 1965, McGraw-Hill Book Co.

Marquardt, M.: Paul Ehrlich, London, 1949, William Heinemann, Ltd.

Milstein, C.: From antibody structure to immunological diversification of the immune response, Science **231:**1261, 1986.

Parish, H.J.: A history of immunization, Edinburgh, 1965, E. & S. Livingstone, Ltd.

Parish, H.J.: Victory with vaccines, Edinburgh, 1968, E. & S. Livingstone, Ltd.

Porter, R.R.: Structural studies of immunoglobulins, Science **180:**713, 1973.

Rains, A.J.H.: Edward Jenner and vaccination, London, 1974, Priory Press, Ltd.

Snell, G.D.: Studies in histocompatibility, Science **213:**172, 1981.

Sourkes, T.L.: Nobel Prize winners in medicine and physiology 1901-1965, New York, 1966, Abelard Schuman, Ltd.

Uhr, J.W.: The 1984 Nobel Prize in medicine, Science **226:**1025, 1984.

Wagner, R.: Clemens von Pirquet, his life and work, Baltimore, 1963, Johns Hopkins University Press.

Yalow, R.S.: Radioimmunoassay: a probe for the fine structure of biologic systems, Science **200:**1236, 1978.

Suggested readings

A listing of supplemental textbooks and journals is provided for those students who wish to consult other sources.

Recent textbooks of immunology

Amos, W.M.G.: Basic immunology, Woburn, MA, 1981, Butterworth Publishers.

Bach, J.F., editor: Immunology, ed. 2, New York, 1982, John Wiley and Sons, Inc.

Barrett, J.T.: Basic immunology and its medical application, ed. 2, St. Louis, 1980, The C.V. Mosby Co.

Bellanti, J.A., editor: Immunology III, Philadelphia, 1985, W.B. Saunders Co.

Bier, O.G., daSilva, W.D., Götze, D., and Mota, I.: Fundamentals of immunology, ed. 2, New York, 1986, Springer-Verlag New York, Inc.

Bigley, N.J.: Immunologic fundamentals, ed. 2, Chicago, 1981, Year Book Medical Publishers, Inc.

Clark, W.R.: The experimental foundations of modern immunology, ed. 3, New York, 1986, John Wiley & Sons, Inc.

Cooper, E.L.: General immunology, Oxford, 1982, Pergamon Press Ltd.

Hildemann, W.H.: Essentials of immunology, New York, 1984, Elsevier Science Publishing Co., Inc.

Hokama, Y., and Nakamura, R.: Immunology and immunopathology, Boston, 1982, Little, Brown and Co.

Hood, L.E., Weissman, I.L., and Wood, W.B.: Immunology, ed. 2, Menlo Park, Calif., 1984, Benjamin/Cummings Publishing Co.

Kimball, J.W.: Introduction to immunology, ed. 2, New York, 1986, Macmillan Publishing Co., Inc.

McConnell, I., Munro, A., and Waldmann, H.: The immune system: a course on the molecular and cellular basis of immunity, ed. 2, Oxford, 1981, Blackwell Scientific Publications, Ltd.

Myrvick, Q.N., and Weiser, R.A.: Fundamentals of immunology, ed. 2, Philadelphia, 1984, Lea and Febiger.

Outteridge, P.M.: Veterinary immunology, New York, 1984, Academic Press, Inc.

Paul, W.E., editor: Fundamental immunology, New York, 1984, Raven Press.

Roitt, I.M.: Essential immunology, ed. 5, Oxford, 1984, Blackwell Scientific Publications, Ltd.

Roitt, I., Brostoff, J., and Male, D.: Immunology, London, 1985, Gower Medical Publishing, Ltd.

Schwartz, L.M.: Compendium of immunology, ed. 2, New York, 1981, Van Nostrand Reinhold Co.

Sell, S.: Immunology, immunopathology and immunity, ed. 3, New York, 1980, Harper & Row, Publishers, Inc.

Stites, D.P., Stobo, J.D., and Wells, J.V.: Basic and clinical immunology, ed. 6, Los Altos, Calif., 1987, Lange Medical Publications.

Unanue, E.R., and Benacerraf, B.: Textbook of immunology, ed. 2, Baltimore, 1984, Williams and Wilkins Co.

Journals and periodicals in english devoted primarily to immunology

Allergy

Acta Pathologica et Microbiologica Scandinavica, Section C: Immunology

Advances In Immunology
American Journal of Reproductive Immunology and Microbiology
Annals of Allergy
Annual Review of Immunology
Cancer Immunology and Immunotherapy
Cellular Immunology
Clinical and Experimental Immunology
Clinical Immunobiology
Clinical Immunology and Immunopathology
Clinical Immunology Reviews
Clinics in Immunology and Allergy
Clinical Reviews in Allergy
Contemporary Topics in Immunobiology
Contemporary Topics in Molecular Immunology
CRC Critical Reviews in Immunology
Current Topics in Microbiology and Immunology
Developments in Immunology
Diagnostic Immunology
European Journal of Immunology
Human Immunology
Hybridoma
Immunogenetics
Immunological Communications
Immunological Reviews
Immunology
Immunology Letters
Immunology Today
Immunopharmacology
Infection and Immunity
Inflammation

International Archives of Allergy and Applied Immunology
International Journal of Immunopharmacology
IRCS Medical Science: Immunology and Allergy
Journal of Allergy and Clinical Immunology
Journal of Biological Response Modifiers
Journal of Clinical Immunology
Journal of Clinical and Laboratory Immunology
Journal of Immunogenetics
Journal of Immunological Methods
Journal of Immunology
Journal of Immunopharmacology
Journal of Interferon Research
Journal of Leukocyte Biology
Journal of Molecular and Cellular Immunology
Journal of Neuroimmunology
Lymphokines
Lymphokine Reports
Molecular Immunology
Monographs in Allergy
Parasite Immunology
Progress in Allergy
Research Monographs in Immunology
Scandinavian Journal of Immunology
Springer Seminars in Immunopathology
Survey of Immunological Research
Thymus
Tissue Antigens: Histocompatibility and Immunogenetics
Transplantation
Transplantation Proceedings
Veterinary Immunology and Immunopathology

Antigens, mitogens, haptens, and adjuvants

≡ GLOSSARY

active immunity   Self-generated immunity.

adjuvant   A substance usually injected with an antigen that improves the immune response.

adoptive immunity   Acquisition of immunity in the form of immunologically competent cells from an immune donor.

alloantibody   An antibody that reacts with an antigen of the same species as the animal synthesizing it.

alloantigen   An antigen present in another member of one's own species.

alloimmunization   The immunization of an individual with antigens from within its own species.

antibody   A globulin formed in response to exposure to an antigen; an immunoglobulin.

antigen   A macromolecule that will induce the formation of immunoglobulins or sensitized cells that react specifically with the antigen.

antigen determinant sites   Unique portions of the structure of the antigen that are responsible for its activity.

antiserum   A serum containing antibodies.

autoantigen   A molecule that behaves as a self-antigen.

autocoupling hapten   One that can combine spontaneously with a carrier.

autoimmunization   Immunization with self-antigens.

concanavalin A   A mitogen that is highly specific for T cells.

conjugated antigen   An antigen covalently joined to a hapten.

cross-reactive antigen   An antigen so structurally similar to a second antigen that it will react with antibody to the second antigen.

epitope   An antigenic determinant.

hapten   A nonantigenic material that, when combined with an antigen, conveys a new antigenic specificity to the antigen.

heteroimmunization   Immunization of an individual with antigens from another species.

heterophil antigen   An antigen that is broadly distributed in nature.

immunodominant region   The most potent epitope in an antigen.

immunogen   Antigen.

immunologic tolerance   A failure or depression in the immune response on proper exposure to antigen.

isoantigen   An antigen present in another member of one's own species.

isoimmunization   Immunization of an individual with antigens of another individual of the same species.

LPS   Lipopolysaccharide, the endotoxic portion of the cell wall of most gram-negative bacteria; mitogenic for B lymphocytes and an adjuvant.

mitogen   A substance that induces cell growth and division (mitosis).

neoantigen   An antigen with a specificity altered by addition of a hapten.

passive immunization   The acquisition of immunity through injection of antibodies or antiserum produced by another animal.

phytohemagglutinin   A mitogen for T lymphocytes.

protein A   A protein found on the surface of *Staphylococcus aureus* that is mitogenic for B lymphocytes.

T cell-dependent antigen   An antigen that requires T and B cell cooperation to induce specific antibody formation.

T cell-independent antigen   An antigen that does not require that T cells assist B cells in the production of its specific antibody.

tolerance   Failure to respond to an antigen.

tolerogen   An immunogen used under circumstances that produce tolerance rather than immunity.

■   ■   ■

No one can define an antigen in exact terms. Rather, antigens are defined in terms of the antibodies they produce; unfortunately antibodies are defined in terms of the antigens that stimulated their formation. Still one can evolve a general understanding of antigens from an admittedly incomplete definition supplemented with descriptions of known antigens.

An antigen is traditionally defined as any substance that, when introduced parenterally into an animal, will cause the production of antibodies by that animal and will react specifically with those antibodies. Because it was feared that this definition emphasized the production of immunoglobulins (the B cell response), the term *immunogen* was introduced to include more definitely the response of T cells to antigens. This term was probably unnecessary, since immunologists had long recognized that the response to antigens was divided into the humoral (immunoglobulin) and cell-mediated (T cell) response. In addition, the term *immunogen* seemed to signify that antigens were always related to immunity (immunogen, that is *generating immunity,* in contrast to antigen, *generating against*). At present most authorities use *antigen* and *immunogen* as synonymous terms, but the latter is more common. This means that we now refer to the response to antigen as the immune response even though it only occasionally refers to immunity as such. Likewise, immunization refers to any productive exposure to an antigen, regardless of whether the antigen is related to disease.

As the term *immunogen* was being popularized, some immunologists began to refer to two classes of antigens: those that could stimulate the immune response (immunogens), and those that could react with immunoglobulins but not stimulate the immune response. The term *hapten* was created for the latter class of molecules nearly 60 years ago, and it seems unfortunate that its definition became confused by

the introduction of immunogen. Haptens are discussed fully in a later section of this chapter.

The traditional definition of antigen or immunogen needs to be dissected so that we can see what is stated, what is implied, and what is omitted from the definition.

First, the word *parenteral* means "outside the digestive tract" and implies that materials given orally are not antigenic. This is not entirely true. What is true is that digestive enzymes often hydrolyze and destroy the antigenic quality of many antigenic subsances. When such an antigen is given parenterally, little can be destroyed before it is carried to the antigen-processing cells. Consequently more antibody results from the parenteral injection. The oral poliomyelitis vaccine is a notable exception. In this instance the virus, an active although attenuated strain, is taken orally, invades the cells lining the intestinal tract, and reproduces itself. For this reason, a larger antigenic dose is produced than in fact was administered. The natural result of this increased antigenic exposure is a heightened antibody response. These same conclusions would hold true for other antigenic materials that actually reproduce in the digestive tract. As a general rule, antigens are much more effective via parenteral routes such as intradermal, subcutaneous, intravenous, intramuscular, or intraperitoneal injection, but parenteral also may be used to refer to inhalation.

Second, even when the immunogen is administered parenterally, it must be given in a correct dose to stimulate the immune response. Obviously too scant an amount will be insufficient, but, surprisingly, too large an amount also may be improper. In young animals especially, but also in adult animals the immune response to an antigen can be temporarily suppressed by exposure to large quantities of antigen. This immune tolerance is antigen specific and does not encompass other antigens. When immune tolerance is the result of a large inoculum of antigen, the antigen may be referred to as a tolerogen.

Third, the definition of an antigen involves animals; plants do not make antibodies. Furthermore only certain types of animals produce true immunoglobulins. Although some invertebrates exhibit resistance to certain pathogens or their toxins, it is not at all certain that they do so through adaptive antibody formation. Consequently a vertebrate animal must be chosen for immunologic studies.

A last and extremely important part of the definition of an antigen is the specific reaction that occurs between the antigen and the antibodies it caused to be produced. Those antibodies do not react with other antigens except within very finite limits. Everyday experience confirms this fact; after all, we are immunized with poliomyelitis vaccine to prevent polio, not to prevent diphtheria or tetanus.

Several factors are omitted from the definition and should be mentioned. The initiation of antibody formation by antigens is not the only change produced in the animal by the introduction of an antigen. One usually can detect concomitant increases in immediate and delayed hypersensitivities. Moreover, many antigens of an infectious or toxic kind provoke their special reaction to this additional biologic activity. If the antigen is administered with an adjuvant, as is often the case, side effects from the adjuvant may be detectable.

All vertebrates are not equally responsive to antigens. The mammals, birds, amphibia, and fishes all have a complex yet similar immune response. The elasmobranchs (sharks and sting rays) have a slightly more primitive response and do not produce as many molecular forms of the immunoglobulins as do the higher life forms. The cyclostomes are the lowest vertebrates that express an immune response. Animals phylogenetically lower than cyclostomes do not respond to antigens and lack lymphocytes or their functional equivalents.

Thus, antigen is secondarily defined as a substance that catalyzes lymphocytes (immunocytes) into specific adaptive responses. In the case of B lymphocytes (so named because they originate in birds, in an organ known as the bursa of Fabricius),

the transformation is to plasma cells that synthesize and excrete immunoglobulins. For T lymphocytes, those lymphocytes that mature in the thymus, this is the elaboration after cell growth and division, of lymphokines, also called interleukins. Antigens also may alter the behavior of phagocytic cells directly during phagocytosis or indirectly in response to lymphokines.

Even if the animal species chosen for active immunization is one that normally has a good antibody-forming capacity to the antigen used, it is possible that the individual selected will not respond or will respond poorly to the antigen. All the reasons that some animals are refractory to antigenic stimulation may yet be unknown, but a specific inheritance is essential before an animal can respond to an antigen.

When injected with a complex antigen, nearly all animals respond with antibody formation. Some animals respond to one or more portions of the molecule, whereas other animals respond to the same or other portions. Thus both groups of animals are labeled as responders, although potentially reacting to completely different portions of the antigen. A different situation exists if feeble antigens are given, a feeble antigen being defined as one with a limited number of antigenic sites. In this case the responding animals are more likely to respond to the same regions of the antigen. Since the capacity to respond is now known to be under genetic control, it can be claimed that the responders share a certain immune response or Ir gene. (These Ir genes and their gene products are described in Chapter 4.)

CHARACTERISTICS OF IMMUNOGENS

The definitions of immunogen previously presented explain what immunogens do but not what they are. In physicochemical terms immunogens are macromolecules that possess a high degree of internal chemical complexity. They are also soluble or easily solubilized by phagocytic cells of the immunized animal and are foreign to that animal.

Macromolecular size

A macromolecule in terms of immunogenicity, is a molecule that has a molecular weight of 10,000 or more. Proteins like insulin (5,700 mol wt), protamines and histones (6,000 mol wt), and low molecular weight fractions of gelatin (10,000 mol wt) are all poor antigens. Polysaccharides of this size are often nonantigenic; heparin (17,000 mol wt), for example, is not immunogenic. In general, polysaccharides are poorer antigens than proteins of the same size because they usually are composed of only four or five monosaccharide units, whereas proteins normally contain 18 to 20 different amino acids.

Large proteins and polysaccharides of natural origin are excellent antigens. Ribonuclease (14,000 mol wt), tobacco mosaic virus protein (17,500 mol wt), egg albumin (40,000 mol wt), tetanus toxin or toxoid (55,000 mol wt), thyroglobulin (669,000 mol wt), and hemocyanin (6,000,000 mol wt) are examples of good protein antigens. Dextrans, ranging from 50,000 to 100,000 mol wt, are antigenic but not for all species. Mice and humans respond well to polysaccharide antigens, but guinea pigs are less responsive.

The greater the molecular weight of a substance, the more likely it is to function as an antigen. Within each molecule there are specific regions of limited size that function as the antigenic determinant sites, also known as epitopes (see section on haptens and antigenic determinant sites). The larger a molecule is, the greater the number of these sites and the greater the variety of antibodies that will be formed.

Molecular complexity

Large molecular size alone is not enough to confer antigenicity on a substance. Organic chemists can produce synthetic polymers of virtually any size, such as polystyrene, nylon, Teflon, Saran, polyacrylamide, and homopolymers of amino acids, all of which are nonantigenic. Various reasons for this nonantigenicity may be cited, but one explanation is that these polymers lack internal molecular complexity. The primary structure of these macromolecules is relatively simple: one or two different monomers are covalently linked into a repetitive structure, which ultimately reaches great size. Most naturally occurring macromolecules are often very complex because they are built from many different low molecular weight constituents; for example, proteins often are

composed of 18 to 20 different amino acids. Variations in amino acid sequence allow a significant internal complexity to be developed in these molecules. Even polysaccharides, which are composed of fewer structurally similar units, are complex compared with the synthetic plastics.

The composition and sequence of the individual structural units in a macromolecule is referred to as its primary structure. When the sequence of these units confers antigenicity upon a molecule, that arrangement is termed a sequential antigenic determinant. By contrast, conformational antigenic determinants are created by the helical coiling (primary structure), bending, and folding of the coil (secondary and tertiary structure) and assembly of multiple primary units (quarternary structure). Certain linear molecules such as silk fibroin have only sequential determinants, more complex molecules have both sequential and conformational determinants.

Solubility

Another argument used to explain the nonantigenicity of synthetic polymers is their insolubility in body fluids and their inability to be converted to soluble forms by tissue enzymes. Complex copolymers of the unnatural D-amino acids are poorly degraded, and that may be the reason for their low antigenicity. The relatively greater immunogenicity of pneumococcal polysaccharides for mice than for rabbits has been related to the greater hydrolytic activity of mouse liver enzymes for these polysaccharides. Practically all cellular antigens, bacteria, viruses, and red blood cells are quickly engulfed by phagocytic macrophages and digested to their soluble constituents. This participation of phagocytic cells is more than casual; if poor antigens are insolubilized or aggregated to ensure rapid engulfment, they become more potent antigens.

Foreignness

To be antigenic, the macromolecule must come from a foreign source, either an entirely different species or an animal of the same species, that is antigenically different from the animal being immunized. The more distant or foreign the antigen source, the better it will be. Duck serum proteins are not good antigens for chickens, but antigens from plant sources are. Plant proteins are usually good antigens in any animal. This concept of foreignness was recognized by Ehrlich and was stated by him as the principle of horror autotoxicus (literally, a fear of self-poisoning); he used this theory to accommodate the observation that molecules that fulfill the characteristics of an antigen already listed but that are a normal part of an animal's circulation are not normally antigenic for that particular animal. Otherwise we would make antibodies against our own erythrocytes, serum proteins, etc. This resulting condition would be incompatible with life, since the ensuing in vivo antigen-antibody reaction would destroy those erythrocytes or other antigens. The body has a built-in protective system that minimizes autoantibody development against normal circulatory antigens.

This is not to say that autoantibodies cannot be formed. They do exist, and their existence is not necessarily in conflict with the concept of horror autotoxicus. There are several mechanisms whereby an individual might produce autoantibodies (see Chapter 20).

From these descriptions of antigens it should be clear that proteins are usually antigenic, within the limits prescribed. Proteins are usually large, have a complex structure, are soluble in body fluids or are easily degraded by proteolytic enzymes to that condition, and can be chosen to meet the restriction of foreignness. Oligosaccharides are frequently but not always antigenic; they ordinarily meet all the criteria except internal complexity. Polysaccharides, through their extensive side branching via glycosidic bonds, do exhibit a secondary and tertiary structural complexity equal to or even greater than that of proteins. Were it not for this complexity, polysaccharides might not be as good antigens as they are.

Despite much literature to the contrary, other biologic polymers in a pure chemical form are not antigenic. Ribonucleic and deoxyribonucleic acids (RNA and DNA) are haptenic, not antigenic. The same is true of lipids. Complexes of lipids or nucleic acids with proteins, or in some cases with polysaccharides, are excellent antigens. In these complexes the nucleic acids or lipids serve as haptens against which antibodies can be formed, provided the hapten is part of a complete antigen.

It should also be clear that many immunogens have nothing at all to do with immunity or disease. In fact, many of the most useful immunogens have been highly purified proteins and polysaccharides of known structure. Likewise, it can be recognized that although we may refer to a bacterium or a virus as an antigen, each is actually composed of several antigens. The singular form antigen is used because the bacterial cell or virus particle is being treated as a single unit.

ANTIGEN NOMENCLATURE
T cell–dependent and –independent antigens

Many adjectives have been used to modify the noun antigen, but few are used as frequently as T cell–independent and T cell–dependent. The importance and meaning of these terms can be clarified by considering some of the cellular events that occur during the immune response.

As described in fuller detail in subsequent chapters, it is believed that phagocytic cells are the first essential cell type encountered by antigen in vivo. These cells ingest and partially digest the antigen and pass the preserved portion to lymphocytes. This activity is designated antigen processing. The two major groups of these lymphocytes, the T lymphocytes and B lymphocytes, are mentioned briefly above. In order for certain of these processed antigens to initiate an immunoglobulin response cooperative events between a phagocytic cell (usually a macrophage), a B cell, and a T cell must occur even though it is the B cell line that eventually produces the immunoglobulin. The antigens that require T cells in order to generate an immune response are obviously called the T cell–dependent (TD) antigens. Antigens that stimulate B cells without the intervention of T cells are the T cell–independent (TI) antigens. Since T cells are required for the high level of immunity that follows booster injections of antigens, only TD antigens are able to initiate the booster or memory response.

☰ SITUATION 1

THE GRANT REQUEST

You attended the first meeting of Microbiology 450—"Host-Parasite Relationships: Pathogenic Mechanisms." The instructor distributed his lecture schedule and course outline, examination schedule, and a page titled "Research Grant Topics." His explanation of these items was routine except for his discussion of the last item. He stated that within 2 weeks each student would be required to select one of the topics and develop a research grant proposal on that subject. To assist in this project, he distributed copies of some of his own research grant proposals and guidelines for the preparation of these proposals.

After some discussion with a couple of predental students at the dormitory and a cursory library search you learned that enzymes of certain streptococci were related to their ability to cause dental caries. For your research grant proposal you selected the subject "Cross-reactive Antibodies to Enzymes and Dental Caries." In this proposal you intend to develop the hypothesis that enzymes in noncariogenic streptococci might be useful in vaccines against dental caries.

Questions

1. Are enzymes as fully antigenic as other proteins?
2. Do antibodies to enzymes neutralize the catalytic activity of the enzymes?
3. Are enzymes with identical substrate specificities but from different species serologically cross-reactive?
4. What kind of immunization routes would favor the appearance of neutralizing antibodies in oral secretions?

Solution

As long as enzymes meet the general criteria of antigens, they are able to elicit an immune response. This was discussed in this chapter in terms of ribonuclease and lysozyme. Lysozyme is especially important because it has a molecular weight of only 14,000. Many enzymes are larger and are globulins with a complicated amino acid sequence and varied composition so that they easily fulfill the requirements of antigenicity. Antisera have been prepared against trypsin, chymotrypsin, pepsin, carboxypeptidase A, carboxypeptidase B, ficin, chymopapain, papain, bromelin, clostridio-peptidase, collagenase, elastase, cathepsins of several types, kallikrein (kininogenase), plasmin, thrombin, streptococcal proteinase, staphylococcal coagulase, and subtilisin, just to list a few antigenic proteases.

Antibodies to enzymes will neutralize the catalytic activity of the enzyme under the proper conditions. Clearly factors such as high salt concentration, acid pH, high temperature, and other physical forces will dissociate antigen-antibody complexes, and enzymes would provide no exception. On the other hand, even under ideal conditions the serologic complex is in a state of constant dissociation and reassociation, with the result that a few molecules of enzyme would be free from its neutralizing antibody at any chosen instant. Thus the recovery of a modicum of enzyme activity in any enzyme-antienzyme mixture is not unexpected. Even within the limits of expectation from these observations, antienzymes are often potent inhibitors of their respective enzymes so that 90% inhibition or more can be achieved. Antienzymes are usually more successful as inhibitors when they combine with an antigenic determinant that is a part of or a neighbor to the catalytic site. In the latter instance steric effects prevent or reduce the opportunity for the substrate to approach the catalytic site. Thus antienzymes are better enzyme inhibitors when the substrate is of great rather than low molecular weight.

Serologic cross-reactions among enzymes follow the same ground rules as with other antigens. Proteins serving similar functions in closely related species are often highly cross-reactive, as has been demonstrated for many serum proteins and hormones and also for enzymes, including trypsins, chymotrypsins, lactic dehydrogenases, galactosidases, and others. By contrast, multiple serotypes of enzymes serving similar functions occasionally are identified within a single species.

In the example considered here it has been recognized that the glucosyltransferase of *Streptococcus mutans* is a contributing enzyme to tooth decay. The enzyme synthesizes extracellular glucose polymers (glucans), which contribute to formation of dental plaques. Within these plaques and under them, dentin-eroding activities lead to the appearance of caries. Serologic types of *S. mutans* are seven in number (a through g), and the glycosyltransferases of types a, d, and g are serologically related, as are the enzymes of types b, c, and e. However, there is little serologic cross-reactivity between the two subgroups. It is potentially possible to use these enzymes, or serologically cross-reactive enzymes from nonpathogenic species, in prophylactic immunization against tooth decay. Since the principal antibody found in saliva is secretory IgA in company with secretory IgM (Chapter 3), immunization routes that favor production of these immunoglobulins should be used. Instillation of killed *S. mutans* into sites near the

major salivary glands and into the parotid gland ducts of monkeys already has been demonstrated as a successful prophylactic for caries in monkeys.

The concept to use cross-reactive glucosyltransferases from nonpathogenic bacteria for this purpose has merit and should result in a high-quality research proposal for the requirement in this course on pathogenic mechanisms.

TABLE 2-1

Comparison of T cell–independent and –dependent antigens

	TI antigen	TD antigen
Require T cells	No	Yes
Initiate memory response	No	Yes
Dose dependency of immune response	High	Low
Structure	Simple, repetitive	More complex
Isotopes of antibody formed	IgM and IgG3	IgM, IgG1, IgG2, IgG3, IgG4, IgA, IgE
Idiotypes of antibody formed	Limited	Varied
Metabolism *in vivo*	Slow	Fast
Induction of tolerance	Easy	More difficult
Antigen processing	May not be required for all	Required

Several other features distinguish TI and TD antigens (Table 2-1). To stimulate an optimal immune response to TI antigens, the antigen dose must be selected carefully. Too little antigen will be inadequate and too much will favor the development of immunologic tolerance rather than immunity.

TI antigens are structurally simpler than TD antigens. Most proteins—diphtheria toxoid, bovine serum albumin, keyhole limpet hemocyanin—and other complex antigens are usually (TD) antigens. TI antigens are often composed of a limited number of structural units that are repeated throughout the molecule. This arrangement limits the variety and complexity of their epitopes. Examples of TI molecules are pneumococcal capsular polysaccharides, dextran, polyvinylpyrollidone (PVP), bacterial lipopolysaccharide (LPS), the polymerized bacterial flagellar protein flagellin, TNP (trinitrophenyl) ficoll, TNP-Sephadex and TNP-*Brucella abortus* (TNP-BA). Though TI antigens are less complex than TD anti-

gens, they are often catabolized more slowly in vivo. It is unclear how these features of TD antigens result in the appearance of several different molecular forms (isotypes or classes) of immunoglobulin (e.g., IgM, IgGs, IgA), but it is known that with few exceptions, only IgM and IgG3 are formed against TI antigens. Although structural variations occur within each immunoglobulin class, these variations (idiotypes) are also more limited in the response to TI than TD antigens.

On the basis of somewhat imperfect criteria, it is possible to subclassify the TI antigens into the TI-1 and TI-2 subgroups. Immature and *xid* (sex-linked immunodeficient) mice will respond to TI antigens. These mice possess the Lyb 3^-5^- or B1 phenotype of B cells but lack 3^+5^+ or B2 cells. Thus, the TI-1 antigens can stimulate the Lyb 3^-5^- class of B cells. These cells are responsible for the synthesis of immunoglobulin M (IgM). In contrast to TI-1 antigens, TI-2 antigens stimulate Lyb 3^+5^+ or the B2 pheno-

≡ SITUATION 2

CROSS-REACTIVE HAPTENS

Henry, a 43-year-old alcoholic, entered the hospital with a temperature of 39.6° C (103.2° F), pulse rate of 140, respiratory rate of 30, and white blood cell count of 23,000 with 99% polymorphonuclear neutrophilic leukocytes. Bilateral respiratory rales and an x-ray film indicated severe lung congestion consistent with pneumonia. Henry was well known to the emergency room personnel for his frequent admissions over the past several years for anaerobic abscess, pneumonia, and a stab wound. Penicillin treatment of these conditions had created a penicillin hypersensitivity. With this knowledge, the attending physician administered sodium cephalothin, a penicillin substitute. The patient had a severe anaphylactic reaction (Chapter 17) in which the blood pressure could not be measured, and respirations were rapid and weak. Epinephrine was administered, and the patient regained consciousness, became well oriented, and seemed almost fully recovered within 30 minutes.

Questions

1. Is cephalothin antigenic or haptenic?
2. How can an allergic reaction follow the first exposure to cephalothin?
3. What, if any, is the relationship between the allergy to penicillin and cephalothin reaction?
4. How do species differences in immunologic responsiveness affect the marketing of potentially antigenic therapeutic agents intended for human use?

Solution

Allergic reactions to penicillin are usually dependent on the development of antibodies to penicillin. Penicillin is not an antigen; it is a hapten of the autocoupling type. The reactive hapten is not penicillin per se, but penicilloic acid, a degradation product that can covalently link to the ϵ-amino groups of proteins to form penicilloyl-protein derivatives. Antibodies to such derivatives are responsible for the allergic reactions to penicillin (see Fig. 2-5).

Allergic reactions to cephalothin are, like those to penicillin, dependent on its haptenic qualities rather than its antigenicity because cephalothin and other simple chemical derivatives of 7-amino-cephalosporanic acid are not antigens. The basis for the development of allergic shock to cephalothin on its first use in a patient who is allergic to penicillin has definitely been determined to result from the structural similarity of the two

7-Aminocephalosporanic acid

6-Aminopenicillanic acid

antibiotics. The thiazolidine ring of penicillin and the dihydrothiazine ring of cephalothin are not unlike chemically and are both fused to a β-lactam ring that emphasizes their similarity. The result is that antibodies formed against the penicillin derivative cross-react with cephalothin or cephalothin derivatives and vice versa. Penicillin-directed antibodies that are already present would thus trigger an allergic reaction to cephalothin or any structurally related compounds on the first exposure to them.

The episode described emphasizes the need for physician awareness of the chemical nature of therapeutic agents. Structural similarities between haptenic compounds of low molecular weight are only one consideration. Materials proven to be nonantigenic in laboratory animals may prove antigenic in humans. It is generally agreed that dextrans with a molecular weight below 50,000 are rarely antigenic for rabbits or humans. Larger dextrans, which were initially thought to be nonantigenic in rabbits and thus presumed to be nonantigenic in humans, were used during World War II as blood volume expanders with unfortunate results. The dextrans proved to be allergenic in humans, possibly because they were cross-reactive with antibodies formed against polysaccharides of the normal human flora. (Dextrans are produced commercially from bacteria of the genus *Leuconostoc*.) It is also probable that certain antigenic impurities in the preparation of these dextrans, plus their own antigenicity for the human species, contributed to these allergic reactions. Because of species differences in responsiveness to antigens and haptens, it is often impossible to prove that humans will tolerate a therapeutic agent that is nonallergenic in several species of laboratory animals.

type of B cells. Immature mice do not possess these lymphocytes and, as a consequence, are unable to respond to TI-2 antigens. In addition to their role as antigens, TI-1 molecules also function as mitogens—that is, they stimulate not only the B cells that will make antibody to the TI-1 antigen, but they also stimulate other, probably all, B cells into a growth and cell-division cycle (mitosis). These TI-1 antigens, because of their effect on a multiplicity of B cells are described as polyclonal antigens. One of the most studied TI-1 antigens is LPS in its native form or as TNP-LPS. Another is TNP-BA. The TI-2 antigens are devoid of mitogenic activity and can be considered as monoclonal B activators since they catalyze only the cells that make specific antibody. Pneumococcal polysaccharide, ficoll, and PVP are examples of TI-1 antigens. Although TI-2 antigens appear to require processing by accessory phagocytic cells, at least some TI-1 antigens may bypass this step.

The evidence is firm that TI antigens do not require T cells to initiate the immune response, but like TD antigens rely on suppressor T cells to slow down this response. Other subclasses of T cells may also influence the response to TI antigens, Thus, the distinction between TI and TD antigens resides in whether they require helper T cells.

Other terms used by immunologists may be confusing. These include *autologous antigen, heterologous antigen, homologous antigen,* and *heterophil antigen*. An autologous antigen is one's own antigen, which under appropriate circumstances would induce autoantibody formation; autologous antigen is thus synonymous with auto- or self antigen. A heterologous antigen is merely an antigen different, from that used in an immunization; it may or may not react with the antiserum depending on its chemical similarity to the immunizing or homologous antigen. The homologous antigen is simply that antigen used in the production of antiserum. In serologic tests a heterologous antigen may be used as a negative control for any nonspecific reaction arising from errors in performing the serologic test or in the preparation of the serologic reactants.

Cross-reactive antigens

Heterophil (heterogenetic) antigens are antigens that exist in unrelated plants or animals but are either identical or so closely related that antibodies to one will cross-react with the other. In many instances heterophil antigens are polysaccharides, which by virtue of their limited chemical complexity are structurally similar even though derived from widely separated taxonomic sources. Two examples of heterophil antigens involve the human blood group antigens. Human blood group A antigen is cross-reactive with antibody to pneumococcal capsular polysaccharide type XIV, and human blood group B antigen reacts with antibodies to certain strains of *Escherichia coli,* the common colon bacillus.

Ordinary cotton is related structurally to both type III and type VIII pneumococcal polysaccharides by virtue of their common cellobiuronic acid content (alternating D-glucose and D-glucuronic acid), and their antisera are mutually cross-reactive. Antisera to pneumococcal antigens III and VIII also cross-react with a polysaccharide from *E. coli* K87 and oat glucan (Fig. 2-1). Capsular cross-reactions have been observed between *Haemophilus influenzae* type a with pneumococcus type 6, *H. influenzae* type b and pneumococcus types VI, XV, XXVIII, and XXXV, and of type c with pneumococcus type XI.

Cross-reactions occur with protein antigens if the antigens are from closely related taxonomic sources. Antisera to hen egg albumin will react with duck egg albumin. Bovine and equine serum albumins, and bovine and human fibrinogens, are also cross-reactive. Cross-reactions of anti-beef insulin with the insulins from pigs, sheep, whales, humans, and other species are known (Table 2-2). These insulins are very low molecular weight proteins with nearly identical structures differing from each other by only a few or by even a single amino acid residue. Sheep insulin, for example, differs from beef insulin only by the replacement of serine with glycine in position 9 of the A chain; pig insulin differs from beef insulin at positions 8 and 10; and horse insulin varies from beef insulin at positions 8, 9, and 10.

The best known of the heterophil antigens is the Forssman antigen, originally described as an antigen

TABLE 2-2

Serologic and sequence relationships of insulins

Species	Amino acid in A chain positions			Reaction with anti-beef insulin
	8	9	10	
Beef	Alanine	Serine	Valine	
Sheep	Alanine	Glycine	Valine	Yes
Pig	Threonine	Serine	Isoleucine	Yes
Whale	Threonine	Serine	Isoleucine	Yes
Horse	Threonine	Glycine	Isoleucine	Yes
Rabbit	Threonine	Serine	Isoleucine	Yes

Data from Moloney, P.J.: Antibodies to insulin. In Young, F.G., editor: The mechanism of action of insulin, Springfield, Ill., 1960, Charles C Thomas, Publisher; and from Pope, C.G.: The immunology of insulin, Adv. Immunol. **5:**209, 1966.

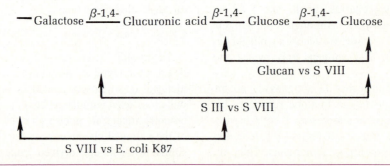

FIG. 2-1

This sequence of galactose, glucuronic acid, and two glucose residues is the basis of serologic cross-reactions, as noted by brackets.

present in most guinea pig tissues (but not red blood cells), which would stimulate the production of sheep red blood cell agglutinins by rabbits. The Forssman antigen is truly heterogenetic, since it is found in human erythrocytes, *Streptococcus pneumoniae,* horses, dogs, tigers, whales, carp, toads, turtles, chickens, and other organisms. It is absent from the rabbit, and it is on this basis that the rabbit is able to make antibodies to the Forssman antigen. Another interesting observation is that it is a hapten, not an antigen, since injections of purified Forssman "antigen" alone will not induce antibody formation. Glucose, galactose, ceramide, and *N*-acetylgalactosamine have been identified in the Forssman haptens.

The generic or class names given to antigens are supplemented by many additional variations. Among these are blood-group antigen, transplantation antigen, tumor antigen, and blocking antigen. It seems that almost any adjective can be used to modify the description of an antigen.

TYPES OF IMMUNIZATION
Active and passive immunization

Now that the nature of antigens has been described, it is appropriate to turn to the responses of the body to these antigens. The response to antigens is known as the immune response; the process itself is immunization, and it can take several forms.

Autoimmunization is the response of one's T or B cells to proteins or polysaccharides that have begun to function as self-antigens (autoantigens) or which serve as targets for immunoglobulins and T cell-directed activities. This process is usually expressed as some form of autoimmune disease or allergy.

Alloimmunization refers to immunization with antigens from an individual within one's own species. The genetic differences between individuals or races or strains within a species dictate the existence of unique antigenic specificities that are not shared by all members of the species. Exposure to these antigens is then an immunizing experience and the basis for blood-transfusion reactions and tissue graft rejection (when these are conducted within one species). The antigens responsible for these reactions are known as alloantigens, and the antibodies are alloantibodies.

The prefix *allo-,* and its use in the terms introduced here, means "other." *Allo-* generally is used when the other is closely related to the term with which it is compared. Alloantigen, alloantibody, alloimmunization, etc. are rapidly replacing other terms where the prefix *iso-* was used in the sense of *equal* or *similar*.

Immunization of one species with antigens from a second species is the usual kind of immunization. Since this is the standard form of immunization, the prefixes *xeno-* or *hetero-* may be used but are usually omitted.

These definitions and explanations of autoimmunization, alloimmunization, and xenoimmunization apply primarily to active immunization, in contrast to passive immunization. In the former situation the individual's own cells respond to the antigen by synthesizing antibodies or producing lymphokines. In the latter case antibodies or lymphokines produced by some donor individual are injected into a recipient who becomes passively immunized. Passive immunization is limited to alloimmunization and heteroimmunization.

Adoptive immunization

A third variety of immunization, more closely related to passive than to active immunization, is adoptive immunization. This term refers to the transplantation of immunocompetent tissue from one individual to an immunologically deficient individual. These tissues may already be in the process of immunoglobulin synthesis, or they may merely be ready for that activity when the recipient is later immunized. In either instance the result is actually a passive immunization, since it is not, strictly speaking, the cells of the recipient animal that synthesize the antibodies.

Adoptive immunization relies on the transplantation of tissue from one animal to another and consequently is subject to the immunologic principles governing transplantation (Chapter 15).

MITOGENS

Mitogens are substances that induce mitosis. Several plant proteins known as phytohemagglutinins because they will agglutinate erythrocytes are mitogenic for lymphocytes. These substances, also called lectins, bind to specific polysaccharide residues on the cells they agglutinate. Mitogens can be considered mimics of antigens because the proliferative response they initiate in lymphocytes causes these cells to engage in the same cellular and chemical activities that follow their exposure to antigens. The availability of mitogens specific for B cells or T cells, or ones that lack specificity and activate both B and T cells has facilitated the dissection of cellular interactions in the immune response and evaluation of lymphocyte-based immunodeficiencies. With few exceptions, these mitogens stimulate all cells in the target population, whether they are B cells, T cells, or both.

B cell mitogens

Lipopolysaccharide (LPS)

The most widely used mitogen for B cells is a lipopolysaccharide (LPS) of bacterial origin. This LPS also functions as an endotoxin. Bacterial endotoxins vary slightly in structure from one species source to another, but all contain a lipid moiety, lipid A, attached to a core polysaccharide. Two of these saccharides are unusual; one is the 8-carbon 2-keto-3-deoxyoctonic acid and the other is a 7-carbon sugar. Attached to the core is a terminal sequence consisting of repeated units of three to five sugars until a lengthy oligosaccharide is formed (Fig. 2-2). This sequence confers antigenicity upon the molecule and allows LPS to be referred to as the somatic (cellular)

antigen or O antigen of the bacterium from which it is derived. Typical sources of LPS include members of the Enterobacteriaceae—gram-negative bacteria that include the *Escherichia* and *Salmonella* among its members.

LPS has two major biologically active portions. Lipid A is the toxic and mitogenic portion that catalyzes cell division in all B cells. The terminal saccharide stimulates those cells destined to respond to LPS as an antigen. Thus LPS has both a monoclonal and polyclonal activity.

Protein A

Protein A is found on the surface of approximately 85% of all strains of *Staphylococcus aureus*. It is a protein with a molecular weight of 42,000 and exists as a single peptide chain devoid of carbohydrate. Protein A is very stable to heat and denaturing agents. Tyrosine residues in the molecule are essential to the ability of protein A to bind to a unique region of immunoglobulins known as the Fc region. Protein A exhibits a preferential binding for the Fc portion of human immunoglobulin G but will bind less actively to other antibody molecules. Four, possibly five, Fc binding areas are present in each molecule of Protein A but steric effects prevent all from functioning simultaneously. Typically the Protein A–IgG complex exists in the ratio of 1:2.

The mitogenic activity of protein A on human lymphocytes has been extensively studied. Only human B cells respond. The basis of this specificity is

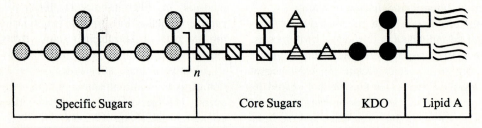

| Specific Sugars | Core Sugars | KDO | Lipid A |

FIG. 2-2

Bacterial lipopolysaccharides tend to share a common structure in which the mitogenic and toxic lipid A portion **(open rectangles)** is linked to 2-keto-3-deoxyoctonic acid (KDO). The core sugars are interposed between KDO and the terminal saccharides that confer antigenic specificity upon the molecule.

that immunoglobulin G is present on the surface of B lymphocytes and serves as the receptor for Protein A. Bridging of two IgGs by Protein A initiates mitosis.

Antiimmunoglobulin

For the same reason that Protein A is mitotic for B cells, antiimmunoglobulin is also mitogenic. Here it must be recognized that an antibody molecule is a large protein that can be antigenic for a second species, thus permitting the production of antiimmunoglobulins.

T cell mitogens
Concanavalin A (Con A)

Concanavalin A (Con A) was first extracted from jack bean *(Canavalia ensiformis)* in 1919 and was identified as a lectin for erythrocytes in 1935. Not until 1970 was it found that Con A would bind to lymphocytes. Con A is a protein existing predominantly as a tetramer above a pH of 7 and as a dimer below a pH of 6 (Table 2-3). The peptide subunits have a molecular weight of 25,500, and each one binds one Mn^{2+} and one Ca^{2+} ion. The presence of the metals is required for Con A binding to saccharides; again, each monomer can bind to one saccharide unit. The amino acid sequence of the monomer units has been determined but is not especially revealing. Salt bridges between 114 and 116 on one

dimer and glutamic acid 192 on the other hold the tetramer together. Succinylation of free amino groups in Con A converts it to the stable dimer.

Both Con A and succinyl Con A are potent mitogens for T lymphocytes, and a dose of 3 μg/ml is optimal. Both B and T lymphocytes bind Con A, and each lymphocyte has about 10×10^6 receptors per cell, but only the T cell is sensitive to Con A-induced lymphocyte transformation. The T cell receptors for Con A are α-D-mannopyranosides and α-D-glucopyranosides. This statement is based on the pronounced ability of methyl-α-D-mannoside and methyl-α-D-glucosides to inhibit Con A binding and mitogenicity.

Phytohemagglutinin (PHA)

PHA is a protein extracted from the red kidney bean, *Phaseolus vulgaris*. It has a powerful hemagglutinating property and in 1960 was discovered to induce lymphocyte activation. The optimal concentration of the reagent needed to demonstrate the maximum amount of mitogenic activity is only 1 to 5 μg/ml.

Most preparations of PHA used as mitogens have been crude extracts of kidney beans. Fractionation of these extracts by ion-exchange chromatography and molecular sieving has separated the lymphocyte-stimulating component, PHA-L, from the hemagglutinin, PHA-H. Both molecules are proteins with mo-

TABLE 2-3

Characteristics of selected mitogens

	Abbreviation	Source	Molecular weight	Lymphocyte receptor	Susceptible cell
Concanavalin A	Con A	*Canavalia ensiformis* (jack bean)	102,000	Mannosides and glucosides	T cells
Phytohemagglutinin	PHA or PHA-L	*Phaseolus vulgaris* (red or yellow beans)	115,000 to 140,000	*N*-acetyl-D-galactosamine	B and T cells; some species predominantly T cells
Pokeweed mitogen	PWM	*Phytolacca americana* (pokeweed)	32,000	Unidentified	T and B cells
Lipopolysaccharide	LPS	Gram-negative bacteria	About 4,000	Unidentified	B cells

lecular weights between 115,000 and 140,000. The PHA-L fraction is a glycoprotein and binds to other glycoproteins, which are its receptors on sensitive cells.

PHA binds to and activates both B and T cells, with some degree of specificity being exhibited in certain species. The ability of PHA to stimulate only 70% of mouse lymphocytes is indicative of a specificity for T cells in this species.

Combined B and T cell mitogens

Extracts from the roots, leaves, stems, and berries of the pokeweed, *Phytolacca americana,* have a feeble erythrocyte-clumping property. These extracts have a potent mitogenic activity for lymphocytes. The active ingredient in these extracts is a protein composed of a single peptide chain with a molecular weight of 32,000. The receptor site on lymphocytes for PWM is not known. PWM activates both B and T lymphocytes of mice.

Lectins extractable from the peanut *(Arachis hypogaea),* soybean *(Glycine max),* pea *(Pisum sativum),* and red and yellow wax bean *(Phaseolus vulgaris)* are all proteinaceous. The peanut agglutinin, soybean agglutinin, and wax bean agglutinin are of tetrameric peptide structure and have molecular weights between 110,000 and 130,000. All are specific for polysaccharides on the surface of cells to which they bind. These mitogens vary in their specificity for T and B cells.

ANTIGENIC DETERMINANT SITES

There is considerable evidence that only a specific, limited part of an antigen molecule is the inducer of B cell and T cell responses. This portion, which is also the part of the antigen with which the antibody reacts, is known as the antigenic determinant site, or epitope. The number of antigenic determinants per molecule of antigen is referred to as the valence of the antigen. In this context valence has absolutely no relationship to the ionic condition of the antigen.

The antigenic valence of a molecule can be considered in two contexts: the total valence and the functional valence. The functional valence of all complete antigens is two or more and for low molecular weight antigens is roughly proportional to the

molecular weight of the antigen, with one valence site existing for each 10,000 or so molecular weight. Functional valence sites are all on the outer surface of the antigenic molecule and can be measured by determining the number of antibody molecules that attach to the antigen. Total valence is the sum of the functional and nonfunctional (hidden) valence sites; this too is undoubtedly related to molecular size.

Since hydrolytic products of the antigen generated by phagocytes contain the epitopes then antibodies can be formed against internal antigenic determinants that are not functional in the parent molecule. These hidden epitopes can be identified only when the antigen undergoes structural alteration, which is possible by enzymatic hydrolysis so that identifiable fragments can be examined for the number of their antigenic determinant sites. Serum albumins, which have molecular weights of about 70,000, contain six functional valence sites, but enzymatic digestion (of bovine serum albumin) produces nine peptides, each of which is capable of precipitating with an antibody. Since it is known that precipitation requires at least two valence sites, a total of 18 (minimum) determinant sites must be present in the original molecule. It is unknown how many additional determinant sites are destroyed by the hydrolysis, but the total valence of bovine serum albumin is at least three times the functional valence.

Efforts to increase our understanding of the nature of antigenic determinant sites have been based on three different approaches: the degradation of antigens, the synthesis of antigens, and the alteration, or haptenic modification, of antigens.

Degradation of antigens

By a careful selection of proteases with restricted peptide-bond specificity, limited proteolysis of protein antigens will generate fragments that can be purified and then analyzed for their capacity to react with antisera prepared against the intact protein. Such studies are rather simply interpreted when linear proteins constitute the antigen; silk fibroin was one of the first to be examined in this manner. In this study ultimately one antigenic determinant site was identified to reside in an octapeptide consisting of Gly $(Gly_3 Ala_3)$ Tyr. (The parentheses indicate that the sequence within them was not determined.) Removal of the carboxyterminal tyrosine halved the antibody-combining power of the peptide; thus this determinant consisted of a linear sequence of about seven or eight amino acids and was dominated by a terminal constituent (Table 2-4).

A similar hydrolysis of tobacco mosaic virus protein produced several peptides with antibody-binding activity, but one, peptide VIII, was far more potent than any of the others. Within this peptide a locus consisting of Leu-Asp-Ala-Thr-Arg seemed to be the immunodominant portion. Synthesis of this peptide readily confirmed this dominance. Analogs that contained a single amino acid substitution revealed that such substitutions seriously affected the binding power. Thus, certain antisera are highly discriminatory, and antigen determinants are small (five amino acids).

Synthesis of antigens

Studies similar to those with degraded antigens have been repeated with synthetic polymers of the L-α-amino acids. The synthetic polyamino acids are much like native proteins but with some striking exceptions; for example, homopolymers containing but a single type of amino acid may be made, and the D isomers of the amino acids are as easily used as the L isomers. A third consideration is that the sequence of synthetic copolymers is exceptionally difficult to regulate and determine after synthesis. Consequently copolymers are discussed in terms of their percentage composition: $Glu_{59} Lys_{41}$ refers to a copolymer of glutamic acid and lysine in which the former accounts for 59% and the latter accounts for 41% of the molecule.

The results of immunochemical studies indicate that neither D nor L homopolypeptides are antigenic, regardless of their molecular weight. This finding is not unexpected in view of the known nonantigenicity of other large molecules that lack internal complexity. A mixture of poly-L-glutamic acid and poly-L-lysine is antigenic for rabbits, although neither polymer alone causes antibody formation. In the case of the mixture it is possible that a noncovalent bonding of these oppositely charged polymers occurs. This bonding could present a physical complexity to the antigen-processing cells that allows them to preserve chemical structures not seen in the individual polymers. A very similar mechanism is used to explain the "antigenicity" of nucleic acids that promote antibody formation when injected in complexes with acetylated bovine serum albumin but that are antigenically inert when injected alone. These studies support the conclusion that an antigenic determinant site

---

TABLE 2-4

Characteristics of antigenic determinants

Antigen or hapten	Molecular weight	Determinant	Determinant size	Important observation
Natural antigens				
Silk fibroin	50,000 to 60,000	Octapeptide	748	Terminal amino acid
Tobacco mosaic virus protein	16,500	Pentapeptide	646	Hydrophobic group
Dextran	50,000 to 100,000	Isomaltose	990	Little internal complexity
Synthetic antigens				
polyamino acids				
$G_{52} A_{38} T_{10}$	4,100			Low molecular weight
$G_{60} A_{30} T_{10}$	13,300	Hexapeptide	792	Noncovalent bonding to form determinant site
Haptens	Generally less than 1,000	Variable	Less than 1,000	End and acid groups, tertiary structure important

need not be entirely a covalently linked structure (Fig. 2-3).

Many copolymers of amino acids are antigenic. Larger molecular weight polypeptides are more antigenic than their lower molecular weight counterparts, even though both have the same qualitative composition. Polypeptides containing only two amino acids are usually poor antigens. The smallest pure polypeptide that is antigenic has a molecular weight of 4,100. Branched and multichain compounds are antigenic by virtue of this increased dimensional complexity. A polylysine, branched through the addition of polyalanine to the ε-amino group of some lysines, with the polyalanines in turn bearing a terminal Tyr-Glu, is antigenic. A polymer of the same composition in which the Tyr-Glu are attached to the polylysine core before the polyalanine is added is not antigenic. Thus, strategic positioning of the amino acids is essential to confer antigenicity on a molecule. Synthetic polypeptides always have low valence, apparently because the same antigenic determinant site recurs periodically in the molecule.

Haptens

From the studies of Karl Landsteiner the concept of haptens emerged. Haptens are nonantigenic compounds, usually of low molecular weight, which could be covalently coupled to existing antigens to create new antigenic determinants. (In some instances it is possible to create antigens by adding many hapten groups to a nonantigen.) These hapten-antigen complexes, or conjugated or neoantigens, generate antibodies with specificity for the haptenic group.

A hypothetical hapten (H) combined with an antigen (Ag-1) forms the new complex H-Ag-1. Immunization of an animal with these substances will result in the formation of antisera (sera containing antibodies), as listed in Table 2-5. Injection of H alone is incapable of raising an antiserum, but the injections of Ag-1 and H-Ag-1 result in the formation of antisera in complete harmony with the fact that these substances are antigens. The reactivity of the antisera to Ag-1 (anti-Ag-1) and to the hapten antigen-1 conjugate (anti-H-Ag-1) is illustrated in Table 2-6. H

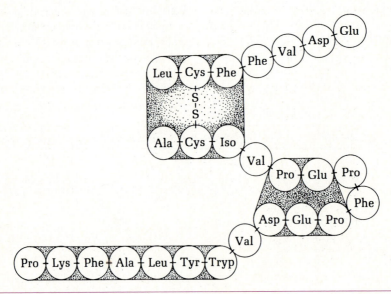

FIG. 2-3

Three antigenic determinants sites, represented by the stippled areas of five to seven amino acids in the peptide fragment shown, indicate that determinant sites may be either linear or nonlinear within a single peptide chain or across two peptide chains. The same features apply to polysaccharide antigens.

will not react with anti-Ag-1 (line 1), but it will react with anti-H-Ag-1 (line 2). The portion of the antiserum reacting is that with a specificity for the hapten. As seen in lines 3 and 4, Ag-1 will react with anti-Ag-1 and anti-H-Ag-1, and in the latter case it is the portion of the antiserum directed against Ag-1 that participates. Occasionally this reaction, although logically expected, does not occur. This may be the situation when the haptenic modification of Ag-1 has been so extensive that every original antigenic determinant site is altered. In such an instance anti-H-Ag-1 actually has a totally new antigenic specificity, which is not similar to that of native Ag-1, and so no reaction occurs between these two. In line 5 we see, as expected, that H-Ag-1 reacts with anti-H-Ag-1. Line 6 again illustrates the specificity of anti-H-Ag-1 for H, since that is the common denominator between the antigen and the antiserum in this instance. Ag-2 can have no bearing on this reaction, as seen by the results of reaction 7.

The selection of haptens with known structures permitted Landsteiner to assess the specificity of the antibody response within very finite limits. Most of Landsteiner's studies involved the use of substituted azoproteins as antigens. Substituted aromatic amines were converted to diazonium salts, which then covalently combined with the tyrosyl residue in any antigenic protein to form the monosubstituted derivative. If the hapten was present in sufficient excess, the disubstituted product would be formed. Antisera formed to one azoantigen, possibly diazoarsanilic acid coupled to bovine γ-globulin, were made to react with diazoarsanilic acid coupled to another carrier such as ovalbumin so that only the hapten specificity would be measured. Then a series of closely related azohaptens coupled to ovalbumin were tested against the antiserum. The reactions were graded on a simple plus-minus basis or estimated in terms of percentage to determine the specificity of the antisera.

A second method used to evaluate the specificity of these antisera was to preincubate them with the related hapten (in its nondiazotized form) prior to an incubation with the original hapten-antigen conjugate. The degree by which the second reaction was inhibited was used as a measure of the specificity of the antiserum for the related hapten.

From these studies several conclusions became evident. Historically it is only fair to state that they have probably been overemphasized. Certainly the following are not conclusions that can be fairly applied to all antigens, but in the framework within which they were developed—the diazohapten-antigen system—they are valid conclusions.

1. Strongly acid or basic groups are usually very decisive in regulating antibody specificity.
2. Nonionic groups of approximately equal size

TABLE 2-5

Effects of hapten-antigen immunization

Material injected	Antibody formed
Hapten (H)	None
Antigen-1 (Ag-1)	Anti-Ag-1
Hapten-Antigen-1 (H-Ag-1)	Anti-H-Ag-1

TABLE 2-6

Reactions of hapten-antigen antisera

Hapten (H) or antigen (Ag)		Antiserum	Reaction	Portion of antiserum reacting
1 H	+	Anti-Ag-1	No	None
2 H	+	Anti-H-Ag-1	Yes	Anti-H
3 Ag-1	+	Anti-Ag-1	Yes	Anti-Ag-1
4 Ag-1	+	Anti-H-Ag-1	Yes	Anti-Ag-1
5 H-Ag-1	+	Anti-H-Ag-1	Yes	Anti-H-Ag-1
6 H-Ag-2	+	Anti-H-Ag-1	Yes	Anti-H
7 Ag-2	+	Anti-H-Ag-1	No	None

and shape are interchangeable without significant losses in serologic activity.

3. Spatial configurations of haptens (D-, L-, ortho-, meta-, para-, and other) are important.
4. Terminal components of an antigen often exert a controlling influence on the specificity of the antibodies formed.

Only one example of these studies is described here. The dominance of acidic groups in determining the specificity of the antibody formed is observable in Table 2-7. In this experiment antisera versus the parapositioned carboxylic, sulfonic, and arsonic acid residues on substituted anilines were prepared. These antisera were tested in mutual cross-reactions with these haptens conjugated to a different carrier protein. In every instance complete specificity for the type of acid was observed, and no cross-reactions occurred.

The basis for this specificity is illustrated in Fig. 2-4 where the acidic groups concerned are depicted in a relative approximation of their sizes—the carboxyl group being the smallest and the arsonic group the largest. Here it can be seen that the sulfonic acid group has the best fit with the anti-sulfonic acid antibody. The carboxyl group can enter the crevice in the antibody built to receive the sulfonic acid moiety but is too small to bind tightly and easily dissociates from it. In contrast, the arsonic acid group is too large to enter the reactive site of the antibody.

Autocoupling haptens

A number of highly reactive low molecular weight compounds, which on the basis of size alone must be considered haptens, will produce antibodies if injected alone into an animal. Representative of such compounds are free diazonium salts, fluoro- and chloro-substituted dinitrophenyl compounds, acid anhydrides, and others. Decomposition products of penicillin have this property, and this is one way antibodies to penicillin are formed (Fig. 2-5). These compounds all have one property in common: the ability to form spontaneous covalent bonds with tissue proteins or polysaccharides to create neoantigens in vivo. These conjugates represent novel antigens to the animal, and the animal responds with antibody. In any discussion of haptens, autocoupling haptens must be considered a unique class of haptens because of their special chemical reactivity.

Unlike the response to the usual hapten-antigen complexes, which are normally no more offensive to an animal's health than the injection of other antigens, the response to autocoupling haptens can have serious consequences. One of these is the anaphylactic reaction based on IgE antibodies formed as a result of the autocoupling hapten's ability to conjugate with tissue macromolecules. Subsequent reinjection of the autocoupling hapten results in an in vivo serologic reaction between the IgE and the hapten that can be fatal or near fatal within minutes after the in-

---

TABLE 2-7

Contribution of acidic radicals to serologic specificity

Antigen conjugated with	Antisera versus			
	NH$_2$ (benzene ring) Aniline	NH$_2$ (benzene ring) COOH PABA	NH$_2$ (benzene ring) SO$_3$H PASA	NH$_2$ (benzene ring) AsO$_3$H$_2$ PAAA
Aniline	+ + +	—	—	—
PABA	—	+ + + ±	—	—
PASA	—	—	+ + + ±	—
PAAA	—	—	—	+ + + ±

From Landsteiner, K.: The specificity of serologic reactions, revised ed., New York, 1962, Dover Press, Inc.

jection. This is the subject of Chapter 17. The application of autocoupling haptens to the skin can induce contact dermatitis, a form of drug allergy related to the sensitization of T cells and the products they release. This subject is dealt with in Chapter 19.

ADJUVANTS

Aside from the intrinsic variations in the immune response governed by the immunized animal and the antigen, the antibody response also can be modified by specific treatments of the animal. Some of these treatments may enhance the antibody response, whereas others may have the exact opposite effect.

Adjuvants (Latin *adjuvare,* to help) are agents used to potentiate the immune response. Although this often is thought of merely in terms of the immunoglobulin response, it is clear that many adjuvants also stimulate the activities of T lymphocytes (cell-mediated immunity [CMI] and activate macrophages. Stimulation of the immune response gen-

erally is measured in terms of a greater antibody response than that produced without adjuvants or in the conservation of the quantity of antigen needed to achieve an optimal immune response. Adjuvants customarily are administered with the antigen; although not an absolute necessity, simultaneous administration generally avoids the need for a second injection of the adjuvant alone. Adjuvants may or may not be antigens in their own right.

Among the repository adjuvants, the aluminum and calcium salts, including aluminum phosphate, aluminum hydroxide, aluminum potassium tartrate (alum), and calcium phosphate, are the best known. When these materials are incorporated with antigen, they form an insoluble complex with the antigen. This complex slows the escape of antigen from a subcutaneous or intramuscular depot (which can be as great as 99% complete in 24 hours without adjuvant); by increasing the physical size of the antigens, they also enhance phagocytosis. The original antige-

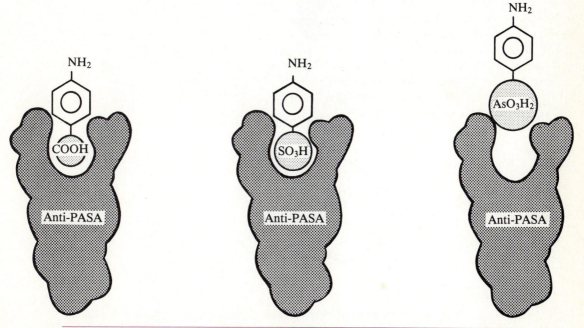

FIG. 2-4

The specificity of an antihapten is represented here by the close physical fit of para-aminosulfonic acid with its antibody, whereas the related carboxylic and sulfonic haptens are respectively too small or too large for a firm combination.

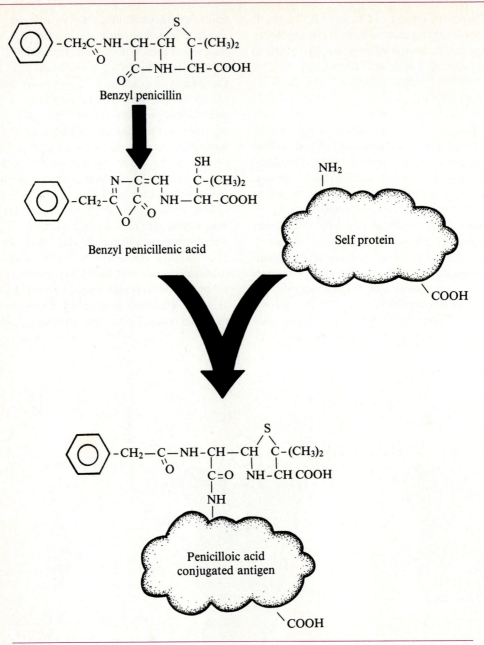

FIG. 2-5

Benzylpenicillenic acid is one of many decomposition products of penicillin G. This acid can form peptide bonds with the amino groups of tissue proteins, creating neoantigens in which the penicillin derivative is most closely related to penicilloic acid. Conjugates of penicillin derivatives can also form easily by —S—S—exchange with the sulfur atom in the thiazolidine portion of the antibiotic structure, but these are less important as allergens.

nic stimulus is prolonged over a period of 3 to 4 weeks because of the gradual dissolution and release of antigen from its insolubilized form. This creates the effect of multiple, microbooster exposures.

Water-in-oil emulsifying adjuvants have had a restricted use in humans, but the prospects for developing new and superior adjuvants of this type are great. The emulsified adjuvants allow only a slow release of the antigen from the oil-covered droplets into the true physiologic milieu of the animal, since the droplets, varying broadly in size, disintegrate at different rates. The second role of water-in-oil adjuvants is to provide microdroplets of antigen in oil to phagocytic cells. Again phagocytes can imbibe these antigen droplets more easily than antigen in solution.

A classic example of the water-in-oil emulsion adjuvant is Freund's adjuvant. The incomplete form of this adjuvant consists of a mixture of a light mineral oil and an emulsifier such as mannide monooleate. To it the antigen in aqueous solution is added, and the emulsion is produced in a pharmaceutical blender or by passing the mixture repeatedly through a small-bore needle-and-syringe assembly. Freund's complete adjuvant contains 0.5 mg/ml killed mycobacteria as a supplement to the incomplete adjuvant. The bacteria available in commercial preparations are either *Mycobacterium butyricum* or *M. tuberculosis*. Experimental formulations often substitute *Corynebacterium parvum (Propionibacterium acnes)* or BCG vaccine for the usual mycobacteria. Freund's complete adjuvant produces such serious granulomas that it is not recommended for human use. The adjuvant property of tubercle bacilli has been identified to reside in an unusual peptide, *N*-acetylmuramyl-L-alanyl-D-isoglutamine, or muramyl dipeptide (MDP) (Fig. 2-6). MDP does not produce granulomas. It and several of its chemical modifications are being compared for their adjuvant effect.

Newer water-in-oil emulsions prepared from highly purified and metabolizable ingredients soon may be sanctioned for human use. Since the ingredients are fully metabolizable, disfiguring granuloma

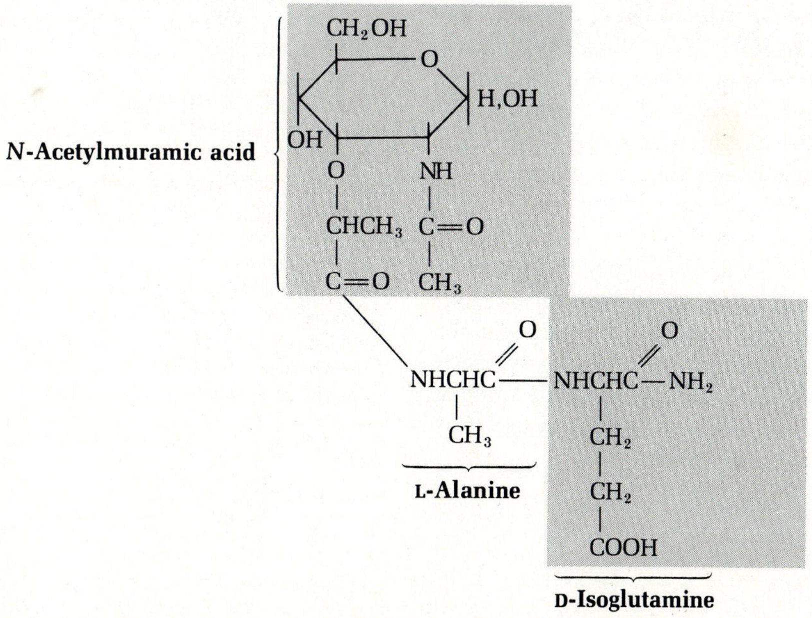

FIG. 2-6

The structure of *N*-acetylmuramyl-L-alanyl-D-isoglutamine, the adjuvant peptide isolated from the tubercle bacillus.

formation is not a complication as it is with other emulsifying adjuvants. Microscopic, uniformly sized water-in-oil droplets are referred to as liposomes. When phospholipids that are normally present in the host's cells are used as the oil base, the liposomes are completely biodegradable.

LPSs from nearly all gram-negative bacilli are stimulants of IgM production. The polysaccharide portion is relatively noncontributory to adjuvanticity, with the dominant biologic activity residing in the lipid A fraction (Fig 2-2). Pure lipid A is pyrogenic and is probably a central cause of the fever observed during infections with gram-negative bacteria. This pyrogenicity is also a handicap to the use of LPS in human medicine as an adjuvant. The primary role of LPS is as a polyclonal stimulant of the IgM class of B lymphocytes.

A bacterium used successfully as an adjuvant is *Bordetella pertussis*. The smooth, or phase I, *B. pertussis* cells contain a lymphocytosis-promoting factor that seems to mobilize both T and B cells. These gram-negative bacteria also contain an LPS.

An additional class of molecules with adjuvant action consists of those that labilize lysosomes. Substances such as vitamin A, beryllium salts, toxic forms of silica, and certain quaternary ammonium salts are all potent activators of macrophages and stimulate lysosomal enzyme release by these cells, which presumably improves antigen processing.

Theoretically adjuvants may act by one or more of the following mechanisms: (1) directly increasing the number of cells involved in antibody formation, (2) ensuring a more efficient processing of the antigen, (3) prolonging the duration of the antigen in the immunized animal, and (4) increasing the synthesis and release of antibody from the antibody-forming cells. There is good evidence that adjuvants may function by the first three methods, but there is no known method of stimulating antibody-synthesizing cells to a greater rate of synthesis. Agents that lyse antibody-containing cells will cause the release of antibody into the serum and temporarily increase the antibody titer, but the long-term effect, resulting from destruction of the cells directly concerned with antibody synthesis, is depression of antibody titers.

REFERENCES

Atassi, M.Z., editor: Immunobiology of proteins and peptides I-III, New York, 1982, Plenum Press.
Atassi, M.Z., vanOss, C.J., and Absolom, D.R., editors: Molecular immunology: a textbook, New York, 1984, Marcel Dekker, Inc.
Berzofsky, J.A.: Intrinsic and extrinsic factors in antigenic structure, Science **229**:932, 1985.
Celada, F., Schumaker, V.N., and Sercarz, E.E., editors: Protein conformation as an immunological signal, New York, 1983, Plenum Press.
Fenichel, R.L., and Chirigos, M.A., editors: Immune modulation agents and their mechanisms, New York, 1984, Marcel Dekker, Inc.
Fudenberg, H.H., and Whitten, H.D.: Immunostimulation: synthetic and biological modulators of immunity, Ann. Rev. Pharmacol. Toxicol. **24**:147, 1984.
Fudenberg, H.H., Whitten H.D., and Ambrogi, F., editors: Immunomodulation: new frontiers and advances, New York, 1984, Plenum Press.
Landsteiner, K.: The specificity of serologic reactions, revised ed., New York, 1962, Dover Press, Inc.
Langone, J.J.: Protein A of *Staphylococcus aureus* and related immunoglobulin receptors produced by streptococci and pneumococci, Adv. Immunol. **32**:158, 1982.
Sela, M.: The antigens, vols. 1–6, New York, 1973–1982, Academic Press, Inc.
Warren, H.S., Vogel, F.R., and Chedid, L.A.: Current status of immunological adjuvants, Ann. Rev. Immunol. **4**:369, 1986.
Westphal, O., Jann, K., and Himmelspach, K.: Chemistry and immunochemistry of bacterial lipopolysaccharides as cell wall antigens and endotoxins, Prog. Allergy **33**:9, 1983.

The immunoglobulins

≡GLOSSARY

α-chain   The H peptide chain of IgA.

Am marker   An allotypic determinant in α-chains.

antibody fragment   A portion of an antibody molecule as created by enzymatic hydrolysis or chemical dissociation.

Bence Jones protein   An immunoglobulin L chain, that is, κ- or λ-chain, often found in urine or blood of patients with a myeloma.

C_H1, C_H2, C_H3, and C_H4   The portions of the H chains of immunoglobulins with constant amino acid sequences.

C_L   The portions of κ- and λ-chains with constant amino acid sequences.

constant domain   A region in an immunoglobulin whose amino acid sequence is homologous to the sequence in another region.

δ-chain   The H chain of IgD.

domain   A section or region in the peptide chain of an immunoglobulin.

ε-chain   The H chain of IgE.

Fab fragment   A fragment of an immunoglobulin consisting of one L chain and half of the H chain.

$F(ab')_2$ fragment   Two Fab fragments plus an additional portion of the H chain of the immunoglobulin joined by disulfide bonds between the H chain portions of the fragment.

Fc fragment   A polypeptide fragment of an immunoglobulin representing the carboxyl half of both H chains joined by disulfide bonds, as after papain treatment of IgG.

Fc′ fragment   The carboxyl half of both H chains after pepsin treatment of IgG.

Fd fragment   That portion of the H chain in an Fab fragment.

Fd′ fragment   The portion of the H chain in the $F(ab')_2$ fragment.

FR   Framework region.

framework region   The section in the V_L and V_H domains between the HV regions.

γ-chain   The H chain of IgG.

γ-globulin   A portion of the serum proteins in which the immunoglobulins are found; characterized by low electrophoretic mobility at pH 8.3.

gammopathy   An imbalance in immunoglobulin concentration.

Gm group   An allotypic group based on antigenic changes in H chain antigens of IgG.

H chain   The heavy chain of an immunoglobulin.

heavy chain   The large polypeptide chain, of which two exist, in the basic four-peptide structure of an immunoglobulin.

hinge region   The region in the H chain of an immunoglobulin between CH1 and CH2 and near the sites of papain and pepsin cleavage.

HV   Hypervariable region.

hypervariable region   A section of intense variability in the V_L or V_H domain.

immunoglobulin A (IgA)   One of five serum immunoglobulins, possessing α H chains.

immunoglobulin D (IgD)   The immunoglobulin in lowest concentration in serum, possessing δ H chains.

immunoglobulin E (IgE)   The serum immunoglobulin with a potent homocytotropic tendency for mast cells, possessing ε H chains.

immunoglobulin G (IgG)   The serum globulin in greatest concentration (75% to 95% of the total) and possessing γ H chains.

immunoglobulin M (IgM)   The serum immunoglobulin of greatest molecular weight (about 900,000) formed earliest after antigen exposure and possessing μ H chains.

isotype   Synonym of class when referring to immunoglobulins.

J chain   A polypeptide chain found attached to secretory IgA and IgM that may function as a joining chain.

ϰ-chain   One of two types of L chain found in an immunoglobulin.

Km   A κ-chain allotypic marker: Km1, Km2, and Km3.

L chain   Light chain of an immunoglobulin.

λ-chain   An antigenic form of L chain of the immunoglobulins.

light chain   The smallest of the two types of polypeptide chains (light and heavy) of immunoglobulins; two exist in the four-peptide unit.

M component   The serum protein produced in excessive concentration in cases of myeloma or macroglobulinemia.

μ-chain   The H chain of IgM.

multiple myeloma   *see* Myeloma.

myeloma   A plasma cell neoplasm resulting in excessive production of one or more immunoglobulins.

SC   Secretory component.

secretory component   A portion of secretory IgA and secretory IgM not present in serum IgA or IgM and not produced in plasma cells.

secretory immunoglobulin   An immunoglobulin found in colostrum, saliva, mucous secretions, etc., as secretory IgA or secretory IgM.

variable domain   A region in an immunoglobulin whose amino acid sequence is inconstant from one molecular species to another.

Waldenström's macroglobulinemia   A myeloma involving IgM or IgM-like molecules.

In the human there are five molecular classes of immunoglobulins, designated IgG, IgA, IgM, IgD, and IgE. In each, Ig refers to immunoglobulin and the third letter to some distinctive property of that immunoglobulin. The immunoglobulin classes also are called isotypes. Within each isotype or class the molecules share antigenic determinants. Thus an antiserum prepared in a rabbit by immunizing it with human IgG would react with all samples of human IgG because they share isotypic determinants.

STRUCTURE AND CHEMISTRY OF IgG

Immunoglobulin G, abbreviated IgG, is the best known and most fully studied of the immunoglobulins. It is the immunoglobulin referred to when reference is made simply to γ-globulin without further specification (Table 3-1). It is also known as γ_2-globulin and 7Sγ-globulin. The γ indicates its position in the serum electrophoretic profile, which is actually a rather broad region compared with that of the albumins. The 7S refers to its $S_{20,w}$ sedimentation coefficient (Svedberg coefficient), a number that indicates its sedimentation rate in the analytic ultra-

TABLE 3-1

Chemical and physical properties of immunoglobulin G

Current designation	IgG
Older names	γ-Globulin, 7Sγ-globulin
Molecular weight	150,000
$S_{20,w}$ value	6.6
Electrophoretic mobility	γ
Carbohydrate content	2.5% to 4%
Resistance to —SH reagents	High
Concentration (mg/dl serum)	1,275 ± 500
Amount of serum immunoglobulins	75% to 85%
Half-life (days)	25 to 35
Rate of synthesis (mg/kg body weight/day)	28
Light chain types	κ or λ
Heavy chain class	γ
General formula	$\gamma_2\kappa_2$ or $\gamma_2\lambda_2$
Light chain allotypes	Km
Heavy chain subclasses	$\gamma_1, \gamma_2, \gamma_3, \gamma_4$
Heavy chain allotypes	Gm
Stable at 56° to 60° C	Yes

centrifuge. The true $S_{20,w}$ value of IgG is closer to 6.6 than to 7. In the human IgG represents about 80% of the total antibody in an antiserum. Expressed in concentration this amounts to 1275 ± 500 mg/dl of serum. This high serum level is a reflection of both the rate of synthesis and the rate of elimination of IgG. It is produced at the rate of about 28 mg/kg body weight/day and has a half-life of approximately a month. IgG has a molecular weight of approximately 150,000, 2.5% of which is in the form of carbohydrate.

Fragments and chains

The history of the chemical structure of the IgG molecule is quite fascinating and is the model after which the study of other immunoglobulins has been patterned. The two studies that contributed most decisively to unraveling the structure of the immunoglobulins were those by Edelman in the United States at Rockefeller University and by Porter at Oxford University in England. In 1972 the Nobel Prize Committee in Physiology and Medicine recognized the contributions of these two scientists by awarding them a joint Nobel Prize. The main observation of Edelman was that purified preparations of IgG were resistant to reductive cleavage by sulfhydryl reagents unless the molecule was unfolded by high concentrations of urea or guanidine. These two compounds at 7M or 8M are known to interrupt hydrogen bonds, which hold globular proteins in their unique shapes. When unfolded by 7M urea, proteins become more linear and expose groupings that were previously situated inside the molecule. This permits compounds such as mercaptoethanol (CH_2OHCH_2SH) to engage in oxidation-reduction reactions with disulfide groups that were previously masked. The —S—S— bonds of IgG are converted to two free —SH moieties while mercaptoethanol is oxidized and dimerized to a disulfide ($CH_2OHCH_2S)_2$. When IgG is examined in an analytic ultracentrifuge after such a treatment, the original 7S protein is absent, and two new peaks are seen. The heavier of these is a 3.5S molecule, and the other is about 2.2S. Calculation of the molecular weights of the heavy (H) and light (L) components indicates that they are about 50,000 and 20,000, respectively. Comparison of these values with the calculated molecular weight of IgG at 150,000 reveals that two H and two L components make up essentially all the original molecule. Each IgG thus has two H chains and two L chains held together by disulfide bonds, and its structure is represented by the simple formula H_2L_2.

The Nobel Prize-winning discovery of Porter was based on his use of the proteolytic enzyme papain and a mild reducing environment to cleave the IgG molecule into three portions, two of which were identical. Papain digestion of IgG reduces it to polypeptides that behave as 3.5S molecules in the analytic ultracentrifuge. No 2.2S peak is observed. This 3.5S product of papain cleavage differs sharply in its immunochemical characteristics from the 3.5S product arising from disulfide reduction in urea. Carboxymethyl cellulose ion exchange chromatography will separate the papain cleavage products in two types of fragments, one of which, the *Fc fragment,* crystallizes spontaneously at 4° C. This fragment is deficient in antigen-binding ability and is now known to represent the carboxyl half of two H chains still held together by one or more interchain —S—S— bonds. The Fc fragment has a molecular weight of approximately 50,000. The sedimentation coefficient of the remaining portion, also 3.5S, indicates that it also should have a similar molecular weight. Since this remaining fragment is antigen-binding, it is called the *Fab fragment.* In the intact IgG molecule it is known that there are two loci capable of binding antigen, and, with the molecular weight borne in mind, it is clear that IgG = 1 Fc + 2 Fab (Fig. 3-1) Each Fab fragment consists of the amino terminal half of the H chain (Fd) plus an L chain. It is thus possible to design a structure that represents these findings (Fig. 3-2).

Pepsin cleavage of IgG yields a fragment that is nearly identical to the Fc fragment, called the Fc′ fragment. The difference between Fc and Fc′ is that the former is slightly larger, retaining somewhat more of the H chain than does the latter. Those amino acids in the region between the Fc and Fc′ cleavage points are termed the *hinge peptides.* This term is more meaningful than it would appear at first. Morphologic evidence indicates that the H chains actually are bent at this position when the antibody combines with antigen.

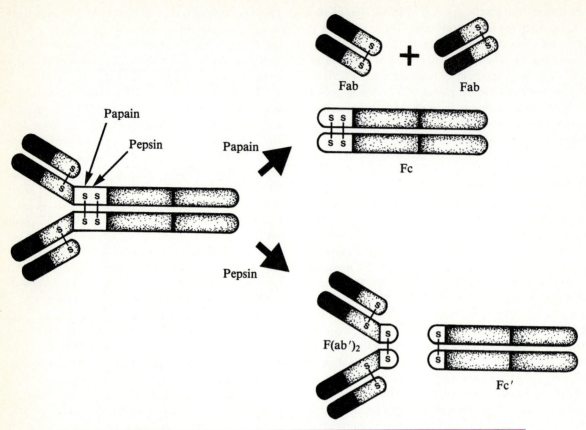

FIG. 3-1

Proteolysis of IgG by papain produces 2 Fab fragments and an Fc fragment whereas pepsin hydrolysis produces one F(ab′)₂ and one Fc′ fragment. Papain and pepsin cleave both H chains.

The remainder of the IgG molecule, after removal of the Fc piece, is basically two Fab pieces held together by an —S—S— bond plus the hinge peptide. It is designated as F(ab′)₂, since it contains a small additional part of the H chain that the Fab fragments lack. That portion of the H chain found in the F(ab′)₂ fragment is Fd′, differing from Fd in that it contains a portion of the hinge region. F(ab′)₂ fragments have an $S_{20,w}$ of approximately 5.

Since the L chains are fairly small, it was thought reasonable to begin amino acid sequence studies with this portion of IgG to unravel some of the mystery of how an antibody combines with an antigen. It had been demonstrated that the total amino acid composition of different antibodies was not identi-

cal, and sequence studies probably would add more understanding to where and how these differences existed.

The possibility of amino acid sequence studies of immunoglobulin L and H chains was greatly increased by the discovery of two unique conditions. The first of these was the availability of human myeloma proteins; the second, the recognition of homogeneous antibodies. More recently hybridomas have been used as a source of pure immunoglobulins.

Multiple myelomas

Multiple myeloma is a neoplasm of proliferating immunocytes or plasma cells. These plasma cell tumors proliferate in the bone marrow and erode away

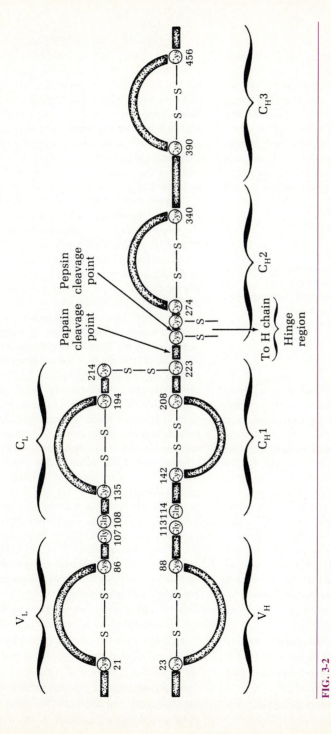

FIG. 3-2

Half of an IgG molecule: the shorter peptide is the L chain, and the longer peptide is the H chain, in this case the γ-chain. At the left, or amino terminal, end a variable domain is present on both the L and H chains. These are the V_L and V_H domains, which consist of approximately 107 amino acids. The next 107 amino acids of the L chain form the constant domain (C_L). The H chain has three constant domains, C_H1, C_H2, and C_H3, with the hinge region situated between C_H1 and C_H2. Each domain contains approximately 107 amino acids. The two H chains are joined where indicated to form the four-chain structure. The points of papain and pepsin cleavage also are indicated.

≡ SITUATION

MULTIPLE MYELOMA

A 60-year-old white man was admitted to the hospital with pains in his back and legs. He had enlarged lymph nodes in the cervical, axillary, and groin areas. His hemoglobulin level was 12.4 g/dl, the white blood cell count was 9,200/mm^3, and the serum bilirubin level was elevated. Urinalysis was 1+ for protein. Serum protein electrophoresis indicated a possible polyclonal gammopathy of the A and G classes. Total serum protein levels were normal. Skeletal x-ray films, bone marrow aspiration, and quantitative immunoglobulin determinations were ordered.

Question

1. What is the probable nature of the proteinuria?
2. How does the total serum level remain normal with a concurrent polyclonal gammopathy?
3. How can a polyclonal gammopathy be suggested only from serum electrophoresis?
4. What is the preferred procedure for immunoglobulin quantitation?

Solution

The proteinuria undoubtedly is caused by Bence Jones protein. To test for Bence Jones protein, it may be necessary to acidify the urine to pH 4.5 with dilute acetic acid. The exact temperatures at which precipitation and dissolution occur vary from patient to patient; some Bence Jones proteins do not dissolve at 100° C. The frequency of Bence Jones protein in urine has varied from as low as 30% to as high as 88% of myeloma cases. This wide range undoubtedly is caused by differences in technique (acidity of urine), protein concentration, and temperature criteria. The electrophoresis of fivefold to tenfold concentrated urine has done much to improve the urinary identification of Bence Jones protein. Systematic investigation indicates an incidence in urine in excess of 50%. The Bence Jones protein is frequently the only protein in the urine, where it is situated in the electrophoretic position occupied by the γ-globulins. It is the L chain of the immunoglobulins or dimeric or polymeric forms of the molecule.

As an aside, it is interesting that the name of Sir Henry Bence Jones has been perpetuated by this protein. Bence Jones was a clinical pathologist who recognized the protein in a urine sample supplied by Dr. Dalrymple, and another physician, Dr. Watson, later cared for the patient. The names of the patient and the two attending physicians have fallen into obscurity.

Polyclonal and monoclonal M components do not necessarily disturb the total γ-globulin concentration of the serum; in fact hypogammaglobulinemia is seen in 12% of all patients with myeloma. This has been interpreted as an elimination of normal plasma cells by cells of the plasmacytoma. Serum electrophoresis may identify the class of the hypogammaglobulinemic as well as the hypergammaglobulinemic protein. Simple serum electrophoresis often will distinguish an IgG myeloma from the others. Mixed IgA and IgM proteins will appear in nearly the same electrophoretic position and obscure the identification of the condition as a polyclonal disease. IgG with either IgA or IgM is more easily identified, although whether the second protein is A or M is often difficult to decide. In the recent past this distinction has been made via immunoelectrophoretic determinations of a crude quantitative nature with specific antisera against IgG, IgA, and IgM with normal strength and diluted serum. If the serum IgG and IgA are no longer detectable with specific antisera tested against diluted serum but the IgM is, then the indication is that the myeloma is of the IgM class. Radial immunodiffusion tests are now preferred because they are more sensitive and quantitative. In the patient described the Mancini test recovered 3.2 g/dl of IgG and 0.6 g/dl of IgA. Normal values should approximate 1.3 g/dl for IgG and 0.3 g/dl for IgA; thus the patient had a combined IgG and IgA myeloma.

the surrounding hard bone. On radiographic examination discrete holes are apparent in the osseous tissue. These can become so extensive that the long bones of the body fracture when moderate weight or stress is applied. Meanwhile plasma cell infiltration of the soft tissues also develops.

In bone marrow or other lymphoid tissue heavy sheets of plasma cells can be detected, accounting for as much as 10% of all cells in the marrow in advanced cases. In the normal individual, plasma cells are relatively uncommon in bone marrow. The plasma cells may be either of two types; the first is

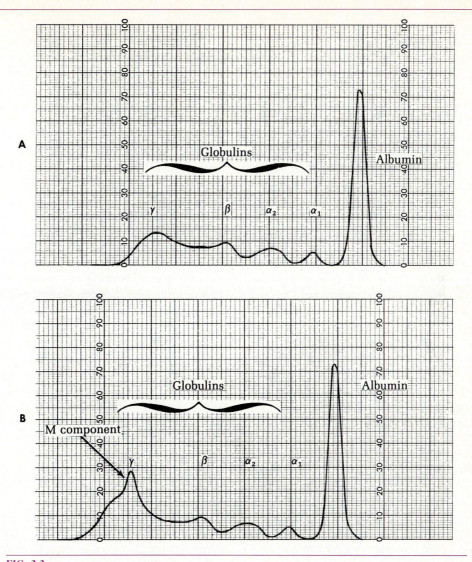

FIG. 3-3

A, Tracing of an electrophoretic separation of a normal serum. **B**, Same type of tracing of a serum from a patient with multiple myeloma. Notice the monoclonal nature of the disease.

the typical plasma cell with sparse cytoplasm and the classic pyroninophilic staining behavior, and the other exhibits a swollen cytoplasm containing globules of protein known as Russell bodies—inclusions of immunoglobulin. Their presence is a reflection of the ambitious protein-synthesizing activity of these plasma cells. The result is an unusually high serum concentration of γ-globulin, which can be detected by ordinary serum electrophoretic analysis. This analysis may reveal that practically all the excess γ-globulin has migrated to a specific point in the γ-β portion of the serum electrophoretic profile (Fig. 3-3). A quantitative tracing of the serum proteins will indicate this point by a pronounced absorption spike.

This nearly monophoretic protein is known as an M (myeloma) component or M protein. When a single spike is seen, it is indicative that the gammopathy (disease of γ-globulin) is related to the excessive replication of a single type of plasma cell to produce a clone of such cells, all of which are excreting the same kind of γ-globulin. This is appropriately described as a monoclonal gammopathy or monoclonal immunoproliferative disease, which indicates the homogeneity of the cells involved and their serum product. In contrast to this situation, when several peaks are seen in the serum profile, or when the entire region is elevated, several different clones of plasma cells are simultaneously engaged in overproduction of immunoglobulin. Accordingly several kinds of γ-globulin are being produced, resulting in electrophoretic heterogeneity. This type of myeloma is referred to as a polyclonal gammopathy.

In certain instances the position of the M component in the electrophoretic profile of the serum will suggest that the M component is of the IgG, IgA, IgM, or other class. If the M component were situated at the far end of the IgG range, it would suggest that it is an IgG myeloma and not an IgA or IgM type, since these latter immunoglobulins typically migrate more toward the β side of the γ-β gulf. However, the electrophoretic positioning of the M components(s) is unreliable in determining the class of immunoproliferative disorder. This can be done only by using antisera that are specific for the different classes of γ-globulin. Only then can one refer to the γG, γA, γM, etc. myeloma. Of these myelomas, 60% are of the IgG class, 16% are IgA, and 14% are IgM. IgD myelomas represent less than 1% of the total.

Waldenström's macroglobulinemia

In the case of the γM myeloma the term *Waldenström's macroglobulinemia* is preferred. This is not because of any gross immunologic difference in this disorder but because of the higher viscosity of IgM compared with other immunoglobulins. Consequently the clinical features of γM myeloma differ from those of the others, and the early descriptions of the disease by Waldenström are honored by continuance of his name.

Bence Jones protein and L chains

Thus in the multiple myelomas and in Waldenström's macroglobulinemia there exist the conditions of hyperimmunoglobulinemia, in some instances from a single plasma cell type. Consequently a source of a single molecular form of immunoglobulin is available from these unfortunate persons. Many of these patients will have in their blood and excrete in their urine a protein termed the *Bence Jones protein*. In fact in about 10% of all myelomas only the Bence Jones protein is produced, with no complete IgG, IgA, or IgM. Bence Jones proteins are unusual in their response to heat. They are soluble at room temperature, become insoluble near 60° or 70° C, and then resolubilize at 80° C. This pattern reverses when the temperature is lowered, so that one can recover Bence Jones protein again. This unique reversible denaturation permits a speedy identification of Bence Jones protein in urine from persons with multiple myeloma. Structurally the Bence Jones proteins are single-peptide chains with a molecular weight of 20,000 or 22,000, but dimerization to a 40,000 or 44,000 mol wt form occurs spontaneously. Serologically the Bence Jones proteins will react with antisera to the L chains of IgG, and L chains will react with antisera to Bence Jones proteins. This stringent serologic test conclusively identifies L chains as Bence Jones proteins. Subsequent serologic tests revealed that all Bence Jones proteins (L chains) are not identical and that there are two types, designated as κ and λ. After the purification of these proteins from urine, amino acid sequence studies were begun with the hope of uncoding the unique antibody behavior of the immunoglobulins.

Early in the studies of the myeloma proteins and the Bence Jones proteins the criticism was offered that the sequence studies were of little value, since false immunoglobulins were being studied. In fact these proteins were termed *paraproteins*, to indicate that, although they were antigenically and structurally related to immunoglobulins, they lacked the antibody function typical of true immunoglobulins.

This problem has been resolved with the discovery that many of the myeloma proteins do react with known antigens. The original problem was simply to identify the antigen, a search that has now been completed for many human myeloma proteins. IgG myeloma proteins have been recognized to neutralize streptolysin O; others have been identified that react with staphylolysin, transferrin, dinitrophenyl hapten, and *Leptospira* and *Brucella* organisms. Serum albumin, human blood group antigens A_1, and I, cardiolipin, *Klebsiella* organisms, and dinitrophenyl groups are among the antigens known to react with different IgM myeloma proteins. Fewer antigens have been identified to correspond with IgA myelomas because the IgA myelomas are rarer, but these include human blood group I and dinitrophenyl groups.

Homogeneous antibody

Among the first antibodies with molecular uniformity to be studied were homogeneous antibodies specific for polysaccharides of the streptococcal cell surface. These immunoglobulins had a uniform electrophoretic mobility that gave them the general appearance of M components on serum electrophoresis. It has now been learned that many polysaccharides situated on the outer surface of bacterial cells, including meningococci, staphylococci, and pneumococci in addition to the streptococci, will encourage formation of homogeneous antibodies. Polysaccharide antigens tend to favor antibodies with restricted heterogeneity because of their limited number of antigenic sites, a factor that forces the response toward molecular constancy.

Hybridoma

One of the best sources for pure immunoglobulins is the cultured myeloma cell, but even this procedure has been improved by the hybridoma technique. The hybridoma technique is described fully in Chapter 9, but in its simplest form spleen cells, which cannot grow continuously in culture, are taken from a mouse immunized with a chosen antigen. These cells are incubated with a mouse myeloma cell, which can grow continuously in culture provided the proper nutrients are present. Mutants of the myeloma cell are selected that no longer secrete immunoglobulin. These cells are incubated in the presence of a chem-

ical, polyethylene glycol (PEG), which causes cell membranes to become destabilized. This destabilization permits some cells to fuse. If the cell mixture is transferred to a tissue culture medium, the spleen cells fail to grow, and the myeloma cells fail to grow because the medium has been adjusted to prevent their growth. The cells that do grow are hybrids or hybridomas. They grow because having some of the nutrient properties of the parental spleen cell, enables them to overcome the composition of the medium, and the property of continuous growth in culture from the myeloma cell. These hybridomas will secrete into the growth medium an antibody with a specificity for the antigen used to immunize the mouse. Moreover this antibody will be specific for a single determinant of that antigen. About 100 μg of this immunoglobulin can be recovered from each milliliter of culture fluid. If the hybridoma is inoculated into the peritoneal cavity of a mouse, it will grow and produce an ascites fluid containing as much as 10 mg of immunoglobulin per milliliter. Such hybridomas have been an important source of a single molecular species of immunoglobulin produced by a single cell. These immunoglobulins are now the starting material for many chemical and genetic studies.

L Chains

One of the most interesting aspects emerging from the L chain sequence studies was the discovery that the carboxyl terminal half of all the λ-type L chains is nearly identical. The κ-chains also have a constant amino acid sequence in their carboxyl half. The constant half of the κ-chain is very similar but not identical to the constant half of the λ-chains. These regions are designated $C_κ$ and $C_λ$, or more generally as C_L (constant light). The amino halves of the λ-chains vary in structure from one to another; the same is true for the κ-chains. These regions are designated $V_κ$ and $V_λ$, or as V_L (variable light). Thus the 214 amino acids of all L chains are arranged in a unique way, with a constant amino acid sequence in the carboxyl half and variable sequence in the amino half. These regions are now customarily referred to as domains, that is, the constant domain and the variable domain. Constant and variable domains of the H chains also are known and are discussed later in the chapter.

Hypervariable regions

Within the first 107 amino acids of L chains the variability of the amino acid sequence fluctuates from residue to residue. Although the sequence of the V_L domain is variable, it is not equally variable at all positions, and the regions of greatest inconstancy are referred to as the hypervariable (HV) regions. Three such HV regions exist in each V_L domain, and these normally encompass amino acids 30 to 35, 50 to 55, and 95 to 100 with slight variations (Fig. 3-4). It is exactly these sequences that serve as part of the antigen-binding site. These regions differ in amino acid sequence according to the specificity of the immunoglobulin. These are the idiotypic regions of immunoglobulins.

These idiotypic regions are separated by the framework (FR) sequences, of which there are four in each V_L domain. These embody the first 29 amino acids from the amino terminal end, the last seven amino acids of the V_L, and the intervening sequences between the three HV regions.

The λ-type L chain has 213 to 216 amino acids,

depending on whether certain additions or deletions of amino acids exist. The penultimate amino acid of the carboxyl terminus is cysteine, one of only five cysteines in this polypeptide (Fig. 3-5). This cysteine is the site of dimerization in Bence Jones proteins and the point at which L chains are covalently linked to H chains in normal IgG. Two of the other four cysteines engage in intrachain disulfide bonding, between residues 135 and 194 in the constant region and between residues 21 and 86 in the variable region. The exact location of the internal disulfide bonds may vary by a few amino residues in different κ- or λ-chains. This double cystine formation creates two nearly symmetric loops of 60 amino acids each in the L chain. The amino terminal acid is serine, but this may be blocked by pyrrolidone carboxylic acid, a cyclized form of glutamic acid.

κ L chains are in many ways similar to λ-chains (Figs. 3-6 and 3-7). They have cysteine as the terminal amino acid on the carboxyl end, and this serves for attachment to the H chain or for dimer Bence Jones protein formation. Two intrachain disulfide bonds occur, between 134 and 194 and between 23 and 88, again creating symmetric loops of approximately 60 amino acids each. These —S—S— bonds and loops are at almost exactly the same posi-

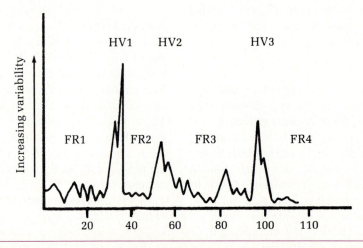

FIG. 3-4

A variability tracing of an L chain. The three major HV regions are identified, with the framework (FR) regions on each side.

tion as those found in λ-chains. This suggests a common genetic origin of the two L chains from which the λ and κ varieties have evolved with the retention of many common structural characteristics. The amino terminal acid is not blocked with pyrrolidone carboxylic acid and is usually aspartic acid.

In a given individual both κ- and λ-chains are produced and found in antibody molecules; however, they are not found simultaneously in a single antibody molecule. Two structural formulas now can be written for IgG: $H_2\kappa_2$ and $H_2\lambda_2$. These two types exist in a ratio of about 2:1 in any one individual.

L Chain allotypes

Human κ-chain allotypes have been identified that permit a finer identification of these L chains. Allotypic proteins are structurally and functionally similar molecules that differ from each other antigenically. The allotypic determinants of κ-chains reside in the C_L domain. The Km1 (κ-marker) L chain has valine at position 153 and leucine at position 191. These are replaced by alanine and valine, respectively, in the Km3 molecule. Km2 has alanine and leucine in positions 153 and 191.

Antigenic variants in human λ-chains have been

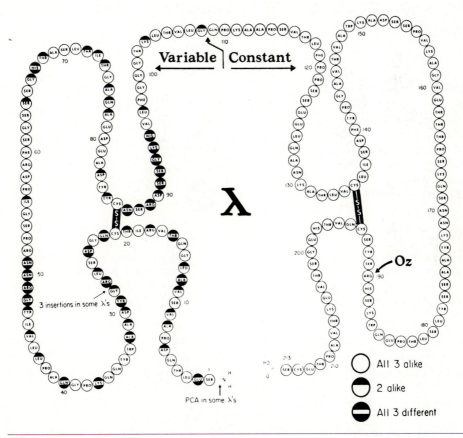

FIG. 3-5

Entire amino acid sequence of three human λ-type L chains. Notice the symmetry of the molecule, in terms of zones of constant and variable sequence, and the placement of disulfide bonds. The location of the Oz determinant at position 190 is noted. (See Fig. 3-6.) (From Putnam, F.W.: Structural evolution of kappa and lambda chains. In Killander, J., editor: Gamma globulins, New York, 1967, Interscience Press.)

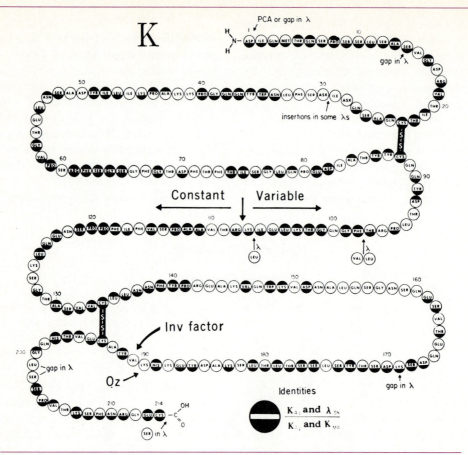

FIG. 3-6

Amino acid sequence of human κ-type L chains. As with the λ-type chain, symmetry of the constant and variable sequence portions and disulfide linkages are apparent. Key at bottom of illustration indicates the homology with human and murine κ-chains and a human λ-chain. (From Putnam, F.W.: Immunoglobulin structure variability and homology, Science **163**:633, 1969.)

identified and were once described as allotypes (Oz, Kern, and Mcg determinants) but are no longer accepted as such. These molecules contained antigenic differences, which can be described as private markers rather than the more general allotypic markers.

γ-Chains

The H chains of IgG are designated as γ-chains to distinguish them from the H chains of the other immunoglobulins. The carbohydrate portion of IgG (2.5% of the total weight of the molecule) is divided equally between the two γ-chains and is situated on the Fc portion of the H chain. Monosaccharide units found in the carbohydrate portions include mannose, galactose, N-acetyl-D-glucosamine, N-acetyl-D-galactosamine, and sialic acid. None of the polysaccharide side chains seems to contain more than five or ten constituent units, although this may be the result of destructive hydrolysis in the preparation of these structures for assay. Attachment of the polysaccharide to the peptide backbone is primarily through asparagine, although one serine-borne unit has been identified.

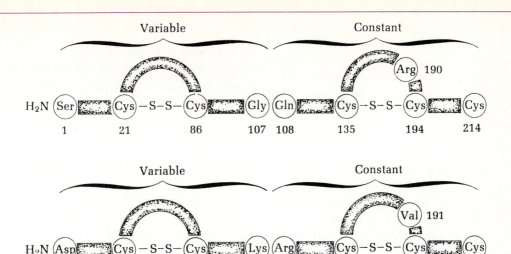

FIG. 3-7

Comparison of κ-*(upper)* and λ-*(lower)* chains. Note that the variable and constant regions are the same size, that the intrachain disulfide loops are comparably positioned, and that the Km factor in the κ-chain is placed at essentially the same location as the Oz factor in the λ-chain, at positions 190 and 191.

Constant and variable domains of γ-chains

The complete amino acid sequence for γ-chains has been determined, and some fascinating parallels to L chain structure have been revealed. The amino terminal portion of the γ-chain, consisting of about 121 amino acid residues and residing in the Fab fragment, is of variable amino acid sequence from one γ-chain to another. This variable domain (V_H or V_γ) is essentially the same length as V_L of κ- and λ-chains. In the first 107 amino acids of the V_H domain are three HV regions at essentially the same positions that hypervariability is located in the V_L domains, that is, near residues 30 to 35, 50 to 55, and 95 to 100. The HV V_L and V_H sequences create a wedge within which determinants of the antigen contact the binding sites of the antibody molecule. The amino acid sequences of the V_H and V_L HV regions are not identical. As with the V_L HV regions, those in the V_H domain are separated by FR sequences.

The HV sequences in the H chain, like those in L chains, may contribute to an antigenic determinant site. These idiotypic determinants are highly unique, since they are present in the antigen-binding site of an antibody that reacts with a single epitope.

The carboxyl terminal region of γ-chains, consisting of about 375 amino acid residues, can be divided into three subregions that have amino acid sequences very similar to each other. These are designated C_H1, C_H2, and C_H3, or $C_\gamma1$, etc. C_H1 is immediately adjacent to V_H, and numbering proceeds toward the carboxyl terminus. The regions 114 to 223, 246 to 361, and 362 to 496 represent the C_H1, C_H2, and C_H3 domains, respectively. Within each is a 60-amino acid disulfide bridge—at 142 to 208 in C_H1, 274 to 340 in C_H2, and 390 to 456 in C_H3. These C_H zones have approximately a 30% to 40% homology with C_L regions of κ- and λ-chains. This configuration has interesting genetic implications, suggesting that genes derived from a common precursor gene have evolved for the C_L and for the separate C_H regions.

Amino acid sequence and enzyme digestion studies indicate that the cleavage point of papain is between threonine 225 and cysteine 226. Cysteines at positions 226 and 229 in IgG1 bridge to the same amino acids in the companion γ-chain to hold them together as the Fc subunit. Cysteines at position 220 serve as the links to the L chains. Pepsin hydrolyzes the γ-chains between two leucine moieties at positions 234 and 235. The disulfide bonds remaining at 226 and 229 enable the Fab units to be preserved as $F(ab')_2$.

The hinge region

The general region of the γ-chains—roughly between cysteine 220 and arginine 241—is known as the hinge region. It is characterized by one interchain disulfide bridge between an L and the H chain and two interchain disulfide bridges between the two H chains. It also contains the unusual sequence Pro-Pro-Pro-Cys-Pro, and the incorporation of proline into an amino acid chain is known to interrupt the normal α-helix configuration and restrict folding of the chain. It is perhaps this interruption that makes the hinge region so sensitive to proteolysis.

γ-Chain subclasses

Four major subclasses of the human γ-chain are detectable by specific antisera. These are designated IgG1, IgG2, IgG3, and IgG4 and occur in the proportions of approximately 65:25:7:1 respectively. The chemical basis for the subclasses is differences in the number and position of disulfide bridges between the two γ-chains. For example, IgG1 has two, IgG2 has four, IgG3 has fifteen, and IgG4 has two inter-γ-chain disulfide bridges. IgG3 has an extended hinge region that gives it a higher molecular weight than the other IgG subclasses. IgG2, 3, and 4 have H-L chain disulfide bonds in a position different from that of IgG1 (Fig. 3-8). These separate subclasses are recognizable by specific antisera; an antiserum prepared against one human γ-chain will react with all other human γ-chains, but the extent of this reaction will not be the same for all chains. There actually will be four levels of reactivity, and on this basis the four subclasses were designated.

γ-Chain allotypes

The discovery of human IgG H chain allotypes arose from the identification of subgroups in the sera of patients with rheumatoid arthritis. These individu-

TABLE 3-2

Subclasses of human IgG

	Percent	**Gm antigens**
IgG1	60.9	Gm1, 2, 3, 17
IgG2	29.6	Gm8, 23
IgG3	5.3	Gm5, 6, 10, 11, 13, 14, 15, 16, 21, 24, 26, 27
IgG4	4.2	Present but not yet correlated with existing Gm system

als commonly have an IgM antibody that reacts with their own IgG. This IgM, also known as rheumatoid factor (RF), will react with pooled human IgG, and indeed this is the serologic device used to identify RF and assist in the diagnosis of rheumatoid arthritis. However, it was found that the IgG of different individuals functioned unequally as the antigen for RF, and subgroups of IgG known as Gm (γ) subgroups or allotypes were created. These Gm allotypes, earlier designated by letters Gma, Gmb, etc., are now numbered, Gm1, Gm2, etc. These Gm allotypes are unequally distributed among the four IgG subclasses (Table 3-2). IgG1 includes four Gm subgroups, IgG2 has but two, and IgG3 includes twelve. IgG4 does have Gm allotypes, but these have not been fully correlated with the other known allotypes. The distribution and terminology of the Gm allotype is in a constant state of revision. The chemical basis for the differences in antigenicity of the Gm allotypes is known in several instances. In IgG3 the Gm5 allotype has phenylalanine at amino acid residues 296 and 436. When tyrosine replaces phenylalanine at both positions, then a different antigenic specificity, Gm21, is created. In IgG1, when the arginine at position 214 is replaced by a lysine, the Gm determinant is lost. Similar exchanges regulate the other Gm determinants as well, and these amino acid substitutions can occur in C_H1, C_H2, or C_H3 domains.

The complications added to the original structure of IgG written as H_2L_2 now can be expanded to include the known variations in H and L chain allotypes. The two major L chain forms of IgG are

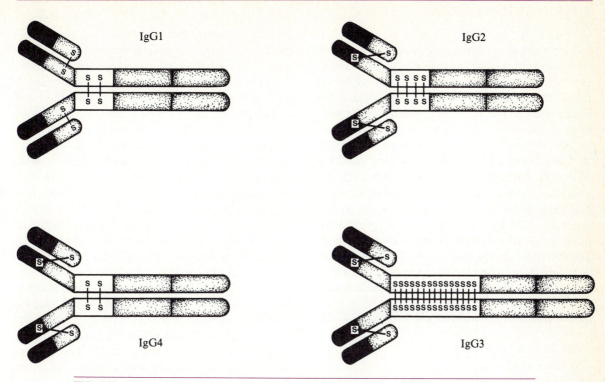

FIG. 3-8

IgG1 and IgG4 each have 2 H-H chain disulfide bonds. IgG2 has 4 such bonds and IgG3 has one extended hinge region that contains 15 S—S bonds. Note also the different placement of the L-H chain S—S bonds in IgG1.

$\gamma_2\kappa_2$ and $\gamma_2\lambda_2$. These formulas indicate that L chains of either the κ or λ type may be present in IgG. We know that further variations in the κ-chain are possible by variations in the Km marker. Thus one could write formulas such as $\gamma_2(\kappa, \text{Km1})_2$ or $\gamma_2(\kappa, \text{Km2})_2$. But these structures do not distinguish between γ-chain variations. For example, $(\gamma\text{Gm1})_2 (\kappa \text{Km1})_2$ and $(\gamma\text{Gm 18})_2 (\kappa \text{Km1})_2$ would be distinguishable by specific Gm antisera. The limit of these variations in one individual is not known, but it is apparent that in the human population many different types of IgG can be produced. It we accept four possible types of L chains and four IgG subclasses and only 18 Gm allotypes, then $4 \times 4 \times 18$, or 288, different forms of IgG could hypothetically be present in one individual. Each of these IgGs would be directed toward a single epitope of the antigen. If the antigen has four epitopes, then nearly 1200 IgGs could theoretically have responded to that antigen. Each would differ from every other in antigenic reactivity and amino acid composition. Further variations could result from amino acid differences in the antigen-combining sites of these antibodies (idiotypic differences) that are not detectable by ordinary H or L chain antisera. It is little wonder that IgG is so electrophoretically heterogeneous. This heterogeneity reflects a vast heterogeneity of the plasma cell population, since only one molecular form of antibody is produced by a single plasma cell. Plasma cell heterogeneity is expanded even further, since the other immunoglobulins yet to be discussed also arise from plasma cells.

STRUCTURE AND CHEMISTRY OF IgA
Serum IgA

IgA of serum is known as γA and β_2A because of its tendency to position between the true γ and β regions on electrophoresis (Table 3-3). It ranges between 7S and 11S in the analytic centrifuge. The predominant portion is 7S, and the cause of the polydispersed behavior is at least partially clarified by the known structures of IgA. IgA represents only 5% to 15% of all serum γ-globulins—equivalent to 225 $\pm$ 55 mg/dl of serum. IgA has a half-life of about 5 days and is synthesized at a rate of about 22 mg/kg body weight/day.

Structural studies have revealed that IgG and IgA possess several common features. Both are composed of four peptide chains, two L chains and two H chains. The L chains in both molecules are identical, that is, κ- and λ-chains, and their known

TABLE 3-3

Chemical and physical properties of immunoglobulin A

Current designation	IgA
Older names	γA, β_2A
Molecular weight	160,000*
$S_{20,w}$ value	7*
Electrophoretic mobility	Fast γ, slow β
Carbohydrate content	10%
Resistance to—SH reagents	Low
Concentration (mg/dl serum)	225 $\pm$ 55
Amount of serum immuno-globulins	5% to 15%
Half-life (days)	5
Rate of synthesis (mg/kg body weight/day)	22
Light chain types	κ or λ
Heavy-chain class	α
General formula	$\alpha_2\kappa_2$ or $\alpha_2\lambda_2$
Light-chain allotypes	Km
Heavy-chain subclasses	α1 and α2
Heavy-chain allotypes	A2m(1) and A2m(2)
Heavy-chain constant domains	3
Stable at 56° to 60° C	Yes
Secretory type exists	Yes

*Polymeric forms of greater molecular weight and S values are known.

subtypes occur in both molecules. The H chains of IgA, the α-chains, differ from the γ-chains of IgG by having a greater carbohydrate content, approximately 10% of the total molecule, and a different amino acid sequence. α-Chains lack the Gm determinants, but two subclasses of α-chains, IgA1 and IgA2, do exist. IgA1 accounts for 90% of the total serum IgA. IgA1 has intrachain and interchain disulfide linkages of the standard type. These are refractory to reductive cleavage except when in high-molarity urea solutions. IgA2 is unique in that it is completely devoid of H-L interchain —S—S— bonding. The two chains are held together by strictly noncovalent linkages. Allotypic variation in the α-chain of IgA2 depends on the presence or absence of two antigens: A2m(1) and A2m(2). α-Chains in IgA1 do not express allotypic variation.

The α-chain of IgA1 contains 472 amino acid residues. This is sufficient to include a V_H and three C_H domains. α-Chains have 34 cysteines, compared with 22 in IgG1. The H chains are joined by cystine formation through the cysteines at 242 and 301. Cysteine 471 is the probable source of the linkage of polymeric IgA to J chain. Oligosaccharide subunits are attached to five serines and three asparagines, and most of this occurs in the hinge region—specifically at serine residues 224, 230, 232, 238, and 239. IgA1 has a duplicated hinge region.

Papain and pepsin digestion of serum IgA yields the expected Fab or F(ab')$_2$ units, but the Fc and Fc' units are difficult to isolate because of their sensitivity to further digestion by papain or pepsin. Certain bacterial proteases cleave only IgA1. Reductive cleavage to release H and L chains is also possible.

Secretory IgA

The ratio of IgG to IgA in serum is 6:1; this is true for synovial fluid, cerebrospinal fluid, aqueous humor, and other internal secretions. In the external secretions—that is, in colostrum and early milk, nasal and respiratory mucus, intestinal mucus, saliva, etc.—IgA is usually present in a much higher concentration than either IgG or IgM. Secretory IgA is a nearly equal mixture of IgA1 and IgA2 in contrast to the IgA composition of serum.

Table 3-4 presents the distinguishing characteristics of human serum IgA, human secretory IgA, and two proteins associated with the latter, termed *secretory component* (SC) and *J chain*. As can be seen, human secretory IgA is a much larger molecule than its serum counterpart, having twice its molecular weight plus about 80,000. The major difference is the addition of SC and J chain and a second IgA unit to secretory IgA. Serum IgA and secretory IgA are not in simple equilibrium. Supporting data for this argument are that radiolabeled serum IgA does not appear in the secretions and that IgA administered to agammaglobulinemic patients does not always elevate the secretory IgA. From this observation it has been deduced that there is a separate cellular origin of serum and secretory IgA. When fluorescent antibody against serum IgA is used as a histochemical reagent, it is found that the plasma cells closely situated beneath the epithelium of excretory glands are stained. If fluorescent antibody against SC is used, the neighboring epithelial cells stain. The fluorescent antibody experiments indicate that plasma cells strategically situated near the body cavities are IgA synthesizers, and epithelial cells produce SC. J chain is produced in the plasma cells.

Secretory component (SC)

The identification of an antigenic difference between serum IgA and IgA in milk is credited to Hanson in 1961, and later studies by Tomasi and others eventually identified this difference as being caused by the SC present in IgA found in secretions. SC is found as a part of the secretory IgA in all species examined, including dog, cow, sheep, goat, rabbit, mouse, and chicken, as well as the human. More recently SC has been identified as a part of human IgM in external secretions. SC bound to secretory IgA or to secretory IgM can be liberated by disulfide reducing compounds (such as 2-mercaptoethanol at a concentration of 0.2M). Free SC exists in secretions of those persons who are hypogammaglobulinemic in regard to IgA.

The molecular weight of SC is 70,000 to 75,000 (Table 3-4). It exists as a single peptide chain with an $S_{20,w}$ of 5. Electrophoretically the molecule moves to the position occupied by the fast β-globulins. Human SC (and presumably that of other species) is lacking in methionine but has a high glycine content. About 11% of the weight of SC is in the form of carbohydrate.

IgA that is destined to become secretory IgA is released from submucosal plasma cells, which neighbor the external mucosal tissue, and diffuses toward the epithelial surface (Fig. 3-9). SC on the epithelial cells serves as a receptor for IgA. On attachment of this IgA to the cell a concentration gradient from the IgA-synthesizing cells is established, which encourages further migration of IgA toward the mucosal surface and its conversion to secretory IgA. The dimeric IgA may enter the epithelial cells (enterocytes, for example) and be transported across the cell in endocytic vesicles. Bile is a rich source of IgA that arises from the blood. Some of this is converted to secretory IgA

TABLE 3-4
Comparison of serum IgA, secretory IgA, SC, and J chain

	Serum IgA	Secretory IgA	Secretory component	J chain
Current designation	IgA	SIgA	SC	J
Molecular weight	160,000	405,000	70,000 to 75,000	15,000 ± 500
$S_{20,w}$ value	7	11	5	About 2
Carbohydrate content (percent)	10	10	9.5	7.5
Comment	Polymeric forms common	Formulas $(\alpha_2\kappa_2)_2 SC \cdot J$ or $(\alpha_2\lambda_2)_2 SC \cdot J$	High glycine content	Prealbumin

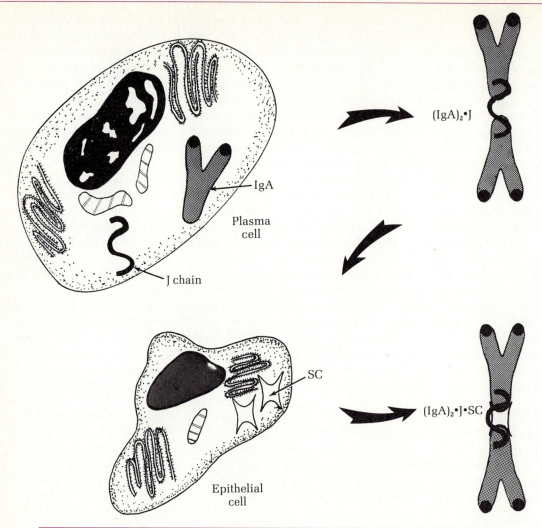

FIG. 3-9

The synthesis of secretory IgA begins in the plasma cell that secretes the J chain combined with two molecules of IgA. This contacts an epithelial cell where it acquires SC to become the complete secretory IgA.

in the liver before being discharged in the bile, where it has been referred to as biliglobulin.

Although 70% to 85% of secretory IgA has SC attached via disulfide linkages, some 15% to 30% of the SC is noncovalently bonded with SC. SC appears to contact the hinge region of both IgA four-peptide units involved in the complex and probably else-

where in the Fc region. Since SC has a high content of glycine, it could easily possess the snakelike flexibility required for this union.

The functional role of SC remains enigmatic. It has not yet been proved to have a secretory role, and it is not required for J chain bonding, since this precedes SC attachment.

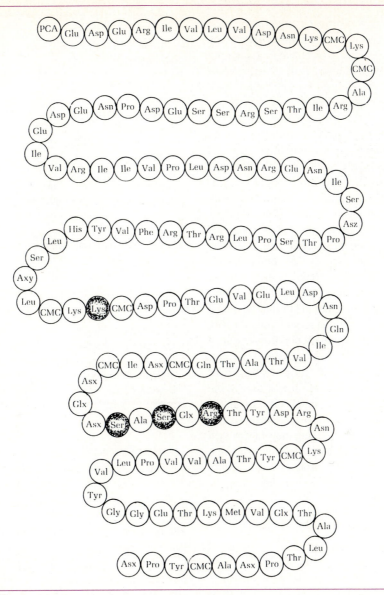

FIG. 3-10

Amino acid sequence of J chain. The numerous aspartic acid residues are apparent, and the shaded amino acids are points of carbohydrate linkage.

J chain

In 1970 it was definitely concluded that a protein originally believed to be a degradation product of SC from secretory IgA was in fact a new, previously undescribed protein. Since this protein is found only in immunoglobulins composed of more than one four-peptide unit, it was named J chain (joining chain).

J chain has a molecular weight of $15,000 \pm 500$ (Table 3-4) and consists of 129 amino acid residues, of which 20 are aspartic acid (Fig. 3-10). This confers a high net negative electrical charge on the molecule, which migrates as a prealbumin. The amino acid composition of J chains of human, rabbit, pig, and dog origin is very similar, and all have about 7.5% carbohydrate. Rabbit and human J chains appear to be immunologically identical and partially related serologically to J chains of lower animals. J chain is attached to the α-chains of secretory IgA by virtue of S—S bonding to the penultimate cysteine at the carboxyl terminus, which is present in these H chains. One J chain links two IgA units. J chain is also found in serum and secretory IgM at one J chain per five IgM 7S units. This stoichiometry suggests that J chain does not merely join the four-peptide units of the immunoglobulins together; if this were the case, IgM should have more J chain units. Plasma cells that synthesize L and α-chains also synthesize the J chain, yet free J chain is scarce in these cells and is almost entirely bound into the immunoglobulin polymer. This is the basis for suggesting that the biologic role of J chain is to initiate polymerization of secretory IgA (and of the IgM globulins as well). Exactly how this polymerization begins and why it ends at different stages for IgA and IgM is not known; but since it is not accomplished randomly, it may be via specific disulfide interchange enzymes. Synthesis of J chain is apparently the rate-limiting step in the synthesis of polymeric IgA and IgM, and this is the reason it is rarely found as a free protein.

The molecular formula for exocrine IgA is $(\alpha_2\kappa_2)_2 SC \cdot J$ or $(\alpha_2\lambda_2)_2 SC \cdot J$.

STRUCTURE AND CHEMISTRY OF IgM

The only immunoglobulin with an $S_{20,w}$ value of 19 is the macroglobulin IgM (Table 3-5). This molecule has a molecular weight of approximately 950,000. The electrophoretic positioning of IgM is in the zone between the clear-cut γ- and β-globulins; IgM has been denoted both as a $\gamma_1 M$ and $\beta_2 M$ molecule. This molecule constitutes about 5% to 10% of the total immunoglobulins in the adult human, or about 125 ± 45 mg/dl of serum. This low serum content of IgM is the combined result of its short half-life (10 days) and low synthetic rate (5 to 8 mg/kg body weight/day). The carbohydrate content of IgM is about 10% to 11%. Because its molecular weight, protein content, and sedimentation value are

TABLE 3-5

Chemical and physical properties of immunoglobulin M

Current designation	IgM
Older names	$19S\gamma$, $\gamma_1 M$, $\beta_2 M$
Molecular weight	950,000
$S_{20,w}$ value	19
Electrophoretic mobility	Fast γ, slow β
Carbohydrate content	10%
Resistance to —SH reagents	Low
Concentration (mg/dl serum)	125 ± 45
Amount of serum immunoglobulins	5% to 10%
Half-life (days)	9 to 11
Rate of synthesis (mg/kg body weight/day)	5 to 8
Light-chain types	κ or λ
Heavy-chain class	μ
General formula	$(\mu_2\kappa_2)_5 \cdot J$ or $(\mu_2\lambda_2)_5 \cdot J$
Light-chain allotypes	Km
Heavy-chain subclasses	μ1, μ2 (M1, M2)
Heavy-chain constant domains	4
Stable at 56° to 60° C	Yes
Secretory type exists	Yes

all five times those of IgG, a structure of IgM consisting of 10 L and 10 H chains was quickly postulated. These peptide chains are held together by disulfide bonds and the J chain, which are easily separated by reducing agents. IgM is very sensitive to dissociation by dilute solutions of —SH reagents such as 2-mercaptoethanol.

When the 19S IgM molecule is treated with reducing agents and the newly formed —SH groups are blocked to prevent recombination, molecules of 6.5S to 7S are formed. This dissociation does not require unfolding of the molecule with urea, since IgM is so sensitive to reducing agents. The 7S fragments (γM_S) have a molecular weight of 190,000 and are similar in structure to IgG in the sense that each is composed of two H and two L chains. The H chains have been isolated and their molecular weight determined as 65,000 to 70,000. The H chains consist of 576 amino acid residues. Cysteine 140 is the link of the H chain to L chains, and cysteines 337 and 575 link the H chains to each other. Five oligosaccharide units have been identified, each being attached to an asparagine. Because of its size and sequence studies, it is agreed that the H chain contains four C domains, rather than three, plus the V domain. Consequently H chains of IgM differ from the H chains of IgG and are referred to as μ-chains. Two IgM subclasses, IgM1 and IgM2, are based on differences in the μ-chain.

The H chains of lymphocyte-bound IgM differ from those of serum IgM by about 40 amino acids at the carboxyl terminal end. These provide the hydrophobic structure needed for anchoring in the cell membrane.

The L chains prepared from IgM are identical to the L chains of the other immunoglobulins, that is, κ- or λ-chains. Since the L chains are identical to those of other immunoglobulins, it is assumed that they are linked to the H chain by the COOH terminal (or penultimate) cysteines.

By enzymatic digestion of the γM_S units, structures corresponding to the Fab and $F(ab')_2$ fragments of IgG are formed. These are designated as the Fab-μ and $F(ab')_2\mu$ fragments. Their molecular weights have been estimated as 47,000 and 114,000, respectively.

The molecular formula of serum IgM is written $(\mu_2\kappa_2)_5 \cdot J$ or $(\mu_2\lambda_2)_5 \cdot J$ (Fig. 3-11). A secretory form of IgM has recently been described. Its distribution in body fluids parallels that of secretory IgA. Its molecular formula is that of serum IgM plus SC.

STRUCTURE AND CHEMISTRY OF IgD

IgD was first identified as a unique immunoglobulin in human serum in 1965 as the result of the discovery of a myeloma protein that was antigenically dissimilar to other immunoglobulins. Since that time several dozen examples of γD myeloma have been reported, and 135 cases were described in one article, although γD myelomas appear at an incidence of less than 3% of all myelomas. The failure to describe IgD earlier can be related to its paucity in normal human serum, where its normal mean level is 0.03 mg/ml. As a further consequence of this, most of the chemical data available on IgD have been derived from the γD myeloma proteins.

IgD is a typical immunoglobulin constructed from two H and two L chains. Both κ- and λ-type L chains are known, but the λ-type myelomas predominate (80%, compared with 20% κ-type). The H chain of IgD is structurally and antigenically different from the H chains of other immunoglobulins and has been designated the δ-chain. The κ- and λ-chains do not differ from their kind found in other antibodies, but the δ-chain has a molecular weight of 70,000 or some 12,000 greater than γ-chains. This led to the suggestion that the δ-chain possessed a fourth C_H unit. The additional size of the δ-chain may be associated with an extended hinge region in the molecule. The δ-chain has been sequenced. It contains 512 amino acid residues, 129 of which are in the V_H domain. The hinge region extends from residue 228 through 291. Because of its large δ-chain, the entire IgD molecule has a molecular weight of 180,000 rather than 160,000. Its average $S_{20,w}$ is 6.5S (Table 3-6).

The H and L chains are easily recovered from the parent molecule after its exposure to 0.1M mercaptoethanol or 0.02M dithiothreitol for 1 or 2 hours at room temperature to reduce the —S—S bonds if the

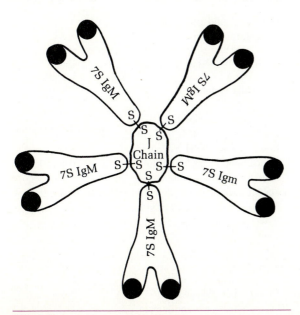

FIG. 3-11

The structure of serum IgM consists of five of the four-peptide or 7S IgM units linked to J chain.

newly formed —SH units are blocked by iodoaceta-mide. Papain releases the expected two Fab and one Fc fragments, but the latter is rapidly degraded further and is difficult to isolate intact.

IgD contains about 12% of its weight in the form of polysaccharide, all of which is attached to the δ-chain. This seems to be divided into three discrete sectors, one located at the Fc-Fd interface, or hinge region, and the other two in the Fc region.

IgD at a level of 30 μg/ml of serum is synthesized at the rate of 0.4 mg/kg body weight/day. This is about 100-fold less than the synthetic rate of IgG. The half-life of IgD is only 2 to 3 days.

Two features that have restricted our understanding of IgD in addition to its scarcity in serum are its heat and acid lability. Holding sera at 56° C for 1 hour reduces its IgD content by 50%, and after 4 hours only 10% is recoverable. This behavior is very like that of IgE, which is also heat labile. A pH of 3 denatures IgD, and this feature means that it cannot be eluted from immunoadsorbent columns by the usual means of acid dissociation without simultaneously destroying the molecule. A third feature that must be held in mind is that IgD aggregates very readily, which can alter its biologic activity as well as its structure.

Membrane-bound IgD differs from serum IgD by having a tailpiece on the end of each H chain. The additional sequence usually consists of about 25 to 30 amino acids of which the majority (20 amino acids) are hydrophobic and insert into the cell membrane.

STRUCTURE AND CHEMISTRY OF IgE

IgE migrates electrophoretically as a fast γ- or $γ_1$-globulin with a molecular weight of 188,000 to 190,000 (Table 3-7). It has a half-life of 2.3 days. It is synthesized at a rate of 2.3 μg/kg body weight/day. Carbohydrate represents about 10.7% to 11.7% of the total weight of the molecule. On the basis of the assumption that IgE is a globular protein, its $S_{20,w}$ value has been reported as 7.92 to 8.2. Reductive mercaptan cleavage followed by alkylation with

TABLE 3-6

Chemical and physical properties of immunoglobulin D

Current designation	IgD
Older names	None
Molecular weight	180,000
$S_{20,w}$ value	6.5
Electrophoretic mobility	Fast γ
Carbohydrate content	12%
Resistance to —SH reagents	Low
Concentration (mg/dl serum)	3
Amount of serum immunoglobulins	<1%
Half-life (days)	2 to 3
Rate of synthesis (mg/kg body weight/day)	0.4
Light chain types	κ or λ
Heavy chain class	δ
General formula	$δ_2κ_2$ or $δ_2λ_2$
Light chain allotypes	Km
Heavy chain subclasses	None
Heavy chain constant domains	3
Stable at 56° to 60° C	No
Stable in dilute acid	No

TABLE 3-7

Chemical and physical properties of immunoglobulin E

Current designation	IgE
Older name	Reagin
Molecular weight	190,000
$S_{20,w}$ value	8.2
Electrophoretic mobility	$γ_1$
Carbohydrate content (percent)	11.7
Resistance to —SH reagents	Low
Concentration (mg/dl serum)	0.1 to 1.0
Amount of serum immunoglobulins	<1%
Half-life (days)	2.3
Rate of synthesis (μg/kg body weight/day)	2.3
Light chain types	κ or λ
Heavy chain class	ε
General formula	$ε_2κ_2$ or $ε_2λ_2$
Light chain allotypes	Km
Heavy chain subclasses	None
Heavy chain constant domain	4
Stable at 56° to 60° C	No

iodoacetamide revealed the presence of λ L chains with a molecular weight estimated as 22,600. Typical κ-chains also have been identified in IgE. This means that the H chain—the ϵ-chain must have a molecular weight of 75,000. It now is accepted that this extra size of the ϵ-chain is a result of its content of a fourth C_H domain. A single disulfide bond unites the ϵ- with the λ-chain. Carbohydrate, previously believed to be shared between the λ- and ϵ-chain, is exclusively restricted to the latter, indicating that the molecular weight of the ϵ-peptide is 61,000. Papain digestion of IgE produces several fragments, including the two Fab units and an Fc unit, but also an L chain fragment, λ C, Fc″, and a $7S_{20,w}$ fragment. Fc has a molecular weight of 98,000 and an $S_{20,w}$ of 5.1S. This Fc fragment is the only papain fragment that inhibits the P-K reaction. This is proof that it contains the cytotropic region of intact IgE. Fc″ is an amino terminal portion of the Fc unit that seems to bear the carbohydrate associated with the ϵ-chain. Two Fab fragments have been identified, one of which has a detectable component of carbohydrate. Tryptic and peptic proteolysis of IgE also have been performed, the latter producing $F(ab')_2$ units of 140,000 mol wt and an $S_{20,w}$ of 6.7. The Fd′ unit has a molecular weight of 45,000.

IMMUNOGLOBULIN GENETICS

Among the dogmas of genetics, the concept that one gene codes for one protein has been among the strongest. This theory became suspect when the amino acid sequence studies of immunoglobulins revealed that each had a series of identical C domains joined to a V domain in the L and in the H chain. In each immunoglobulin within a class, regardless of its specificity, the C domains were the same, but the V domains all differed. Thus for an L chain of the κ type the C_κ domain must be joined with a vast array of V sequences to construct globulins specific for the vast number of antigens that stimulate antibody synthesis. This logic also applies to the C_λ and C_H domains. A variation in the amino acid sequence of one portion of a molecule that is always joined to the same amino acid sequence in its remainder can be explained by several genetic hypotheses.

The germ line theory

The hypothesis known as the germ line theory, in harmony with the one gene–one protein dogma, envisioned one structural gene for each peptide in an immunoglobulin. This would consist of a V-C gene, and, to provide the variation in immunoglobulin structure that a cell can display, the cell would need to have a large library of V-C genes. Each V region would differ, but the C region would be identical to the C regions in all other pairs. One problem with this hypothesis is related to the amount of DNA a lymphocyte would require to make immunoglobulins by this method. The problem of DNA mass was resolved on the basis of a few assumptions and some mathematics. One early calculation suggested as little as 15% of the available nuclear DNA was needed to synthesize an antibody to each (potentially) existing antigenic determinant. More recent calculations indicate that 10^8 different antibodies could be generated from only 0.25% of the available DNA. Even so it seems uneconomic that a cell would carry so much excessive V-C gene baggage when only half of the gene set will be varied.

The somatic mutation theory

The uneconomic aspect of the germ line theory was met by the somatic mutation theory, which recognized the constancy of the amino acid sequences in the C domain as requiring but a single C gene and the demand for variations in the V gene as being met by a mutable behavior of this gene. Thus from any germ line V-C pair a series of gene paris (V_1C, V_2C, V_3C . . . V_nC) would arise spontaneously. This theory obviously requires a large number of mutations to achieve the many immunoglobulins that would be needed to correspond with all antigens; but this mutation rate is not impossible. Based on a population of 10^8 B lymphocytes in an animal, approximately 1,000 V gene mutants emerge each day.

The somatic recombination theory

A modification of the germ line theory suggests that a series of V genes exists but not in an unlimited series as in the germ line theory. Recombinational events during cell growth would reorder the codons within the V genes to expand the library of V genes.

These events would not transpire in the C genes, and the diversity of antibodies needed thus could be generated.

Because the existing models of one gene–one protein did not seem compatible with immunoglobulin structure, Dreyer and Bennett hypothesized that the V and C genes (whatever their origin) were not in tandem but were independent. A large series of V region genes could be joined to one or a few C region genes. Modern chemical and genetic techniques have been coupled to support this hypothesis.

Mapping immunoglobulin genes

Myeloma cells have the ability to grow readily in culture. Since these cells have focused on the production of a single immunoglobulin, it is possible to harvest their mRNA in substantial quantity with little contamination from mRNA contributing to the synthesis of other proteins. Immunoglobulin mRNA can be used in several ways as a probe for the structural immunoglobulin genes. By one method the mRNA is taken from cells grown in the presence of radiolabeled constituents. The mRNA is then fragmented and added to DNA taken from lymphocytes. Hybridization occurs between the complementary sequences in the mRNA and the DNA, and the isotope in the mRNA localizes the immunoglobulin gene sequences. These DNA sequences can be recovered, purified, and sequenced to confirm that they contain the correct triplet codons for the sequence of amino acids as they appear in the L or H chain. These DNA sequences then can be joined to a vector that will infect a bacterial cell, and multiple copies of the gene then can be recovered from the bacteria. This abundant DNA supply can be sequenced and either analyzed with probes that are specific for sectors of the immunoglobulin chain or be used as a probe itself.

Alternatively the mRNA can be used as a template for the enzyme reverse transcriptase to synthesize a copy DNA (cDNA). Fragmentation of the cDNA with restriction endonucleases will yield fragments that can be identified by sequencing to contain the codons for specific regions of the immunoglobulin molecule. Fragments of a radiolabeled cDNA fragment will bind to whole single-stranded DNA (ssDNA) from lymphocytes and localize the codons

in the native DNA. By these methods specific probes for V_L, C_L, V_H, and C_H genes have been generated.

The use of probes for the mouse V_L and C_L domains has identified four to ten copies of the V_κ gene on chromosome 6 but only one copy of the C_κ gene. This finding eliminates the germ line theory as the basis for immunoglobulin diversity, since it predicted an equal number of V and C genes would be present.

There are actually many more than four to ten V_L genes in a mouse cell. First of all the probe used was a single V_κ probe. It is known that mice produce in excess of 50 V_κ chains, each differing slightly but regularly from the others in amino acid sequence. Thus there are 200 to 500 V_κ genes in the cell. Mouse V_λ chains are less variable, but adding some reasonable number of these to the V_κ genes would result in an excess of 500 or 600 V_L genes in mouse DNA.

The germ line theory also hypothesized that V and C genes would be adjacent to each other, and this was widely assumed to be the case, in harmony with the one gene–one protein dogma. However, the V_L probes applied to mouse embryo DNA were bound at several sites, each a definite distance from the C_L probes. When the same probes were applied to DNA from a mouse plasmacytoma, the V_L and C_L probes were positioned adjacent to each other.

The import of this discovery extends far beyond immunology. It indicates that clearly separated, multiple genes are required for the synthesis of a single peptide, and these genes are not expressed by a simple on-off switch but are expressed only after gene rearrangement. This space between the genes in the embryonic cell which has no known protein product is defined as an intron (intervening sequence), whereas the expressed sequence is known as the exon (see discussion on Tonegawa, p. 22).

When the DNA that had been identified to contain the exon for the C domain was sequenced, all the triplets needed to account for the 107 amino acids in the C_L domain seemed to be present. However, when the V_L gene sequence was completed, it accounted for only the first 95 amino acids. This gap has been accounted for by locating a nucleotide sequence (in what was earlier thought to be an intron region) that accounts for the remaining amino acids. This is now referred to as the J (joining) gene. Thus the genes for the κ-chain consist of a DNA segment that codes for the first two HV regions—the V gene—a J gene segment that codes for the third HV region, and the C_L gene (Fig. 3-12). Antibody diversity is arranged by the selection of one of the several hundred V_L genes, and one of the five different J genes. These are translocated, placed in a linear sequence with the C_L gene, transcribed into mRNA, and translated into protein.

The gene arrangement for λ chains differs from that for the κ chains. For the λ chain V gene–J gene pairs precede the C gene. Since there are a larger number of V compared with J genes, it is not likely that the V–J gene pairs are transcribed as a unit.

The mechanism of the translocation and excision of the introns and unification of the exons must be very complex. One recognition system for determining the location of introns may reside in the sequences known as palindromes. A palindrome is a base sequence in DNA that reads the same in both directions from a base pair when read according to its respective 5' to 3' orientation. These palindromes create loops in the DNA strand. If an endonuclease breaks the DNA on both sides of the palindrome, when reannealing occurs, the intron is removed, and the exons are joined. Any error in this cleavage by the enzyme, at one or two bases away from its normal excision site, would cause a shift in the triplet reading frame. This shift would create deletions (or

additions) in the amino acid sequence of the immunoglobulin chain and would be a mechanism for somatic mutation to occur.

The biogenetic analysis of H chains (which are located on mouse chromosome 12) has revealed several parallels to the conclusions about the L chains, with slight differences in terminology. A library of V_H genes is available that codes for the first two HV regions much the way the V_L genes do for the L chain. These may be preceded by an L or leader sequence. The genetic unit coding for the third HV region is called the D (diversity) gene. The exact number of these on the chromosome is not yet known but probably would be large. A separate exon codes for the final J gene region of the V_H domain. Thereafter a library of C genes is present in the sequence $C\mu$, $C\delta$, $C\gamma_3$, $C\gamma_1$, $C\gamma_{2b}$, $C\gamma_{2a}$, $C\epsilon$, and $C\alpha$. (Coding of the human H genes also follows the sequence μ, δ, γ, ϵ, and α.) Thus in the construction of the H chain gene, introns between these segments are excised to juxtapose the selected V_H, D, J, and C_H domain genes (Fig. 3-13).

The present view is that each C_H gene actually consists of a large sequence encoding for the C_H1, the hinge region, the C_H2, and the C_H3 domains. An additional C_H4 sequence would be needed for certain immunoglobulins, for example, IgM. These subloci may be separated by short spacer introns, but this is uncertain.

It is interesting that the C_H domain genes are in the order which has been deciphered, since gene

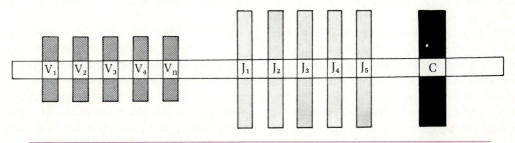

FIG. 3-12
Genetic analysis of the mouse κ-chains indicate the sixth chromosome contains a large library of V genes (V_1 to V_n), five J genes, and a single C gene. One of each gene set is translocated to place one V, one J, and the C gene in immediate sequence before being transcribed to form the mRNA. The genetic arrangement for λ chains has alternate V–J gene segments.

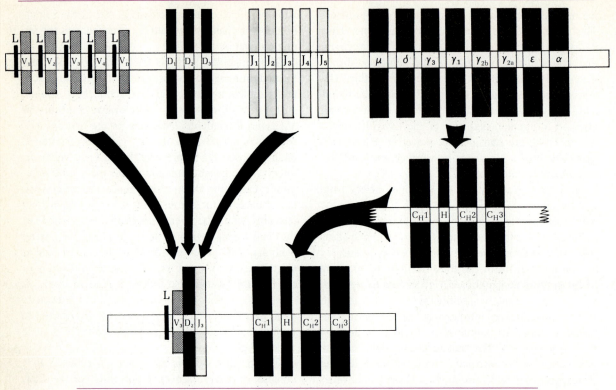

FIG. 3-13

The murine chromosome 12 contains the genes for the H chains. From the series of V genes one is selected and placed next to one D gene, which is placed next to a J gene. When one of the gene sets for an H chain class is chosen, the domain sequences are properly aligned. In this example the γ_1 H chain gene sequence is shown to contain individual genes for the C_H domains and the hinge (H) region.

switching is in agreement with this order. The immature lymphocyte first has IgM on its surface, later often accompanied by IgD. Mature lymphocytes that synthesize IgM may later switch from IgM to IgG synthesis. The stimulus for such switching has not yet been identified, but a chemical basis for it has been suggested. Sequence analysis of the space between the H gene codons for μ, δ, γ, etc., has identified two sequences that are repeated. One of these is TGGGG, and the other is CAGCTG. These are hypothesized to represent switch sequences (S or SS) which, when recognized, cause the next H chain genome to be transcribed.

Progress in the mapping of human genes has trailed behind the studies in the laboratory mouse,

but the data that are available follow the pattern of the earlier studies.

Allelic exclusion

Some of the data derived from immunoglobulin gene mapping has been used to explain the phenomenon known as allelic exclusion. When the immunoglobulin allotype of two parents is different, the immunoglobulin allotype of individual cells of the F_1 is always that of one parent, never a blend of the two. One of the parental alleles is never expressed. This is unlike the inheritance of other characters, such as blood groups, where heterozygous A and B parents produce AB children. Thus only one of the immunoglobulin genes is read. How this choice is made is uncertain. It is possible that, when gene translocations occur in one chromosome, genes in the other chromosome are in some way blocked from relocating. The genes in the other chromosome could persist but in a disconnected, nonexpressible configuration. Some data indicate that the unexpressed alleles are deleted or rearranged into a nonexpressible order. It will not be possible to decide whether stabilization of the original germ line configuration, rearrangement, or deletion is the end state of the excluded allele until further studies have been reported.

BIOLOGIC FUNCTION RELATIVE TO IMMUNOGLOBULIN STRUCTURE

The behavior of immunoglobulins follows the general tenets of protein behavior since fragments and domains are easily prepared that simultaneously preserve certain structural elements and biologic activities.

The early separations by Porter and Edelman clearly demonstrated that the antigen-binding property of an immunoglobulin resided in its amino terminal end. Eventually the HV regions in the V_L and V_H domains were identified as the exact loci.

The constant domains were recognized as the loci for allotypic variations in both L and H chains that could not reside in the variable regions because the allotypic markers were regularly expressed.

Although the Fc fragment initially was described in terms of its ease of crystallization, it is emphasized now as the site of receptors for molecules of the complement system and cell surfaces. Only certain subclasses of IgG and IgM have receptors for the complement system, and the exact sequences essential to this function are not entirely agreed on but are probably in or near the hinge region and C_H2. Likewise the C_H2 domain is associated with the binding of IgG and IgM to the cell surfaces of phagocytic cells, of IgM and IgD to lymphocytes, and of IgE to mast cells and basophils.

The hinge region has a unique amino acid composition containing several prolines, which renders this section uncoiled and exposes it to enzymatic attack. This region actually flexes when antigen combines with the antibody molecule and is the hinge for joining the L and H chains.

IMMUNOGLOBULINS OF LOWER MAMMALS

In general, the higher mammals reflect closely the immunoglobulin variations of humans. As one progresses to the lower vertebrates, IgA and IgE are lost, then IgG is lost, and finally IgM is preserved. All vertebrates synthesize secretory IgA.

The mouse, which is said to be the experimental animal in 70% of all occasions when a mammal is used, has eight distinct serum immunoglobulins. In addition to IgA, IgM, IgD, and IgE, four varieties of IgG exist: IgG1, IgG2a, IgG2b, and IgG3. The numbering of the mouse IgG subclasses is not intended to reflect a homology with human IgG. Except for the lack of IgG3, the rat immunoglobulin profile is the same as that of the mouse. Canines have IgA, IgM, and IgE but no IgD. Four IgGs also exist in dogs but are numbered IgG1, IgG2a, IgG2b, and IgG2c. Horses have four IgG-like globulins, labeled IgGa, IgGb, IgGc, and IgGT.

PURIFICATION OF IMMUNOGLOBULINS

There are basically two different methods by which immunoglobulins can be purified. The general, or nonspecific, methods simply treat the immunoglobulins as γ-globulins and separate them from other serum proteins on the basis of their unique biophysical properties. In the specific methods the separation of the antibody globulins is accomplished through procedures that take advantage of the special antigen- or hapten-combining powers of immunoglobulins.

Nonspecific methods

The general methods for the purification of immunoglobulins are based on the discovery of Kabat over 40 years ago that antibodies are found in the γ-globulin fraction of the serum proteins. Although some of the antibodies are more properly called β-globulins, their chemical behavior is sufficiently like that of the γ-globulins to permit their isolation by many procedures designed for the latter class of proteins.

The γ-globulins are insoluble in half-saturated ammonium sulfate solutions; thus mixing of antiserum in equal proportions with saturated ammonium sulfate produces a globulin precipitate. Sodium sulfate may be used as the precipitant instead of ammonium sulfate. This precipitate is soluble in distilled water and can be reprecipitated for additional purification. Dialysis or gel filtration to remove sulfate ions yields a purified antibody preparation. γ-Globulins may also be precipitated from serum by lower concentrations of heavy metal ions than needed to precipitate other proteins. Rivanol at 0.4% concentration will precipitate most serum proteins other than the γ-globulins, which remain in the supernatant.

In addition to the solubility differences displayed by γ-globulins and other serum proteins, differences in ionic behavior also permit purification of antibodies. Preparative zone electrophoresis, ion-exchange chromatography, isoelectric focusing, and related techniques are examples of methods used to purify the immunoglobulins or their fragments.

Specific methods

All the specific methods for the purification of antibodies depend on a specific serologic reaction of the antibody with its antigen or hapten, after which the antibody is separated from the complex. This is easiest when the antigen in question is a polysaccharide, since polysaccharides have chemical properties grossly different from those of globulins. Certain haptens also present unique opportunities for the purification of antihaptens.

Antisera may be purified by first preparing the antigen–antibody precipitate, harvesting it by centrifugation, and washing it free of contaminating serum proteins. The antigen-antibody aggregate may be dissociated by increasing the salt concentration, raising the temperature, or altering the pH. Either acid or alkaline pH may result in dissociation, depending on the system. Dissociation is followed by a chemical or physical procedure adapted to the separation of the antigen from the immunoglobulin, or it may take place in a medium designed to hold one of the reactants in an insoluble condition. For example, dissociation in acid followed by salt precipitation of the globulin with $(NH_4)_2SO_4$ has been used. A hapten or antigen, which remains in the supernatant, is washed from the antibody. The dissociated antigen–antibody complex can be subjected to electrophoresis, gradient centrifugation, gel filtration, or ion-exchange chromatography to separate the two reactants, provided that they differ appreciably in size or ionic charge.

The most recent innovation in the purification of antibodies is the use of immunoadsorbents in affinity columns, which may be of several types: gels in which the antigen is entrapped but that have pores large enough for some physical contact between the antigen and antibody; inert polymers to which the antigen is bound covalently; or cellulose derivatives or other chemicals to which the antigen is bound covalently. One of the first cellulose immunoadsorbents used was p-aminobenzylcellulose. If diazo-

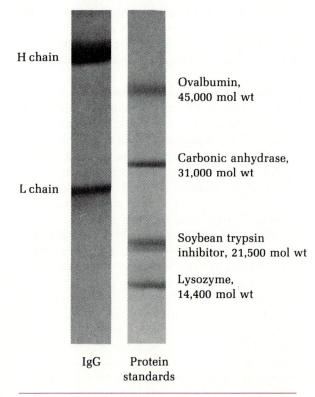

FIG. 3-14

An IgG purified from a protein A immunosorbent column was reduced to separate the H and L chains. These then were electrophoresed in a polyacrylamide gel under conditions that prevented reassociation. The positions of the H and L chains can be identified relative to the position of proteins of known molecular weight. (Courtesy Dr. C. Parker).

tized, this substituted cellulose will bond to any protein containing tyrosyl residues. If such a cellulose-protein is mixed with an immune serum to the protein, the antibody will attach to it. The cellulose derivative is then removed and washed, and the antibody is eluted, usually by lowering the pH. In this way *p*-aminobenzylcellulose diazotized to bovine serum albumin was used to prepare rabbit anti-bovine serum albumin that was 89% pure. A similar procedure using *p*-aminobenzyloxymethylcellulose will produce antibodies between 90% and 100% pure to protein antigens such as rabbit globulin, human serum albumin, and hen egg albumin. Protein A columns will bind IgG regardless of its antigen specificity, and the immunoglobulins can be eluted later. This is a useful method for purifying IgG from a hyperimmune serum (Fig. 3-14).

REFERENCES

Alexander, A., Rosen, S., and Buxbaum, J.: Human immunoglobulin genes in health and disease, Clin. Immunol. Rev. **4**:31, 1985.

Calame, K.L.: Mechanisms that regulate immunoglobulin gene expression, Ann. Rev. Immunol. **3**:159, 1985.

Davie, J.M., Seiden, M.V., Greenspan, N.S., Lutz, C.T., Batholow, T.L., and Clevinger, B.L.: Structural correlates of idiotopes, Ann. Rev. Immunol. **4**:147, 1986.

Davies, D.R., and Metzger, H.: Structural basis of antibody function, Ann. Rev. Immunol. **1**:87, 1983.

Honjo, T.: Immunoglobulin genes, Ann. Rev. Immunol. **1**:499, 1983.

Honjo, T.: Origin of immune diversity: genetic variation and selection, Ann. Rev. Biochem. **54**: 803, 1985.

Kindt, T.J., and Capra, J.D.: The antibody enigma, New York, 1984, Plenum Press.

Koshland, M.E.: The coming of age of the immunoglobulin J chain, Ann. Rev. Immunol. **3**:425, 1985.

Lerner, R.A.: Antibodies of predetermined specificity in biology and medicine, Adv. Immunol. **36**:1, 1984.

Perlmutter, R.M., Crews, S.T., Douglas, R., Sorenson, G., Johnson, N., Nivera, N., Gearhart, P.J., and Hood, L.: The generation of diversity in phosphorylcholine-binding antibodies, Adv. Immunol. **35**:2, 1984.

Rajesky, K., and Takemori, T.: Genetics, expression, and function of idiotypes, Ann. Rev. Immunol. **1**:569, 1983.

Solari, R., and Kraehenbuhl, J.P.: The biosynthesis of secretory component and its role in transepithelial transport of IgA dimer, Immunol. Today **6**:17, 1985.

Thorbecke, G.J., and Leslie, G.A, editors: Immunoglobulin D: structure and function, Ann. N.Y. Acad. Sci. **399**:1, 1982.

Yancopoulos, G.D., and Alt, F.W.: Regulation of the assembly and the expression of variable-region genes, Ann. Rev. Immunol. **4**:339, 1986.

The major histocompatibility complex

GLOSSARY

β₂ microglobulin   A protein associated with H-2 and HLA antigens.

class I gene or protein   Genes, or their products, of the H-2 or HLA region of the MHC.

class II gene or protein   Genes, or their products, of the Ir region of the MHC.

class III gene or protein   Genes, or their products, of the MHC that contribute to the complement system.

H-2   The major histocompatibility system of mice.

HLA   The major histocompatibility system in humans (HLA = human leukocyte antigen).

Ia protein   Immune-associated protein, found on B lymphocytes and macrophages.

I-A   A gene, or its gene product, the latter being an Ia protein, of the immune associated region of the MHC.

Ir gene   Immune response gene.

major histocompatibility complex (MHC)   A collection of structural genes associated with the immune response transplantation antigens, and proteins of the complement system.

All species of animals so far examined devote a portion of one chromosome pair to a segment that codes for three functionally different proteins: those that regulate the immune response, those that determine the acceptance or rejection of transplanted tissues between individuals within that species, and those that are a part of the complement system. This gene segment is referred to as the major histocompatibility complex (MHC) because its original discovery was based on transplantation experiments, and only later were the other two properties identified as a part of this complex. Understanding the role of the MHC in the immune response has done much to clarify the significance of the MHC. Immediately after it was initially described, the MHC was viewed only as a regulator of graft acceptance. The question was posed as to why an animal would devote so much DNA to regulate an event-tissue transplantation—that would never occur in nature. The revelation that both the immune-response segment and the histocompatibility segment of the MHC govern cell-cell recognition and interaction has clarified the purpose of the MHC.

THE MURINE MHC
Discovery of the H-2 system

The MHC of mice was described serologically in 1936 by Gorer, who was studying mouse blood-group antigens. Of the four antigens under investigation, Gorer noted that antigen II was related to transplant survival; grafts between animals that shared antigen II were usually successful. Snell suggested that such antigens be called histocompatibility antigens, and the nomenclature system was born. H-2 antigens in mice and the genetic basis for their inheritance were clarified by the use of inbred, congeneic mouse strains developed by Snell. Ultimately more than 50 alloantigens were described that controlled

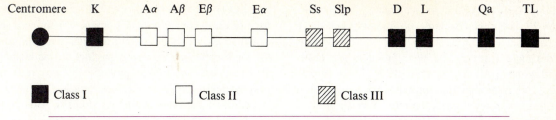

Class I   Class II   Class III

FIG. 4-1

Structural genes for the murine major histocompatibility are situated on chromosome 17. The class I H2-K histocompatibility genes are separated from the H2-D and H2-L genes by the class II immune response genes I-A and I-E and by the class III genes Ss and Slp of the complement system.

graft rejection, and the genes determining these antigens were linked to those that regulate the immune response and the complement system (Fig. 4-1).

Discovery of the Ir system

Several early observations had suggested a genetic basis for the immune response. The familial tendency toward susceptibility to infectious disease or allergy had been recognized for many years. Immunologists had encountered experiments in which certain strains of animals responded poorly or not at all to certain antigens, but it was not until the studies of Benacerraf, McDevitt, and a few others, that a genetic basis for this tendency was proven. Benacerraf examined the immune response of guinea pigs to synthetic polypeptides of limited antigenic potency. In fact, it is only by using antigens with a small number of epitopes that a genetic restriction of the immune response can be recognized.

When many functional epitopes are present in an antigen, one animal may respond to one set of epitopes, and a second animal to a different set. The conclusion is that both animals are responders even though their inheritance has dictated their response to different epitopes. When an animal is challenged with an antigen that has a limited number of epitopes, either it responds or it doesn't. When two animals respond, it is likely they are responding to the same epitopes. Since the capacity to respond to a certain antigenic determinant is an inherited characteristic, it can be claimed that the responders have the same immune response (Ir) genes. Any animal failing to respond lacks the necessary Ir gene.

Three separate forms of antigenic challenge have been used to analyze the Ir genes. The most successful have been synthetic polypeptides, but allogenic proteins that usually present very few novel epitopes to an animal have also been used. A third and less frequently used technique has been immunization with a minimal dose of antigen so that only vigorous responders could be identified.

By immunizing guinea pigs with a polymer of glutamic acid and alanine it was possible to show that Ir genes are transmitted as a single dominant trait. Strain 2 guinea pigs are high responders to the polymer but strain 13 animals are poor responders. All the first generation progeny (F1) of strain 2-strain 13 matings were high responders. F1-strain 13 matings yielded progeny that were 50% high and 50% low responders. F1 mating with strain 2 animals produced 100% high responders. These facts are proof of a simple mendelian inheritance of a single dominant gene.

An identical genetic relationship was recognized in mice. The CBA mouse is a low responder to a tripolymer of glutamic acid, lysine, and alanine that is highly immunogenic for the C57BL strain. Breeding of these two strains produced mice that were all high responders. Back-crosses of the F1 generation with either parent produced mice characteristic of a single dominant gene transmission of an immune response gene.

Mapping the location of the Ir genes was possible in the mouse because Snell and his associates had developed many inbred strains in a continuation of their studies on histocompatibility. The genes controlling histocompatibility were located on chromosome 17, the same chromosome that harbored the Ir genes. The histocompatibility genes are referred to as the class I genes, and their products are designated variously as the class I proteins, histocompatibility, or transplantation proteins. (Because these proteins are also antigens, the terms can be used interchangeably.) The Ir genes, since they were the second discovered, are known as the class II genes, or sometimes as the immune associated (Ia) genes. The gene products, in addition to having specific names, are usually referred to as the Ir or Ia proteins (or antigens).

Class I genes and their products

In the mouse three genes or gene clusters, the H-2K, H-2D, and H-2L genes, situated on chromosome 17 are the structural genes that determine the composition of the histocompatibility antigens. The K gene locus is separated from the juxtaposed D and L loci. The K, D, and L loci are very polymorphic and have been identified to result in the production of more than 50 antigenically distinct proteins. Allogeneic immunization and adsorption experiments have yielded highly purified sera, which can be used to identify these antigens on cells. More recently hybridoma antibodies have become available for this same purpose.

These histocompatibility antigens have been identified on the surface of all nucleated cells. It is the immune response of a transplant recipient against these antigens that dominates the graft rejection process; hence these are defined as the major transplantation antigens. Less potent or minor histocompatibility antigens also may contribute to graft rejection.

The H-2 antigens can be removed from cell membranes by detergents or potassium chloride salt extraction procedures, which disturb the lipid bilayer of the membrane. The free H-2 antigens are glycoproteins with a molecular weight near 45,000 (Fig. 4-2). These proteins can be described as possessing five domains; three extracytoplasmic domains, $\alpha 1$, $\alpha 2$ and $\alpha 3$, each consisting of approximately 90 amino acids, a transmembrane segment of approximately 40 amino acids, and a cytoplasmic anchor of about 30 amino acids. The complete H-2 protein

consists of 345 amino acids. The observation that each of the three α domains contains 90 amino acids and that two of them contain internal disulfide linkages presents an interesting parallel to the domain structure of the immunoglobulins. Two units of polysaccharide are present, one attached to the $\alpha 1$ domain and the other to the $\alpha 2$ domain. This polysaccharide consists of galactose, mannose, fucose, and glucosamine. The polysaccharide side chains do not contribute to the antigenic specificity of the H-2 proteins.

The most exterior of the extracytoplasmic domains, the $\alpha 1$ and $\alpha 2$ segments, contain amino acid sequences that provide most of the antigenic specificity for the H-2 antigens. Amino acid-sequencing of these proteins from different sources and with varying specificity has confirmed this fact as well as demonstrated a near constant sequence in the $\alpha 3$, the transmembrane segment and the cytoplasmic portions. Ionically associated with the $\alpha 2$ and $\alpha 3$ domains is a β_2-microglobulin with a molecular weight of 12,000.

In addition to the murine H-2K, H-2D, and H-2L class I proteins, a series of two other proteins are considered class I proteins. These proteins are related to the Qa and TL structural genes, each of which contains numerous alleles. Whereas the H-2 proteins are important in cell-cell interactions including transplantation, the function of the Qa and TL proteins is uncertain. Despite their similar size, domain structure, and association with the β_2-microglobulin like the H-2 proteins, neither the Qa or TL proteins contributes significantly to graft rejection. The TL protein, also known as the Tla (thymic leukemia antigen) is found on normal, immature thymocytes and neoplastic thymocytes. Upon maturation of the thymocyte in the thymus gland, synthesis of the TL protein ceases. This event does not occur in thymic leukemia.

β_2-Microglobulin

Noncovalently bonded to the H-2 protein is the β_2-microglobulin, a unique protein containing 99 amino acids with a molecular weight of approximately 12,000 (Fig. 4-2). This identical β_2-microglobulin is ionically associated with all the antigeni-

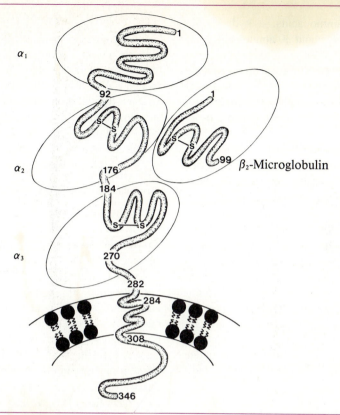

FIG. 4-2

The H2-K, -D, and -L gene products, the histocompatibility or transplantation antigens are similar in their basic structure to the human HLA-A, -B, and -C gene products. All are composed of a protein of 45,000 molecular weight that is divisible into three extracellular domains, a transmembrane segment, and a cytoplasmic tail. The β_2-microglobulin is noncovalently associated with the antigen specific transplantation protein.

cally diverse H-2 proteins. Structural genes on mouse chromosome 2 encode for this protein. The β_2-globulin is of interest because early in the study of the human histocompatibility antigens it was recognized that they functioned as cross-reactive antigens with antisera to IgG. This cross-reactivity now has been related to the close amino acid sequence homology of the constant domains of immunoglobulins (Chapter 3) and the β_2-microglobulin. In fact amino acid sequencing of several β_2-microglobulins has revealed only one with a single amino acid substitution that differed from the others. Thus this protein does not contribute to the antigenic specificity of the transplantation antigens.

Class II genes and their products

Situated between the H-2K and H-2D genes are a cluster of structural genes known as the Ir or Ia genes. Although it was once believed that as many as five major loci resided in this region of chromosome 17, it is now thought there are only two, the I-A and the I-E regions. The Ia proteins related to these genes consist of two peptide chains. Of these, the α chain with a molecular weight of approximately 30,000 appears to be slightly larger than the β chain with a molecular weight just under 29,000. Each of the two peptides that are ionically and not covalently associated can again be described in terms of domains. Each has two extracytoplasmic domains of approximately 90 amino acids, a hydrophobic transmembrane domain of about 30 amino acids, and a cytoplasmic anchor of 10 to 15 amino acids. There is a single disulfide bridge in the α chain but two such linkages in the β chain (Fig. 4-3). The α and β peptides also differ in that the α chain contains two polysaccharide side chains whereas the β chain bears but one.

The I-A and I-E gene products are found on the surfaces of macrophages and B lymphocytes. I-A or I-E receptors are located on the surfaces of T lymphocytes. Thus these Ia proteins function in the immune response to TD antigens by fostering a cooperation between macrophages, B cells, and T cells with the same antigenic specificity. This cooperation demands that there be an extensive variation in the structure of the Ia proteins (and their receptors) equivalent to the variation in the specificity of antigens. Amino acid sequencing of a few Ia proteins supports this concept, and the needed variation appears to be located in the α chain; the β chains demonstrate very little variation in sequence from one molecule to another.

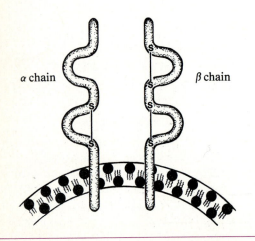

α chain   β chain

FIG. 4-3

The I-A and I-E proteins consist of two ionically associated peptides. The α chains contain one internal disulfide bridge and display considerable diversity in amino acid sequence. The β chain has two disulfide bridges and shows less sequence diversity. Both proteins are near 30,000 molecular weight.

Class III genes and their products

On the mouse chromosome 17 two genes (Ss and Slp) are present between the Ir region and the D gene locus. The Ss gene is the structural gene for protein C4 of the murine complement system. The Slp (sex-limited protein) also codes for a C4 protein, but this molecule is mutated and nonfunctional. These and their gene products in the complement system are described in Chapter 10.

THE HUMAN MHC
Discovery of the HLA system

The human histocompatibility antigens are present on all nucleated cells of the body, including leukocytes. Antibodies to human leukocytes were discovered in people who had undergone several transfusions and were found to function independently of the antibodies to the ABO antigens. Beginning in about 1958 several groups of workers began a serious study of these antibodies, each group adopting a nomenclature system of its own and in some instances reporting some observations about the transmission or grouping of these antigens. For example, Dausset indicated in 1958 that monozygotic (identical) twins had identical leukocyte agglutination patterns and that dizygotic twins did not. By 1962 van Rood and van Leeuwen arranged a simple leukocyte antigen-grouping system from the examination of the agglutinating susceptibility of leukocytes from 100 individuals tested against a panel of antisera. By 1967 it was obvious that many antigens existed on the white blood cell surface; a special workshop of experimenters on this subject accepted HL-A1, HL-A2, etc. as the symbols to refer to human leukocyte antigen 1, 2, and so on. This was later changed to HLA. At the same time studies of transplantation antigens of mice revealed that they were located on the surfaces of leukocytes, and by the early 1960s it was learned that injections of human leukocytes resulted in accelerated graft rejection. Thus the HLA antigens came to be synonymous with the human transplantation or histocompatibility antigens.

Class I genes and their products

Three gene sets of the HLA systems have been identified on human chromosome 6 and are desig-

Dausset J.

Iso-leuco-anticorps.
Acta Haematol. **20**:156-66, 1958.   [Centre National de Transfusion Samguine, Paris, France]

This paper provides a description of the first human leucocyte (tissue) group. Polytransfused patients' sera agglutinated some but not all leucocytes. This group, initially called 'Mac,' is now known as HLA-A2. This work opened up the understanding of the human major histocompatibility complex HLA, a key to the immune system. [The SCI® indicates that this paper has been cited in over 165 publications since 1961, making it the 5th most-cited paper ever published in this journal.]

Jean Dausset
Unité INSERM U. 93
Hôpital Saint-Louis
75475 Paris
France

January 19, 1983

"In 1952, when only the red blood cell groups were known, I mixed on a glass plate the serum of an agranulocytic woman with the bone marrow of another individual. I observed a massive macroscopic agglutination. I soon understood that it was not due to autoantibodies but to alloantibodies (at that time called isoantibodies)

"This paper gathered together all the work that had been done since 1952, in collaboration with Gilbert Malinvaud. Hélène Brécy, and later, Jacques and Monique Colombani. (This work was also described in a book.[1])

"During this time, we organised the systematic detection of leucoantibodies in the sera of polytransfused patients tested against a panel of leucocytes from volunteers from the National Blood Transfusion Centre. The agglutinations were sometimes obvious and sometimes weak, of very dubious reproducibility. There were no computers at that time and our results were exposed on a large poster on the laboratory wall. We almost lost hope of ever making sense of it, so numerous were the different patterns. However, we noticed, after numerous repetitions, that the leucocytes from three panel donors were less often agglutinated than others. This gave us the idea that they lacked a certain antigen which is otherwise frequent in the population. Six sera did not agglutinate these three individuals, but agglutinated 11 others, thus dividing the population into two groups: one bearing the Mac antigen (not a Scottish name, but the initials of the surnames of the three non-agglutinated individuals) and the other without this antigen. An important fact was that these sera were unable to agglutinate their own leucocytes (they were not autoantibodies) nor the leucocytes of the other patients who produced similar antibodies.

"Formal proof was obtained when we observed that among the patients systematically transfused with Mac-positive blood, only the Mac-negative recipients developed an anti-Mac antibody.

"These leucocyte antigens are genetically determined since the pattern of agglutination with a battery of anti-leucocyte sera was strictly identical in monozygotic twins and different in dizygotic twins. Lastly, we demonstrated that leucocyte antibodies were responsible for the transfusion reactions.

"Thus, this work gathers together all the principles and first fruits of leucocyte immunohaematology. This was the starting point of an extraordinary biological adventure and is the reason why this paper has been highly cited. Two laboratories followed in our footsteps: J.J. Van Rood soon afterward described a supertypic antigen, 4a4b (Bw4,Bw6);[2] Rose Payne with W. Bodmer described the first two alleles: LA1 and LA2 (LA2 being identical to Mac).[3]

"Soon there were more than three musketeers: B Amos, R Ceppellini, F Kissmeyer-Nielsen, P Terasaki, and R Walford joined the game, rapidly followed by numerous scientific communities. A unique collaborative research study was undertaken and has continued ever since. Thanks to ambitious international workshops which allow the exchange of reagents and information, the extraordinary skein of the human HLA complex was unraveled.[4-10] Its essential role in transplantation and, generally speaking, in immunology is well known, as well as its association with numerous diseases.

"Starting with the first serological data, it has been possible, in the space of 20 years, to decipher the biological composition and function of these molecules, protruding like antennae from the surface of our cells. We are now beginning to study the genes which govern these cells, and can expect still more marvels to come."

1. Dausset J. *Immuno-hématologie biologique et clinique.* Paris: Flammarion, 1956. 718 p.
2. Van Rood J J & Van Leeuwen A. Leukocyte grouping. A method and its applications. *J Clin Invest* **42**:1382-90, 1963.
3. Payne R, Trip M, Weigle J, Bodmer W & Bodmer J. A new leukocyte iso-antigen system in man. *Cold Spring Harbor Symp* **29**:285-95, 1964.
4. Videbaek A, ed. *Histocompatibility testing, 1965.* Copenhagen: Munksgaard, 1965. 4288 p.
5. Curtoni E S, Mattiuz P L & Tosi R M. eds. *Histocompatibility testing, 1967.* Copenhagen: Munksgaard, 1967, 458 p.
6. Terasaki P I, ed. *Histocompatibility testing, 1970.* Copenhagen: Munksgaard, 1970. 658 p.
7. Dausset J & Colombani J, eds. *Histocompatibility testing, 1972.* Copenhagen: Munksgaard, 1973. 778 p.
8. Kissmeyer-Nielsen F, ed. *Histocompatibility testing, 1975.* Copenhagen: Munksgaard, 1975. 1035 p.
9. Bodmer W F, Batchelor J R, Bodmer J G, Festenstein H & Morris P J, eds. *Histocompatibility testing, 1977.* Copenhagen: Munksgaard, 1977. 612 p.
10. Terasaki P I, ed. *Histocompatibility testing, 1980.* Los Angeles, CA: UCLA Tissue Typing Laboratory, 1980. 1227 p.

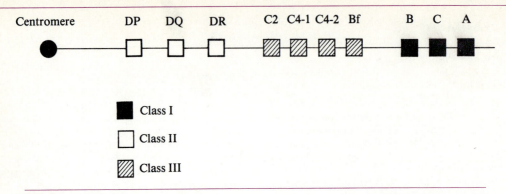

FIG. 4-4

The structural genes for the human major histocompatibility complex are on chromosome 6. The class I genes HLA-A, -B, and -C are grouped, unlike the murine MHC. The class II or immune response genes are separated from the histocompatibility genes by the class III genes of the complement system.

nated HLA-A, HLA-B, and HLA-C (Fig. 4-4). These gene regions are clustered, as is the case in all species studied except the mouse. Each gene is highly pleomorphic. The A gene is currently recognized to have at least 23 specificities, the B gene 50 specificities, and the C gene 8 specificities. Because of serologic cross-reactions between some products of the A gene and to a lesser extent with products of the B gene, these numbers are not exact. This discrepancy is also true because an annual workshop of scientists engaged in studying the genetics and serologic behavior of these proteins frequently reassigns the position of a certain specificity that in turn alters the number of specificities within the A, B, or C loci. At the present time, all eight of the C gene specificities are considered provisional and subject to reassignment.

The chemistry of the HLA-A, -B, and -C proteins is reflective of the structure of the H2-K, -D, and -L proteins. Each consists of a peptide chain of 345 amino acids associated with the human β_2-microglobulin. The larger protein is divisible into five domains, parallel in structure to that seen in the murine system. Variations in the amino acid sequence of the most external domains, the $\alpha 1$ and $\alpha 2$ domains, contribute most importantly to the antigenic specificity of these molecules.

The role of these proteins in tissue transplantation is described in Chapter 15, but these proteins also have an interesting application in genetics and autoimmune disease.

Class II genes and their products

The immune-response region of human chromosome 6 is separated from the HLA region by the class III genes. The exact number of genes in this, the D region (a letter selected to separate it from the HLA A, B, and C loci) is uncertain, but three are widely accepted. These are DR, DP, and DQ. DP and DQ replace the earlier designations SB and DC, respectively. DQ has also been known variously in the past as MB and DS. The number of alleles for each gene is not known but, in view of the function of the gene products, must be quite large. At least six different specificities for each of the DP and DQ genes are known.

The class II human proteins, sometimes described as the HLA-D proteins, again reflect the structure of the murine class II proteins. Each protein consists of two peptides, an α chain with a molecular weight of about 30,000 and a β chain that is slightly smaller. These two peptides are ionically associated on the surfaces of macrophages and β cells. The evidence indicates that, whereas in the murine system there is a single pair of genes at each locus, one for the α and one for the β peptide, in the human system there are two pairs, α1 and α2, and β1 and β2.

Class III genes and their products

Four gene loci situated between the HLA and the HLA-D loci on chromosome 6 are associated with the complement system. These Class III genes are the structural genes for proteins C2, C4, and factor B of the complement system. The C4 gene is duplicated in the human system, and both products are active unlike the case of the murine system and the inactive Slp protein.

SUMMARY

The term *major histocompatibility complex* (MHC) is now in many ways a misnomer. Although genes of the MHC are very important in the regulation of transplant success or failure, the transplantation of tissues is still a comparatively rare medical event. In contrast, the immune response is a regular event in every living mammal, and we now know that this event is genetically restricted. The common theme for the class I and class II genes and their products is the control of cell interactons. They provide a system for intercellular communication. In transplant rejection this is most simply viewed as the attack of the recipient cells on donor cells that carry foreign class I MHC proteins on their surface. In the immune response, the ability of macrophages and B cells to cooperate in the immunoglobulin response is based on their sharing the identical class II protein. The helping T cell must have the appropriate receptor for this protein.

The role of the class III genes and the complement proteins in direct cell-cell interaction is less evident, nevertheless the molecules of the complement system are very important in many cellular events.

REFERENCES

Accolla, R.S., Moretta, A., and Carrel, S.: The human Ia system: an overview, Semin. Hematol. **21**:287, 1984.

Cohen, I.R., and Friedman, A.: Processed antigen and MHC molecules, Prog. Allergy **36**:190, 1985.

Colten, H.R.: Molecular genetics of the major histocompatibility linked complement genes, Springer Semin. Immunopathol. **6**:149, 1983.

deVries, R.R.P., and van Rood, J.J., editors: Immunobiology of HLA class-I and class-II molecules, Prog. Allergy **36**:1, 1985.

Fey, G., Domdey, H., Wiebauer, K., Whitehead, A.S., and Odink, K.: Structure and expression of the C3 gene, Springer Semin. Immunopathol. **6**:119, 1983.

Figueroa, F., and Klein, J.: The evolution of MHC class II genes, Immunol. Today **7**:78, 1986.

Giles, R.C., and Capra, J.D.: Biochemistry of MHC class II molecules, Tissue Antigen **25**:57, 1985.

Giles, R.C., and Capra, J.D.: Structure, function, and genetics of human class II molecules, Adv. Immunol. **37**:1, 1985.

Gonwa, T.A., Peterlin, B.M., and Stobo, J.D.: Human Ir genes: structure and function, Adv. Immunol. **34**:71, 1983.

Kaufman, J.F., Auffray, C., Korman, A.J., Shackelford, D.A., and Strominger, J.: The class II molecules of the human and murine major histocompatibility complex, Cell **36**:1, 1984.

Kimball, E.S., and Coligan, J.E.: Structure of class I major histocompatibility antigens, Contemp. Top. Molec. Immunol. **9**:1, 1983.

Klein, J., and Figueroa, F.: The evolution of class I MHC genes, Immunol. Today **7**:41, 1986.

Lafuse, W.P., and David, C.S.: Ia antigens: genes, molecules and function, Transplant **38**:443, 1984.

Mallory, D., Hackel, E., and Fawcett, K., editors: HLA techniques for blood bankers, Arlington, VA, 1984, Amer. Assoc. Blood Banks.

Mellor, A.: The class I MHC gene family in mice, Immunol. Today **7**:19, 1986.

Mengle-Gaw, L., and McDevitt, H.O.: Genetics and expression of mouse Ia antigens, Ann. Rev. Immunol. **3**:367, 1985.

Porter, R.R.: The complement components of the major histocompatibility complex, CRC Crit. Rev. Biochem. **16**:1, 1984.

Steinmetz, M., and Hood, L.: Genes of the major histocompatibility complex in mouse and man, Science **222**:727, 1983.

Steinmuller, D.: Tissue-specific and tissue-restricted histocompatibility antigens, Immunol. Today **5**:234, 1984.

Schwartz, R.H.: T-lymphocyte recognition of antigen in association with gene products of the major histocompatibility complex, Ann. Rev. Immunol. **3**:327, 1985.

Macrophages and antigen-processing and -presenting cells

≣ GLOSSARY

activated macrophage Macrophage from antigen-sensitized or otherwise stimulated animals.

alveolar macrophage An aerobic macrophage of the lung.

APC antigen-presenting cell.

bacteriotropin An immune opsonin that stimulates phagocytosis of a bacterium, other cell type, or particle.

basophil A blood granulocyte whose granules release histamine during anaphylactic reactions.

chemotaxis Attraction of leukocytes or other cells by chemicals; synonymous with *leukotaxin* in reference to white blood cells.

dendritic cell A nonphagocytic, antigen-presenting cell.

eosinophil A white blood cell that contains cytoplasmic granules with an affinity for acid dyes; synonymous with *acidophil*.

granulocyte A collective term for leukocytes with pronounced cytoplasmic granulation.

HETE Hydroxyeicosatetraenoic acid, a chemotaxin derived from arachidonic acid.

HHT Hydroxyheptatrienoic acid, a chemotaxin derived from arachidonic acid.

hydroxyl radical A toxic form of oxygen produced by phagocytes; $\cdot OH$.

IL-1 Interleukin 1.

interleukin A monokine that acts on other leukocytes.

interleukin 1 A monokine that activates T cells and possibly B cells.

Kupffer cell A macrophage of the liver.

Langerhans' cells Macrophages found in the skin.

macrophage Tissue or blood phagocytes, 20 to 80 μm in diameter, containing lysosomes, vacuoles, and partially digested debris in their cytoplasm.

monocyte White blood cell, 12 to 30 μm in diameter, with rounded nucleus, precursor to macrophage.

monokine A protein elaborated by a monocyte or macrophage that acts on other host cells.

myeloperoxidase An enzyme in lysosomes that aids intraphagocyte killing.

neutrophil A leukocyte with granules that are not predominant in their affinity for acid or basic dyes.

opsonin An antibody that attaches to a cellular or particulate antigen and which "prepares" it for phagocytosis.

phagocytosis The engulfing of cells or particulate matter by leukocytes, macrophages, or other cells.

polymorphonuclear neutrophilic leukocyte (PMN) A white blood cell with a granular cytoplasm and multilobed nucleus that is very active in phagocytosis.

reticuloendothelial blockade Malfunction of phagocytic cells by prior exposure to phagocytosable particles.

reticuloendothelial system (RES) A collective term for actively phagocytic cells of varying morphology and tissue residence.

singlet oxygen A toxic form of oxygen produced by phagocytes $^1O_2$.

superoxide radical A toxic form of oxygen produced by phagocytes: $\cdot O_2$.

TBX$_2$ Thromboxane 2, a chemotaxin derived from arachidonic acid.

tuftsin A chemotactic tetrapeptide derived from a γ-globulin.

The cells of the body that respond to antigens are variously categorized as belonging to the hematopoietic, the reticuloendothelial, the phagocytic, or the lymphoid system. The organs and tissues that make up these systems are not as well defined as those of the nervous, skeletal, endocrine, or other systems, which exist as distinct structural organs and have a clear, often singular, physiologic role. The organ systems of interest to immunologists are often dispersed and may have multiple functions, as do cells of the mononuclear and granulocyte phagocytic system described in this chapter.

THE HEMATOPOIETIC SYSTEM

For most purposes the hematopoietic system is an appropriate beginning study for the immunocytologist. Cells of the immune response system are formed and mature and are dispersed from the bone marrow. They are then reclassified as cells of the phagocytic, lymphoid, or other system according to the new functions they acquire or express outside the bone marrow (Fig. 5-1).

In mammals the bone marrow, if considered as a single tissue, is the largest tissue of the body. In the average human adult the total weight of the bone marrow is about 3 kg. Marrow fills the central core of all long bones, but other bones, especially in the cranium, contribute significantly to total marrow mass. Marrow is divisible into two parts: the vascular and adipose portion and the portion directed to hematopoiesis, or blood-cell formation. The vascular tissue is simply the circulatory system that supplies nutrients and removes wastes from these actively growing cells. This tissue plus the fat represents about half the weight of bone marrow.

The remaining half of the bone marrow is the source of erythrocytes, platelets, granulocytes, monocytes, and lymphocytes. These arise from a primitive, undifferentiated stem cell, the reticulum cell, which differentiates into a separate precursor for each cell line. Within each of these cell lines or systems a further developmental series of cells, intermediate between the precursor and the end cell, has been recognized. Of these cells, only those of the granulocytic, monocytic, and lymphocytic series are effector cells of the immune response. Cells of the erythroid and megakaryocytic (platelet) series often are affected by the immune response and may serve as targets for it. In bone marrow the white blood cells surpass the red blood cells in number by a ratio of 3:1.

THE RETICULOENDOTHELIAL SYSTEM

The term *reticuloendothelial system (RES)* is nearly archaic and lacked a satisfactory definition even when it was a more useful and timely term. At present the RES can be considered a collection of cells of different origin and morphology that are united by their common property of phagocytosis. Two major subdivisions exist within the RES: the mononuclear phagocytic system and the granulocytic phagocytes. The mononuclear cells are the more active of the two phagocytic systems.

Mononuclear phagocytic system

The mononuclear phagocytic cell system consists of the blood monocytes and the free (motile) and fixed (nonmotile) macrophages of the tissues. Monocytes arise from precursor promonocytes of the bone marrow, from which they are released into the blood, although monocytes also can be found in the marrow. Most, if not all, of the tissue macrophages arise from the blood monocytes.

Monocytes

The monocytes represent 1% to 3% of the circulating leukocytes in the adult human, or about 300 cells per cubic milliliter of blood. Monocytes have a circulating half-life of only 8 to 10 hours. They must be synthesized at a rate of about 1.7×10^8 cells per kg of body weight per day to maintain their normal circulating population. These cells range from 10 and 20 μm in diameter; the monocytic nucleus is large and usually occupies about half the space within the cell. The nucleus may be oval or indented or shaped like a crude horseshoe or a kidney. The abundant cytoplasm has a fine granular texture as a result of its generous content of lysosomal granules (Fig. 5-2).

Macrophages

Monocytes that disappear from the blood are not removed from the body as dead or damaged cells.

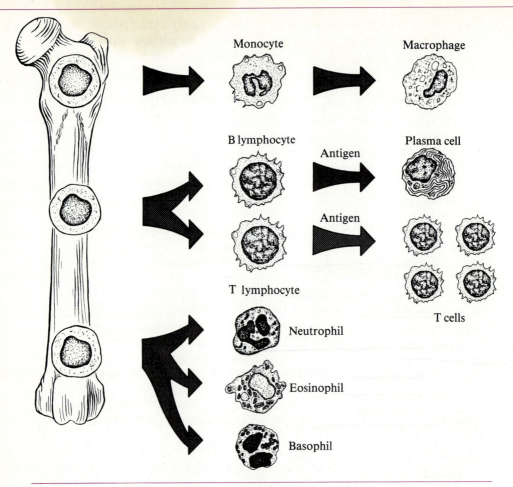

FIG. 5-1

The bone marrow is the source of the immunologically active effector cells. Promonocytes of the bone marrow generate the blood monocytes that then enter tissues to become macrophages. An undifferentiated reticulum cell serves as the progenitor of cells in the lymphoid series, the B and T lymphocytes. The B cells mature to become immunoglobulin secreting plasma cells. T cells mature and divide without a significant morphologic alteration. A myeloid stem cell is the source of the polymorphonuclear neutrophils, eosinophils, and basophils. Of these cells, the monocytes, macrophages, and neutrophils are the most active phagocytes. The macrophages are the most important antigen presenting cells.

Instead these cells enter the tissues and become macrophages where they may have a life span of many months or years. There are more macrophages per gram of tissue in the spleen than in any other organ, but there are more total macrophages in the liver because of its larger size. Macrophages have specific tissue names that vary according to their tissue location (for example, histiocytes in connective tissue, Kupffer cells in liver, alveolar macrophages or dust cells in lung, and microglial cells in the neural system). The tissue macrophages do not have an identical morphology, even though they all arise

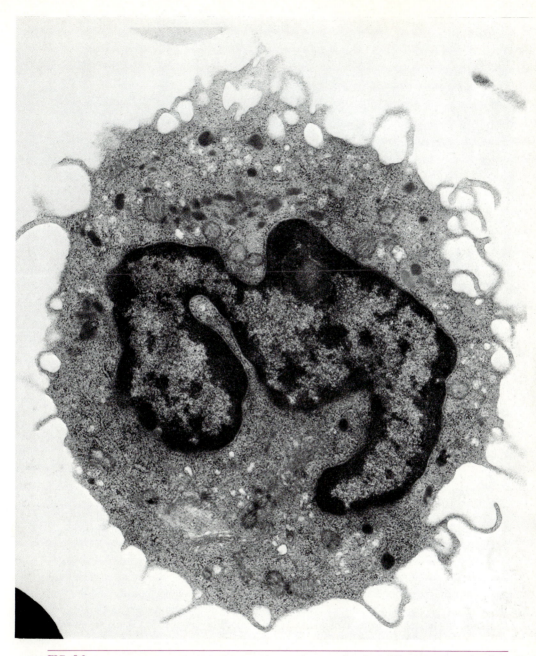

FIG. 5-2

This electron microscopic view of a blood monocyte was cut at a plane which reveals a large cleft in the dark nucleus. Notice the many different types of cytoplasmic inclusions. (Courtesy Dr. E. Adelstein.)

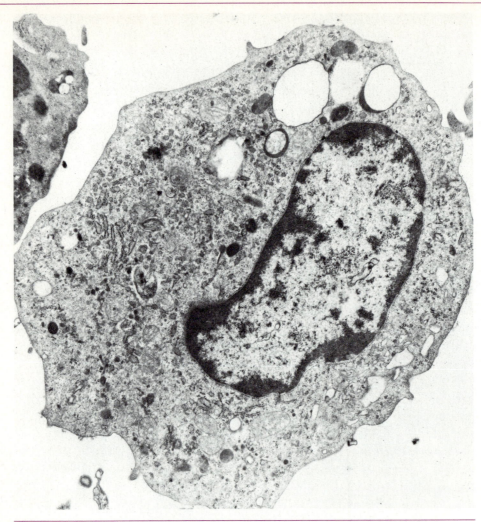

FIG. 5-3

Electron micrograph of a macrophage. Note the large cytoplasmic space and the numerous types of granules. (Courtesy Dr. E. Adelstein.)

from a common precursor, the peripheral blood mono-cyte. When the monocyte enters tissues, it undergoes a metamorphosis, during which there is a rapid in-crease in size, in protein synthesis, and in lysosome content. The extent of these changes is modified by the tissue in which the alteration takes place, thus leading to individual characteristics and separate names for the macrophages that arise in the different tissues. The appearance of macrophages is regulated

by the cell's ameboid motility and the exact moment that fixed preparations are made in relationship to this motility (Fig. 5-3). Because macrophages will attach to glass or plastic surfaces they are easily sep-arated from other cells of the immune system, such as the lymphocytes, that lack this adherent quality.

Macrophages serve many roles. They are the most active of the body's phagocytic cells and are impor-tant in antigen processing (Fig. 5-4). Macrophages

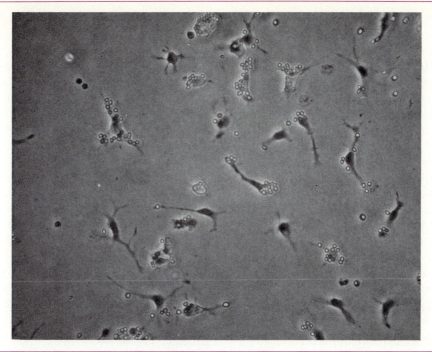

FIG. 5-4

Macrophages in culture. Note their elongated form, indicative of their motility. The clear refractile bodies are erythrocytes that the macrophages are phagocytosing. (Courtesy Dr. E. Leonard.)

cooperate with B cells and T cells in the immune response to T cell–dependent antigens. Macrophages are important secretory cells, producing and secreting components of the complement system, hydrolytic enzymes, toxic forms of oxygen, and the monokines described later. The macrophage surface bears unique proteins that serve as identifying markers.

Within germinal centers where clones of T cells or B cells develop after exposure to antigen, macrophages and dendritic cells are also present. The former can receive, ingest, and process free antigens. The latter can receive antigen in the form of antigen-antibody complexes but do not seem to ingest or process antigens. Dendritic cells are not ameboid, either, and thus are not macrophages. The exact function of dendritic cells is uncertain, but their presence seems essential to the perpetuation, if not the initiation, of the germinal center.

Peritoneal macrophages. Macrophages (resident macrophages) washed from the untreated peritoneal space, along with other cells normally present there, approach twice the diameter of the monocyte and have an oval or indented nucleus and a lightly granular cytoplasm. Rough endoplasmic reticulum also can be seen in electron micrographs of these cells. These cells adhere readily to surfaces over which they move by ameboid motion. Unstimulated, or resident, peritoneal macrophages are active phagocytes and cytodestructive to cells they ingest.

Irritation of the peritoneal cavity with suspensions of agar, starch, mineral oil, and the like stimulates the immigration of macrophages into the peritoneal cavity. The "stimulated" macrophages are basically the same as the resident macrophages. The activated macrophage represents the most motile, most actively phagocytic, most enzyme laden, and most cytocidal of the macrophages. It is known variously as the activated, armed, angry, or professional macrophage. It is a third-level cell, exceeding the monocytes and ordinary macrophages in activities associated with phagocytosis. Generation of activated macrophages relies on a message from antigen- or mitogen-exposed T cells.

Kupffer cells. Macrophages of the liver are represented by Kupffer cells. These cells attach to or embed themselves within the endothelial lining of the small blood vessels. Here they are ideally situated for clearance of foreign particles that enter the blood. Their cytoplasm, already granular because of its lysosome content, becomes even more uneven in appearance as engulfed particles in various states of decomposition reflect their phagocytic activity. These characteristics enable an easy identification of Kupffer cells despite variations in shape and size, which is usually in the range of 40 to 50 μm in diameter.

Alveolar macrophages. Alveolar or pulmonary macrophages are unique among their kind because they roam freely on the outer surface of the lung in a fully aerobic atmosphere where they are exposed to constant supply of inhaled phagocytosable particles. Somewhere between 3 million and 15 million of these cells are present in each gram of lung, depending on the animal species studied. The alveolar macrophage is 15 to 50 μm in diameter and contains many types of intracytoplasmic inclusions, some of which are lysosomes. These cells move over the alveolar surface scavenging dust particles, microorganisms, and other debris. Their aerobic metabolism and enzyme content indicate that these bone marrow–derived cells, like macrophages in other tissues, contribute significantly to body defenses and immunity.

Langerhans' cells. Langerhans, who first described the pancreatic islet cells that secrete insulin, also discovered cells in the epidermis, since named for him. These Langerhans cells represent 3% to 8% of the cells in the epidermis, or approximately 500 to 1,000 per square millimeter. In tissues Langerhans' cells are irregular, even branching in profile, are about twice the diameter of monocytes, and have a deeply indented nucleus. Rod-shaped granules are present in the cytoplasm and on electron microscopy are seen as laminated structures swollen at one end like a tennis racket. This granule is a reliable marker for Langerhans' cells. Langerhans' cells arise from the bone marrow and are distributed largely to the skin but are found at other sites: lymph nodes, tonsils, and mucous membrane, for example.

Langerhans' cells sequester and present antigen after its intradermal injection and are a prime source of haptens (dinitrochlorobenzene) that have been deposited on the skin. Exposure of the skin to ultraviolet light depletes it of Langerhans' cells, after which the provocation of contact dermatitis with haptens is virtually impossible.

Giant and epithelioid cells. Variants of giant cells may be seen in granulomas provoked by different irritants, but the typical giant cell is a polykaryon containing multiple nuclei. The number of nuclei present represents the number of macrophages that have fused to form the giant cell. These nuclei are typically 2 to 10 in number, but cells with 30 or more nuclei have been observed. These nuclei are arranged as a peripheral ring enclosing lysosomal granules, mitochondria, and other cellular substructures. Giant cells may be 100 μm or more in diameter and have numerous fine cytoplasmic processes extending from their surface with which they interdigitate with other cells.

Within human granulomas a secretory form of macrophage known as the epithelioid cell is often seen. Only phagocytosing macrophages become epithelioid cells; the inactive macrophages do not.

MACROPHAGE SURFACE MARKERS

The traditional means of identifying cells through their morphologic and staining characteristics loses its utility when cells to be categorized have aberrant features, or when cells as yet immature fail to express the features typical of their mature form. Some cells are so morphologically heterogeneous that their identity or developmental position cannot be determined precisely without recourse to techniques more subtle than microscopy.

Within the past decade, it has become apparent that antigenic proteins situated on the exterior surfaces of cells often provide a convenient marker for identifying these cells. Macrophages possess several such markers, the best known being the Ia proteins, the Mac 1 protein, the Fc receptor, and the CR3 receptor.

The Ia or immune-associated protein exists in two major forms, the I-A and I-E proteins with an infinite number of variations in the amino acid sequence of each. The I-A and I-E proteins are found on the surfaces of macrophages that cooperate with T lymphocytes in the immune response to TD antigens. The Ia marker is recognized by a receptor on the T lymphocyte that facilitates the needed cooperation between these cells. Ia proteins are also found on B lymphocytes. A third marker, the I-J characteristic, is present on macrophages that cooperate with suppressor T lymphocytes to diminish the immunoglobulin response. (The chemistry and genetic origin of these markers is described in Chapter 4.) Since there is a multitudinous number of TD antigens there must be a multitude of specificities in the I-A, I-E, and I-J characteristics.

Macrophages may also bear immunoglobulin molecules on their exterior surfaces. The antibody molecule is attached by noncovalent binding forces to the Fc receptor. In the order of 10^5 to 10^6 Fc receptors are present on a single macrophage. The Fc receptor is so named because the antibody molecule attaches to the macrophage via the structural portion designated Fc. The specificity of the Fc receptor is directed toward immunoglobulin G (IgG) and, since several subtypes of IgG exist, it is not entirely unexpected that mouse macrophages have separate Fc receptors for IgG1, IgG2a, IgG2b and IgG3.

Mac 1 is a protein antigen found on the surfaces of mouse monocytes and macrophages but not on B or T lymphocytes. A protein with a similar distribution on human cells has been designated the M1 marker. The Mac 1 protein is identical to the cell receptor (CR3) for several forms of the C3 molecule of the complement system that are produced during serologic reactions. Another interesting feature of the Mac 1-CR3 receptor protein is its structural relationship to two other surface glycoproteins, the leukocyte functional antigen (LFA), and a third protein designated only gp 150/95. Each of these three proteins consists of a noncovalently joined dimer of an α and a β peptide, the latter of which always has a molecular weight of 95,000 and is identical in each of the three molecules. The α chain of LFA has a molecular weight of 180,000, of Mac 1 a weight of 170,000, and of gp 150/95 a weight of 150,000. Whereas the distribution of Mac 1 and gp 159/95 is highly restricted to cells of the monocytic cell line plus a population of large granular lymphocytes (LGL) also known as natural killer (NK) cells, LFA is found on both these cells plus T lymphocytes and granulocytes. The function of LFA is to improve cell adhesion with other cells. Mac 1 binds C3b and improves phagocytosis via its opsonic property. The role of gp 150/95 is unknown. A deficiency of these proteins by virtue of a loss in synthetic ability for the β chain is characterized by recurrent bacterial infections.

An additional receptor for C3b and C4b of the complement system known as CR1 is found on macrophages. Because of the ubiquitous nature of the CR1 marker—it is found on granulocytes, B and T lymphocytes, and even erythrocytes—its function is uncertain and presumably differs on the different cell types. CR1 has a molecular weight of 25,000.

THE GRANULOCYTIC PHAGOCYTES
Neutrophils

The polymorphonuclear neutrophilic leukocytes (PMN) represent about 60% to 65% of the 5,000 to 10,000 circulating white blood cells in each cubic milliliter of blood. This amounts to about 3 to 6×10^3 PMNs per milliliter of blood. PMNs are easily recognized in stained blood smears by their multilobed nucleus composed most often of three lobes connected by thin strands of nuclear material. These cells are about 11 to 14 μm in diameter, or about twice the size of erythrocytes. The abundant cytoplasm is filled with small granules that do not stain intensely with either acidic or basic dyes (Fig. 5-5). The granules are seen as neutral-staining, violet-hued structures.

PMNs originate from the bone marrow through a series of mitotic divisions that begin with the myeloblasts, which are transformed first to promyelocytes and then to myelocytes. This conversion requires about a week and is followed by another week of postmitotic maturation. During this phase nuclear changes permit the recognition of the metamyelocyte, the band cell, and the mature neutrophil. These nucleated cells represent approximately two

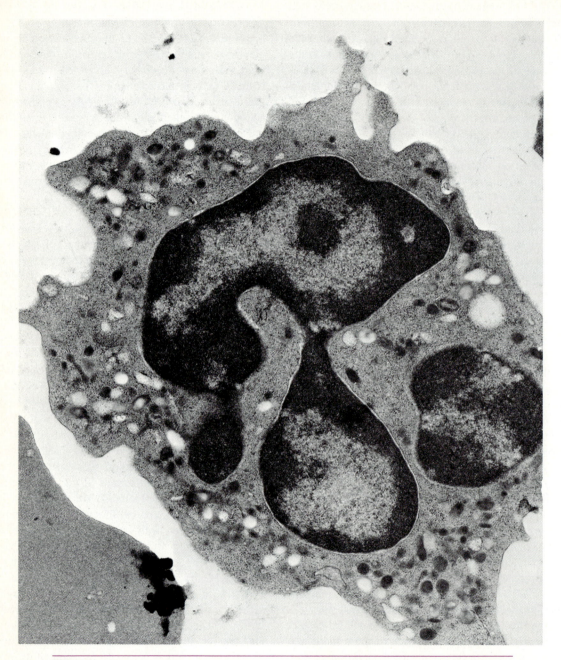

FIG. 5-5
Cytoplasmic granulation and a multilobulated nucleus are visible in this electron micrograph of a neutrophil. (Courtesy Dr. E. Adelstein.)

thirds of all nucleated cells in the bone marrow. More than 10^{11} neutrophils leave the bone marrow and enter the blood of a 70-kg individual each day. In the blood the neutrophils have a half-life of only 4 to 10 hours. Many cells are lost from the blood into urine, oral, and pulmonary secretions, the gastrointestinal tract, and tissues that they enter in response to inflammatory stimuli. By virtue of their ameboid motion, PMNs penetrate between the endothelial cells of the venules and collect in the inflammatory exudate, where they may live for an additional 1 or 2 days.

The granules in PMNs are of two different types. The primary granules are so named because they are the first recognized at the promyelocyte stage. These are also known as the azurophilic granules because they stain light blue with Wright's blood stain. These represent about one third of the granules in the mature neutrophil. Myeloperoxidase, neutral proteinases, lysozyme, acid hydrolases, β-glucuronidase, and several other classes of enzymes characteristic of lysosomes are found in these granules, in addition to the cationic protein. The secondary or specific granules become numerous during the promyelocyte-myelocyte stage and are characterized by their inclusion of lysozyme, neutral proteinases, and lactoferrin and by their lack of myeloperoxidase. During phagocytosis the granules of the neutrophil disappear (degranulation), and the enzymes stored within them are discharged.

Eosinophils

Acidophilic leukocytes also are called eosinophils because eosin, an acid dye used in staining blood smears, stains their granules intensely. Eosinophils represent about 3% of the circulating white blood cells, or 70 to 450/ml. These cells are about 10 to 15 μm in diameter. The eosinophil's nucleus is eccentrically located within the cytoplasm and is usually bilobed or ellipsoid.

The granules of eosinophils are unlike those of neutrophils. By light microscopy one notices the difference in their staining properties. By electron microscopy the larger granules can be seen to have a distinct crystalloid core composed largely of the major basic protein. This protein (with a molecular weight of about 6,000) is found as a cross-reactive antigen common to eosinophils of different animal species. Smaller granules lacking the crystalloid bar also are seen in eosinophils (Fig. 5-6).

Eosinophil granules contain many enzymes, including acid phosphatase, peroxidases, histaminase, aminopeptidase, ribonuclease, deoxyribonuclease, and proteinases.

Eosinophils possess ameboid motility and are phagocytic, but less so than neutrophils. Degranulation and oxidative metabolism are associated with phagocytosis, but these are less cytocidal than those of neutrophils.

Basophils

The basophils of human blood are 14 to 18 μm in diameter and are so named because their cytoplasm contains granules that are receptive to the basic dyes. Basophils constitute 1% or less of the white blood cells; there are perhaps 40 to 50 per cubic milliliter of human blood. The nucleus of basophils is not always well segmented and may be obscured by its numerous cytoplasmic granules (Fig. 5-7). The granules are 0.3 to 0.8 μm in diameter and round or oval in profile. On electron microscopy an indentation of the limiting membrane of the granules is noticeable. The inner structure of the granule is fine grained and consists of minute particles about 100 Å in diameter. These granules are very important because they are delicate structures whose outer membrane is easily disrupted. When granulolysis occurs, the contents of the granule are released into the surrounding tissue and bloodstream. Among the important contents of the granule are heparin and histamine. Heparin is a powerful anticoagulant, and histamine is a vasoactive amine that contracts smooth muscle. These products also are found in tissue mast cells. The histamine of blood basophils and mast cells contributes to the severity of the IgE-dependent allergies. Basophils are also important in basophilic cutaneous hypersensitivity reactions but have little or no phagocytic capacity.

COLONY STIMULATING FACTORS (CSF)

Stem cells of the monocyte-macrophage cell line, as well as those of granulocytic lineage, can be stimulated to proliferate and mature into their "adult" form upon exposure to proteins known as colony stimulating factors (CSF). These factors are produced

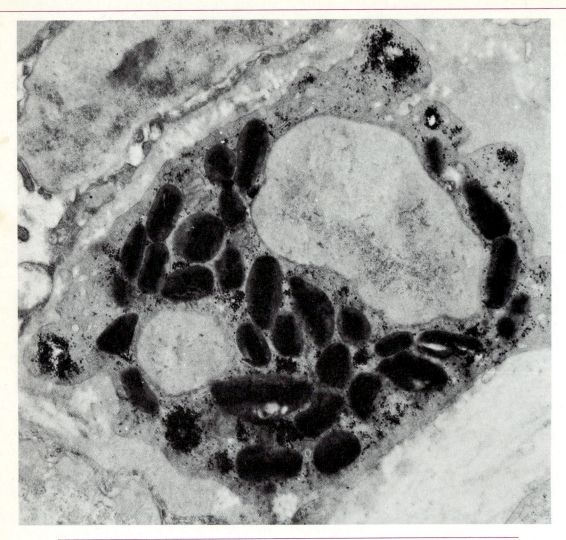

FIG. 5-6
Crystalloid bars can be seen by electron microscopy in many of the granules of this eosinophil.
(Courtesy Dr. E. Adelstein.)

by several cell types, including T lymphocytes, fibroblasts, macrophages, and epithelial cells. Stem-cell specificity is characteristic of some but not all CSFs (Table 5-1). The pluripotential multi-CSF acts upon precursor cells of both macrophages and granulocytes and may act on precursors of other blood cells. GM-CSF also stimulates granulocytes and macrophages whereas G-CSF and M-CSF are specific for granulocytes and monocytes as their designation indicates.

Despite the observation that three CSFs act on the monocytic lineage, it is clear that each is a unique chemical entity. Molecules with molecular weights between 19,000 and 30,000 contain multi-CSF activity and bind to a receptor with a molecular weight of 70,000 on early stem precursors to monocytes (and polymorphonuclear granulocytes) to force their appearance as adult cells. M-CSF has a molecular weight near 70,000 and attaches to a receptor of

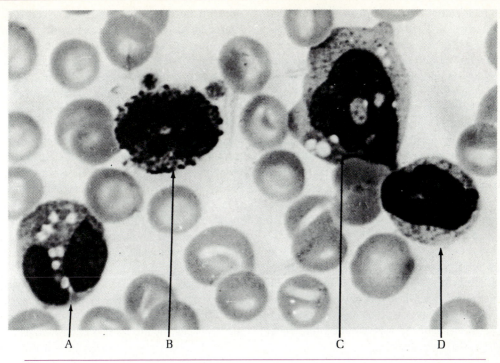

FIG. 5-7

The nucleated cells in this stained blood film illustrate their relative size and structure. *A*, Eosinophil; *B*, basophil; *C*, monocyte; *D*, lymphocyte. (Courtesy Dr. E. Adelstein.)

TABLE 5-1

Characteristics of the colony stimulating factors

	Molecular weight	Receptor size	pI	Source
Multi-CSF	19,000-30,000	70,000	—	T lymphocytes
M-CSF	70,000	150,000	3.7-4.9	Fibroblasts
GM-CSF	23,000	50,000	5	Macrophages, fibroblasts, etc.
G-CSF	25,000	150,000	—	Macrophages

150,000. M-CSF is electrophoretically heterogeneous and displays pI values ranging from 3.7 to 4.9. GM-CSF is the smallest of these three CSFs with a molecular weight near 23,000. It has a pI of 5 and binds to a receptor with a molecular weight of 50,000. Although fibroblasts are a source of M-CSF and GM-CSF, T lymphocytes are the best source of multi-CSF. Macrophages secrete G-CSF, a molecule whose molecular weight is 25,000 that uses a large receptor molecule of 150,000.

Although these four CSF differ from each other in important ways, there is evidence that each has a core size of about 13,000 to 15,000 that is modified by glycosylation and polymerization to achieve the sizes recorded.

ANTIGEN PROCESSING
History of phagocytosis

The Russian-born immunologist Metchnikoff is credited with the discovery of phagocytosis and clarifying the relationship of phagocytosis to natural immunity. Metchnikoff's theories evolved from his observation in 1882 that starfish larvae possessed a group of highly mobile ameboid cells that congregated at points of inflammation, which he induced by inserting thorns into the animals. He also observed that these cells would engulf carmine particles and immediately suspected that they might devour other types of particles, such as microbes, and digest them. This supposition was supported by his observations of an infectious disease in the transparent water flea of the genus *Daphnia,* caused by the yeast originally known as *Monospora bicuspidata.* The outcome of this disease was directly related to whether phagocytic cells of the flea could destroy the yeasts, as was the case when the yeast inoculum was kept small. Overpopulation by yeasts after large inoculations resulted in the death of the fleas. Metchnikoff quickly expanded his research to higher animals and found phagocytosis to be an effective natural defense mechanism; he was awarded the Nobel Prize in 1908 for these studies.

The phagocytic process

The ingestion and destruction of living cells by phagocytes is divisible into the separate stages of chemotaxis or attraction, attachment or opsonization, engulfment, intracellular killing, and digestion.

Chemotaxis

The first consideration in phagocytosis is how the phagocytic cell and the victim cell or particle make contact. This process requires little explanation if the victim cell is injected into the bloodstream, since immediate contact with the circulating granulocytes is possible. Moreover, as the blood passes through the internal organs, the fixed macrophages will have an opportunity to contact and engulf their prey. Because motile phagocytes do migrate toward bacteria and accumulate at inflammatory loci in tissues even if microorganisms are not present, it is thought that bacteria and injured tissue cells excrete chemoattractants for phagocytes. Such substances are called chemotaxins or leukotaxins.

Although some chemotaxins stimulate several different types of phagocytic cells, others act on only one or a few types of cells. This selectivity may be caused by the absence of receptors for the chemotaxin on the cell surface, failure of the chemotaxin to penetrate the cell surface, or other factors.

Two chemotaxins are generated from the complement system, a result of the combination of antigens with certain isotypes of IgG or with IgM, which then activates the complement system. A cleavage product of the fifth component of complement is chemotactic for macrophages, neutrophils, eosinophils, and basophils. This molecule, C5a, is an example of a chemotaxin derived from a chemotaxinogen, C5. C5a is a protein with a molecular weight of approximately 16,000 that consists of 77 amino acids in a linear sequence. Its amino terminal arginine is critical to the anaphylatoxic role of C5a but not to its chemotactic role.

The characteristics of a second chemotaxin originating in the complement system somewhere in the C5, C6, C7 complex are still vague. It is active on macrophages, neutrophils, and eosinophils. It is not C5a, but its chemistry has not been defined yet.

Although a substantial amount of scientific literature ascribes a chemotactic function to C3a, a peptide derived from the third component of complement, this conclusion is now believed to be in error. The similarities of C3a and C5a did not allow purification of C3a without trace contamination by C5a, which is now considered the cause of chemotactic activity in C3a preparations.

Tuftsin is the name assigned in 1974 to a tetrapeptide discovered by researchers at Tufts University that was chemotactic for both granulocytes and macrophages. Tuftsin is a tetrapeptide consisting of Thr-Lys-Pro-Arg derived from a unique globulin described as leukokinin. The amino acid sequence of tuftsin is found at or near residues 289 through 292 in the C_H3 portion of the crystallizable fragment (Fc) region of most γ-globulins. Tuftsin is released from globulins first by a cleavage at the carboxyl terminal side of the arginine, followed by hydrolysis of a lysine-threonine bond by the enzyme leukokininase present on the outer membrane of macrophages and neutrophils.

Receptors for tuftsin present on neutrophils and macrophages bind the chemotaxin prior to its internalization. It has been suggested this is the same as the receptor for LPS. Tuftsin not only stimulates phagocyte motility but also improves antigen processing and aids oxidative metabolism of the cells, thus making them more cytocidal.

Peptides of low molecular weight in which the amino group on an amino terminal methionine is formylated are also chemotactic for human, rabbit, and guinea pig granulocytes. Formyl Met-Leu-Phe and formyl Met-Met-Phe are examples of these substituted tripeptides. The presence of the formyl group is critical, since the unsubstituted peptides are not chemotactic. These molecules stimulate the secretion of lysosomal enzymes and oxidative metabolism within granulocytes, in addition to being chemotactic. The presence of the formyl Met residue at the amino terminal end of these peptides suggests that they are peptides or portions of proteins whose synthesis was interrupted, or that they are peptides that represent the first, possibly leader sequences, of proteins.

Mast cells that undergo degranulation during allergic reactions release the eosinophil-specific ECF-A (eosinophilic chemotactic factor of anaphylaxis). Two tetrapeptides, Val-Gly-Ser-Glu and Ala-Gly-Ser-Glu from mast cells, demonstrate ECF-A activity. These peptides exist preformed in mast-cell granules and are not synthesized just at the time of the allergic reaction. Because of their low molecular weight and amino acid structure, the ECF-A peptides are resistant to several proteases.

Fatty acids contained within the phospholipids of mammalian cell membranes are released by various stimuli. One of these fatty acids is a 20-carbon acid with four unsaturated bonds, that is, an eicosatetraenoic acid, better known by its common name, arachidonic acid. Arachidonic acid is further metabolized by two separate pathways (Fig. 5-8). In the lipoxygenase pathway hydroxyl groups are added to form the hydroxyeicosatetraenoic (HETE) acids. Of these, the 12 hydroxy and 5 hydroxy (12-HETE and 5-HETE) are powerful chemotaxins for granulocytes. The leukotrienes in the B series are also chemotactic. (Leukotrienes [LT] C, D, and E are anaphylatoxic. See Chapter 18.) In the cyclooxygenase pathway both oxidative and cyclization reac-

tions occur to produce the prostaglandins (PG), thromboxanes, and related compounds. Thromboxane B_2 and hydroxyheptatrienoic acid (HHT) both are derived from platelets, and both are chemotactic for neutrophils and eosinophils.

Antigen or mitogen stimulation of T lymphocytes causes them to release a chemotaxin that is active on macrophages. This chemotaxin has the electrophoretic mobility of an albumin and a molecular weight between 35,000 and 55,000. These characteristics separate this chemotaxin from lymphocyte-derived chemotactic factor (LDCF), which may be produced by either B or T lymphocytes and has a molecular weight of only 12,500. Another T cell-derived chemotaxin is also a low molecular weight (about 25,000 to 50,000) protein and is referred to as ECF-L, since it is an eosinophilic chemotactic factor from lymphocytes.

Many bacteria produce chemotaxins during growth in culture or during infection. Several different capsular serotypes of *Streptococcus pneumoniae* produce a chemotaxin with a molecular weight of about 3,600. Unrelated bacteria such as those in the genus *Proteus* apparently produce the same leukotaxin. This substance obviously is not related to the capsular antigens of the diplococcus, which have long been accorded a negative or antichemotactic activity. *Staphylococcus aureus* produces a molecule whose molecular weight is less than 10,000, that is chemotactic.

A wide array of other compounds are also chemotactic. These include fibrin, collagen, lysosomal enzymes, kallikreins (proteases), bacterial endotoxin (LPS), and plasminogen activator.

BIOCHEMICAL MECHANISMS IN CHEMOTAXIS

The biochemical events that stimulate motility and aggression in macrophages have come under intense scrutiny but are still incompletely understood. These events are divisible into two parts, the messenger system and the contractile system.

In its messenger role, the chemotactic receptor is thought to be modulated by a nucleotide regulatory protein and guanosine triphosphate (Fig. 5-9). Binding of this receptor with the chemotaxin activates en-

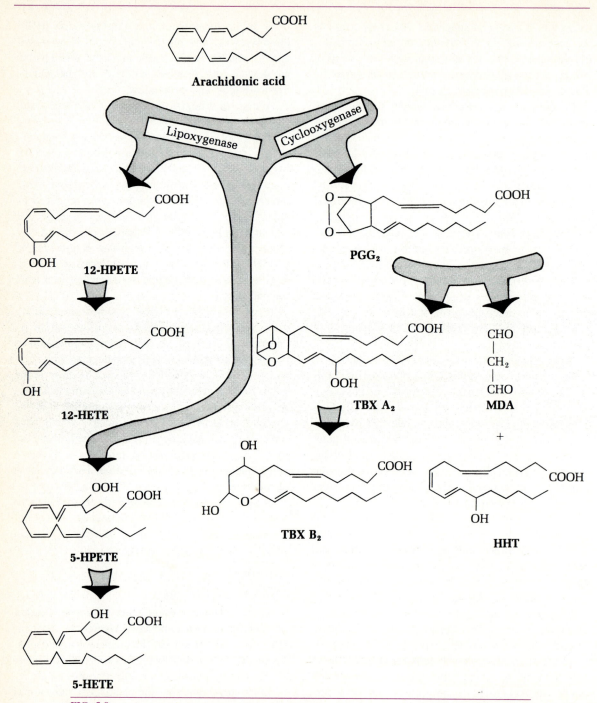

FIG. 5-8

In the metabolism of arachidonic acid by the lipoxygenase pathway two chemotaxins *(5-* and *12-HETE)* are produced. By the cyclooxygenase pathway, thromboxane B₂*(TBX B₂)* and HHT are the chemotaxins produced.

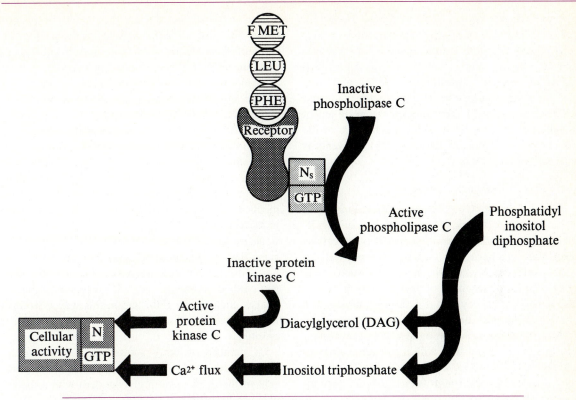

FIG. 5-9

One model for the transmission of the chemoattractant signal theorizes that the receptor, in this case for tuftsin, is anchored to a nucleotide regulatory protein, N, that is in its resting or stable state. The N protein then associates with guanine triphosphate (GTP) rather than the diphosphate normally present at rest. The stabilized N_S, GTP complex activates phospholipase C. This enzyme degrades phosphatidyl inositol diphosphate to diacylglycerol and inositol triphosphate. The former activates protein kinase C and the latter promotes a calcium flux into the cell. These, possibly through the N protein, and GTP catalyze further intracellular events that initiate cell motility.

zymes that convert guanine from its diphosphate form to its triphosphate form and also stimulate transmethylation reactions. Subsequently, phospholipase C is activated and inositol triphosphate and diacylglycerol (DAG) are liberated from cell-membrane lipids by the action of this enzyme. These compounds mobilize intracellular Ca^{2+} and activate protein kinase C. Through the phosphorylation of proteins by protein kinase C and other unknown events directional cell motility, increased oxygen consumption, and increased synthesis of lysosomal enzymes are initiated.

Certain but not all portions of the contractile sys-

tem, the system that provides the cytoskeleton for cell locomotion, are understood. The flux of Ca^{2+} into the cell plus the mobilization of Ca^{2+} from intracellular stores are the key features of this process since calcium is required for the conversion of actin from its monomeric globular form into its filamentous form. Actin is a protein of 42,000 molecular weight that accounts for 10% of the cytoplasmic protein of macrophages where it exists largely in its gel (G) or monomeric form. A role for myosin is suspected in the conversion of G actin into its filamentous (F) form. The actin filaments may then be drawn into contact with gelsolin, a calcium-sensitive protein that cuts actin filaments. Thus, there is a conversion of globular actin to filamentous actin, cell motility over the cytoskeleton, actin cleavage, and the renewed conversion of G to F actin. Two regulatory proteins—profilin and acumentin—are also involved. Acumentin stabilizes actin filaments, whereas profilin prevents actin monomer-filament transitions. It is clear that a delicate balance in the timing and magnitude of these agents and events is required for cell locomotion.

Attachment and opsonization

Contact between the phagocytic cell and its victim is not always sufficient to cause phagocytic engulfment; some intended victims escape. If phagocytosis takes place in a fibrin clot, on a blood vessel wall, or on another surface where the ameboid motion of the phagocyte favors recontact of the two cells, escape is less possible. Phagocytosis is a surface phenomenon and is much less efficient in a fluid medium.

Molecular factors that promote attachment of phagocytes and the object they will engulf are called opsonins (from the Greek word that means *to prepare for eating*). The earlier term *bacteriotropin,* once almost synonymous with opsonin, is outdated.

The most potent opsonins are immunoglobulins, which can be considered from two viewpoints. The immunoglobulins that bind to the surfaces of neutrophils, macrophages, and eosinophils are predominantly IgG1 and IgG3. These cytophilic antibodies, when possessed with specificity for an engulfable antigen (such as bacteria, yeast, virus, and erythrocyte), bind its exposed antigenic determinants and hold the antigen only one molecule in length from the phagocyte surface. This binding is possible because the Fc portions of IgG1 and IgG3 are the parts held to the phagocyte, leaving the immunoglobulin's antigen-binding fragments (Fab) free to attach to antigen.

Humoral antibodies that attach to bacteria encourage phagocytosis by neutralizing ionic charges on the bacterial cell surface; thus, they are more approachable by the phagocyte. The negative chemotactic force of encapsulated bacteria such as the pneumococcus, *Klebsiella pneumoniae,* and *Hemophilus influenzae* clearly is related to their capsule; nonencapsulated variants are easy prey for phagocytic cells. But when the capsules of the pathogenic form of these bacteria are coated with antibodies, they are no longer able to repel phagocytes and are as easily engulfed as the nonencapsulated forms.

The opsonic activity of circulating antibodies is caused largely by IgG and IgM, the latter being about 500- to 1,000-fold more potent than the former in stimulating phagocytosis of bacteria. This potency may reflect only the tendency of polysaccharide capsular and somatic antigens to favor IgM formation, since gram-negative bacteria and encapsulated pneumococci often were used as the phagocytic subjects in these studies.

When complement component C3 is split to release the anaphylatoxin C3a during serologic reactions, the residue C3b remains attached to the antigen-antibody complex. The CR3 receptor on macrophages engages the C3b, and in this way C3b links the phagocytic cell with its victim as an important opsonin.

A number of other substances have been described as opsonins. Fibronectin, one of the most recent of these, is a serum glycoprotein with a molecular weight of about 200,000 to 250,000. Fibronectin can exist also in a dimeric form. Macrophages synthesize fibronectin, and this is believed to aid their phagocytosis. When serum levels of fibronectin fall, after surgery or burns, phagocytic activity falls. Many other proteins, when added to simple buffers used to study phagocytosis in vitro, will stimulate phagocytosis and could be described as opsonins, although their activity is far below that of the molecules previously described.

Engulfment

Exactly how the phagocytosed particle is taken into the cell without rupturing the cytoplasmic membrane of the phagocyte continues to be a mystery. The phagocyte cell cytoplasm apparently flows completely around the engulfed cell and fuses with itself. The victim cell is held inside this phagocytic vesicle, or phagosome, which is surrounded by an everted cell membrane cover. This phagosome is displaced centrally, and contact with cytoplasmic lysosomal granules occurs. Fusion of the lysosome and phagosome follows, and the lysosome disintegrates, releasing a multitude of hydrolytic enzymes into what is now referred to as the phagolysosome.

Intracellular killing

The original concept that hydrolytic enzymes released from lysosomes were responsible for the cytocidal events within phagocytes now has been abandoned. Instead attention has been directed at oxygen-dependent and oxygen-independent avenues for cell death, with the former being the most fully explored.

Oxygen-dependent reactions

The resting phagocyte, with the exception of the alveolar macrophage, uses anaerobic glycolysis as its major energy source. In this pathway of carbohydrate metabolism sugars are converted to lactic acid, and no oxygen is consumed. During and after the phagocytic act the phagocytes begin to consume oxygen as they shift their pathway of carbohydrate metabolism to the greater energy-yielding hexose monophosphate (HMP) shunt (Fig. 5-10). Phagocytes may increase their rate of oxygen consumption 100-fold when challenged to engage in phagocytosis.

Associated with this pathway is the enzyme nicotinamide-adenine dinucleotide phosphate (NADPH) oxidase. This enzyme may be physically associated with receptors for chemoattractants, immune complexes, lectins, and adjuvants that stimulate the oxidative pathway of oxygen metabolism in phagocytes. NADPH oxidase reduces normal oxygen O_2 to the superoxide radical $\cdot O_2^-$ through the addition of one electron, e.g., $\cdot \ddot{O}{:}\ddot{O} \cdot$ is converted to $:\ddot{O}{:}\ddot{O}\cdot$. Since the superoxide ion has an unpaired electron it is highly reactive and carries a negative charge. The superoxide anion is itself only weakly toxic but it is very easily converted to more lethal reagents. The enzyme superoxide dismutase (SOD) scavenges the superoxide radical and through the addition of hydrogen protons produces hydrogen peroxide (H_2O_2) and single oxygen ($^1O_2$). This reaction is written:

$$\cdot O_2^- + \cdot O_2^- + 2H^+ \xrightarrow{\text{SOD}} H_2O_2 + {}^1O_2$$

The position of the electrons in hydrogen peroxide is $H{:}\ddot{O}{:}\ddot{O}{:}H$ so that each oxygen atom has a complete

electron shell. Singlet oxygen has the same number of electrons as normal oxygen, but the unpaired electrons rotate in opposite directions to each other $\downarrow\cdot\ddot{O}{:}\ddot{O}\cdot\downarrow$. When singlet oxygen returns to ground state or normal oxygen, light is emitted. This chemiluminescence is detectable in scintillation counters during phagocytosis. Certain dyes and carotenoid pigments will absorb this energy and quench the luminescence. It is interesting that microorganisms that contain a high concentration of carotenoid pigments are more resistant to intraphagocytic death than cells deficient in these pigments.

Hydrogen peroxide has long been considered a bactericidal agent but the evidence is not always convincing, since many aerobic and facultative bacteria rapidly decompose H_2O_2 by means of catalases and peroxidases. These enzymes are also present in macrophages and protect these cells against whatever toxic activity H_2O_2 may possess.

Conversion of hydrogen peroxide to the hypochlorite ion through the agency of the enzyme myeloperoxidase (MPO) may be a more likely explanation of its role within macrophage. This reaction is:

$$H_2O_2 + Cl^- \xrightarrow{\text{MPO}} H_2O + OCl^-$$

MPO is present in the primary or azidophilic granules of phagocytes where it can represent as much as 5% of the cell weight. During phagocytosis, MPO is released into the phagolysosome and adheres to the bacterial surface. Radioactive iodine substituted for chlorine in the above MPO reaction is found on dead bacteria recovered from phagocytes, good evidence for a toxic role of the hypochlorite ion and MPO.

One other toxic form of oxygen is produced within phagocytes when hydrogen peroxide reacts with the superoxide radical in the presence of iron. The products are oxygen, hydroxyl ions, and the hydroxyl radical ($\cdot OH$).

$$\cdot O_2^- + H_2O_2 \rightarrow O_2 + OH^- + \cdot OH$$

The hydroxyl radical is a one electron–reduction product of hydrogen peroxide and is the most potent oxidizing agent produced in biologic systems. Thus it is considered an important contributor to intraphagocytic killing.

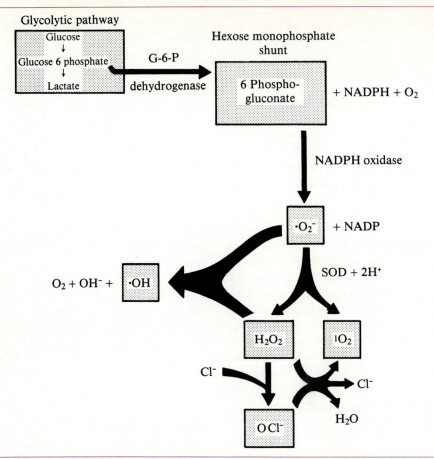

FIG. 5-10

Cytotoxic forms of oxygen arise from the hexose monophosphate, aerobic pathway for carbohydrate metabolism, which replaces the glycolytic pathway used by the resting cell. Nicotinamide dinucleotide phosphate oxidase generates the superoxide ion from which four other potent oxidizing agents, the hydroxyl radical ($\cdot OH$), singlet oxygen ($^1O_2$), hydrogen peroxide (H_2O_2), and hypochlorite ion ($OCl-$) are produced.

Oxygen-independent reactions

The intracellular accumulation of lactic acid and the lowering of the pH to about 4.5 within the phagosome create a definite bacteriostatic if not bactericidal pH. The enzyme lysozyme that can hydrolyze the cell wall of gram-positive bacteria is present within phagocytic cells. Cationic proteins within these cells may bind to the surface of microorganisms, most of which are negatively charged, and interfere with cell transport functions. Transferrin that is contained within phagocytes and lactoferrin bind iron and remove it from the nutrient supply of microbes, thus preventing their growth.

Intracellular digestion

Nonviable antigens within phagocytes are quickly digested within the phagolysosome. Viable cellular antigens are digested after their death from exposure to toxic forms of oxygen and the oxygen-independent pathways. Many living microbes are resistant to lysosomal enzymes and become sensitive to them only after cell death.

CITATION CLASSIC

Klebanoff S. J.

Antimicrobial mechanisms in neutrophilic polymorphonuclear leukocytes.
Semin. Hematol. **12:**117-42, 1975.   [Dept. Medicine, Univ. Washington Sch. Med., Seattle, WA]

The antimicrobial systems of neutrophils are divided into those dependent on oxygen and those which are not. The former include the myeloperoxidase-H_2O_2-halide system and highly reactive oxygen radicals, and the latter include granule cationic proteins, lysozyme, lactoferrin, and possibly a fall in intraphagosomal pH. [The SCI® indicates that this paper has been cited in over 355 publications since 1975.]

Seymour J. Klebanoff
Department of Medicine
School of Medicine
University of Washington
Seattle, WA 98195

August 23, 1982

"From 1957 to 1962, I was at Rockefeller University, an endocrinologist by trade and a thyroidologist by research interest. I had two projects under way with a graduate student, Cecil Yip, both involving peroxidases. One dealt with the mechanism of action of the thyroid hormones; thyroxine by virtue of its phenolic hydroxyl group was found to greatly stimulate reactions catalyzed by peroxidase.[1] The second project dealt with the biosynthesis of thyroxine, a reaction which required a thyroid peroxidase to iodinate the tyrosine residues of thyroglobulin.[2] This interest in peroxidases and their role in the mechanism of thyroxine action prompted a search for biologically important peroxidases which could be stimulated by thyroxine. Granulocytes are rich in peroxidase. We purified this enzyme (myeloperoxidase) and found that it, like horseradish peroxidase, was stimulated by thyroxine and, like thyroid peroxidase, iodinated proteins. Another peroxidase, lactoperoxidase, present in milk and saliva, was purified and found to react similarly.

"At the same time that this work was going on, Zanvil Cohn and James Hirsch at Rockefeller University had characterized the cytoplasmic granules of rabbit granulocytes[3] and demonstrated the release of their contents into the phagosome as a prelude to the death of the ingested organisms. I therefore approached Hirsch with a tube of green myeloperoxidase and a proposal that we determine if this granule enzyme could kill bacteria. If so, this biological action of a peroxidase might be stimulated by thyroxine. We found that myeloperoxidase was ineffective alone or when combined with H_2O_2. It was, however, known from thyroxine synthesis that peroxidase and H_2O_2 oxidize iodide to iodine, a well-known germicidal agent. So we added iodide; the solution turned light yellow and the bacteria were killed, all according to expectation. However, the key experiment, the stimulation of this reaction by thyroxine, was negative. We lost interest.

"The next several years were spent at the University of Washington on other things until I was made aware by Ray Luebke, an endodontics trainee; of an incompletely understood antimicrobial system in saliva, which required a heat-stable dialyzable component (thiocyanate ions) and an unknown heat-labile nondialyzable component. We demonstrated that the latter was salivary peroxidase and that H_2O_2 was an additional requirement.[4] This rekindled an interest in the antimicrobial properties of myeloperoxidase, which was found to have potent antimicrobial activity when combined with H_2O_2 and a halide (iodide, bromide, chloride). Evidence was found implicating this as one of the antimicrobial systems of phagocytes. Unfortunately, we were unable to come full circle and demonstrated a stimulation of this peroxidase-dependent reaction by thyroxine. Over the years these studies have been punctuated by reviews of the antimicrobial systems of phagocytes. The paper indicated here is one of these, and has been highly cited as it appeared at a time of exploding interest in the role of oxygen metabolites in the cytocidal mechanisms of phagocytes (see reference five for a more recent review of this area)."

1. Klebanoff S J. An effect of thyroxine and related compounds on the oxidation of certain hydrogen donors by the peroxidase system. *J. Biol. Chem.* **234:**2437-42, 1959.
2. Klebanoff S J, Yip C & Kessler D. The iodination of tyrosine by beef thyroid preparations. *Biochim. Biophys. Acta.* **58:**563-74, 1962.
3. Cohn Z A & Hirsch J G. The isolation and properties of the specific cytoplasmic granules of rabbit polymorphonuclear leucocytes. *J. Exp. Med.* **112:**983-1004, 1960.
4. Klebanoff S J & Luebke R G. The antilactobacillus system of saliva. Role of salivary peroxidase. *Proc. Soc. Exp. Biol. Med.* **118:**483-6, 1965.
5. Klebanoff S J. Oxygen-dependent cytotoxic mechanisms of phagocytes. (Gallin J I & Fauci A S, eds.) *Advances in host defense mechanisms.* New York: Plenum Press, 1982. Vol. 1. p. 111-62.

Lysosomes contain a vast array of hydrolytic enzymes, including those that are active on proteins, polysaccharides, nucleic acids, lipids, and other biopolymers. Among these enzymes and substances are β-acetylglucosamine hydrolase, acid phosphatase, acid ribonuclease, acid deoxyribonuclease, arylsulfatase, cathepsin, collagenase, cytochrome c reductase, elastase, esterases, β-galactosidase, α-glucosidase, β-glucuronidase, hyaluronidase, lipase, lysozyme, α-mannosidase, neuraminidase, and phagocytin.

These enzymes ultimately digest the phagolysosomal contents until they are unrecognizable debris (Fig. 5-11). These residual bodies at different stages of digestion are seen within active phagocytes. Meanwhile the phagocyte regenerates its lysosomes in preparation for the next phagocytic event.

Antigen presentation

Although several types of phagocytic cells may be instrumental in the degradation of antigens, it is quite probable that only cells of the mononuclear system can be considered antigen-processing cells. Extracts of these cells prepared during their attack on antigens yield a highly potent form of antigen, sometimes referred to as a super antigen. The forces that direct the elimination of the nonessential portions of an antigen coupled with a sparing of the antigen's epitopes are unknown.

Just as all phagocytes are not antigen-processing cells, neither are all macrophages antigen-presenting cells. Only macrophages with the I-A or I-E protein on their surface can cooperate with T_H cells in the immune response. Since the structure of these Ia proteins is regulated by genes present in the MHC, the immune response is genetically restricted at the MHC level. The T cells and antigen-presenting macrophages must be of the same genetic background.

Dendritic cells

A more recently described second cell type—the dendritic cell—is also capable of antigen presentation. Dendritic cells are highly pleomorphic with a central cell body of 6 μ to 12 μ from which six to ten needlelike processes, each 10 to as much as 50 μ in length radiate. Thus, the dendrite body can achieve a total diameter of 100 μ but this is uncommon, 50 μ is a more representative figure. Dendritic cells are found in germinal areas of lymphoid tissues, particularly spleen and lymph nodes. It is believed these cells are responsible for the long-term retention of antigen in follicles.

The dendritic cells, so easily distinguished from macrophages morphologically, can also be separated from them by a number of other features. Dendritic cells are not phagocytic, the antigen present on their surface appears to be in a complex with antibody. Fc receptors on the dendritic cell surface may thus be responsible for its ability to bind and then present antigen. Dendritic cells are Ia^+, Mac 1^- but Den 1^+. Den 1 refers to a protein unique to dendritic cells. Dendritic cells do have complement receptors.

As mentioned above, Langerhan's cells in the skin have a morphology very similar to that of dendritic cells. These cells have both Fc receptors and Ia proteins on their surfaces and are believed to be antigen-presenting cells.

The stimulation of T lymphocytes by antigen has often been described as requiring two signals. The first of these is clearly the transmission of the antigen in the context of the Ia protein. Increasing evidence that a single receptor on T cells simultaneously recognizes the antigen and Ia protein emphasizes that this pair of proteins behaves as the first signal.

Interleukin 1

The second signal is interleukin 1. Interleukin 1 (IL-1) is the first of several hormonelike substances to participate in the immune response. Since IL-1 is produced by one type of white blood cell and is active on a second type of white blood cell, the term interleukin is appropriate. Since IL-1 functions with antigen to stimulate T lymphocytes, the term lymphokine is equally appropriate.

Although macrophages and dendritic cells are important sources of IL-1, keratinocytes and other cells may produce IL-1. Antigens, lectins, lymphokines from T cells (macrophage activating factor) and agents that perturb the macrophage cell membrane (LPS, phorbol myristate acetate, muramyl dipeptide, latex particles) stimulate IL-1 secretion. IL-1 is a protein of about 15,000 molecular weight that easily aggregates to form larger polymers. Human and murine IL-1 may be a collection of molecules because

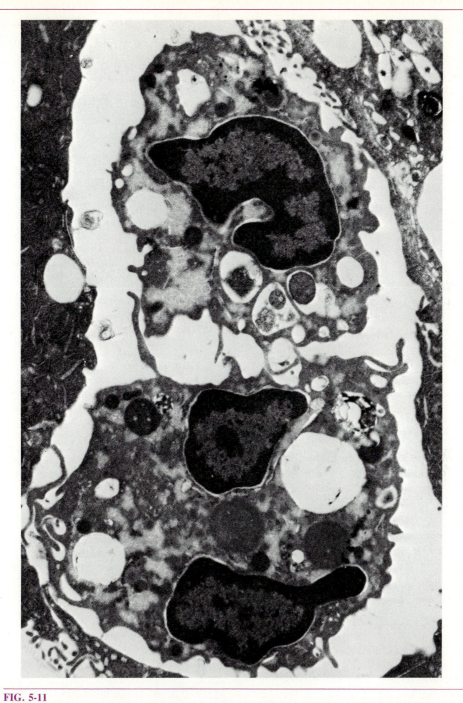

FIG. 5-11

These two neutrophils seen in an electron microscopic photograph have depleted their cytoplasmic granules during phagocytosis. The upper cell contains bacteria at different levels of destruction in the phagolysosomes just below its nucleus.

several variants with different isoelectric points have been recognized. Multiple copies of DNA that code for IL-1 have also been identified. Although IL-1 induces fever (it is the endogenous pyrogen) and stimulates an increase in acute-phase serum proteins, its most important role appears to be in the immune system where it augments T lymphocyte proliferation and activation. By this means, it is instrumental in immunoglobulin production.

Macrophages as secretory cells

In addition to IL-1, macrophages synthesize and secrete a large number of other substances with great biologic significance. The several cytotoxic forms of oxygen and the numerous lysosomal enzymes have already been mentioned. To this must be added a second lymphokine, interferon, complement molecules 1, 2, 3, 4, and 5, properdin, factors B and D; fibronectin, prostaglandins, coagulation factors, $\alpha 2$ macroglobulin, plasminogen activator, erythropoietin, and the colony-stimulating factors.

REFERENCES

Adams, D., Edelson, P., and Koren, H., editors: Methods for studying mononuclear phagocytes, Orlando, 1981, Academic Press, Inc.

Bellanti, J.A., and Herscowitz, H.B., editors: The reticuloendothelial system, vol. 6, Immunology, New York, 1984, Plenum Publishing Corp.

Butterfield, J.H., Maddox, D.E., and Gleich, G.J.: The eosinophil leukocyte: maturation and function, Clin. Immunol. Revs. 2:187, 1983-1984.

Chestnut, R.W., and Grey, H.M.: Antigen presenting cells and mechanisms of antigen presentation, CRC Crit. Rev. Immunol. 5:263, 1985.

Dinarello, C.A.: Interleukin-1 and the pathogenesis of the acute-phase response, N. Engl. J. Med. 311:1413, 1984.

Dougherty, G.J.: Macrophage heterogeneity, J. Clin. Lab. Immunol. 14:1, 1984.

Durum, S.K., Schmidt, J.A., and Oppenheim, J.J.: Interleukin 1: an immunological perspective, Ann. Rev. Immunol. 3:263, 1985.

Gallin, J.I.: Neutrophil specific granule deficiency, Ann. Rev. Med. 36:263, 1985.

Gleich, G.J.and Loegering, D.A.: Immunobiology of eosinophils, Ann. Rev. Immunol. 2:429, 1984.

Goldstein, E.: Hydrolytic enzymes of alveolar macrophages, Rev. Infect. Dis. 5:1078, 1983.

Goldstein, I.M.: Neutrophil degranulation, Contemp. Top. Immunobiol. 14:189, 1984.

Goodwin, J.S., editor: Prostaglandins and immunity, Boston, 1985, Martinus Nijhoff Publishing.

Griffin, F.M., Jr.: Activation of macrophage complement receptors for phagocytosis, Contemp. Top. Immunobiol. 13:57, 1984.

Kay, A.B.: Eosinophils as effector cells in immunity and hypersensitivity disorders: a review, Clin. and Exp. Immunol. 62:1, 1985.

Keller, H.U., and Till, G.O., editors: Leukocyte locomotion and chemotaxis, Basel, 1983, Birkhäuser Verlag Basel.

Kluger, M.J., Oppenheim, J.J., and Powander, M.C., editors: The physiologic, metabolic, and immunologic actions of interleukin-1, New York, 1985, Liss.

Lipsky, P.E.: Role of interleukin-1 in human B-cell activation, Contemp. Top. Molec. Immunol. 10:195, 1985.

Mosser, D.M., and Edelson, P.J.: Mechanisms of microbial entry and endocytosis by mononuclear phagocytes, Contemp. Top. Immunobiol. 13:71, 1984.

Najjar, V.A., and Fridkin, M., editors: Antineoplastic, immunogenic and other effects of the tetrapeptide tuftsin: a natural macrophage activator, Ann. N.Y. Acad. Sci. 419:1-273, 1983.

Pastan, I., and Willingham, M.C., editors: Endocytosis, New York, 1985, Plenum Publishing Corp.

Poulter, L.W.: Antigen presenting cells in situ: their identification and involvement in immunopathology, Clin. Exp. Immunol. 53:513, 1983.

Snyderman, R., and Pike, M.C.: Transductional mechanisms of chemoattractant receptors on leukocytes, Contemp. Top. Immunobiol. 14:1, 1984.

Spitznagel, J.K.: Nonoxidative antimicrobial reactions of leukocytes, Contemp. Top. Immunobiol. 14:283, 1984.

Steinman, R., and Nussenzweig, M.: Dendritic cells: features and functions, Immunol. Revs. 53:127, 1983.

Streilein, J.W., and Bergstresser, P.R.: Langerhans cells: antigen-presenting cells of the epidermis, Immunobiol. 168:285, 1984.

Unkeless, J.C., and Wright, D.D.: Structure and modulation of Fc and complement receptors, Contemp. Top. Immunobiol. 14:171, 1984.

vanFurth, R., editor: Mononuclear phagocytes, characteristics, physiology, and function, Dordrecht, 1985, Martinus Nijhoff Publishers.

Volkman, A., editor: Mononuclear phagocyte biology, New York, 1984, Marcel Dekker, Inc.

Wilkinson, P.C.: Chemotaxis and inflammation, edition 2, Edinburgh, 1982, Churchill Livingstone.

Wilkinson, P.C.: The measurement of chemotaxis, J. Immunol. Meth. 51:133, 1982.

Yoshida, T., and Torisu, M., editors: Immunobiology of the eosinophil, Amsterdam, 1983, Elsevier Biomedical Press.

See related **Reading 1,** page 411.

The B lymphocytes

≣ GLOSSARY

ADCC   Antibody-dependent cell cytotoxicity.

B cell   A lymphocyte that matures in the bursa of Fabricius or its mammalian equivalent.

B cell differentiation factor (BCDF)   A lymphokine derived from T cells needed for the transformation of B cells to plasma cells.

B cell growth factor (BCGF)   A lymphokine derived from T cells needed for B cell proliferation.

bursa of Fabricius   A cloacal organ in fowl where the immunoglobulin-producing B cells mature.

capping phenomenon   The movement of dispersed antigens on the surface of the B cell to a single locus.

central lymphoid tissue   Bone marrow, thymus, and bursa of Fabricius.

GALT   Gut-associated lymphoid tissue.

LAK   A lymphokine-activated cell.

LGL   Large granular lymphocyte, active in target-cell killing.

lymphocyte   An agranular leukocyte with a sparse cytoplasmic rim surrounding a rounded nucleus.

NK cell   Probably a synonym or subgroup of LGL cells.

perforins   A group of cytolytic proteins produced by LGL cells.

plasma cell   The end cell of B cell differentiation that is an active immunoglobulin-synthesizing cell.

T cell   A lymphocyte that matures in the thymus.

thymus   A gland situated near the thyroid in which T cells mature.

THE LYMPHOID SYSTEM

The lymphocyte is the dominant cell of the lymphoid system, which is generally discussed in terms of the central and peripheral lymphoid tissues. The two central lymphoid tissues of mammals are bone marrow and thymus. Lymph nodes, spleen, tonsil, intestinal lymphoid tissue (Peyer's patches), and other collections of lymphocytes constitute the peripheral lymphoid tissues. In addition to marrow and thymus, fowl have a third central lymphoid organ, the bursa of Fabricius, which is critical to the development of immunoglobulin-producing cells.

The central lymphoid organs
Bone marrow

The structure of bone marrow is described in the section on hematopoietic tissue in Chapter 5. The bone marrow contains precursor stem cells of the lymphocytes that later mature in the thymus or bursa. These prolymphocytes enter the blood and "home in on" the tissue required for their maturation.

Thymus

The human thymus is a flat, bilobed organ situated below the thyroid gland along the neck and extending into the thoracic cage. In the mouse it is also bilobate and lies over the heart (Fig. 6-1). In some species the thymus tissue is distributed along the neck and thorax in several small lobules. In the chicken and other fowl the thymus is a multilobed structure rarely extending into the thoracic cavity and usually lying along the neck (Fig. 6-2). Likewise the guinea pig thymus is basically extrathoracic, but it exists as a single major lobe. The thymus emerges from the third and fourth branchial pouches during embryonic development and is a fully developed organ at birth. At this time the human thymus will weigh 15 to 20 g. By puberty it will reach 40 g, after which it will atrophy, becom-

ing less significant structurally and functionally. Atrophy of the thymus with age is a characteristic of all species.

Anatomically the thymus may be considered as a pouch of epithelial cells filled with lymphocytes (the thymic, or T, lymphocytes), nourished and drained by the vascular and lymphatic systems. The epithelial cells and other structural cells divide the thymus into a complex assembly of continuous lobes, each of which is heavily laden with thymocytes. The lymphocyte population is greatest in the cortex, or outer portion, of each lobule, whereas the inner section, the medulla, is relatively free of these important cells. The cortical thymocytes are

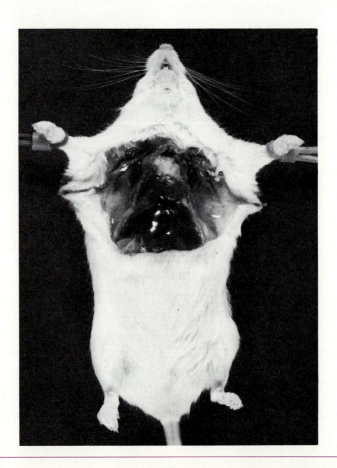

FIG. 6-1

The mouse thymus is the light-colored tissue that lies directly over the heart. The bilobed nature of the mouse thymus is not easily seen here, since the left lobe is lying over the right lobe. (Courtesy T. Ellis.)

not as mature as those that have moved to the medulla. The medullary portion is continuous from one lobe to another, and, in addition to its content of vascular structures, reticulum cells, and lymphocytes, it is the most common site for Hassall's corpuscles. These are concentric, cellular structures that stain lightly and have as yet no functional identity; however, they are a histologic hallmark of thymus tissue.

The thymic cortex, between the septa, is rich in lymphocytes of all sizes. These thymocytes are not morphologically distinguishable from lymphocytes in other tissues, but they are antigenically identifiable by the presence of the Thy 1 antigen, a distinctive surface marker antigen that separates them from B lymphocytes.

The nude mouse

The nude mouse is a hairless mouse with the combined genetic fault of an inability to grow hair and to develop a thymus (Fig. 6-3). In 1968 this strain of mouse was observed to produce paired thymus sacs in the normal anatomic position, but the glands were devoid of lymphocytes. Thymus grafts into nude mice will restore the normal T cell population, and it has been determined that these are of nude mouse, not donor mouse, origin. Bone marrow grafts from nude mice to normal mice that have had the thymus irradiated will repopulate the recipient with T cells. These experiments indicate there is no stem-cell defect in the nude mouse, only a defect in the maturation of these stem cells.

The nude mouse has been a primary resource for determining the role of T cells in many aspects of the immune response. As can be deduced from Chapter 2, TD antigens are ineffective in nude mice that are better able to respond to TI antigens. The role of "third population lymphocytes," those that are neither T nor B cells, in immunity to cancer, in the rejection of transplants, and in resistance to virus infection has been elucidated in a large part by experimental use of this mouse strain.

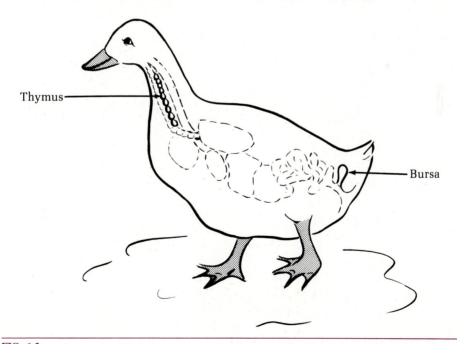

Thymus

Bursa

FIG. 6-2

The bursa of Fabricius is present in the cloacal region. The avian thymus is a multilobed structure laying along the esophagus.

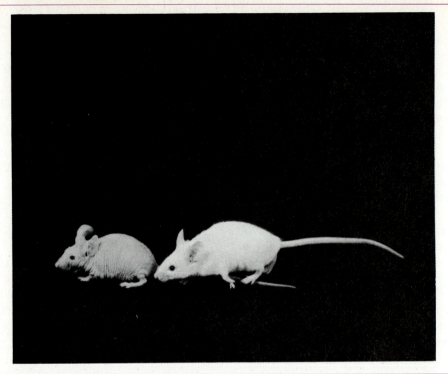

FIG. 6-3

The nude mouse *(left)*, here compared with a normal mouse, has been an excellent source of information about the role of the thymus in immunology, since it lacks this organ. (Courtesy Dr. H. Mullen.)

Bursa of Fabricius

The bursa of Fabricius is a lymphoid organ situated near the terminal end of the gut in fowl; higher animals do not possess a bursa (Fig. 6-2). It is a sac-like structure about 3 cm in diameter at the time of its maximal development, when the bird is about 4 months of age. After that time the bursa begins to atrophy.

A cross section of a young bursa reveals that it, like the thymus, is subdivided into follicles. Within each follicle there are cells of many types, among the most prominent being macrophages, lymphocytes, and plasma cells. The lymphocytes are morphologically similar to the lymphocytes seen in the thymus but differ significantly from them in function. These are the B (bursal) cells, which have their own unique antigen, the β, or B, antigen, which they acquire in the bursa. B cells lack the Thy 1 antigen. The bursa relies on the bone marrow as the source of the precursor cells that will eventually become B cells.

Mammals do not have a bursa, yet they have lymphocytes that perform the same functions as B lymphocytes and which are given the same name. As one might imagine, there has been a considerable research effort toward identifying the bursal equivalent in mammals. One line of inquiry assumed that the bursal equivalent, like the bursa, might reside along the gastrointestinal tract. Removal of gut-associated lymphoid tissue (GALT) early in the life of experimental animals will impair the immunoglobulin response. Because of this severe effect on the physiologic homeostasis of the animal, it remains somewhat uncertain if GALT is the bursal equivalent. Bone marrow is used as a source of B cells in most experimental studies.

The bursaless bird

Glick's experiment in which young, surgically bursectomized chickens were unable to muster an immunoglobulin response to a bacterial vaccine was one of the first to indicate a division of the immune response into a thymic compartment and a bursal compartment. Experiments to confirm this finding were simplified by the anatomical division of the immune system in birds. Whereas bursectomized birds could not produce immunoglobulins, thymectomized chickens were soon demonstrated to lack what we now recognize as T cell-dependent responses—delayed type hypersensitivity and cell mediated cytotoxicity, for instance. Not all of these early experiments with bursectomized or thymectomized birds were successful; it was necessary to perform the required surgery before the peripheral tissues became seeded by lymphocytes from these central lymphoid organs. To some extent seeding could be avoided by applying 19 nortestosterone to the eggshell of the developing chicken embryo. Absorption of this hormone through the shell has a pronounced inhibitory effect on bursal development. Due to an interference with the maturation of other lymphoid tissue, including the thymus, early surgery, that is, surgical bursectomy is generally preferred to chemical bursectomy.

The peripheral lymphoid organs

The central lymphoid organs are not a repository of lymphocytes. These cells leave the thymus and bursa, pass through the bloodstream, and enter the tissues, reentering the thymus and bursa. Some of these tissues are dominated by a lymphoid structure and are collectively termed the *peripheral lymphoid organs*. The most prominent organs of this group are the spleen and lymph nodes, but others, including the tonsils and appendix, have a pronounced lymphocytic character.

Lymph nodes

Lymph nodes are complex, cellular stations situated along the lymphatic ducts, which lead from the tissue to the thoracic duct that empties into the circulatory system just as the vessels enter the heart. Each node serves as a central collecting point for the lymph from a discrete, adjacent anatomic region.

Lymph nodes are numerous near the joints and where the arms and legs join the body. Some animals, notably fowl, are almost totally lacking in lymph nodes.

All lymph nodes are irregular spheres surrounded by a tough capsule and often embedded in adipose tissue (Fig. 6-4). Afferent ducts carry lymph into the gland that serves partially as a filtering or settling basin. The macrophages, granulocytes, and lymphocytes flow slowly through the gland because of the reduction in flow created by the vast spongelike meshwork of the gland. This reticular meshwork provides the surface on which macrophages may impinge and phagocytose antigens arriving from the tissue. The lymphocytes are gathered into follicles or nodules in the cortex.

Lymphocytes are also present in the medullary portion of the gland, but here the septa between the follicles are inapparent. This anatomic similarity of thymus, bursa, and lymph nodes is very striking. The T lymphocyte is more apt to reside in the medullary region and the B lymphocytes in the cortical region of lymph nodes. The T lymphocytes proliferate on antigenic stimulation and create germinal centers after antigenic stimulation, but these are situated nearer the center of the node than are B cell germinal centers, which are cortical or far cortical in location.

Spleen

The spleen, situated in the abdominal cavity, may be ovoid or rather fingerlike in shape, depending on the species. It is a vital organ early in the life of an animal, but may be removed from adults without much influence on normal health. Nevertheless the spleen does contribute to several important body functions, particularly the removal of aged cells of most classes but especially erythrocytes, the phagocytosis of blood-borne particles and antigens, and the synthesis of immunoglobulins. Except for the splenic removal of erythrocytes, these same functions are performed by the lymph nodes. What the lymph node is to the lymphatic system, the spleen is to the circulatory system.

A fibrous outer capsule encloses the body of the spleen. Traditionally the spleen is considered to be composed of two parts: the red pulp and the white

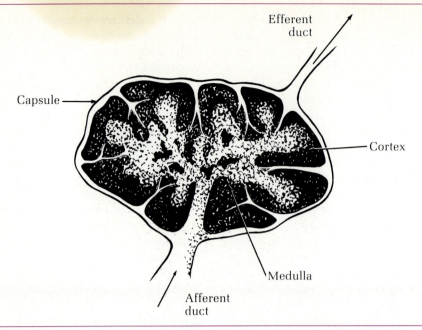

Capsule

Efferent
duct

Cortex

Medulla

Afferent
duct

FIG. 6-4

The lymph node receives lymph through the afferent duct. The cells enter the spongelike lobules and concentrate according to their specificity for the cortex (B cell region) or medulla (T cell region) and then leave by way of the efferent duct.

pulp. The red pulp is well supplied with arteries and is that portion of the organ in which injured erythrocytes are engulfed by phagocytic cells and destroyed. The red pulp constitutes about 50% of the organ, but this and the size of the spleen can change dramatically in disease states. The white pulp contains nodules or follicles of lymphocytes surrounding the lymphatic sheaths. On repeated antigenic stimulation germinal centers develop in the white pulp, where lymphocytes, plasma cells, and their important cell products are fabricated. Although T lymphocytes may be found in the spleen, its function as a B cell organ is more evident.

Other lymphoid organs

The tonsils are lymphoid tissues that, like the thymus, are rather large in childhood and tend to diminish in size with age. The internal structure of tonsils is very reminiscent of the thymus, bursa, and lymph nodes, being divided into follicles that are more lymphoid in nature near their outer, cortical perimeter.

Tonsillar lymphocytes are largely B cells. Other potentially important collections of lymphoid tissue exist in the appendix, lamina propria, and Peyer's patches of the intestine. The lymphocyte population of Peyer's patches is a mixture of B and T lymphocytes. The lamina propria contains T cells and a large population of plasma cells.

Lymphocytes

The important cell common to all lymphoid tissue is the lymphocyte. Lymphocytes are derived from lymphoblasts in bone marrow and are dispersed into the blood where they represent 20% to 30% of the circulating leukocytes. Lymphocytes carried by the blood course through many organs, but critical events take place in the thymus and bursa of Fabricius (or its mammalian equivalent) that appear to imprint the lymphocytes with special functions and regulate the response of the lymphocytes, as either T or B lymphocytes, to antigens.

Lymphocytes are traditionally classified according

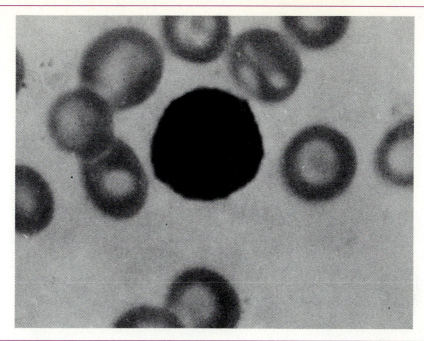

FIG. 6-5
The large nucleus and small rim of cytoplasm are characteristic of lymphocytes as they appear in blood films. (Courtesy Dr. E. Adelstein.)

to their size. The smaller variety usually ranges from 6 to 10 μm in diameter and the large class from 10 to 20 μm in diameter (Fig. 6-5). An intermediate class also is sometimes designated. All lymphocytes have a rounded nucleus or a nucleus that has a single indentation. The nucleus is large in comparison to the cytoplasm, which may appear as a mere fringe about the nucleus. In the large lymphocytes the cytoplasm is a more significant portion of the total cell volume. The nucleus of lymphocytes is characterized by an irregular clumping of chromatin into darkly staining linear arrangements, which may give the nucleus a vague cartwheel appearance. The cytoplasm is slightly basophilic because of its content of ribosomes, but the arrangement of ribosomes into polysomes or into the rough endoplasmic reticulum typical of cells endowed with active protein-synthesizing capabilities is not prominent. A few cytoplasmic mitochondria and lysosomes are visible in electron micrographs of lymphocytes (Fig. 6-6).

Lymphocytes are feebly motile. A pseudopodlike structure, the uropod, is the means by which lymphocytes are motile and is used to establish contact with macrophages, tumor cells, or other cell types. The uropod sometimes is seen as a long, narrow projection and at other times as a more blunt, footlike structure.

Life-span studies of lymphocytes of most mammalian species divide them into two fractions: those with a short span (mostly large lymphocytes) of 5 to 7 days and the small lymphocytes with a life span measured in months or even years. The former are B cells, and the latter are T cells. This is only one of the many differences between B and T cells.

B lymphocytes

Ontogeny and surface markers. B line stem cells are present in the bone marrow and are the source of the pre–B cell. The pre–B cells, even in the animal not yet stimulated by an antigen, synthesize the heavy-chain portion of IgM, the μ chain. The μ

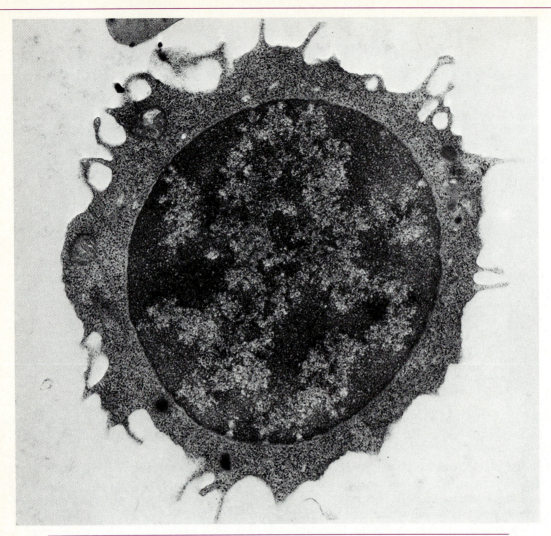

FIG. 6-6

A lymphocyte seen by electron microscopy. The lymphocyte tends to lack a well-developed endoplasmic reticulum; biochemically this must be interpreted as a handicap to protein (antibody) synthesis by this cell. Note the cytoplasmic extensions. (Courtesy Dr. E. Adelstein.)

chain is retained in the cytoplasm—it is not secreted nor combined with the light chain of IgM. The formation of the complete IgM molecule categorizes a B cell as an immature B cell. The IgM produced by the immature B cell is not secreted, it is held at the cell surface. This IgM is structurally distinct from IgM found in the blood by having several additional amino acids on its heavy chains that anchor it in the cell membrane. This surface IgM is of the type described as 7S IgM, a form of IgM that represents only one fifth of the complete IgM found in blood.

The immature B cell also usually has an Ia protein, the Fc receptor, and the CR1 and CR3 receptors of the complement system on its exterior. These do not appear simultaneously and, in fact, the appearance of the complement receptors is often delayed.

☰ SITUATION

A VISIT TO THE ANIMAL QUARTERS

You are on your way through the animal quarters to check your rabbits when the animal caretaker stops you in the hall and asks for your advice. A litter of mice has recently been born in which each animal had a malformed hind leg. One of the young was born dead and was given to a professor of comparative anatomy for examination. In his report he described the anatomy of the limb malformation and the results of his examination of other organs and tissues. The striking result of his study was the detection of a total absence of splenic tissue in the afflicted mice. The animal caretaker was aware that the spleen had something to do with immunity and asked you if the loss of a spleen meant that the rest of the litter would die from infectious disease. He was curious, if the animals could be kept alive and bred with a perpetuation of the spleenless condition, whether the animals would be valuable in immunologic experimentation.

Questions

1. What is the role of the spleen in the immune defense system, and what would be the life expectancy of a spleenless animal?
2. What experiments come to mind as potential immunologic adventures with these unique mice?

Solution

The spleen is a lymphoid organ that is often divided for purposes of discussion into the white pulp and the red pulp. The latter is important in the clearance of defective or aged erythrocytes from the bloodstream and plays no significant role in immunity. The white pulp is the lymphoid portion of the organ, and it is divided into sectors or lobules of lymphocytes surrounded by connective tissue. The lymphocyte population of the spleen is dominated by cells of the B type. In the human about 55% of splenic lymphocytes are of the B type and 15% of the T type, with the remainder unidentified. A slightly higher percentage of T cells is found in rat and mouse spleen.

As with other peripheral lymphoid tissues, the spleen is seeded with B and T lymphocytes before the birth of an animal. Since numerous other peripheral lymphoid tissues are present in mammals, including lymph nodes, tonsils, appendix, Peyer's patches, and other more diffuse tissues, the loss of the spleen generally has little influence on the resistance of adult animals to infectious disease. The removal of a ruptured spleen from human beings is not really a rare medical event and is not associated with an increased incidence of infectious disease, perhaps because other tissues may become seeded by cells escaping through the rupture. "Clean" surgical splenectomy of children does carry some risk for an increased incidence of infectious disease, perhaps because of the containment of splenocytes during clean surgery. Congenitally spleenless mice should be examined regularly for disease but are not under extreme risk for disease.

This discussion does not imply that immunologic experiments with spleenless animals would be fruitless. These unusual animals would be useful in evaluating the spleen as a source of immunologically active hormones; for example, extracts of splenic lymphocytes could be injected into spleenless animals to determine if the spleen influenced their immune response. Purified B and T lymphocytes from the spleens of congenic donors could be injected into spleenless animals for the same purpose. Purified B and T lymphocytes from the spleens of congenic donors could be injected into spleenless mice to determine the tissue homing pattern of these cells. The capacity of spleenless mice to perform phagocytic functions could be evaluated, since an important role of the spleen is phagocytosis. The immunoglobulin class or subclass distribution IgG1 versus IgG2 versus IgM might differ between normal and spleenless mice. Other experiments are without doubt of value to those with special areas of interest.

The mature B cell retains the complement receptors, Fc receptor, and surface IgM and adds surface IgD. The IgM and IgD have been identified as having the same idiotype. The quantity of surface IgD has been equated with the extent of B cell maturation. These early forms of the B cell have and execute their capacity to synthesize immunoglobulins prior to any exposure to antigen.

Other surface markers are also found on B cells. Certainly class I proteins of the MHC complex are found on very early B cells. In contrast, the Lyb 3 and 5 proteins are found quite late and are considered a feature only of mature B cells. Mature B cells respond to TI-2 antigens, whereas the younger Lyb $3^-,5^-$ cells do not. Other Lyb (lymphocyte B) proteins such as Lyb 6, Lyb 17, Lyb 19 have been recognized on these cells, but their function is unknown.

The pre–B cells are first found in the fetal liver and later in the bone marrow, as early as the ninth gestational week in the human being and at the end of the second week in mice. The immature B cell also may be found in the bone marrow and is detectable in the peripheral lymphoid organs and blood. Mature B cells are located in the blood and peripheral lymphoid tissues by the 14th week after conception, presumably after a differentiating pass through the bursa or its equivalent. In the latter site they will be accompanied by plasma cells, but these cells are not found in blood or normal bone marrow.

Approximately 30% of the lymphocytes circulating in the blood can be identified as B cells on the basis of their surface immunoglobulin marker. Nearer to 50% of tonsillar and splenic lymphocytes are B cells.

It should be emphasized that, whereas these B cells may have many common features, they can be subdivided into major subsets on the basis of the isotype of immunoglobulin that they are patterned to synthesize. Thus from the pre–B cell, separate B cell lineages are derived that synthesize only IgM as adult cells (Bμ lineage), IgG (Bγ lineage), etc., to create Bα, Bδ, and Bε lineages. Within each major B cell line, subdivisions depend on two features: the type of light chain that is present in the immunoglobulin, either κ or λ, and the subclass of the heavy chain. (See Chapter 3.) In this way Bμκ and Bμλ, and Bγκ and Bγλ, can be distinguished from each other. Since there are four separate γ-chains known, the Bγκ actually exists as Bγ1κ, Bγ2κ, Bγ3κ, and Bγ4κ. Beyond this a B cell recognizes only one determinant on an antigen, so the B cell lineage expands to a vast number of such cells.

Immunoglobulin on the B cell surface behaves as the specific receptor for antigen. Histochemical techniques reveal that this immunoglobulin is randomly distributed over the B cell surface. When antigen is added, the immunoglobulin begins to accumulate in distinct foci that further blend into one agglomerate. This process is referred to as lymphocyte capping; it precedes a gradual disappearance as the antigen-immunoglobulin complex is internalized.

Lymphocyte capping is a B cell phenomenon not demonstrated by T cells. It signals a phase of cell differentiation into actively secreting plasma cells and memory cells. Memory cells cannot be described in cytologic terms, but they are functionally responsible for the recognition of antigen on reexposure and the rapid antibody response that follows this second as compared with the first exposure. Plasma cells are easily recognized both morphologically and functionally.

The initial trigger for the conversion of B cells to plasma cells is the reaction of surface immunoglobulin specific with antigen. However, the activated B cell does not proliferate until its receptor for B cell growth factor (BCGF now also known as B cell stimulating factor or BSF) is satisfied. BCGF is derived from T cells. Once BCGF ensures B cell growth, the B cells begin to express a second receptor, one for B cell differentiation factor (BCDF). This molecule, also from T cells, permits differentiation of the B cell to the plasma cell level with the concomitant secretion of immunoglobulin. Artificial initiators of B cell activities that substitute for antigen include mitogens (LPS, PWM) and protein A, which mimic antigen by cross-linking surface immunoglobulin, or anti-immunoglobulin.

BCGF has not yet been biochemically characterized. It is not IL-1 nor IL-2, but is a T cell product. It may be a family of proteins with molecular weights near 15,000 to 30,000. Isoelectric points ranging from 6.4 to 8.5 have been reported. These values appear to represent different degrees of glycosylation. The molecule is trypsin-sensitive and is inactivated upon reduction by 2 ME. Likewise, the chemistry of BCDF is in its primitive stages. Molecular weights between 30,000 and 50,000 and pI values between 4.3 and 5.0 have been cited for this protein.

The plasma cell. The plasma cell is about the same size as the small lymphocyte (6 to 10 μm) and can be confused with it in simple stains of tissue preparations. Confusion is less likely with blood stains, since plasma cells are quite scarce in blood. All plasma cells are not the same size; some can approach 20 μm in diameter. Plasma cells have a centrally placed nucleus, and the cytoplasm, which is usually sparse in relation to that of other cells, is often gathered at one side. The nucleus stains intensely, and the lumpy strands of chromatin give the nucleus a cartwheel appearance. This pattern is much more prominent in the plasma cell than in the lymphocyte, where the chromatin also may be unevenly distributed within the nuclear membrane. The cytoplasm of the plasma cell has a strong affinity for basic (cationic) dyes such as pyronin. When used in combination with methyl green, pyronin is an excellent stain for plasma cells. The plasma cell nucleus takes on a blue-green color and its cytoplasm an intense red because of the binding of methyl green and pyronin to these cell structures. This pyroninophilic character of the plasma cell cytoplasm results from its highly acidic nature, which in turn results almost entirely from its content of RNA. This statement is amply supported by electron microscopy, which reveals that the cytosol of plasma cells is literally filled with rough endoplasmic reticulum (Fig. 6-7). This complex intracellular system consists of two serpentine, parallel membranes heavily laden with ribosomes. The ribosomes contain considerable RNA of their own and serve as the site of messenger RNA attachment during protein synthesis. It is here that immunoglobulin synthesis proceeds.

"Third" population lymphocytes

It may seem discordant to discuss the so-called third population of lymphocytes before a complete description of the T cells introduced earlier in this chapter, but so much is known about T cells that they deserve an entire chapter to themselves. In addition, at least some of these third-population cells have characteristics nearer those of B rather than T cells.

Large granular lymphocytes (LGL) and natural killer (NK) cells

A population of less than 3% of the peripheral blood lymphocytes has been categorized as large granular lymphocytes. These cells have a more granular cytoplasm than B or T cells, are nonphagocytic and nonadherent to surfaces despite being Mac 1^+. There is not yet complete agreement on the nature of the surface markers borne by these cells, but they are generally thought to be surface immunoglobulin negative and Fc^+; it is thought that they bear asialoganglioside M1. Some are reported to be Thy 1^+ ($T11^+$ humans) and $CR3^+$. Rosettes formed with sheep red blood cells are easily dispersed; such is not true of the firmer rosettes formed with T cells. The probability exists that either these cells change their surface features as they mature or that subpopulations exist. LGL probably include cells formerly known as natural killer (NK) cells. The role of the Fc and CR3 markers on these cells is mysterious because these cells kill target cells without the aid of antibody or complement. As their name—natural killer cell—implies, they also destroy their target without prior training, as is required of T_C cells. Like T_C cells, however, LGL have IL-2 receptors and at least one report indicates T_C cells may be derived from LGL. IL-2 and IFN both activate LGL.

The granules in LGL are essential to the ability of these cells to kill tumor cells, virus-infected cells, and allogeneic cells. The chemistry of the target molecule on these victim cells may indeed vary with the target or the subtype of LGL. Cell killing is not MHC class I or class II restricted. It requires direct contact of the LGL with the target, during which time the target is programmed for lysis. Afterward the cells can be separated, and the target cell will continue in its cytocidal path. After separation from the first target cell the LGL can "recycle" its lytic machinery and effect a lethal hit on a second cell.

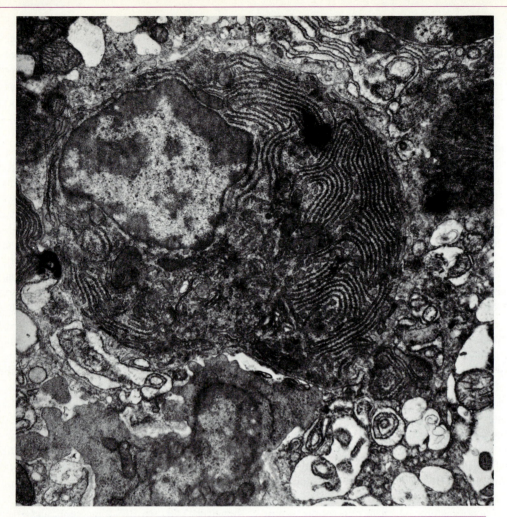

FIG. 6-7
Electron microscopic view of a plasma cell. The cytoplasm is literally filled with endoplasmic reticulum, which is seen as parallel curving lines. This is the site of immunoglobulin synthesis. (Courtesy Dr. E. Adelstein.)

It is believed that upon LGL-target cell contact, the cytoplasmic granules in the LGL cell orient in the direction of the cellular interface (Fig. 6-8). The granules translate, possibly along the Golgi microtubules, toward the cell surface from which they are discharged. This directional nature of the granule displacement accounts for the failure of neighboring target cells to escape this LGL attack. Five separate glycoproteins contribute to LGL cytotoxicity, since an antiserum to this mixture is protective. It is uncertain if one of these proteins is the lymphotoxin (LT) produced by T_C cells since LT is not a rapid-acting toxin. Tumor necrosis factor (TNF) is a protein with a molecular weight of 17,000 that has been found in LGL cells. It has a delayed killing time. Protracted killing is also characteristic of NKCF (natural killer cytotoxic factor) a trypsin-sensitive protein with a molecular weight of 20,000 to 40,000. The most

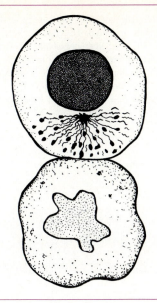

FIG. 6-8

The cytoplasmic granules in the large granular lymphocyte (LGL) have moved toward the cell perimeter where contact with a tumor cell has been established. Cytotoxic proteins including lymphotoxins, tumor necrosis factor, perforins and others are released from the granules and contribute to the death of the target cell.

prominent candidates for LGL killing are a group of perforins, of molecular weight varying from 20,000 to 80,000, that, like LGL cells, destroy target cells within a few minutes. It is interesting that the perforins are serologically cross-reactive with C9, the last component of the complement system that is required for the dissolution of cellular antigens.

The role of LGL in immunity has been underscored by the discovery that the beige mouse, a mutant strain deficient in LGL, is very sensitive to transplanted tumors. In contrast, the nude mouse lacks T_C cells but has LGL cells and is quite resistant to tumors.

Antibody-dependent cell cytotoxicity (ADCC)

Several morphologically distinct cells have been assigned a key role in antibody-dependent cell cytotoxicity, or ADCC. Macrophages and neutrophils participate in ADCC, but they are easily distinguished from a population of lymphocyte-like cells that also cooperate with antibody to destroy cellular targets. These cells are not T cells, since they are present in neonatally thymectomized and nude mice. Anti–Thy 1 sera do not deplete their numbers in vivo. ADCC-active cells, sometimes referred to as K cells have been described as null cells (non-T and non-B) despite the presence of surface receptors for immunoglobulin. ADCC cells have receptors for IgG that, when this is specific for cell surface antigens, serve as a focal point for a cytolytic destruction of the target cell. Though ADCC cells do not require complement and are not MHC restricted they are unable to kill target cells except in the presence of antibody.

Other related cells

Within the last two years, two other cellular activities have been described for cells that are more T cell-like than B cell-like. The first is a population of cells that infiltrates tumors and has a greater tumor-killing potency than do cells isolated from other tissues. Lymphokine-activated killer (LAK) cells, activated by exposure to IL-2 are also potent tumoricidal agents. A more complete description of these cells will clarify their relationship to the cells described in this chapter.

REFERENCES

Baum, C.M., Davie, J.M., and McKearn, J.P.: B-cell subsets: functional and structural characteristics, CRC Crit. Rev. Immunol. **5:**349, 1985.

Calvert, J.E., Maruyama, S., Tedder, T.F., Webb, C.F., and Cooper, M.D.: Cellular events in the differentiation of antibody-secreting cells, Semin. Hematol. **21:**226, 1984.

Cambier, J.C., Monroe, J.G., Coggeshall, K.M., and Ransom, J.T.: The biochemical basis of transmembrane signalling by B lymphocyte surface immunoglobulin, Immunol. Today **6:**218, 1985.

Fauci, A.S., and Ballieux, R.E., editors: Human B-lymphocyte function, New York, 1982, Raven Press Books, Ltd.

Goldfarb, R.H., and Herberman, R.B.: Characteristics of natural killer cells and possible mechanisms for their cytotoxic activity, Adv. Inflamm. Res. **4:**45, 1982.

Hamaoka, T.: T-cell-replacing factors and its acceptor site on B cells: molecular properties and immunogenetic aspects, Contemp. Top. Molec. Immunol. **10:**231, 1985.

Hamaoka, T., and Ono, S.: Regulation of B-cell differentiation: interactions of factors and corresponding receptors, Ann. Rev. Immunol. **4:**167, 1986.

Herberman, R.B., editor: NK cells and other natural effector cells, Orlando, 1984, Academic Press, Inc.

Howard, M.: Soluble-factor induction of B-cell growth, Contemp. Top. Molec. Immunol. **10:**181, 1985.

Ingils, J.R., editor: B lymphocytes today, New York, 1983, Elsevier Biomedical Press.

Kincade, P.W.: Formation of B lymphocytes in fetal and adult life, Adv. Immunol. **31:**177, 1981.

Kishimoto, T.: Factors affecting B-cell growth and differentiation, Ann. Rev. Immunol. **3:**133, 1985.

Klinman, N., Mosier, D.E., Scher, I., and Vitetta, E.S., editors: B lymphocytes in the immune response: functional, developmental and interactive properties, New York, 1981, Elsevier/North-Holland, Inc.

Melchers, F., and Andersson, J.: B cell activation: three steps and their variations, Cell **37:**713, 1984.

Melchers, F., and Andersson, J.: Factors controlling the B-cell cycle, Ann. Rev. Immunol. **4:**13, 1986.

Ortaldo, J.R., and Herberman, R.B.: Heterogeneity of natural killer cells, Ann. Rev. Immunol. **2:**359, 1984.

Ratcliffe, M.J.H.: The ontogeny and cloning of B cells in the bursa of Fabricius, Immunol. Today **6:**223, 1985.

Rogers, J., and Wall, R.: Immunoglobulin RNA rearrangements in B lymphocyte differentiation, Adv. Immunol. **35:**39, 1984.

Schreier, M.H., and Smith, K.A., editors: Growth and differentiation of B cells, Lymphokines **10:**1, 1985.

Swain, S.L., and Dutton, R.W.: T-cell factors that promote B-cell proliferation and differentiation, Contemp. Top. Molec. Immunol. **10:**219, 1985.

Waldmann, T.A., and Broder, S.: Polyclonal B-cell activators in the study of the regulation of immunoglobulin synthesis in the human system, Adv. Immunol. **32:**1, 1982.

See related **Reading 2,** page 416.

The T lymphocytes

≡ GLOSSARY

CD1, CD2, CD3, etc.   Cluster of differentiation of T cells.

contrasuppressor cell   A subclass of T cells (Tcs) whose function is opposite that of a suppressor cell.

CTC   Cytotoxic T cell.

CTL   Cytotoxic T lymphocyte.

helper cell   A subclass of T cells (T_H) that aids in the activation of other T cells and B cells.

interferons (IFN)   A series of three related lymphokines α, β and γ, the last with an immunoregulatory role.

interleukin 2 (IL-2)   A lymphokine produced by T_H cells that aids the activation of other T cells.

Leu 1, Leu 2, Leu 3, etc.   A series of antigens found on human T cells.

lymphotoxin (LT)   A cytolytic protein produced by T_C cells.

Lyt marker   An antigenic marker on T cells.

macrophage chemotaxin   A chemotaxin produced by T_{DTH} cells.

macrophage migration inhibitory factor (MIF)   A product of T_{DTH} cells that arrests macrophage motility.

rosetting   The adsorption of sheep erythrocytes to T cells in such a way as to resemble a flower.

suppressor cell   A subclass of T cells (T_S) whose function is opposite that of T_H cells.

Tac   An antigen on activated T cells that serves as the IL-2 receptor.

T1, T2, T3-T11   A series of antigens found on human T cells.

T3   A T cell marker intimately associated with Ti.

T_C   Cytotoxic T cell.

T_{CS}   Contrasuppressor T cell.

T_{DTH}   A T cell that participates in delayed type hypersensitivity reactions.

T_H   Helper T cell.

Thy1   An antigen found on murine T cells.

Ti   The antigen receptor on T cells.

T_S   Suppressor T cell.

TSF   T cell suppressor factor.

■   ■   ■

As was described in Chapter 6, the bone marrow is the source of two functional groups of lymphocytes. Those that mature in the bursa of Fabricius or its mammalian equivalent are the B cells. These cells are ultimately responsible for the synthesis of the immunoglobulins, specific subsets of these B cells being devoted to the synthesis of only one molecular form of immunoglobulin. In this chapter, the T cells will be described. These, too, originate from precursor cells of the bone marrow but mature in the thymus. As with the B cells, several subsets of the T cells arise during this maturation process, each becoming focused upon a specific function.

T LYMPHOCYTE ONTOGENY
AND SURFACE MARKERS

Immature B cells and T cells are recognized in the bone marrow by the presence of the enzyme terminal deoxynucleotidyl transferase (Tdt). This enzyme adds deoxynucleotides to the growing biopolymer of DNA. The immature B cells and T cells leave the bone marrow via the blood stream (Chapter 6).

The maturation of the T lymphocytes is best described by reference to surface proteins that appear and are either retained or lost during different phases of the maturation process. Unfortunately, four different nomenclature systems for these proteins are in use—the murine system, two human systems and an additional human scheme proposed by the World Health Organization (WHO).

The murine system

The immature murine T cell found in the blood in its passage from the bone marrow can be recognized by the presence of the surface Qa2 and TL (or Tla) proteins. These proteins are coded for in the MHC. Both are class I proteins with a molecular weight of 45,000, associated with the β2 microglobulin. Perhaps as many as 30 alleles of the Qa gene exist, and there may be several alleles of the TL gene. When the young T cell enters the cortical region of the thymus, it loses its Tdt enzyme, its TL protein, and the Qa2 protein but begins to express the Qa3 protein and the universal marker of all mouse T cells, the Thy 1 antigen. These changes are associated with the movement of the T cell from the thymic cortex to the medulla.

The Thy 1 glycoprotein was first described in the 1960s, but its function is still not known. The peptide portion of the molecule has a molecular weight of 12,500, and its oligosaccharide is nearly half that size resulting in a total molecular size of 17,500. The two alleles, Thy 1.1 and Thy 1.2, are identifiable by a single amino acid substitution at position 89 in the gene products.

The Lyt (lymphocyte T) marker proteins 1, 2, and 3 are found on all Thy 1^+ cells in the thymus. Again, two alleles exist for each gene. The structures of the Lyt proteins is not known. Although Lyt 1, 2, and 3 refer to three separate proteins, segregation of these markers during maturation of the T cell always co-associates protein 2 and 3. For this reason Lyt 2^+3^+ cells are sometimes designated simply as Lyt 2^+ cells. The other population arising from the parent Lyt 1^+2^+ cell is, of course, the Lyt 1^+ cell. In the adult mouse, about 50% of the Thy 1^+ cells remain Lyt 1^+2^+, about 35% are Lyt 1^+ and 15% Lyt 2^+; thus, the normal proportion of Lyt 1^+ to Lyt 2^+ cells is roughly 2:1.

The origin of two populations of T cells, identifiable by the presence of either the Lyt 1 or Lyt 2,3 proteins has an important relationship to T cell function. Lyt 1^+ cells tend to be cells that assist B cells and other T cells in their response to antigen (helper or T_H cells) or contribute to delayed hypersensitivity (T_{DTH} cells). In contrast, the Lyt 2^+ cells demonstrate cytotoxic activities against virus-infected tumor cells or transplants (T_C cells) or tend to suppress the immunoglobulin response (T_S cells).

For several years Lyt 1 was considered specific for T_H and T_{DTH} cells, but more recently it has been identified on B cells. Consequently, the Lyt 1 marker can no longer be considered a functional marker for those two groups of T cells. Fortunately, another surface protein, L3T4, has been identified on the surfaces of several T cell subsets and has not been found on B cells. It is now clear that the newly described L3T4 marker is a better marker than Lyt 1 for T_H and T_{DTH} cells. The Lyt 2 protein continues to be a useful marker for T_C and T_S cells.

The human system

The maturational sequence of T cells in all mammals parallels that described for the mouse. In the human system, the enzyme Tdt is present in bone marrow precursors of the T cells. These early cells, as they leave the bone marrow have proteins like Qa and T1a on their outer surfaces. From this point on, the nomenclature system deviates for the human cells.

An extensive panel of monoclonal antibodies has been used to recognize surface antigens given the letter T followed by numerical designations ranging 1 through 11. Few of these markers have, as yet, any relationship to T cell function. Thus, virtually all mature lymphocytes have proteins T1, T3, T10 and T11, of which only T3 and T11 have identified roles. Marker T1 is equivalent to the mouse Thy 1

Raff M C.

Two distinct populations of peripheral lymphocytes in mice distinguishable by immunofluorescence.
Immunology **19**:637-50, 1970. [National Institute for Medical Research, Mill Hill, London, England]

In immunofluorescence studies using anti-θ (now called Thy-1) and anti-immunoglobulin (Ig) antibodies on cell suspensions prepared from mouse peripheral lymphoid tissues, thymus-dependent T lymphocytes were shown to be Thy-1+ and Ig−, while thymus-independent B lymphocytes were shown to be Ig+ and Thy-1− [The SCI® indicates that this paper has been cited in over 570 publications since 1970.]

Martin C. Raff
MRC Neuroimmunology Project
Department of Zoology
University College London
London WC1E 6BT
England

May 7, 1984

"In 1968, I went to the National Institute for Medical Research at Mill Hill, London, to work on the immune system with Avrion Mitchison. I had just completed my training in clinical neurology in Boston, and this was my first real taste of science. It was an exciting time in cellular immunology: it was becoming clear that there were two classes of lymphocytes—now called T and B cells—and several laboratories, including Mitchison's, were gathering evidence that T and B cells collaborated with each other in making antibody responses. Since the two types of lymphocytes looked the same and were always found together in lymphoid tissues, methods were badly needed for distinguishing and separating them. Mitchison pointed me toward the θ (Thy-1) antigen as a possible marker for T cells.

"Reif and Allen had discovered Thy-1 in 1964 and showed that it was on the surface of mouse thymus lymphocytes by killing these cells with anti-Thy-1 antibodies and complement.[1,2] I[3] (and, independently, Schlesinger and Yron[4]) used a similar approach to show that T cells, but not B cells, in peripheral tissues were also Thy-1+. In order to visualize Thy-1 on T cells, I turned to indirect immunofluorescence, using fluorescent anti-Ig antibodies to detect the binding of anti-Thy-1 antibodies. The method worked beautifully but turned up an unexpected result: in control experiments where the anti-Thy-1 antibodies were omitted, the fluorescent anti-Ig labelled a substantial proportion of lymphocytes on its own. Roger Taylor and Michel Sternberg, working across the hall from me, independently found the same thing using radiolabelled anti-Ig antibodies, and we published our observations together in *Nature* in 1970.[5] These findings were exciting because they provided strong support for an important corollary of the clonal selection hypothesis—that lymphocytes have antibodies on their surfaces that function as receptors for antigen. On the other hand, they raised the question of why most lymphocytes were Ig−. Interestingly, in 1961, Möller had observed that fluorescent anti-Ig antibodies labelled a small number of lymphocytes but, since the concept of antibody-like receptors on lymphocytes was not at the forefront of immunological thinking, the implications were missed.[6,7]

"In the paper published in *Immunology* in 1970, I showed that the Ig+ lymphocytes were B cells whereas the Ig− lymphocytes were T cells. The paper has been widely cited, I suspect, because it was the first direct demonstration that B cells but not T cells have detectable Ig on their surfaces. Since the publication of this paper, the presence of surface Ig has been the defining characteristic of B cells. Although not often cited in this regard, the paper also raised the possibility for the first time that T cell receptors for antigen may not be classical antibody molecules. This began a prolonged and heated controversy concerning the nature of T cell receptors, which has only been resolved recently with the demonstration that these receptors are homologous to, but distinct from, Ig molecules (reviewed in reference 8).

"It is ironic that both the *Nature* and *Immunology* papers on cell-surface Ig were originally rejected by *Science* and by the *Journal of Experimental Medicine*, respectively, because they were not considered sufficiently important."

1. Reif A E & Allen J M V. The AKR thymic antigen and its distribution in leukemias and nervous tissues. *J. Exp. Med.* **120**:413-33, 1964.
2. Reif A E. Citation Classic. Commentary on *J. Exp. Med.* **120**:413-33, 1964. *Current Contents/Life Sciences* **26**(5):17, 31 Januray 1983.
3. Raff M C. Theta isoantigen as a marker of thymus-derived lymphocytes in mice. *Nature* **224**:378-9, 1969. (Cited 415 times)
4. Schlesinger M & Yron I. Antigenic changes in lymph node cells after administration of antisera to thymus cells. *Science* **164**:1412-14, 1969. (Cited 80 times.)
5. Raff M C, Sternberg M & Taylor R B. Immunoglobulin determinants on the surface of mouse lymphoid cells. *Nature* **225**:553-4, 1970. (Cited 470 times.)
6. Möller G. Demonstration of mouse isoantigens at the cellular level by the fluorescent antibody technique. *J. Exp. Med.* **114**:415-34, 1961.
7. ------------. .Citation Classic Commentary on *J. Exp. Med.* **114**:415-34, 1961. *Current Contents/Life Sciences* **27**(27):20, 2 July 1984.
8. Williams A F. The T-lymphocyte antigen receptor—elusive no more. *Nature* **308**:108-9, 1984.

marker. Markers T6 and T9 are found on thymocytes, but these markers are lost when the cells enter the blood stream. As the thymic T cells mature, T4 and T8 appear and are retained on separate functional subsets of these cells.

Thus, of the many T proteins, four are of definite importance. T3 is closely associated with the antigen receptor, Ti, that is described below. T11 is the receptor for sheep red blood cells. T4 is a marker for helper T cells and the T_{DTH} cells. Approximately 60% of mature T cells possess this protein. The T8 protein is a positive marker for T_C and T_S cells. In man as in other animals, the T_H to T_S ratio is 2:1.

A second panel of monoclonal antibodies has been applied to the identification of the different functional subsets of T cells using the abbreviation Leu. Leu2 cells are equivalent to T8 cells and Leu3 cells are equivalent to T4 cells.

In an effort to prevent an expansion of the names applied to human T cells, an expert committee of the WHO has suggested the abbreviation CD be used. CD refers to cluster of differentiation. At this time, the numbering system for CD is equivalent to T so that CD4 cells are T4 whereas CD8 cells are T8 cells.

Thymic hormones. The differentiation and maturation of cells from the bone marrow that terminate in the recognition of a mature T cell are regulated by a number of peptides, which have been described as thymic hormones.

Many different preparations from thymus glands, from purified T cells, and even from serum have been identified to contain a thymic hormone. Only a few of these hormonelike molecules have been purified sufficiently to permit the assignment of a specific biologic activity to a specific compound (Table 7-1).

Thymic humoral factor is prepared from calf thymus where it is present as a heat-labile protein consisting of 31 amino acids. Its isoelectric point is between that of thymulin, previously known as thymic serum factor (facteur thymique serique, or FTS) and that of thymosin α_1 at 5.6. Thymic humoral factor has been demonstrated to repair T-cell deficits in thymectomized mice, to augment T_H cell activity, to stimulate the mixed leukocyte culture (MLC) response, and to stimulate responsiveness to T cell lectins.

Thymosin is a mixture of 15 or more proteins, of which one, thymosin α_1, has been fully described. Thymosin α_1 is a peptide with a molecular weight of 3,108 and an isoelectric point of 4.2. The amino acid sequence of thymosin is unlike that of any other known protein. Immunologic and biochemical evidence indicates that it is synthesized in the thymus, possibly in the form of a precursor approximately fivefold its own size. Thymosin is heat stable, possibly because it contains no cysteine and lacks disulfide bonds. It is also free of aromatic or heterocyclic

---

TABLE 7-1

Characteristics of thymic hormones

	Source	Molecular weight	Isoelectric point	Major activities
Thymosin α_1	Calf thymus	3,108	4.2	Increases Con A response, sheep red blood cell rosettes, Thy 1–positive cells
Thymic humoral factor	Calf thymus	About 3,300	5.6	Enhances T_H numbers and response to Con A
Thymulin	Serum	859	7.3	Enhances sheep red blood cell rosettes, Thy 1–positive cells
Thymopoietin II	Calf thymus	5,562	—	Induces Thy 1– and Lyt–positive cells
Serum factor	Serum	<500	—	Several T cell–enhancing activities

amino acids. Thymosin restores T cell characteristics to T cell–deficient mice, as measured by an increase in rosetting with sheep red blood cells, increase in the response to T cell lectins, increased number of T_H cells, enhanced MLC activity, induction of Thy 1–positive and Lyt-positive cells, and the induction of T_{DTH} activity. Additional active molecules present in the original thymosin preparations, such as thymosin α_7, have been less well characterized, but thymosin β_4 has been sequenced. It is unlike thymosin α_1 in structure. Thymosin β_4 consists of 43 amino acids and contains one residue of phenylalanine and three of proline. It induces T_{DTH} in prolymphocytes.

Thymulin is the smallest of the chemically characterized thymic hormones. It has a molecular weight of only 859 and is composed of only 9 amino acids. Its isoelectric point is 7.3. This small peptide is apparently synthesized in Hassall's corpuscles, the round refractile structures regularly seen in the thymus. When injected into T cell–deficient animals, thymulin induces the appearance of the Thy 1 antigen, increases sheep-cell rosetting by lymphocytes, and diminishes the T_S cell population.

Thymopoietin II, the largest of the well-characterized thymic hormones, has a molecular weight of 5,562; it is a heat-stable protein composed of 49 amino acids. Among its activities is the ability to induce Thy 1 and Lyt antigen expression on immature lymphocytes. These cells are positive for Tdt activity until thymopoietin binds; then the cells mature and lose this enzyme while expressing the typical antigens of mature T cells. Thymopoietin is a product of the thymus epithelium and not of thymocytes or other cells. Thymectomy removes this hormone from the blood within hours.

Other factors have been described that have thymic-replacing activity. These include serum factor, a small peptide with a molecular weight of less than 500 from human blood, and lymphocyte-stimulating hormones from calf thymus.

T CELL RECEPTORS
Erythrocyte receptor

In addition to surface components on T lymphocytes that are useful in identifying cells with unique functions there are other important molecules on the exterior of these cells. One is the receptor for sheep red blood cells—the T11 protein in the human nomenclature system. Incubation of sheep erythrocytes with human T cells results in the formation of rosettes in which the T cell is surrounded by a cluster of the erythrocytes (Fig. 7-1). The enumeration of T cells, which is very simple by this technique, indicates that approximately two thirds of all peripheral blood lymphocytes are T cells. Of the remaining lymphocytes about 30% are B cells, and the remainder are LGL and third-population cells. In thoracic-duct fluid nearly 90% of the lymphocytes will form rosettes with sheep erythrocytes. The T cell density of lymph nodes is greatest in the medulla.

The Ia protein receptor

A second important receptor on certain T cells is specific for Ia proteins. The chemical nature of this receptor is still obscure, however, it is able to recognize the Ia protein on B cells and macrophages and enable the cooperative events between these cells that allow the immune response to TD antigens. In mixed cultures of B and T cells from genetically different donors, the T cells pass through repeated growth and differentiation cycles known as lymphocyte transformation. This cycling is known variously as the mixed lymphocyte reaction (MLR) or mixed lymphocyte culture (MLC). The response of the T cell to the I-A or I-E proteins (DP, DQ, or DR proteins in man) on B cells is an important part of this reaction.

The T cell antigen receptor

The antigen receptor on T cells escaped identification for many years despite the facile demonstration of antigen specificity in these cells. Some of the early evidence suggested that only a portion of immunoglobulin molecules could be found on the T cell surface and that these functioned as antigen receptors. Because of the parallel between this and IgM and IgD as the antigen receptor on B cells the conclusion seemed logical. Recent experiments employing recombinant DNA technology have failed to find any sequences of DNA in T cells that code for immunoglobulins. Separate experimentation has

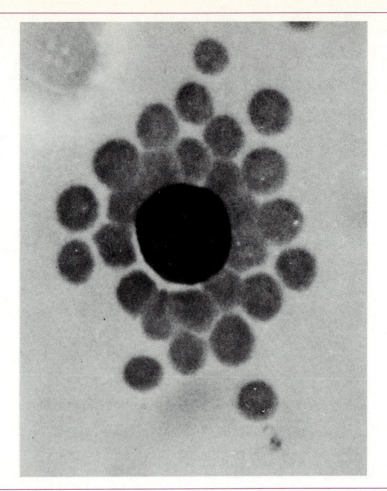

FIG. 7-1
This rosette reveals how large the number of sheep erythrocytes that attach to lymphocytes can be. (Courtesy Dr. E. Adelstein.)

identified a human T cell protein, Ti, as the antigen receptor. The murine molecule is known simply as the antigen receptor. Molecular parallels among the chemistry and genetics of the antigen receptor in man and mouse have already been confirmed, though there are still important areas of uncertainty.

The Ti molecules consists of two definitely accepted peptides, the α and β chains with the probable participation of a third, the γ chain (Fig. 7-2). The Ti protein and the T3 protein are intimately associated, and antisera to either will prevent antigen recognition because peptides of the T3 molecule,

though more interior on the cell membrane than the Ti peptides, are interlaced with peptides of the Ti molecule. As a consequence, antibodies to either molecule would physically mask the true antigen receptor.

The two accepted Ti peptides α and β, exist as a disulfide-linked heterodimer with a molecular weight of approximately 90,000. The murine α-β chain combination appears to be smaller, with a molecular weight of perhaps only 75,000. Both the α and β peptides can be divided into four major domains. The most exterior, encompassing some 90 amino ac-

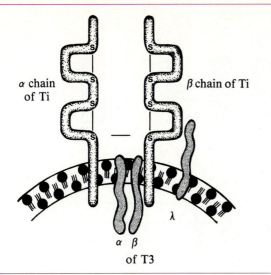

α chain of Ti

β chain of Ti

λ

α β of T3

FIG. 7-2

The T cell receptor for antigen Ti, is closely associated with the T3 protein. Ti consists of two peptides, α and β, shown here as strippled structures with internal disulfide bonds. A third, the γ peptide, may also be a part of Ti. The T3 protein is composed of three peptide chains (shaded) that are more deeply imbedded in the cell membrane than the Ti peptides.

ids is the variable domain. Nearer the cell surface is another segment of approximately 90 amino acids; the constant domain. Both the variable and constant domains contain internal disulfide bonds. The terms *variable* and *constant* as used here have the same connotations as in the structure of the immunoglobulins, that variation in the amino acid sequences of the Vα and Vβ domains provide the antigenic specificity of the receptor where as the Cα and Cβ potentially provide effector functions. A transmembrane sequence of 25 and a cytoplasmic portion of only 5 to 10 amino acids completes the structure.

The T3 protein consists of three peptides α, β and γ, each with a molecular weight of 20,000 to 25,000. The T3 protein isolated from genetically nonidentical sources is not polymorphic, thus does not appear to have a direct role in antigen recognition. Nevertheless, the intimate association of Ti and T3 suggests a cooperative interaction. Perhaps T3 serves as a transmembrane messenger after the combination of Ti with its ligand.

The genetics of the T cell receptor are already quite well understood and mirror the genetics of the immunoglobulins (Fig. 7-3). The structure of the α chain is derived by a combination of one of several variable genes (Vα) with a joining gene (Jα) sometimes designated as a diversity (D) gene and then a constant-domain gene. The V and J genes code for the exterior 90 amino acid region of the protein and the C gene for the next 90 amino acids. The genetic arrangement of the β chain involves several Vβ genes, diversity genes (Dβ), and Jβ genes, before the Cβ gene. This sequence is followed by additional segments of Dβ, Jβ, and Cβ genes. Recent evidence indicates the γ peptide genes include a set of Vγ genes followed by pairs of JγLγ genes repeated several times.

IL-1 and IL-2 receptors

The macrophage interleukin 1 combines with a receptor on T cells as part of the initial events catalyzing the T cell response. The T_H cell then produces interleukin-2, which stimulates the other functional subsets of T cells. Receptors for IL-1 and IL-2 are discussed below.

T CELL SUBSETS AND THEIR FUNCTIONS

Neonatal thymectomy of experimental animals causes a number of immunodeficiency symptoms. One of the most easily demonstrated is a marked inability to form immunoglobulins against the structurally complex T-dependent antigens. Such animals may reject tissue transplants more slowly than untreated controls and some allergic responses, notably the delayed-hypersensitivity response, may not develop to its fullest. These functions are acquired by adoptive immunization with T cells from genetically identical donors.

The purification of T lymphocytes by the use of antisera directed against surface proteins has revealed that there are five major functional subsets of these cells. Some of these cells have been grown as clones (Fig. 7-4) by incorporating IL-1 and the thymic lymphokine IL-2 into the growth medium. Analysis of the medium after the growth of these cells has identified products that are associated with the unique activity of the T cell subset. The prospect

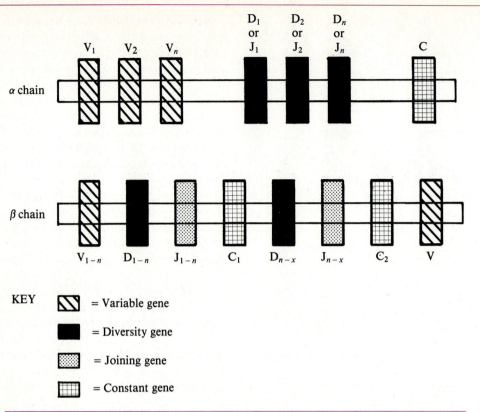

KEY

◫ = Variable gene

■ = Diversity gene

▦ = Joining gene

▦ = Constant gene

FIG. 7-3

Although the genetics of the Ti protein are incompletely known, differences in the gene distribution for the α and β chains have already become apparent. Several variable and diversity (also called joining) genes prefix the constant gene for the α chain. For the β chain, the gene order has irregularly placed duplicates of variable, diversity, joining and even of the constant gene.

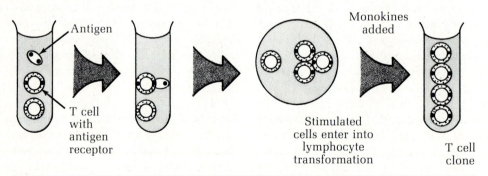

FIG. 7-4

A clone of T cells can be generated only with difficulty, unlike that of macrophages and B cells. Antigen-stimulated T cells will reproduce for several generations if supplied with monokines or lymphokines. Unstimulated cells slowly die.

that protein-free growth media can be developed that will sustain these cells certainly exists, and when attained will facilitate isolation and characterization of these lymphokines. Although this goal has been achieved to some extent through recombinant DNA technology, some of the "engineered" products may lack properties of the natural product because they have no polysaccharide side chains.

Helper T cells (T_H)

The helper-cell function of T cells for the immune response has been demonstrated in several animal models; the most commonly used is perhaps the nude mouse. Neonatally thymectomized animals, or animals lethally irradiated and reconstituted with B cells have also been used to identify the need for T cells in several aspects of the immune response.

The classic experiment to prove the need for T cells as helper T cells is that of Claman, Chaperon, and Selner (Reading 2). Lethally irradiated mice failed to make antibody against sheep erythrocytes, as determined by a lack of plaque-forming cells, unless reconstituted with B cells and T cells. These T cells were later proven to be Lyt 1^+ cells. Upon the discovery of the L3T4 marker, it too was found on these cells. T_H cells are thus Lyt 1^+, L3T4$^+$ cells. These are equivalent to T4$^+$ (CD4 or Leu3) human cells.

The molecular basis for T_H cell assistance of B cells in the immunoglobulin response has only recently come under rewarding study. BCGF and BCDF have both been implicated in this effect (Chapter 6). The helper T cells also provide assistance, probably to all the other T cell subsets for their activities as well. Interleukin 2 (IL-2) is the lymphokine responsible for this activity.

Interleukin 2 (IL-2)

The ability of products found in cultures of antigen- or mitogen-stimulated T cells to perpetuate the growth of T cells in these cultures led to the acronym TCGF (T cell growth factor) for these products in 1976. Later the term interleukin 2 was adopted. IL-2 has the capacity to convert T cells from the G1 stage of the cell cycle to the S and then subsequent growth stages. Thus, one assay for IL-2 is to observe for an increase in a specific T cell activity, such as the number of T8$^+$ cells and cytotoxic activity in a culture. Human IL-2 is a protein with a molecular weight of 15,400, and other species produce a molecule of similar size. The secreted IL-2 contains 133 amino acids after losing the signal peptide of 20 amino acids. Isoelectric heterogeneity results from differences in the amount of glycosylation. The structural gene is on chromosome 4 and contains 4 introns.

Two signals are required to stimulate IL-2 production—one can consist of either antigen or mitogen and the other of IL-1 from macrophages. (Macrophages were present in the cultures used for the original descriptions of TCGF.) Thus only activated T cells secrete IL-2. Although all T cell subsets are capable of IL-2 production, the major source is the T4$^+$ cell.

A major function of IL-2 is to cause activated T cells to proliferate. T cells not activated fail to absorb IL-2. An antibody specific to activated T cells (anti-Tac) binds to these cells and blocks IL-2 binding. Monoclonal anti-IL-2 has the same effect. Thus the Tac antigen is all or part of the IL-2 receptor. Several studies have incriminated a surface glycoprotein with a molecular weight near 50,000 as the IL-2 receptor, and the DNA for the Tac antigen has been cloned. The first 21 amino acids represent the signal peptide, the next 220 amino acids represent the extracellular portion, and the remaining 35 amino acids are nearly equally divided between the transmembrane and cytoplasmic portions of the molecule.

In addition to the response of activated T cells to IL-2, NK cells are a major responding cell. That B cells also have IL-2 receptors may account for the production of antibody in T cell-depleted systems exposed to IL-2.

The clinical use of IL-2 preparation in cancer patients or those with acquired immune deficiency syndrome (AIDS) or other T cell-compromised immune deficits has been disappointing, presumably because of a diminished expression of IL-2 receptors on the existing T cells.

Interleukin 2 receptor

The resting T cell has perhaps 100 molecules of an IL-2 binding protein, i.e., an IL-2 receptor. The antigen and IL-1-stimulated cell has 10,000 to 12,000 molecules of the IL-2 receptor. This molecule was originally described as the Tac antigen, an antigen that was enhanced on T cell activation.

The IL-2 receptor is a protein with a molecular weight of about 50,000, although some estimates are as great as 65,000. Neither figure agrees very well with information derived from the cloned DNA of this molecule unless one accepts that IL-2 is about 50% oligosaccharide and 50% protein. The cloned DNA predicts a protein of 251 amino acids, not including a signal peptide of 21 amino acids. The external portion of the molecule encompasses the first 220 amino acids, of which the most external 50 or 60 are the active site for IL-2 binding. The transmembrane sequence of the IL-2 receptor has 18 amino acids, and the cytoplasmic portion contains only 12 amino acids.

Interleukin 3 (IL-3)

A peptide product of T_H cells not as well described as IL-2 is interleukin 3 (IL-3). The peptide has a molecular weight between 28,000 and 40,000 and stimulates the growth and maturation of many cells of hemopoietic origin. B cells, T cells, basophils, and mast cells respond to IL-3, a response that, in addition to cell growth, activates the enzyme 20 α steroid dehydrogenase. The relationship of the appearance of this enzyme and cell maturation is unknown.

Delayed type hypersensitivity T cells (T_{DTH})

The early discovery of Landsteiner and Chase that lymphoid cells from animals with contact dermatitis or an allergy of infection would transfer those conditions was the first indication that lymphoid cells were engaged in delayed type hypersensitivity. Approximately 30 years later it was possible to show that Lyt 1^+ T cells were responsible for this activity. Again the L3T4 marker is present; in fact, it is not yet possible to distinguish the T_H cell from the T_{DTH} cell on the basis of surface markers. Cloned T_H cells demonstrate the characteristics of T_{DTH} cells. One

difference may be in the kind or quantity of interleukins they secrete, the T_H cell secreting primarily IL-2, and the T_{DTH} cell primarily the macrophage chemotaxin and macrophage migration inhibition factor.

Macrophage chemotaxin

T_{DTH} cells produce chemotaxins that are active on different cell populations. The chemotaxin that attracts monocytes and macrophages is an important contributor to the infiltration of these cells into tissues where a delayed type hypersensitivity reaction is occurring (Chapter 18). The chemical nature of this interleukin is related to its species origin. The molecule of human origin has a molecular weight of 12,500 but the guinea pig chemotaxin is more than twice that size, possibly as great as 55,000, although dimerization may be the explanation for activity in molecules in this size range. Both chemotaxins are heat stable at 56° C for 30 minutes and are unrelated to chemotaxin C5a of the complement system.

Migration inhibition factor (MIF)

Antigen- or mitogen-stimulated T_{DTH} cells secrete a factor that is able to inhibit the migration of macrophages (Fig. 7-5). Obviously the combined secretion of a chemotaxin and a migration inhibitor for the same cell indicates that the molecules act at different concentrations, or as it may also be stated, at different distances. Clearly the chemotaxin acts at the greatest distance from the T_{DTH} cell to attract the cell to a region where the MIF can arrest cell motility.

MIF from one species is biochemically quite different from that of another. Murine MIF is a β globulin whose activity is found in the molecular-weight range of 48,000 to 68,000. Human MIF activity is contained in molecules with a molecular weight near 32,000. Two separate kinds of MIF are produced by guinea pigs. Though both behave electrophoretically as albumins, one has a molecular weight near 65,000, and the other's is between 25,000 and 40,000.

In the past, MIF was also described as having MAF-macrophage-activating or macrophage-arming-

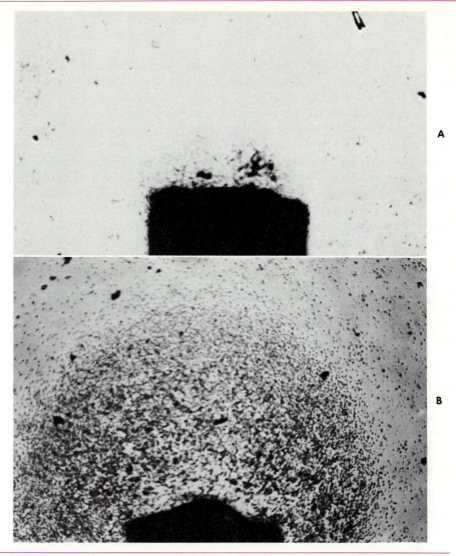

FIG. 7-5

A macrophage migration inhibition test. Peritoneal exudate cells from a guinea pig possessing a delayed hypersensitivity to histoplasmin were used. **A,** Little or no migration is seen in the presence of histoplasmin. **B,** Abundant migration in the presence of tuberculin. (Courtesy Dr. W. Irvin.)

factor activity. MIF does have macrophage-agglutinating activity also sometimes abbreviated MAF. Currently, the activation of macrophages is believed to be another property of interferon, in addition to that of MIF.

Transfer factor (TF)

Extracts of antigen-exposed T_{DTH} cells are able to convert unexposed cells to the response characteristics of the donor cells. Analysis of transfer-competent extracts from human cells has identified the transfer factor (TF) or factors in molecules of different sizes. One fraction with a molecular weight between 700 and 4000 has been partially characterized. Its absorption spectrum is typical for a complex of nucleic acid and peptide. Putative structures have been forwarded but none has been fully proven.

Because the molecular weight of TF is much lower than that of even the smaller interleukins, and because TF seems to be composed of largely nucleic acid in composition, it does not fall within the usual descriptive boundaries for these molecules. Other features also separate TF from the usual lymphokines. When the T_{DTH} cell is exposed to antigen, it secretes TF and no longer itself is active as a source of TF. Thus it appears the T_{DTH} cell synthesizes TF slowly, and establishes a TF store, which, when exhausted, is only slowly replenished—such is not the case in the synthesis of the interleukins where no significant cell storehouse exists.

Another distinguishing feature of TF is its ability to confer the properties of the donor cell on other lymphocytes. These newly acquired properties are not permanent but do persist for several weeks or months. At first TF appeared to be a messenger RNA or even a natural recombinant DNA, but structural studies have been unable to confirm that TF is either kind of nucleic acid.

This persistence in a recipient of the newly acquired delayed type hypersensitivity is a medically useful feature of TF. Because the molecular weight of TF places it below the range of antigenicity, injections can be repeated. Thus a person with a deficiency of T_{DTH} cellular activities can have this function restored by receiving TF from a competent donor. Since the macrophage chemotaxin and migration inhibition factor are so intimately associated with immunity, TF injections can help a person developing immunity to a few pathogenic agents, particularly the fungi (see Chapters 18 and 20).

Interferons (IFN)

The discovery of interferons (IFN) in 1957 by Isaacs and Lindenmann revealed for the first time that animals have a second means of acquired immunity, other than immunoglobulins, that is based on an excreted cell product. IFN was found in the serum of animals within a few hours after exposure to a virus, much before immunoglobulins were present. To measure IFN's protective activity, these sera were transfused into a normal animal that was subsequently challenged with an infectious virus. It was soon learned that IFN was protective against not only the inducing virus, but also against many antigenically unrelated viruses.

Viruses, especially the myxoviruses and arboviruses, are potent inducers of IFN, but other intracellular parasites are also effective. The initial efforts to identify the inducer molecule led to the identification of double-stranded RNA (dsRNA) as among the most potent. Synthetic RNA pairs, such as polyinosinic-polycytidylic acid (poly IC), or other anionic polymers are good inducers. Later it was found that mitogens—phytohemagglutinin and concanavalin A—and even many common antigens functioned as IFN inducers. While these studies were being carried out, parallel efforts were made to identify the best IFN-producing cells. As a result, T lymphocytes, fibroblasts, macrophages, and several other cell types could produce IFN. Not all inducers and responding cells, however, produced IFN of equal potency. Then in 1978 it was learned that there are three separate interferons, IFN α, β and γ.

The three IFNs share a few common features but also differ from each other in important ways (Table 7-2). The molecular weights of α and β IFN are similar. Both types are inducible by viruses or dsRNA and are relatively stable at pH2. IFN γ is slightly smaller, induced by antigens and mitogens but less stable at pH2. Considerable information about the genetics, chemistry, and activity of these three IFNs is now available.

The active gene products differ by only one or two amino acids in most instances. Thirteen α genes and six pseudo-α IFN genes are situated on human chromosome 9. The DNA contains no introns; it codes for a product containing 188 (in some variants, 189) amino acids, the first 23 of which create a hydrophobic leader that splits off when the remaining 165 are secreted as α IFN. This protein has a molecular weight of 17,000, is stable at pH2, and is derived from T cells after exposure to dsRNA or viruses.

TABLE 7-2

Distinctive characteristics of the IFNs

Current designation	Type	Cell source	Inducer	Molecular weight	Acid stability (pH 2)	Number of variants
α-IFN	I	T cells	Viruses, dsRNA	17,000	Yes	13
β-IFN	I	Fibroblasts	Viruses, dsRNA	17,000	Yes	5
γ-IFN	II	T cells	Antigens, mitogens	15,000	No	Unknown

IFN β has a similar chromosomal origin; its DNA contains no introns and it codes for 187 amino acids. Only one natural β gene is known but several variants have been produced artificially. IFN β has a 29% homology with IFN α and, like it, is acid-stable and inducible from fibroblasts by dsRNA and viruses.

Human chromosome 12 is the location of the structural gene for IFN γ, and this DNA contains three introns. The gene product contains 166 amino acids. Numerous artificial variants have been produced. T cells stimulated with antigens or mitogens are a good source of the acid-labile IFN γ. IFN γ binds to a cell receptor different from the receptor common to both IFN α and IFN β.

Many activities are shared by these IFNs, though they are not equally potent. The production of antiviral immunity is primarily related to the α and β molecules. IFN γ is a potent immune regulator and is approximately 100-fold more active than α in inducing increases of class I MHC antigens, the receptor for IL-2 on T cells, in activating NK, T8$^+$ cells, and macrophages, and increasing the density of Fc receptors for IgG on the last cell type. Its ability to inhibit cell growth prompted trials of IFN α as an anticancer agent.

Interferons from other species are very similar to the human proteins, though rat and mouse IFN α are glycosylated. Each animal species is most receptive to IFN of its own species source, but IFNs from closely related species are mutually protective against viruses. Of course, the initial virus-infected cell, the one that produces the IFN, is not protected. During a viral infection, it secretes IFN that may subsequently destroy it, but this secreted IFN protects neighboring cells. This protection is related to the activities of new enzymes that appear in the IFN-exposed cell. One of these which has been identified is a protein kinase that adds phosphate groups taken from adenosine triphosphate (ATP) to proteins. When IFN is present, the kinase "erroneously" phosphorylates the small subunit of eIF-2, the protein-initiating factor. Phosphorylation of the initiating factor interrupts synthesis of the proteins needed for viral replication.

A second target molecule proved to be a nuclease that is activated by a molecule derived from ATP. The current hypothesis is that dsRNA or IFN activates a 2′5′-adenosine polymerase that degrades ATP to form short chains of adenosine linked by 2′5′-phosphodiester bonds (Fig. 7-6). The polymerase is active only after viral derived dsRNA is present. The product, 2′5′-adenosine, or 2′5′A, reacts with an endonuclease that cleaves RNA, and the newly synthesized messenger that arises after viral infection and is needed for viral replication is destroyed. The failure of the protein kinase, the 2′5′-adenosine polymerase, and endonuclease to halt host-cell growth is attributed to the operation of these three enzymes in a microenvironment near the viral invader.

Suppressor T cells (T$_S$)

The identification of the T$_S$ cell emerged from several different experiments. In one, it was discovered that thymectomy enhanced the B cell response to a T cell-independent antigen. In another study, large doses of antigen were used to thwart the immunoglobulin response through the phenomenon of immune tolerance. T cells transferred from such ani-

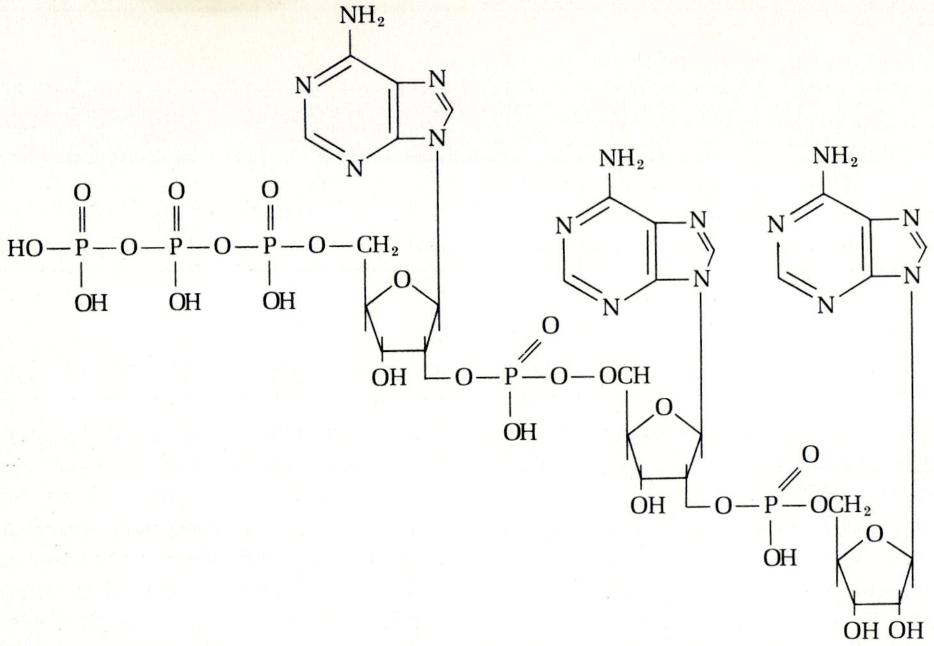

FIG. 7-6

2'5'-Adenosine or 2'5'-oligoadenylate is the first new compound detected in a cell exposed to IFN, and it catalyzes a sequence of reactions that prevent viral replication.

mals to normal animals that were then given the customary immunizing dose of antigen penalized the antibody response in the recipients. It could also be demonstrated in a variation of these experiments that an animal cannot be made tolerant except when T cells are present.

Fractionation of the T cells used in these studies revealed the suppressing cell to be Lyt 1$^-$ but Lyt 2$^+$. The corresponding human cell is T8$^+$ (CD8$^+$) or Leu 2$^+$. Convincing evidence now exists that there are several subsets of T_S cells. The interaction of these cells is described in Chapter 8. The T_S cell referred to here is the final suppressor or the effector T_S cell. Kinetic studies reveal that the level of T cell suppressor activity remains low after normal doses of antigen. At this time, T_H cell activity is foremost, encouraging an immunoglobulin response. Subsequently, T_S cell activity increases and remains high, in mice for as long as 2 months. It is also possible to create tolerance in B cells but more antigen is re-

quired and the tolerance persists for a shorter time than does T-cell tolerance. Consequently T cell tolerance is described as *long term-low dose tolerance*.

Specific T suppressor factors have been difficult to isolate, but several have been partially described. One is a protein with a molecular weight of 30,000 that has an antigenic relationship to the I-J protein. The I-J protein itself is poorly characterized. Another soluble immune-response suppressor molecule has a molecular weight of 21,000. A third factor, also related to the I-J protein has a size of 90,000 and binds to antigen. It appears unlikely from these results that there is but a single suppressor factor unless these size differences relate to an association of antigenic determinants with the factor.

Cytotoxic T cells (T_C)

The ability of mouse T cells exposed to cellular antigens to destroy these cells on a second exposure enabled the identification of a second population of

TABLE 7-3

Characteristics of the B and T lymphocytes

	B Lymphocyte	T Lymphocyte
Tissue origin	Bone marrow	Bone marrow
Tissue where maturation occurs	Bursa of Fabricius or bursal equivalent	Thymus
Surface markers	1. Fc receptor	1. Thy 1 or T1
	2. Immunoglobulin	2. Lyt or CD markers
	3. CR3	3. IL-1 and IL-2 receptors
	4. Ia protein	
Antigen receptor	IgM and IgD	Ti aided by T3
Functional subsets	B_μ, B_γ, B_α, B_δ, B_ϵ	T_H, T_{DTH}, T_C, T_S, T_{CS}
Subset variants	κ and λ chain variants	T_S and T_{CS}, possibly T_H
Cell products	Immunoglobulins	Interleukins
Tissue distribution	Low in blood, high in spleen	High in blood, thoracic lymph
Sensitivity to lectins, etc.	PWM, LPS, Protein A	ConA, PHA, PWM
Response to conjugated antigens	Mostly to hapten	Mostly to carrier
Immune tolerance	High dose, short term	Low dose, long term

Lyt 2^+ cells. (The corresponding human cells are again $T8^+$, Leu 2^+.) These cytotoxic T cells, now usually referred to as CTC or T_C cells, differ from the T_S cell in an important characteristic. T_S cells require assistance from a population of macrophages that are I-J^+ and are believed to function via a lymphokine that contains the I-J marker. In contrast, the T_C cell may not require assistance from antigen-processing macrophages of any type. Instead, the T_C cell responds to antigen in association with class I proteins of the MHC. This difference is amplified in Chapter 8.

The basis for destruction of target cells by T_C cells is ascribed to a series of molecules known as lymphotoxins (LT). As originally described, these molecules originated from a macromolecule that was degraded from its original size (molecular weight of 200,000) through a series of lymphotoxic intermediates of diminishing size to the smallest active molecule (molecular weight about 25,000). Now this cascade has been reversed, and the opinion is that the parent lymphotoxin is the smallest molecule. Aggregation of this monomer into polymers of various multiples accounts for the dispersion of activity across a large range of molecular weights. Other cytotoxic agents such as the perforins are also pro-duced by T_C cells; the perforins, however, affect target cells very quickly after cell contact. By comparison, the T_C cell or LT requires several hours to kill the target cell.

Contrasuppressor cells (T_{CS})

Experiments completed in the last few years have indicated that a population of Lyt 1^+ cells can negate the role of the T_S cell. Unlike T_H cells, these cells lack the L3T4 marker. Since they are not simply another population of T_H cells, they have been designated as contrasuppressor T cells (T_{CS}). The biochemical basis for their activity is presumed to reside in soluble contrasuppressor factors yet to be described. These cells also function with macrophages that are I-J positive. Human T_{CS} cells are $T8^+$.

As was the situation with the other T cell that interacts with the I-J protein, i.e., the T_C cell, the T_{CS} cells actually consist of a network of cells. The interactions of these cells is described in Chapter 8. The T_{CS} described here can be considered the effector countersuppressor.

SUMMARY

The B, T, and third-population lymphocytes are a critical collection of cells necessary for the development and regulation of the immune response. As yet, the third-population cells are not well understood. The distinguishing features of B and T cells, by comparison, have been gradually recognized over the past two decades. Table 7-3 presents a review of the many differences and similarities of B and T cells.

REFERENCES

Altman, A., and Katz, D.H.: The biology of monoclonal lymphokines secreted by T cell lines and hybridomas, Adv. Immunol. **33**:73, 1982.

Came, P.E., and Carter, W.A., editors: Interferons and their applications, Berlin, 1984, Springer-Verlag, Berlin, Heidelberg.

Davis, M.M.: Molecular genetics of the T cell-receptor beta chain, Ann. Rev. Immunol. **3**:537, 1985.

Dinarello, C.A.: Interleukin 1, Rev. Infect. Dis. **6**:51, 1984.

Durum, S.K., Schmidt, J.A., and Oppenheim, J.J.: Interleukin 1: an immunological perspective, Ann. Rev. Immunol. **3**:263, 1985.

Friedman, R.M.: Interferons: a primer, Orlando, 1984, Academic Press, Inc.

Gillis, S.: Interleukin 2: biology and biochemistry, J. Clin. Immunol. **3**:1, 1983.

Goldstein, A.L., editor: Thymic hormones and lymphokines. In Basic chemistry and clinical applications, New York, 1984, Plenum Press.

Greene, W.C., and Leonard, W.C.: The human interleukin-2 receptor, Ann. Rev. Immunol. **4**:69, 1986.

Henry, K., and Farrer-Brown, C.: Color atlas of thymus and lymph node histopathology, Chicago, 1982, Year Book Medical Publishers, Inc.

Ihley, J.N., Lee, J.C., and Hapel, A.J.: Interleukin 3: biochemical and biological properties and possible roles in the regulation of immune responses, Lymphokines **6**:239, 1982.

Katz, D.H., editor: Monoclonal antibodies and T cell products, Boca Raton, 1982, CRC Press.

Kirkpatrick, C.H., Burger, D.R., and Lawrence, H.S., editors: Immunology of transfer factor, New York, 1983, Academic Press, Inc.

Kronenberg, M., Siu, G., Hood, L.E., and Shastri, N.: The molecular genetics of the T-cell antigen receptor and T-cell antigen recognition, Ann. Rev. Immunol. **4**:529, 1986.

Lengyel, P.: Biochemistry of interferons and their actions, Ann. Rev. Biochem. **51**:251, 1982.

Owen, M.J., and Collins, M.K.L.: The molecular biology of the T cell antigen receptor, Immunol. Let. **9**:175, 1985.

Paetkau, V., Bleackley, R.C., Riendeau, D., Harnish, D., and Holowachuk, E.W.: Toward the molecular biology of IL-2, Contemp. Top. Molec. Immunol. **10**:35, 1985.

Rocklin, R.E.: Properties and mechanism of action of human leukocyte migration factor, Lymphokines, **2**:163, 1981.

Robb, R.J.: Interleukin 2: the molecule and its function, Immunol. Today **5**:203, 1984.

Schader, J.W.: The panspecific hemopoietin of activated T lymphocytes (Interleukin 3), Ann. Rev. Immunol. **4**:205, 1986.

Schwartz, R.H.: T-lymphocyte recognition of antigen in association with gene products of the major histocompatibility complex, Ann. Rev. Immunol. **3**:237, 1985.

Smith, K.A.: Interleukin 2, Ann. Rev. Immunol. **2**:319, 1984.

Stutman, O.: Ontogeny of T cells, Clin. Immunol. Allergy **5**:191, 1985.

Stutman, O.: Postthymic T-cell development, Immunol. Rev. **91**:159, 1986.

Taylor-Papadimitriou, J., editor: Interferons, Oxford, 1985, Oxford University Press.

Waldmann, T.A.: The structure, function, and expression of interleukin-2 receptors on normal and malignant lymphocytes, Science **232**:727, 1986.

Webb, D.R.: The biochemistry of antigen-specific T-cell factors, Ann. Rev. Immunol. **1**:423, 1983.

Weiss, A., Imboden, J., Hardy, K., et al.: The role of the T3/antigen receptor complex in T-cell activation, Ann. Rev. Immunol. **4**:593, 1986.

See related **Reading 3,** page 418.

Cellular interactions in the immune response

≡ GLOSSARY

Contrasuppressor cell circuit   Relief of immunoglobulin suppression by T_{CS1}, T_{CS2} and T_{CS3} cells.

Suppressor cell circuit   Feedback inhibition of immunoglobulin synthesis via T_{S1}, T_{S2} and T_{S3} cells.

T_{CS1}, T_{CS2}, T_{CS3} Inducer, transducer, and effector contrasuppressor cells.

T_{S1}, T_{S2}, T_{S3} Inducer, transducer, and effector suppressor cells.

•   •   •

It would be very satisfying if the complexities of cell communication in the immune response were more completely understood than it is now. Each new intricacy of the immune system and the wealth of information about the interactions of immunoactive cells that has appeared in the last decade, have only served to remind us how complex the system is. Fortunately, a large number of immunologists are devoted to unraveling the mysteries of immunity, and the pace of discovery in this area of immunology is destined to continue its surge.

PURIFICATION OF ACTIVE CELLS

Numerous methods have been employed to harvest and separate macrophages, B cells, and T cells. Reconstitution of these cells into artificial mixtures allows investigators to identify the cellular requirements for the basic immunologic functions, examine behavioral alterations these cells exhibit when subjected to various stimuli, evaluate the separate cell subsets, and perform other important experiments.

Since macrophages have several properties not shared by lymphocytes, they can be prepared relatively free from these cells as contaminants. The in

vivo chemotactic response of macrophages facilitates their accumulation in the peritoneal cavity when it has been inoculated with irritants such as glycogen, starch, or mineral oil. Use of the last of these has been abandoned, since macrophages engulf droplets of the oil, and oils may interfere with subsequent assays. Macrophages collected under these conditions are activated and display the heightened responses of such cells. Resident macrophages can be collected by peritoneal lavage without prior stimulation, but the cell harvest is smaller. Bronchopulmonary lavage can be used to collect alveolar macrophages.

Depending on the procedure, the macrophage population will be contaminated with neutrophils, mast cells, and a few other cell types, including lymphocytes. The macrophages' ability to adhere to surfaces, which they use so efficiently in phagocytosis, leaves most contaminating cells free in the suspending fluid, with which they can be decanted (Fig. 8-1). The phagocytic activity for bacteria, yeasts, or other particles is useful in the enumeration of macrophage but also can be used to purify them from a mixed population. Macrophages that have ingested iron filings can be held in place by a magnetic force

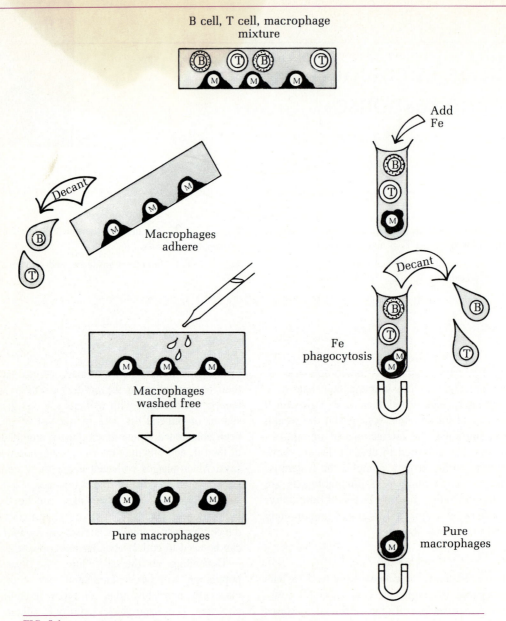

B cell, T cell, macrophage
mixture

Decant

Macrophages
adhere

Macrophages
washed free

Pure macrophages

Add
Fe

Decant

Fe
phagocytosis

Pure
macrophages

FIG. 8-1

The purification of macrophages is relatively simple, since they adhere to surfaces and engulf particles that aid in their recovery.

while other cells are washed away. Unfortunately iron-laden phagocytes are not useful in all studies.

Because B and T cells are so similar, they are more difficult to separate physically from each other than from macrophages. Purified B cell preparations

can be achieved by adding cytotoxic anti-Thy 1 sera and complement to B and T cell mixtures. The T cells will be lysed, and the B cells will remain free. Sheep cell rosetting by T cells likewise produces aggregates that can be separated physically from B

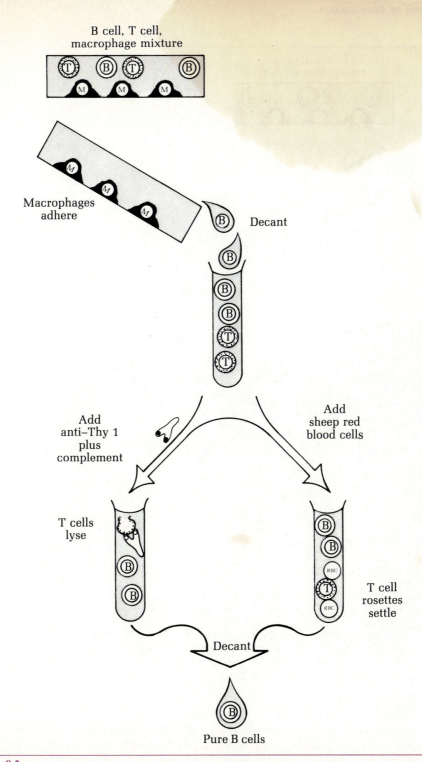

FIG. 8-2

One avenue toward the preparation of pure B cells is to eliminate the macrophages by adherence and then lyse the T cells with anti–Thy 1 sera and complement. A second approach is to sediment the T cells in rosettes, which leaves the B cells in suspension.

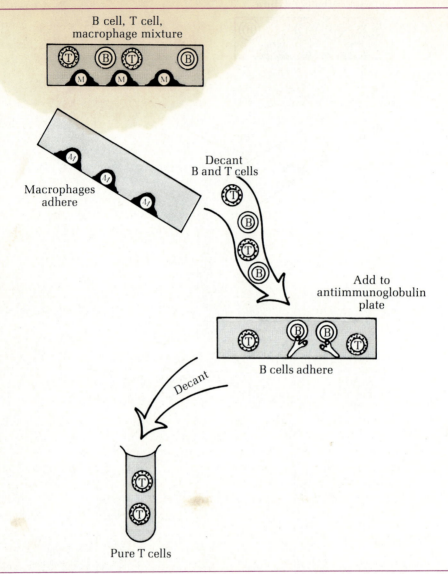

FIG. 8-3

Pure T cells can be prepared from macrophage-free preparations by panning B cells. In panning the immunoglobulin on the B cell surface is held to an antiimmunoglobulin on the pan. This holds the B cells firmly to the pan, facilitating recovery of the T cells.

cells (Fig. 8-2). The simplest procedure for securing pure T cells is "panning" (Fig. 8-3). Antibody molecules adhere spontaneously to glass or plastic surfaces, and B cells have immunoglobulins on their surfaces. If a dish is coated with an antibody to glob-

ulins, it will bind B cells to the dish so that pure T cells can be collected by decantation.

Harvesting functional subsets of B and T cells is also possible. Immunoadsorbent columns with antigen attached to an insoluble matrix bind B cells and T cells with a specificity for that antigen. The B cells bind quite avidly, but the T cells are easily displaced and become mixed with T cells that, lacking specificity for the antigen, passed through the column. Elution of the B cells is possible by percolating through the column small molecules that represent part of an antigenic determinant site. This is most simply done when hapten-antigen conjugates are used. B cells bound to a dinitrophenyl-antigen adsorbent column can be eluted with dinitrophenyl lysine, for example.

Hybridoma technology is an alternative approach to isolating antigen-specific B cells. Normally hybridomas responding to several epitopes can be recovered from cell fusions of plasmacytomas and immune spleen cells. Although heterogeneity is expressed in terms of epitopes this expression is more limited in terms of immunoglobulin class where IgM- and IgG-producing hybridomas far outnumber those producing the other immunoglobulins.

Hybridoma technology has had some success in providing clones of the functional subsets of T cells, and clones of T_H, T_{DTH}, and T_C cells, specific for a few antigens, are available. More usual is the sorting of T cells according to their surface markers after panning to remove macrophages and B cells. Anti Lyt 1^+ sera plus complement eliminates those cells and allows recovery of Lyt 2^+, T_C and T_S cells. Differences in sensitivity to cyclophosphamide has also been useful in enhancing the population of some cells. In the suppressor cell circuit, the final acting cell is more sensitive to cyclophosphamide than its precursor cells.

MACROPHAGE INTERACTIONS

Antigen processing and the transfer of antigenic determinants is a primary event in most B and T cell-regulated responses, though exceptions are known. Macrophages are usually responsible for this alteration in antigen structure.

With B cells

B cells have the important antigen receptors IgM and IgD on their exterior surfaces. Experiments have been reported in which the B cells used these immunoglobulins to capture free antigen and continue through antigen capping, interiorization, and processing without relying on the macrophage for these events. The immunologic dogma is contrary to this finding—surface immunoglobulins on B cells are used to effect the transfer of antigenic determinants from macrophages into its own sphere of activity. In addition to receiving antigen from macrophages, the B cell may respond to the monokine IL-2, though this response is more commonly seen in T cells.

Too often the reciprocal influence of the B cell on the macrophage is ignored, possibly because it is so well understood. It is simply the ability of immunoglobulins, especially the IgG isotypes, to bind to Fc receptors on macrophages. The importance of this in antigen processing is quite obvious.

With T cells

Activation of T cells is a multisignal event in which macrophages play a critical role. The type of macrophage involved depends on the nature of the T cell.

The communication of T_H and T_{DTH} cells with macrophages relies again on the presentation of processed cells by the latter to the Ti, antigen receptor. The human T3 and T4 proteins and the murine L3T4 protein are believed to participate in this communication—perhaps only by transducing the membrane signal but also possibly by strengthening the antigen bond to the Ti molecule.

This cooperation of T_H, T_{DTH} cells with macrophages is class II restricted. The antigen receptor on the T cell has the ability to recognize compatible I-A or I-E proteins simultaneously (Fig. 8-4). But even this acceptance of antigen and recognition of the proper Ia protein must be supplemented by the monokine IL-1 before T cell activation is complete. Only then do the T_H and T_{DTH} cells initiate IL-2 production, expand their bank of IL-2 receptors, proliferate and secrete other lymphokines.

Several of these lymphokines modify the behavior of macrophages. The macrophage chemotaxin, migration inhibition factor, and γ interferon function cooperatively to further enhance antigen processing. This bidirectional assistance of T cells and macrophages is thus self-amplifying as was the macrophage–B cell partnership.

The influence of macrophages on T_C cells is less

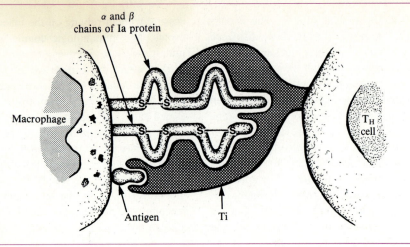

α and β
chains of Ia protein

Macrophage

T_H cell

Antigen   Ti

FIG. 8-4

The T_H cell has a single receptor, the Ti protein that simultaneously recognizes antigen and class II MHC proteins on an antigen-presenting macrophage.

clear. The need for antigen processing by these T cells is clouded. The antigen receptor on T cells differs from that on T_H cells by recognizing class I proteins of the MHC in the context of antigen (Fig. 8-5). Yet even this needs further clarification. The T_C cell responsible for the elimination of allografted cells must see in the class I protein both its nature as a foreign antigen and its position as a class I protein. It could if there are two functions of this class I receptor—a portion that potentially recognizes the α1 and α2 domains of the molecule as the foreign antigen and the α3 domain as its restricting domain. Such a view is compatible with sequence variation within these domains.

This possibility does not exist for the T_C cell that eliminates self cells that express viral antigens, tumor antigens, or other foreign, non-MHC antigens on their surfaces. The receptor on this T_C cell must recognize antigen as a structure altogether different from the class I protein and still be restricted by it, again possibly by its α3 domain.

Suppressor and contrasuppressor T cells interact with macrophages that carry, as these T cells themselves do, the I-J marker. Some of these macrophages may also have the Ia markers, particularly the macrophages that cooperate with T_{CS} cells. Thus there remain several unresolved aspects of T_S and

T_{CS} communication with macrophages. Foremost is the need for clarification of the nature of the I-J characteristic. What is a structure? Wherein resides its antigen specificity? Is the dual presence of Ia and I-J trivial or meaningful? The genetics of this marker is still not understood but is certainly not resident in the MHC as originally believed.

B cell interactions
With B cells

As yet, B cells exhibit no unequivocal need for cooperative stimuli from other B cells. This need may exist in terms of antibody feedback control or anti-idiotypic control, but these are self-control mechanisms and are not interactive between B cells. It is uncertain whether antigen presentation by B cells to other B cells is a significant event even though B cells may present antigen to T cells.

With T cells

If T cells do receive antigen from antigen-presenting B cells, it must be presented, as from macrophages, in association with I-A or I-E class II proteins. The activated helper cell presumably receives IL-1 from macrophages and produces IL-2, BCGF, BCDF and other essential soluble factors required by other T cells and B cells.

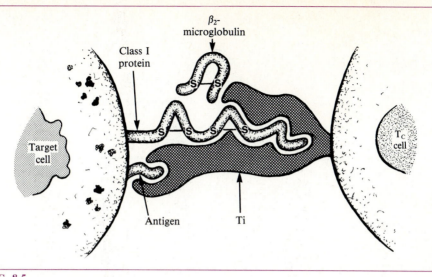

FIG. 8-5

The T_C cell recognizes antigen in the context of a class I MHC protein. The T_C cell may require an antigen presenting macrophage for its initial sensitization, but not for its subsequent cytolytic attack on the cellular antigen.

T cell interactions with other T cells

The reactions of T cells with each other can be thought of as directional, from the T_H to the T_{DTH}, T_C, T_S and T_{CS} cells, and within the network of T_C and T_{CS} cells.

From T_H cells

The role of IL-2 as a critical product of the T_H cell is seen in the need, of probably all other classes of T cells for this interleukin, though critical evidence for an effect of IL-2 on T_S and T_{CS} cells is still lacking. T_C cells, in contrast, after recognizing their target begin to develop IL-2 receptors, which must be satisfied by IL-2 before the cell becomes fully cytolytic.

The suppressor cell circuit. As briefly mentioned in Chapter 7, an integrated network of T_S cells is involved in the regulation of the T_H cell (Fig. 8-6). The initial cell in this network is T_{S1}, the first-order suppressor or suppressor inducer. Antigen from I-A$^+$ and I-J$^+$ macrophages plus IL-1 activate this T cell. This cell, though Lyt 1$^+$, differs from the T_H cell by the absence of L3T4 and the presence of I-J$^+$. The nature of this interaction by two I-J$^+$ cells is pre-sumably not based on the usual ligand-receptor interaction. The T_{S1} cell activates the second-order or suppressor transducer, the T_{S2} cell, by means of a soluble substance that is acted upon by an I-J$^+$ macrophage. This intervention by the macrophage is apparently an oxidative event necessary for the full expression of the suppressor substance or suppressor factor activity.

The T_{S2} cell is I-J$^+$ and Lyt 1$^+$2$^+$; it has an anti-idiotype receptor on its surface. These features distinguish the T_{S2} cell from other cells. A soluble factor acts directly on the final cell in the series, the effector or third-order suppressor cell, T_{S3}. This cell is Lyt 2$^+$, I-J$^+$ and responds to antigen presented by I-J$^+$ macrophages and the signal from T_{S2}. This cell is quite sensitive to cyclophosphamide. The T_{S3} cells suppress T_H, T_{DTH}, and T_C cells, but it is unknown if a single T_{S3} cell can affect all three of these. The suppression of B cells is believed to be mediated by the failure of T_H cells to continue production of BCGF and BCDF.

The human T_S system apparently functions in the same manner as the murine system with T4$^+$ inducers eventually generating T8$^+$ suppressors.

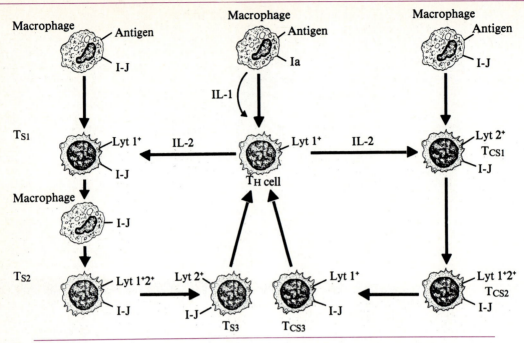

FIG. 8-6

The suppressor and contrasuppressor circuits involve I-J$^+$, antigen presenting macrophages. On the left, the suppressor circuit of T_{S1}, macrophage, T_{S2} and T_{S3} are shown, on the right, the T_{CS1}, T_{CS2} and T_{CS3} are illustrated. Note that an intermediate Lyt 1^+2^+ cell is common to both pathways. The T_H cell (center) stimulates one or the other circuit depending on the strength of its message from the effector T_S or T_{CS} cell.

The contrasuppressor cell circuit. A contrasuppressor circuit that incorporates inducer, transducer, and effector (or first-, second-, and third-order) cells with different surface markers closely parallels the T_S circuit. The contrasuppressor pathway is initiated by an Lyt 2^+, I-J$^+$ cell. Its message, presumably a soluble factor, acts without the intervention of a macrophage on the transducer Lyt 1^+2^+, I-J$^+$ lymphocyte. Notice that the suppressor inducer and the contrasuppressor inducer have identical features. Whether it becomes an Lyt 1^+ (L3T4$^-$) I-J$^+$ contrasuppressor or an Lyt 2^+, I-J$^+$ suppressor depends on the comparative strength of the suppressor and contrasuppressor inducer signals. When the latter is more potent, the T_{CS2} produces a soluble factor that creates the Lyt 1^+, I-J$^+$ effector cell. This T_{CS3} cell is L3T4$^-$ (a few experiments report otherwise, how-

ever) and is not a T_H cell. It also differs from T_H cells by binding to *Vicia villosa* lectin. The T_{CS3} cell does not inhibit T_S cells but rather T_H, T_{DTH}, and probably T_C and B cells.

CONCLUSION

The suppressor and contrasuppressor cell circuits both have an Lyt 1^+2^+ lymphocyte as a central intermediary. As we know this is the cell that, when lacking the I-J characteristic, is the precursor cell of T_H and T_{DTH}, both Lyt 1^+, and the Lyt 2^+ T_C cell. It is curious that the I-J protein should have such a powerful influence on a cell's activity, in essence converting a Lyt 1^+ T_H cell to a contrasuppressor, or a T_C cell to a T_S cell. It seems likely that the true lineage of cells bearing or lacking the I-J marker will differ and that the difference in the behavior of these cells will not be explained by the simple addition or removal of a protein from the cell surface.

It is also clear that there are many other details within the suppressor and contrasuppressor circuits that still must be understood before we can use these pathways in the repair of immunodeficiencies or treatment of autoimmune disease. At least a half dozen soluble factors, none of which has yet been adequately described, must participate in these pathways. There is already evidence that two classes of T_H cells exist, one being $L3T4^+$ and the other $L3T4^-$ but bearing an Ia protein. Which of these is most influenced by the contrasuppressor or suppressor factors? Where do the Lyb 5 B cells fit into this scheme? The old axiom remains true, the more we know, the more we need to know.

REFERENCES

Asherson, G.L., Colizzi, V., and Zembala, M.: An overview of T-suppressor cell circuits, Ann. Rev. Immunol. **4:**37, 1986.

Dingle, J.T., and Gordon, J.L., editors: Cellular interactions, Amsterdam, 1981, Elsevier/North-Holland, Biomedical Press.

Dorf, M.E., and Benacerraf, B.: Suppressor cells and immunoregulation, Ann. Rev. Immunol. **2:**127, 1984.

Fathman, C., and Fitch, F.W., editors: Isolation, characterization and utilization of T lymphocyte clones, New York, 1982, Academic Press, Inc.

Feldman, M., and Mitchison, N.A.: Immune regulation, Clifton, NJ, 1985, The Humana Press, Inc.

Green, D.R., Flood, P.M., and Gershon, R.K.: Immunoregulatory T-cell pathways, Ann. Rev. Immunol. **1:**439, 1983.

Kapp, J.A.: Antigen-specific suppressor T-cell factors, Hosp. Pract., August 1984.

Krensky, A.M.: Lymphocyte subsets and surface molecules in man, Clin. Immunol. Rev. **4:**95, 1985.

Resch, K., and Kirchner, H., editors: Mechanisms of lymphocyte activation, Amsterdam, 1981, Elsevier/North-Holland Press.

Smith, K.A., and Ruscetti, F.W.: T-cell growth factor and the culture of cloned functional T cells, Adv. Immunol. **31:**137, 1981.

vanBoehmer, H., and Haas, W., editors: T cell clones, Amsterdam, 1985, Elsevier Sciences Publishers, B.V. (Biomedical Division).

Biologic aspects
of the immune response

alkylating agent An agent that reacts with electronegative centers in another compound and forms covalent
bonds with it during the reaction; such compounds are
often immunosuppressants.

anamnestic response The rapid rise in immunoglobulin
following a second or subsequent exposure to antigen;
synonymous with *booster* or *secondary response*.

antigen competition Failure of a mixture of antigens to
produce an antiserum as highly titered to one or more of
the antigens, as when the antigens are administered singly.

antilymphocyte serum (ALS) An antiserum prepared
against lymphocytes of either the B or T type, or (usually) a mixture of them.

booster response *see* Anamnestic response.

clonal selection theory A theory of immunoglobulin formation suggesting that an antigen causes the replication
of a cell to form a clone of cells producing antibody to
that antigen.

corticosteroids Natural (or synthetic) compounds from
the adrenal cortex that are antiinflammatory and immunosuppressive.

folic acid antagonist Structural analogs of folic acid that
function as immunosuppressants, such as aminopterin
and methotrexate.

germinal center A discrete cellular structure in lymphoid organs of antigenically stimulated animals containing macrophages, T or B lymphocytes, and plasma
cells.

immunologic tolerance A failure or depression in the
immune response on exposure to antigen, especially
massive doses.

immune suppression Suppression of an immunologic
response by chemical, physical, or biologic means.

memory cell A cell that responds more quickly to the
second exposure to antigen than to the primary exposure; responsible for the anamnestic response.

purine and pyrimidine analog Structural analogs of the
bases of DNA and RNA that function as immunosuppressants.

The primary focus of this chapter is immunoglobulins and the kinetics of their response to antigen. It
also considers theories about their formation and
about immunosuppression, elaborating on the chemistry and genetics of the immunoglobulins discussed
in Chapter 3.

IMMUNOGLOBULIN RESPONSE

The injection of an antigen into an animal may
initiate several important changes. The immunoglob

ulin response is to some extent preceded by a period
of antigen elimination. These two topics introduce us
to other biologic aspects of the immunoglobulins.

Antigen elimination curve

For intravenously injected antigen, three phases
of antigen removal are easily detected (Fig. 9-1).
The first phase occupies only 10 to 20 minutes if
particulate antigens are used and represents the time
required for equilibration of the antigen with tissues

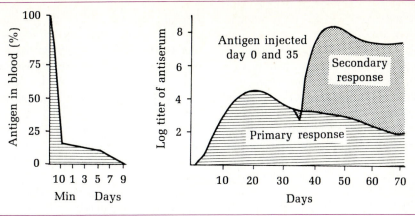

FIG. 9-1

Antigen decay (elimination) and primary and secondary immunoglobulin formation curves. The antigen elimination curve shows the three phases of equilibration, metabolic elimination, and immune elimination, the last beginning at about the fifth day. Circulating immunoglobulins are not detectable until about the fifth day. Notice how the secondary immunoglobulin response following the readministration of antigen at the thirty-fifth day reaches a very high titer compared with the primary response.

and fluids. Because of extensive phagocytosis in the liver, lung, and spleen, nearly 90% of the antigen is removed from the circulation in its first passage through these organs. Examination of sections from these tissues shortly after antigen administration will reveal that the macrophages have become engorged with antigen. Soluble antigens are not removed from the blood quite so quickly because of their slower pinocytic uptake by cells. If the antigen is aggregated, it is removed more quickly, indicating that size is important in phagocytosis and pinocytosis.

The second phase of antigen elimination is a phase of gradual catabolic degradation and removal of the antigen. This phase lasts for 4 to 7 days, and represents the gradual enzymatic hydrolysis and digestion of the antigen. Consequently, the limits of this period are regulated by the enzymatic capability of the host for the particular type of substrate that the antigen represents. Polysaccharide antigens survive for fairly long periods in rabbits. The extended half-life of poly-D amino acids is explained by the fact that most animals are deficient in enzymes that can degrade unnatural stereoisomers of amino acids. In animals that fail to produce antibody (that is, they become tolerant to the antigen), this second phase is

extended for several weeks and represents the last phase of the antigen elimination curve.

The third portion of the curve, in which there is again an accelerated removal of antigen, is the immune elimination segment. This phase is the result of the combination of newly formed antibody molecules with the antigen, enhancing phagocytic engulfment, digestion, and removal of the antigen. Although the antigen decay shown in Fig. 9-1 progresses to zero between the fifth and fourteenth days, this is meant to reflect only the quantity of detectable antigen in blood. The absolute removal of all antigen from an immunized animal can take many months or years. Certainly, as serologic and chemical tests of greater and greater sensitivity have been applied to the detection of antigen in vivo, antigen has been recovered for longer periods of time after injection.

Immunoglobulin formation
Primary response

By restricting this discussion to the appearance and total quantity of antibodies in the blood, and by not considering the individual immunoglobulins, the antibody response plotted against time will approximate the curve seen in Fig. 9-1. After the first injection of antigen, there is a lag of several days before antibody is detectable. This latent period, or induction period, varies from several hours to several days, depending on the kind and amount of antigen given, the route of administration, the species of animal and its health, and the sensitivity of the test used to measure the antibody. Antibody should appear sometime between the fifth and the tenth day.

The latent period is not a reflection of the time it takes to begin antibody production at the cellular level. When antibody-forming cells are removed from the immunized animal, antibody synthesis can be detected within 20 minutes after the exposure to antigen. Since only a few cells are producing antibody at this time, it may take several days before antibody is measurable in the blood. Another important consideration is that the first antibody molecules to appear in the blood usually react with residual antigen still in the circulation. Excretion of these antigen-antibody complexes will be rapid, so the first evidence of free antibody is not seen until a few days after the first antibody molecules are introduced into the bloodstream.

As the latent period ends, the primary antibody response becomes visible. The titer of antibody gradually increases over a period of a few days to a few weeks, plateaus, and begins to drop. The general shape of the primary response curve is the typical sigmoid curve, with an extended decay phase. The exact shape of the response curve is dictated by many variables.

Secondary response

If the same animal is subsequently exposed to additional antigen, the antibody response differs dramatically from the primary antibody response. This secondary response first consists of a sharp drop in circulating antibody because it complexes with the newly injected antigen. Immediately thereafter, certainly within 2 or 3 days under ordinary circumstances, a marked increase in the antibody content of the blood becomes evident. This increase continues for several days, and ultimately the titer far surpasses that of the primary response. The secondary response is often called the memory, anamnestic (without forgetting), or booster response. It is as though the previously immunized animal becomes primed for that antigen and is prepared to respond to it in an accelerated way. All the variables that regulate the primary response also influence the booster response to some degree, but the booster response has an abbreviated latent period, a heightened titer, and an extended duration of detectable antibody, when compared with the primary response curve (Fig. 9-1).

Several interesting facts about the anamnestic response should be cited.

1. The anamnestic response is not the result of a sudden release of preformed antibody that has been stored; it is the result of the bulk synthesis of new antibody. This theory has been proven in experiments in which a radiolabeled amino acid is injected at the same time as the antigen. When the antibody is studied after a few days, it is found to be heavily labeled with isotope, indicating that it was produced recently.

2. The anamnestic response may be induced at almost any time after the primary response. Even many years after the primary response, when the primary titer has dropped to zero, the anamnestic response is still inducible. It may not be quite as striking as a booster nearer in time to the initial response, but the true secondary response will develop.

3. The secondary response is repeatable many times until the physiologic limit of that particular animal to that particular antigen is reached.

4. Cross-reactive antigens will induce the response. In this case the degree of anamnesis will be correlated with the sameness of the two antigens; the more they are alike, the better the response.

5. Nonspecific anamnesis may occur. Antibody originates in lymphoid tissue. Any treatment of the immunized animal that causes lysis or hyperplasia of the antibody-forming cells will cause a (minimal) anamnestic response.

6. The decrease in antibody titer after the secondary response is more gradual than the decrease after the primary response. One reason is that more cells are involved in antibody production in the secondary antibody response. If some of these cells are rela-

tively long lived and continue functioning, then anti-body will be formed over a longer period after the secondary than after the primary response. Another reason is that the antiserum seen in the secondary response is qualitatively different from that seen after the initial response. It contains relatively more IgG, which has a half-life of 25 to 35 days. The primary antiserum is relatively rich in IgM, which has a half-life of only 8 to 10 days. The relative contribution of IgG and IgM to the primary and secondary response is illustrated in Fig. 9-2. The IgM secondary response in only one tenth that of IgG; for this reason hyperimmune sera are predominantly IgG in nature. IgG has been referred to as the memory component, implying that IgM anamnesis does not occur. This is true in a relative sense only, since secondary IgM levels are in fact somewhat greater than primary levels.

7. Reactivation of the immunoglobulin response is not entirely without danger, especially when soluble antigens or autocoupling haptens are employed. Immunoglobulin E formed in response to the primary injection of antigen is distributed through the blood stream from which it enters into the tissues where it adsorbs to the surface of mast cells. Since soluble antigens given in the booster injection can also diffuse readily into tissues, this antigen can com-bine with the mast cell–bound IgE, with disastrous consequences. This effect is due to the release of pharmacologic agents from the mast cell, as the result of the serologic reaction on its surface. If a sufficient concentration of these reagents is achieved, the animal may die of anaphylactic shock (Chapter 17).

8. The anamnestic response and the primary response are blended when adjuvant is combined with antigen in the primary immunization. Antibody will appear after about the same latent period and will rise at about the same rate, but will continue to rise over an extended period compared with the usual primary response. Enhancing the immune response by incorporating the antigen into an adjuvant-antigen mixture is a very practical way to spare expensive antigens, since small quantities of the mixture will ensure high-titer antisera. The application of adjuvant-antigen mixtures in immunization against infectious diseases creates a better and longer-lasting immunity.

REGULATING IMMUNOGLOBULIN SYNTHESIS—THE IDIOTYPIC NETWORK

How does the body control the synthesis of immunoglobulins? Certainly there is a physiologic limit to antibody synthesis that an animal will not exceed, and further booster doses of antigen will prove non-

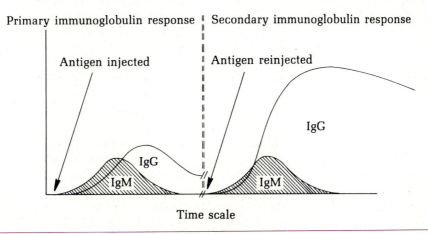

Primary immunoglobulin response   Secondary immunoglobulin response

Antigen injected

Antigen reinjected

IgG

IgG

IgM

IgM

Time scale

FIG. 9-2

Difference in the IgG response to primary and secondary exposure to antigen indicates why it is termed the memory antibody. IgM, illustrated to exhibit no "memory" usually shows a slight anamnestic response.

productive. Several explanations have been forwarded to account for the slowdown in antibody synthesis.

One possibility is that the high concentration of circulating antibody itself functions as a feedback inhibitor to cause a halt in antibody synthesis. This is described more fully later in this chapter. A better understood mechanism is the adjustment of the population of functionally different T cells during the course of the immunoglobulin response, as described in Chapter 7. This brings us to the third method, known as *the idiotypic network*.

When an antibody is produced in response to an antigen, the antibody contains HV regions with unique amino acid sequences, which create the combining site for that antigen. These idiotypic HV regions are unique antigenic determinants which the animal has not previously confronted; therefore the animal responds with an antiidiotypic antibody. But even the antiidiotypic antibody contains unique idiotypic regions, and these stimulate a second generation of antiidiotypic antibody. In this process, a sequence of antiidiotypic globulins are formed, each capable of reacting with the previous one in the sequence. This sequence of serologic reactions serves to slow or halt antibody synthesis, as first suggested by Jerne. Support for Jerne's network theory emerged over the past decade, and contributed to his Nobel award in 1984. The presence of autoreactive immunoglobulins, specific for one's own immunoglobulin, was originally described by Oudin during his studies of rabbit globulins. Jerne foresaw the antiidiotypic response as a means of self-regulation of the antibody response. Thermodynamic principles indicated that each subsequent antiidiotypic antibody would be less potent—either by loss of specificity or diminished concentration—than its predecessor, thus ensuring a gradual decay in the system.

The antigenicity of idiotypic determinants has found a practical expression in the use of antiidiotypic molecules as a replacement for antigen for use as immunizing agents to control infectious diseases (Chapter 14).

ANTIBODY PRODUCTION BY SINGLE CELLS

Study of antibody formation at the cellular level has been very informative in several ways; it has identified the cells involved in this unique kind of protein synthesis, has helped to estimate the time after antigen stimulation that antibody synthesis begins, has aided in evaluating how adjuvants function at the cellular level, has indicated the limitations on the kinds of antibody synthesized by a single cell, and has contributed to the solution of other immunobiologic problems.

Single cell techniques for studying antibody synthesis have come and gone, but the agar plaque technique of Jerne for identifying plaque-forming cells (PFCs) remains in use. The development of this technique also contributed to Jerne's recent Nobel Prize.

PFCs

The agar plaque technique devised by Jerne is the most widely applied single cell technique. In this method, individual cells from lymphoid tissue or from the spleen of the immune animal are plated in a nutrient agar with erythrocytes of the type used in the immunization. The tissue culture medium supports the growth and excretion of antibody by the antibody-synthesizing cells. These antibodies diffuse radially from their originating cell and attach to the neighboring erythrocytes. Serum complement in the form of normal guinea pig serum is added; this promotes lysis of the red blood cells which have become coated with antibody. Consequently a clear area, or plaque, develops around the antibody-forming cell against the light red, erythrocyte-laden background (Fig. 9-3). The PFC is usually a plasmacyte, but lymphocytes sometimes are seen. Macrophages or other antibody-absorbing cells are rarely seen.

By the original Jerne procedure only IgM-forming cells are detected; this is because of the feeble complement-binding and lytic activity of IgG antibody. However, IgG PFCs can be observed by flooding the plate with an antibody to γ-globulin prior to the addition of complement. This antiglobulin, or indirect, procedure actually detects both IgM and IgG plaques, so duplicate plates must be prepared. The IgG cells then must be calculated by computing the difference.

Nonerythrocytic antigens can be used if they are adsorbed onto erythrocytes. There are many techniques for coupling soluble antigens to erythrocytes,

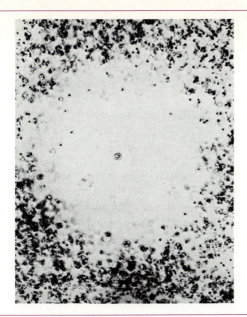

FIG. 9-3
A PFC in the center of a cleared area resulting from anti-body from the PFC and complement lysis of the surrounding erythrocytes. (From Jerne, N.K. In Amos, B., and Kaprowski, H.: Cell-bound antibodies, Philadelphia, 1963, Wistar University Press.)

so this is not a severe handicap. Bacterial cells of the gram-negative type can be used, since they too are lysed by antibody and complement. In one such study, after immunization of human subjects with *Salmonella typhi* vaccine, peripheral blood leukocytes produced 57 direct plaques and 570 indirect plaques per 10^6 leukocytes. From animal spleen cells, 10 to 100 times more plaques are often recovered.

The plaque-forming method has been used to determine the time that cells become primed for antibody formation. Within a few hours after the injection of polysaccharides, rabbits have PFCs in abundance. The influence of immunosuppressant drugs can be examined at the cellular level by the PFC procedure. The opposite effect, that of adjuvanticity, has also been studied. Kinetic studies of antibody-forming cells in culture indicate that spleen cells produce about 10μg of antibody per gram of spleen per hour; this is roughly equivalent to two molecules per second per lymphoid cell.

Monoclonal hybridomas

In 1965, the first report of an immunoglobulin-secreting hybridoma was published. Since that time, it has been recognized as one of the most significant advances in modern immunology. This was acknowledged by the fact that Köhler and Milstein received the Nobel Prize in 1984 for developing this technique. The improvements in creating hybridomas have relied primarily on the selection of the myeloma cells to be used; otherwise the procedure is much the same as originally described.

The hybridoma cells are created by a fusion of spleen cells from an immunized mouse with a mouse myeloma cell line (Fig. 9-4). The myeloma cells grow in normal culture media but fail to grow in a HAT (hypoxanthine, aminopterin, and thymidine) medium. The myeloma cells fail to grow in this medium because they lack the enzyme hypoxanthine phosphoribosyl transferase. The spleen cells fail to grow in HAT medium or other media because they are not a continuous cell line. Approximately equal numbers of spleen and myeloma cells are fused in the presence of PEG (polyethylene glycol). This has replaced the viruses previously used as the fusing agent. Electrofusion as a technique for forcing cell combination is superior to, but has not yet replaced, the PEG method because it requires a special apparatus to achieve fusion. PEG allows the cytoplasmic membranes of the two cell types to become more liquid. Contiguous cells may "melt," and when the PEG is removed, the membranes "freeze" again. The cell mixture is then plated on HAT medium. The spleen cells and any spleen-spleen doublets die a natural death. The myeloma cells (or myeloma-myeloma doublets) fail to grow because they lack the hypoxanthine transferase needed to overcome the medium. The hybridomas have the needed hypoxanthine transferase derived from the spleen cells, plus the growth capacity of the myeloma cell; consequently, only the hybridoma cells grow. The clones that develop are screened for antibody production, and these may represent 10% of all the clones. Positive clones are propagated from single cell preparations and reexamined to ensure that they have not lost their immunoglobulin-producing capacity. During growth in culture, approximately 10 to 100 μg/ml of specific antibody may be formed. The hybridoma

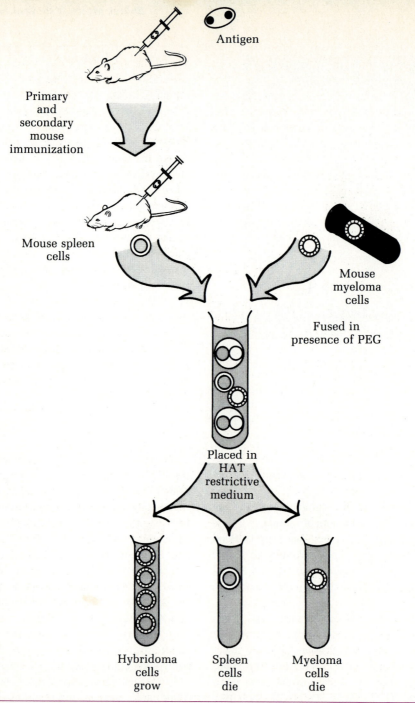

Antigen

Primary
and
secondary
mouse
immunization

Mouse spleen
cells

Mouse
myeloma
cells

Fused in
presence of PEG

Placed in
HAT
restrictive
medium

Hybridoma
cells
grow

Spleen
cells
die

Myeloma
cells
die

FIG. 9-4

The construction of a hybridoma begins with a primary immunization of a mouse, followed by a
booster injection to ensure that a high density of antibody-forming cells will be present in the
spleen. These are fused with nonsecreting myeloma cells and then plated in a restrictive medium.
Only the hybridoma cells grow in this medium, where they synthesize and secrete a monoclonal
immunoglobulin specific for a single determinant on the antigen.

cells will produce tumors in mice, since they are derived from plasmacytomas, and in the ascites fluid (or serum) 5 to 20 mg/ml of specific antibody may be present. These hybridomas may be perpetuated by transfers in mice or frozen as stock cultures.

In the original experiments both the spleen cells and myeloma cells were antibody producers, so it was necessary to examine the hybridoma not simply for the production of γ-globulin, but also for the production of antibody-specific for the antigen used to immunize the mouse. Later it was possible to use mutant myeloma cells that had lost their immunoglobulin-synthesizing function. Hybrids produced from these cells secrete a single molecular form of antibody, specific for the antigen used in the immunization.

Hybridoma antibodies provide many advantages for immunologic research. Of major importance is the ability to get pure antibody from a crude antigen preparation. The hybridomas can even make antibodies to antigens that are not detectable by conventional means. Heretofore, it was always necessary to purify the antigen to secure a pure antiserum. Moreover, the hybridoma antibody is of a single immunoglobulin class and specific for a single epitope, since it arises from a single cell. Depending on the nature of the antigen, an antiserum normally contains antibodies of many different classes and specificites. The class composition of an antiserum fluctates with the intensity and time of immunization, whereas the hybridoma product is constant. In addition, by selecting and analyzing the several hybridomas secured from one fusion, it is possible to recover antibodies that are specific for different determinants of the antigen so that antigen mapping can be done.

Another advantage of the hybridoma antibody is that it is always available from stock cells whenever needed, and it will be exactly the same as it was before. A new antiserum, even though prepared in the same species with the same immunization program, rarely will be the same as that produced in an earlier phase of the study.

Since the hybridoma cell line can be manipulated after pure cloning, one can study mutations in antibody-producing cells as they are expressed in terms of rate, antibody structure, antibody specificity, binding affinity, biologic activities such as cytotropism and complement activation, class switch, and other mutations.

Human lymphoblastoid cell lines have been fused with mouse myeloma cells to produce human immunoglobulin-secreting hybridomas. By careful selection of the lymphoblastoid cell line and examination of the hybridoma for the expression of immunoglobulin synthesis coupled with chromosome analysis, it has been demonstrated that human chromosome 14 contains the genes for heavy-chain synthesis. The human κ-chain gene is on chromosome 2 and the λ-chain gene on chromosome 22. In mice the κ-chain genes are on chromosome 6 and the H chain genes on chromosome 12.

The hybridoma technique provides a novel avenue for investigating the antigenic nature of infectious agents, tumor antigens, histocompatibility antigens, and maturation of differentiation antigens and provides reagents of a purity never before available to immunologists for research and routine serology.

THEORIES OF IMMUNOGLOBULIN FORMATION
The clonal selection theory

The current theories of antibody formation are modifications of either Ehrlich's original receptor theory or of the template theory. The template theory is an example of an instructive theory which assumes that the antigen can inform a cell in some way to make an antibody against that antigen. However, few immunologists support the instructive theory. The contrasting assumption is that a cell is naturally endowed with the ability to make the specific antibody. This is a selective type of theory; its modern form is known as the clonal selection theory.

The earliest form of the selective theory, Ehrlich's receptor hypothesis, supposed that certain cells possess specific surface receptors for antigens. These are present in the normal, nonimmunized animal. When an antigen is injected and reaches the proper fitting receptor, it will combine with that receptor. The receptor then breaks off the cell, enters the blood, dissociates from the antigen, and exists as the free-circulating antibody molecule. A new receptor is formed in its place, and the process is repeated, the result of which is the appearance of antibody in the blood following the injection of antigen. The discovery of surface IgM and IgD on immature B cells, plus the presence of PFCs in animals not previously exposed to antigen provides contemporary support for the selective theory. Again, Jerne's name must be mentioned as an important contributor to the modern form of the selective theory.

Burnet gradually evolved a modification of this selective theory of antibody formation, which became the clonal selection theory. (A clone is a population of cells arising from a single parent cell.) The present form of the clonal theory is essentially the following: in the mature animal the lymphocyte is genetically endowed with the capability of synthesizing immunoglobulins. At rest, unstimulated by antigen, only small amounts of immunoglobulin are made. This is found as surface IgM and IgD on the lymphocyte. On contact with the corresponding antigen, lymphocyte capping heralds a change of that lymphocyte to reproduce and differentiate into a clone of immunoglobulin-secreting plasma cells. The resulting clone of cells would consist of a large enough population that the antibody produced would become measurable in the blood.

What are the sources of support for the clonal theory? (1) Morphologically, there is strong support. When antibody-forming cells are identified in highly stimulated animals, either by fluorescent antibody or by plaque-forming tests, the cells tend to be clustered in groups. By light microscopy, these clones are seen as a part of typical germinal centers with dividing cells in the center, and lymphocytes, immunoblasts, and plasma cells situated at the periphery (Fig. 9-5). (2) Clonal theories are harmonious with the kinetics of the immune response in both its primary and anamnestic phases. The latent period of the primary phase represents the time required for the transformation of lymphocytes into plasma cells and memory cells. Separate clones of cells corresponding to each type of antibody (IgG, IgA, and IgM) and for each determinant of the antigen must be generated. (3) Cell transition, so vitally a part of the clonal theory, explains the different effects of immunosuppressant drugs on the immune response before and after antigen stimulation and on the pri-

mary and secondary responses. The precursor cell is sensitive to these chemicals, but after contact with antigen it transforms to a resistant cell. The survival of this resistant cell until a subsequent antigenic exposure, followed by another reproductive spurt, would account for the known resistance of the anamnestic response to immunosuppression. (4) The recognition that B cells from normal, nonimmunized animals have IgM and IgD molecules scattered over their surface has been taken as physical evidence of the receptors first postulated by Ehrlich and incorporated into the selective theories of antibody formation. (5) A recent source of support for the clonal theory has been the discovery that embryonic cells do contain structural genes for immunoglobulins prior to exposure to antigen, and that mature cells use the same biochemical processes to synthesize immunoglobulins which they use for the synthesis of other proteins.

The instructive theory

The principal contrasting theory to the clonal theory of antibody formation is the instructive, or template, theory. Several forms of this theory appeared almost simultaneously from 1930 to 1932. The basic tenet of all instructive theories is that the antigen enters a cell that is routinely engaged in normal γ-globulin synthesis. The antigen interferes with this process, possibly by complexing with mRNA in the polysome. The result is an adjustment in protein synthesis so that the globulin becomes molded into a complementary form with the antigen and therefore becomes an antibody globulin. The antibody dissociates from the antigen and is excreted into the blood. The antigen is retained and serves as the template for continued antibody synthesis.

Some of the arguments for and against instructive theories are the following.

1. How does each antigenic determinant have the same mRNA-binding ability when some 10^4 to 10^8 such determinants exist? Why fragments of all proteins and polysaccharides should bind to DNA or RNA and stimulate antibody formation cannot be readily explained by currently known biochemical reactions. On this basis, template theories tend to be incompatible with biochemical knowledge.

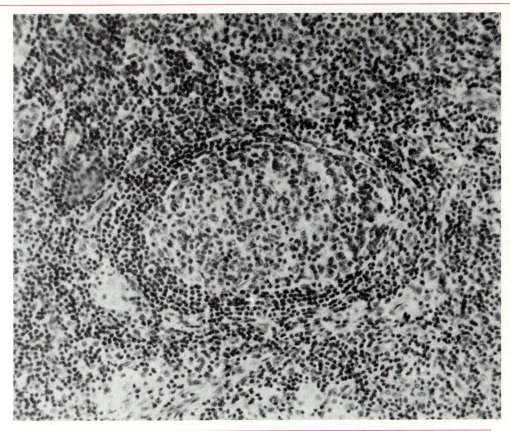

FIG. 9-5
This view of a germinal center clearly illustrates the self-containment of a clone of immunoglobulin-secreting cells within a perimeter of aligned cells.

2. Experimental immunologic tolerance is not explained by the template theory. In this condition, an abundance of antigen is present. Thus one might expect that a prime immune response would follow, yet the opposite is the case; antibody synthesis is impaired.

IMMUNOSUPPRESSION

A reduction in the activities of macrophages and B and T lymphocytes, measured as a lowered capacity to phagocytose or to produce immunoglobulins or lymphokines, is the property of immunosuppressives. These functions can be limited by three types of action: physical, chemical, or biologic means.

Physical immunosuppression
Radiation

Radiation immunology began in 1908 when it was discovered that the primary antibody response of rabbits to injections of whole serum was depressed by x rays.

Many variations of the initial experiment have been performed to measure the effects of x rays on the primary immune response. The two immunosuppressing effects observed are an extended latent period, associated with a prolonged antigen elimination curve, and decreased antibody titers. B cells have proven to be more sensitive to irradiation than T cells. Protection of the major lymphoid organs by lead shields preserves the animals immune capacity. Sublethal doses of x rays, which amount to 400 to 500 R for most laboratory animals, impair the immune response when given not more than 4 days prior to the antigen. X rays are less effective if given with the antigen and have a much reduced effect if given after the antigen. The irradiation is best given as a single dose rather than in fractionated doses. This impairment of antibody synthesis is transient; partial recovery is obvious after 1 week, and recovery is complete at 2 months.

Surgery

Antibodies are produced by the joint action of macrophages and lymphoid tissues; the physical removal of these tissues from an animal will impair its response to antigen. Because macrophages are widely dispersed, it is physically impossible to locate and remove all these cells. Lymphoid tissue also is widely distributed throughout the body but tends to exist in concentrated packets in special organs: lymph nodes, bone marrow, tonsil, appendix, thymus, Peyer's patches, spleen, and elsewhere. As a consequence of this clustering, it is more feasible to extirpate it, or sizable parts of it, than to remove phagocytic cells. When such removal is performed, an impairment of the immune response is noted.

Surgical extirpation of the mammalian thymus has a pronounced effect on the immune status of the animal, provided the surgery is properly timed with the maturation of the animal. In general, this means that surgery must be performed as soon after the birth of the animal as possible, although with slowly developing species (rabbits, hamsters) surgery after a few days will still illustrate the immunologic deficit. Care must be taken to remove the thymus without damaging the thyroid and parathyroid glands.

Among the most notable results of neonatal mammalian thymectomy is the wasting disease syndrome. This can be described simply as a failure to thrive. Young mice display a decreased growth rate and become listless, their hair becomes coarse and dirty, and premature death often associated with diarrhea ensues. Wasting disease reflects a novel and marked susceptibility to infectious disease, since germ-free mice do not exhibit wasting disease, and antibiotic treatment and good animal care procedures reduce the incidence of wasting disease.

Young bursectomized birds also develop wasting disease. This is clearly a result of the loss of B cells, which are the parents of the immunoglobulin-forming plasma cells. The earlier the bursa is removed from the chick or chick embryo, the greater is the deficit in the immunoglobulin response. If the developing chick embryo is treated with 19-nortestosterone, the bursa fails to develop during embryogenesis. Such hormonally bursectomized birds fail to develop an adequate immunoglobulin response. Bursectomy does not seriously affect any aspect of the immune response other than immunoglobulin synthesis.

Surgical or hormonal inhibition of the bursal equivalent centers is not possible in mammals as it is in birds, although a combination of x radiation and cyclophosphamide treatment is known for its central attack on B cell centers.

Chemical methods

A chemical that depresses any aspect of the immune response may be defined as an immunosuppressive. The application of the definition is not difficult when the activities of B and T lymphocytes are being examined, but becomes confused when the influence of chemical substances on factors related to natural resistance, such as iron concentration, action of ciliated cells in the respiratory tract, synthesis of the components of complement, motility of phagocytes (chemotaxis), and similar factors are considered. This conflict is avoided if the definition is restricted to the adaptive phases of the immune response.

Many variables can influence the success of immunosuppressant therapy: the drug, the amount of the drug used, the route of administration, the schedule of administration, the time in relation to the exposure to antigen, the form of the antigen (soluble versus aggregated versus cellular), and the species of animal, to name a few. Even when the desired effect is reached, the general cytotoxic nature of many of the compounds demands the careful observation of the individual for the emergence of infectious diseases or tumors, since host resistance to these decreases in the immunosuppressed condition.

By this time the question, "What is the benefit of immunosuppressants?" is often posed. It is obvious that their use will provide no survival benefit to the normal animal; however, for the abnormal animal suffering from an autoimmune disease or undergoing a graft rejection reaction, immunodepressants are of considerable benefit. They may not be totally curative, but a clearer understanding of their action eventually may lead to the discovery of a totally effective and safe immunosuppressive therapy.

Corticosteroids

The glucocorticoids, so named because of their pronounced effect on glucose metabolism and their origin from the adrenal cortex, are more generally known as the corticosteroids because of their tissue of origin and typical steroidal chemical structure (Fig. 9-6). Cortisol is the major natural corticoste-

roid of humans and corticosterone that of rodents. These are the primary natural steroids which have been used in immunologic experimentation. A large number of synthetic or semisynthetic steroids, including prednisone, prednisolone, methylprednisolone, triamcinolone, and dexamethasone, has been used in immunologic experiments.

The immunosuppressive action of corticosteroids on lymphocytes may be related to several factors. One of these is lymphocytolysis, which can be demonstrated in vivo and in vitro with concentrations of the drugs that are used in immunologic experiments. This effect has been noted with human, guinea pig, mouse, and rat lymphocytes, although cells of the first two species were much more resistant than those of the latter two. Evidence of in vivo lymphocytolysis is based on the development of a lymphopenia and a shrinkage of the thymus gland, both of which are evidence of an attack on T lymphocytes. B cells are more resistant to the steroids than T cells. Even though lymphocytes may not be lysed by the

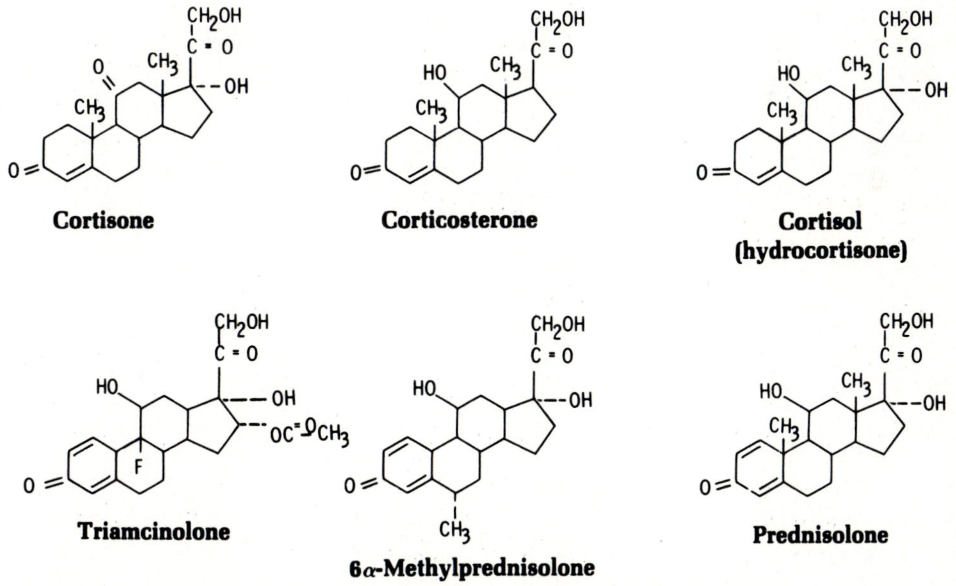

FIG. 9-6

Chemical structures of some steroidal immunosuppressants. The differences in structure reside primarily in the side chains and the oxidation state of carbon 11 in the C ring.

steroids, their inhibition of DNA synthesis, RNA synthesis, and protein synthesis is sufficient to explain the capacity of these compounds to impair immunoglobulin and lymphokine synthesis. Among the latter, an impairment of IL-1 synthesis by T cells is a recognized property of steroids.

Steroids also have pronounced effects on macrophages and neutrophils, probably more so than on lymphocytes. Steroids stabilize macrophage lysosomes, reducing their ability to release hydrolytic enzymes. Cytolysis of monocytes by steroids can also occur, and this would impair antigen processing. A depression of oxidative metabolism, a feature of neutrophil metabolism closely related to intraphagocytic killing of bacteria, is characteristic of the steroids. Steroids also affect Langerhans' cells, by reducing their Fc and CR receptor functions.

As a result of these multicellular effects, the corticosteroids have become useful immunosuppressants. They reduce the primary IgG response, but have little effect on IgM or on the secondary IgG response. They prolong graft survival, minimize both immediate and delayed skin reactions, reduce lymphokine synthesis, and may predispose the patient to infection.

Purine and pyrimidine analogs

Purine analogs such as 6-mercaptopurine, 6-thioguanine, 8-azaguanine, 6-thioinosine, and azathioprine have been repeatedly confirmed as inhibitors of the immunoglobulin response in many species of animals including chickens, mice, rabbits, dogs, monkeys, and humans. The activity of the purine analogs of course is based on their antimetabolite effect on the normal purines adenine, guanine, xanthine, and hypoxanthine. The analogs, including azathioprine, which bear the additional substituted imidazole ring, all have a close structural resemblance to the natural purines (Fig. 9-7). The addition of this moiety to 6-mercaptopurine to create azathioprine actually improves its immunosuppressive activity. This is rather surprising, since the side group is eliminated in vivo to liberate 6-mercaptopurine. One possible explanation is that the blocked sulfhydryl group alters cell

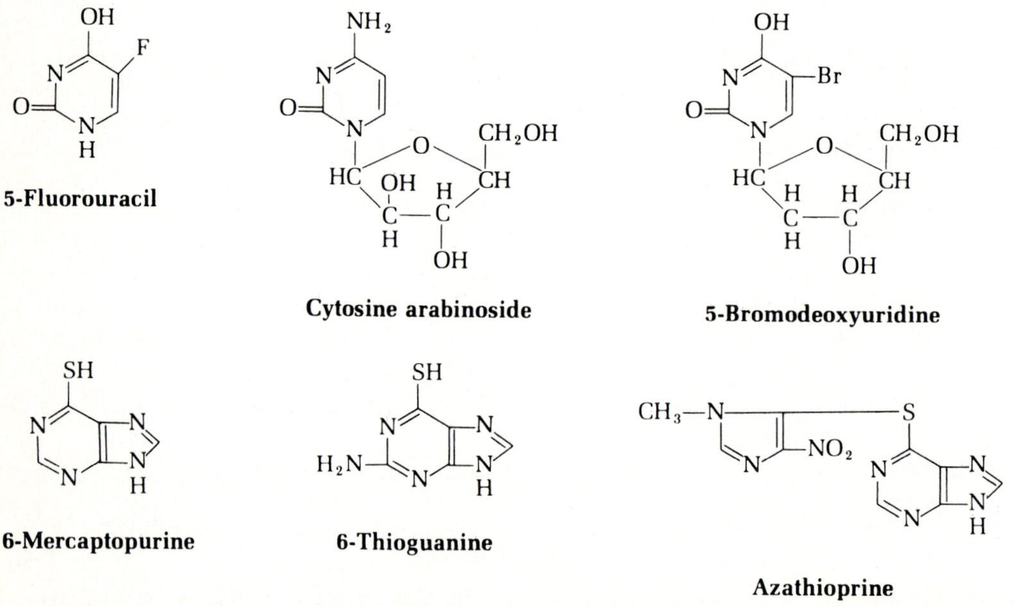

FIG. 9-7

Pyrimidine analogs (upper row) and purine analogs (lower row) with B and T cell–suppressing activity. A large number of similar compounds are available for human use.

permeability, allowing greater access of the drug to the immunoglobulin-synthesizing ribosomes. Another possibility is that detoxification may occur at the SH group, and, if temporarily blocked, the half-life of the inhibitor in vivo may be extended.

These purine analogs may function at more than one biochemical level: simple competitive inhibition of purine compounds in the biosynthetic pathway to other purine bases, inhibition of purine synthesis from low molecular weight precursors, and possibly analog incorporation into nucleotides as substitutes for the natural purine bases. Azathioprine and 6-mercaptopurine, the most widely used purine analogs, block the synthesis and conversion of inosinic acid to adenylsuccinate, and thus function directly via the first mechanism; however, their most important inhibitory effect is their eventual incorporation into 6-methylthiopurine ribonucleotide, which is a potent inhibitor of purine synthesis. Incorporation of these purine analogs into mRNA to create a "nonsense messenger," which would result in the synthesis of defective proteins and antibodies, has now been conclusively demonstrated. The most "purine-sensitive" cell appears to be the immunoblast, an early cell in the sequence of cellular maturation of antibody-forming cells. This is consistent with the opinion that cells in the S phase, or phase of active DNA synthesis, are most susceptible to the purine analogs.

Pyrimidine analogs are structural mimics of uracil, thymine, cytosine, and other forms of cytosine such as 5-methylcytosine or 5-hydroxymethylcytosine, which have a more limited biologic distribution. Several of these pyrimidine compounds are halogen-substituted in the 5 position; 5-fluorouracil and 5-bromouracil are examples. Other cytotoxic chemicals based on the structure of pyrimidine are nucleotides of the halogenated pyrimidine with D-ribose, such as 5-iodo-2-deoxyuridine, 5-iodo-2-deoxycytidine, and 5-trifluoromethyl-2-deoxyuridine. At least some of these halogenated compounds are incorporated into DNA and interrupt the basic genetic capabilities of the afflicted cell. False pyrimidine nucleotides such as cytosine arabinoside may function through their inhibition of DNA polymerase.

Folic acid antagonists

Aminopterin and amethopterin (methotrexate) are both antagonists of folic acid metabolism. Amethopterin is different from aminopterin by only one methyl group. These two antimetabolites are actually inhibitors of tetrahydrofolic acid, which is a carrier of one-carbon units essential to the synthesis of purine (Fig. 9-8). Folic acid antagonists interfere with this process and consequently impair DNA and protein synthesis. Cell division is halted at the S phase in the cell reproduction cycle—the period of DNA formation just prior to cell division. The mouse, rat, guinea pig, and human are all more sensitive to these compounds than is the rabbit, the animal most often used in these experiments. As with other suppressing chemicals, the IgG and primary antibody responses are more sensitive to folic acid analogs.

Alkylating agents

Alkylating agents are compounds that have an affinity for nucleophilic (negatively charged) zones in other molecules. Typical nucleophilic centers in biomolecules include amino acid and sulfhydryl groups. Intracellularly, the most critical point of attack for the alkylating agents is DNA, although obviously RNA and proteins also would be alkylated. Alkylation of the amino groups of guanine and adenine, of which guanine is probably the most sensitive, may result in several critical effects. The alkylated base may not be properly read in the transcription to RNA, forming fraudulent proteins. The same result occurs if the alkylated purine is excised and the depurinated DNA is falsely transcribed. Potentially, the alkylated DNA can be repaired, but errors in the repair mechanism also could lead to the synthesis of nonfunctional proteins. Depurinization also is known to induce breaks in the DNA, and shortened DNA strands would result in the synthesis of incomplete proteins. The affected proteins may be the immunoglobulins or lymphokines themselves, or enzymes responsible for their synthesis. Direct alkylation of the lymphokines and immunoglobulins easily could render them nonfunctional if their nucleophilic centers are required for combination with antigen or cell receptors.

Difunctional and polyfunctional alkylating com-

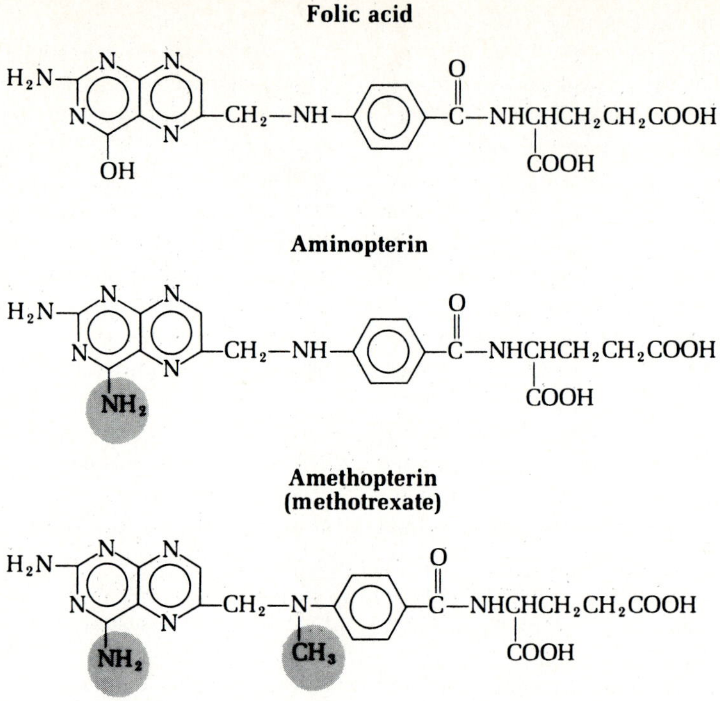

Folic acid

Aminopterin

Amethopterin (methotrexate)

FIG. 9-8

Structural analogs of folic acid—aminopterin and methotrexate—differ from the vitamin by the substituents in the stippled circles. These differences confer an immunosuppressant function on the analogs.

pounds create bridges between natural biopolymers, thus rendering them inactive. In the case of DNA, the two strands cannot separate as required in normal cell division (Fig. 9-9). As a result, the affected cells continue to enlarge but do not divide. Cell clones cannot form. Prolymphocytes, immunoblasts, or other cells in the maturation pathway of lymphocytes cannot escape their premitotic condition. This accounts for the severe lymphopenia that accompanies the administration of alkylating drugs.

The biologic effects of therapy with alkylating reagents so closely parallels the changes produced by x rays that these reagents are known as radiomimetic drugs. Like x rays, these drugs are more effective against the primary and IgG responses than against the secondary response or that of other immunoglobulin classes.

Although literally dozens of alkylating agents have been synthesized and tested for an immunosuppressive function, only a half dozen have had widespread use. The relationship of the structure of these compounds to that of mustard gas is readily apparent except for triethylenemelamine and thiotepa. Most of the information about the immunosuppressive action of alkylating agents stems from experiments with cyclophosphamide.

A single injection of cyclophosphamide drastically reduces the number of lymphocytes in the spleen, thymus, and blood. Both B and T cells are reduced in number, but cyclophosphamide is especially active against B lymphocytes. When it is given to newly hatched chicks, an involution of the bursa resulting in an agammaglobulinemia is induced.

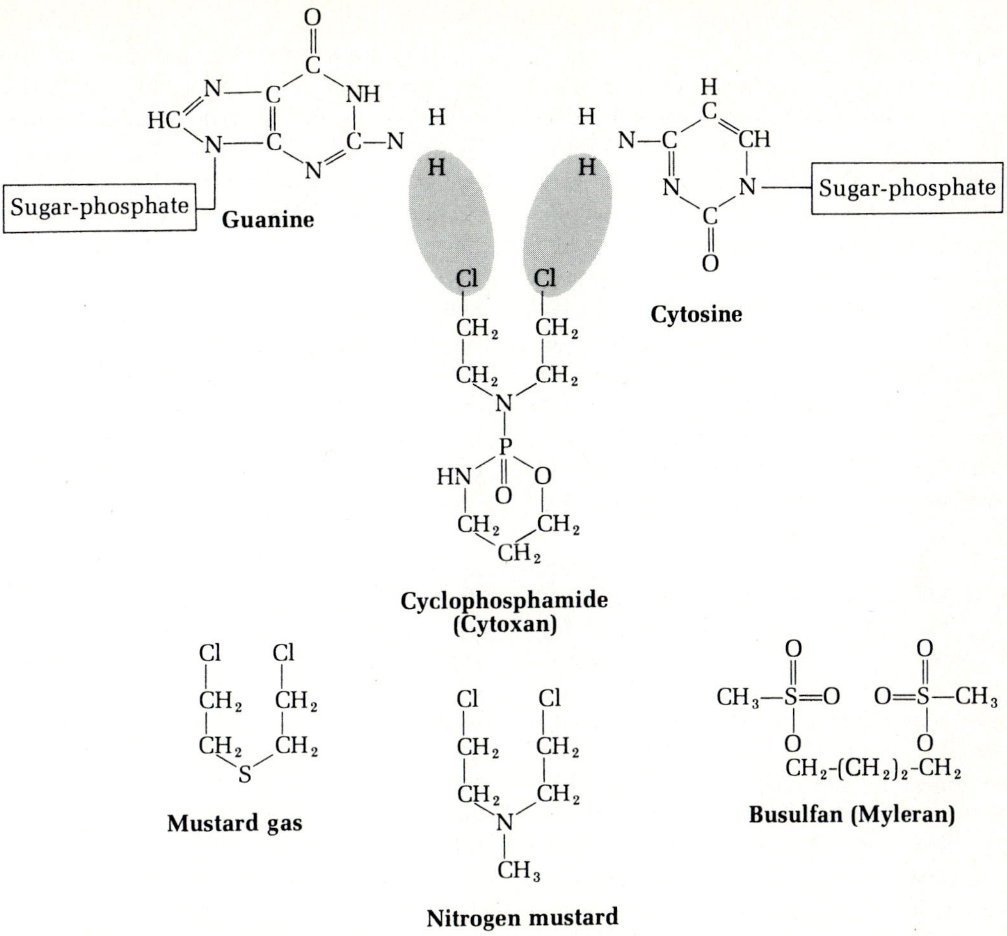

FIG. 9-9

Structures of cyclophosphamide and busulfan, which are alkylating immunosuppressants, clearly are related to the structure of mustard gas. The alkylating reaction of cyclophosphamide with nucleic acids also is illustrated.

An important sidelight to the use of cyclophosphamide as opposed to other alkylating agents is its ability to enhance immunologic tolerance to several antigens. A specific protocol may need to be developed for specific antigens or certain animal species, but generally the antigen is given 1 or 2 days prior to the administration of the drug. This timing apparently is essential because it allows the antigen to induce immunoblast formation. The immunoblast is presumed to be more sensitive to cyclophosphamide than the unstimulated lymphocyte. Another aspect of the capacity of cyclophosphamide to aid tolerance probably lies in the differential susceptibility of the T_C subsets to this compound.

Miscellaneous agents

A number of other cytotoxic agents display immunosuppressive activity, but because of variations in their chemical structure or mode of action, they cannot always be placed with other discrete classes. Several are antibiotics, others are enzymes, and still others are plant alkaloids. In the antibiotic category are actinomycin D, mitomycin C, puromycin, cyclo-sporin, and chloramphenicol.

Puromycin, excreted by *Streptomyces alboniger,* functions at the RNA level and acts by impairing the transfer of the activated amino acids from transfer RNA (tRNA) to the ribosomal protein. *Streptomyces parvullus* is the source of actinomycin D, a third antibiotic operating on RNA, in this instance by preventing the movement of mRNA from the nucleolus to the cytoplasm, where the message for protein synthesis is "read." At doses lower than necessary for this effect, inhibition of RNA polymerase and DNA binding at guanine residues interfere with protein synthesis. Mitomycin C from *Streptomyces caespitosus* acts as an alkylating agent and tends to depolymerize nucleic acid.

Cyclosporin, a cyclic peptide consisting of eleven amino acids, is ineffective as an antibiotic but has exhibited a pronounced immunosuppressive function on lymphocytes. T_H and T_C cells are greatly inhibited and there is some effect on B cells as well. Macrophages and neutrophils are quite resistant to cyclosporin. The powerful influence of this unique peptide on T_H cells and the T_H cells' production of IL-2 has resulted in its incorporation into the immunosuppressive regimen applied to human transplant patients. Animal experimentation with rats, dogs, mice, and rabbits has conclusively proved the benefits of cyclosporin treatment for the prolongation of grafts.

Two enzymes also have had immunosuppressive functions ascribed to them: ribonuclease and asparaginase. Ribonuclease could conceivably function on the RNA and RNA-antigen fragments from macrophages, should these ever exist free extracellularly on their way to "instruct" the lymphoid cells to initiate antibody formation. Asparaginase from *Escherichia coli* produces a marked lymphopenia, and causes a reduction in the size of most lymphoid organs, which results in diminished immune responses. The basis for this effect is the high nutritive demand of lymphocytes for asparagine. Colchicine, vincristine, and vinblastine are plant alkaloids that act on phagocytic cells and halt cell division, both of which are important in the sequence of events leading to antibody synthesis.

Biologic methods

There are five biologic means by which the production of antibodies can be hindered. One of these is nature's own experiment, a deficiency in the ability to synthesize γ-globulins: hypogammaglobulinemia or agammaglobulinemia. The other four methods are competition of antigens, antilymphocyte serum (ALS), feedback inhibition, and immunologic tolerance. The latter two of these techniques display immunologic specificity; that is, it is possible to predetermine on immunologic grounds which antibodies will be inhibited. With hypogammaglobulinemia and ALS, like the physical and chemical methods, there is a generalized diminution of the immunoglobulin response.

Immunologic tolerance

Immunologic tolerance is a state of specific nonreactivity to a normally effective antigenic challenge, induced by a prior exposure to the antigen concerned. As a consequence, immunologic tolerance is significantly different from other forms of immunosuppression, which are unlimited in spectrum and represent a nonspecific rupture of antibody-synthesizing systems against all antigens. The immunotolerant condition is restricted to one antigen and follows the rules of serologic specificity.

The existence of immune tolerance was postulated by Burnet and Fenner in 1949 in the self-marker aspect of their clonal theory on antibody formation. They hypothesized that there were recognition centers on self-antigens which caused them to be ignored as antigens by one's own antibody-making machinery. It was suggested that this self-identification occurred in embryonic life when the antigens were first formed, and at a time before the immune mechanism was functioning. Fetal tolerance was thus postulated to result from an inactivation of immunoreactive cells by the presence of antigen at a time when the cells were immature. Chimeric blood groups in cattle (see related Reading 4, page 423) were a natural expression of these events. Medawar, Billingham, and Brent, in their Nobel Prize winning studies, produced an experimental tolerance in fetal mice by in utero injection of antigens. After birth, these mice would not respond to the antigens they encountered during their fetal life, but were able to respond to other antigens. This experiment ably supported Burnet's hypothesis.

This type of immune tolerance; that is, the inactivation of immune reactive cells in fetal animals, may differ in its basic mechanism from the type of tolerance discussed in the previous chapter. Certainly in adult animals, in which all subpopulations of T cells are active, tolerance is due to the emergence of T_S cells that nullify the immune response.

Antigen competition

The competition of antigens refers to an inhibition of the immune response to one antigen by the injection of a second antigen. Antigenic competition functions best when the inhibiting antigen is given prior to or concurrently with the primary antigen. There are virtually no criteria available to determine if an antigen is a good competitor or not. Unfortunately little more can be stated about this phenomenon.

ALS

ALS, antilymphocyte globulin (ALG), or antithymocyte serum or globulin (ATS or ATG) is prepared by immunization of a heterologous species with cells from the lymph nodes, blood, thymus, or spleen of the donor. To produce its immunosuppressive effect, it is administered as a passive immunization of the donor species before, at, and after the exposure to antigen. Because the antigen preparation used to produce ALS is often impure and contains cells of several types, ALS contains antibodies to these cells (granulocytes, erythrocytes, reticulum cells, and structural cells). Most of these antibodies can be removed by adsorption of ALS with homologous kidney or liver powder. More specific antisera can be prepared by using purified preparations of the antigen; for example, ATS or ATG can be prepared using thoracic duct lymphocytes.

ALS usually induces a transient lymphopenia. Repeated injections may extend this condition for several weeks; however, lymphocyte populations return to normal about 2 weeks after the last treatment. The size and structure of the thymus is not significantly altered by ALS, but it is by ATS. The white pulp of the spleen is reduced by ALS, and a similar cell loss is seen in lymph nodes and other peripheral lymphoid organs. In fowl, antibursa sera have a pronounced influence on the bursal lymphocyte population but little effect on thymocyte numbers. The reverse is true of antithymus sera administered to fowl.

The preferential elimination of lymphocytes from the blood and the thymus-dependent centers of peripheral lymphoid tissues appears to be a logical explanation for the capacity of ATG and even ALS to impair both the cell-mediated and immunoglobulin arms of the immune response. Lymphocytopenia is never total, and its degree does not always correlate with the extent of immunosuppression observed. Comparatively low doses of ATS will deplete the IL-2 producing T helper cells, whereas higher doses are required to affect T_C cells.

Among the in vitro assays used to estimate the immunosuppressive property of ALS are leukoagglutination, cytotoxicity for lymphocytes in the presence of complement, mitogenic effect on lymphocytes, inhibition of the mitogenic effect of Con A or PHA on lymphocytes, inhibition of PFCs, and inhibition of rosette formation by lymphoid cells. There is no correlation of leukocyte agglutination with in vivo activity of ALS, possibly because impure antigen preparations of mixed granulocytes and agranulocytes have been used most often in the test and in the preparation of the ALS. Most immunosuppressive sera are lymphocytotoxic with complement, but the reverse is not always true.

Feedback inhibition

It is almost an axiomatic part of modern biochemical thinking that the regulation of a biochemical pathway is partially controlled by the end product of that pathway. It is not surprising to find this idea of feedback inhibition applied to immunologic experiments, the results of which have paralleled those in other biochemical investigations.

Passively administered antibody depresses the synthesis of new antibody when injected just prior to, simultaneous to, or up to 5 days after the injection of the antigen. This inhibition is immunologically specific; that is, only the corresponding antibody against the antigen can suppress antibody formation against that antigen. Heterologous antibody is relatively ineffective. Injection of only that portion of the antibody molecule which combines with the antigen (Fab or F(ab')$_2$ fragments) is almost as inhibitory as injection of the entire molecule. Feedback inhibition of the primary response is much easier than for the secondary response; even though the primary response is inhibited, the animal becomes primed for a secondary antibody response that can be demonstrated on reexposure to the antigen. Feedback inhibition can be demonstrated at the cellular level by the PFC technique.

The application of feedback inhibition has provided an effective means of preventing hemolytic disease of the newborn (HDN) caused by Rh incompatibility. This is discussed fully in Chapter 18. Briefly, most cases of HDN are caused by maternal antibodies to the Rh antigen present on fetal erythrocytes. These antibodies pass the placental barrier and combine with and promote destruction of the fetal red blood cells. The pregnant woman usually has these antibodies as the result of earlier pregnancies with Rh-positive children. With this information at hand it was rightly theorized that, if women were given anti-Rh sera at childbirth, by virtue of feedback inhibition, they would be prevented from synthesizing the unwanted antibodies. This is such an effective procedure that it is considered a required part of perinatal care and, where practiced as described, essentially has eliminated Rh-dependent HDN.

Genetic immunodeficiencies

A primary genetic inability to form mature cells of the B, T, or phagocytic lineage can result in a permanently immunosuppressed condition unless corrected by medical intervention. These conditions are the subject of Chapter 20.

REFERENCES

Anderson, R.E., and Standefer, J.C.: Radiation injury in the immune system, In Patten, C.S., and Hendry, J.H., editors: *Cytotoxic insult to tissue,* Edinburgh, 1983, Churchill Livingstone.

Bennett, W.M., and Norman, D.J.: Action and cytotoxicity of cyclosporin, Ann. Rev. Med. **37:**215, 1986.

Bona, C., and Cazenave, P.A., editors: Lymphocytic regulation by antibodies, New York, 1981, John Wiley & Sons, Inc.

Cooper, D.A., and Penny, R.: Glucocorticoid action on human immune and inflammatory responses, Clin. Immunol. Update 1, 1985.

Fabris, N., Garaci, E., Hadden, J., and Mitchison, N.A., editors: Immunoregulation, New York, 1983, Plenum Press.

Faney, N., Guyre, P.M., and Munck, A.: Mechanisms of anti-inflammatory actions of glucocorticoids, Adv. Inflamm. Res. **2:**21, 1981.

Fenichel, R.L., and Chirigos, M.A., editors: Immune modulation agents and their mechanisms, New York, 1984, Marcel Dekker, Inc.

Fudenberg, H.H., Pink, J.R.L., Wang, A.-L., and Ferrara, G.B.: Basic immunogenetics, ed. 3, New York, 1984, Oxford University Press, Inc.

Hraba, T., and Hasek, M., editors: Cellular and molecular mechanisms of immunologic tolerance, New York, 1981, Marcel Dekker, Inc.

Humphrey, J.H.: Regulation of *in vivo* immune responses: few principles and much ignorance, Ciba Found. Symp. **119:**6, 1986.

Nydegger, U.E.: Suppressive and substitutive immunotherapy: an essay with a review of recent literature, Immunol. Let. **9:**185, 1985.

Shevach, E.M.: The effects of cyclosporin A on the immune system, Ann. Rev. Immunol. **3:**397, 1985.

Zaleski, M.B., Dubiski, S., Niles, E.G., and Cunningham, R.K.: Immunogenetics, Marshfield, MA, 1983, Pitman Publishing, Inc.

See related **Reading 4,** page 423.

The complement system

≡GLOSSARY

alternate complement pathway A system for activating complement beginning at C3 and not involving a serologic reaction.

Ana INH Anaphylatoxin inhibitor.

anaphylatoxin Originally believed to be a substance that caused histamine release; now regarded as specific peptides from complement fractions 3, 4, and 5, which release histamine from mast cells and basophils.

anaphylatoxin inhibitor An enzyme that destroys the biologic activity of C3a, C4a, and C5a.

angioneurotic edema A sporadic edematous condition related to a genetic deficiency in C1 esterase inhibitor.

C1, C2, etc. Components of serum complement numbered sequentially from 1 through 9.

C1 esterase An esterase formed from activation of the C1s component of complement.

C1s INH The serum inhibitor of the activated first component of complement.

classic complement pathway A system for activating all nine components of complement that is initiated by a serologic reaction.

complement fixation Binding or use of serum complement in a reaction with antigen and antibody.

conglutination A type of complement fixation test incorporating bovine conglutinin that clumps sheep red blood cells in the presence of nonhemolytic complement.

conglutinin A protein normally present in bovine serum that reacts with C3.

CR1, CR2, and CR3 Designations for complement receptors on cells.

HANE Hereditary angioneurotic edema.

hemolysis Lysis of erythrocytes by specific antibody and serum complement.

immune adherence The adhesive nature of antigen-antibody complexes to inert surfaces when complement is bound.

immunoconglutinin An antibody to antigenic sites of C3 revealed or created by antigen-antibody binding of complement.

kinins Peptides or polyamines released during anaphylaxis that possess vasodilating and muscle-contracting activity.

COMPLEMENT
Its discovery: the Pfeiffer phenomenon

The discovery of complement is credited to Pfeiffer and resulted from his studies in 1894 on experimental cholera infections in guinea pigs. Pfeiffer observed that a reinoculation of cholera bacilli *(Vibrio cholerae)* intraperitoneally into guinea pigs that had recovered from an earlier infection of the organism resulted in the rapid dissolution of the bacteria within the peritoneal cavity. Pfeiffer determined three facts from a further study of this system:

1. The immunity was specific and could not be induced by injections of antigenically unrelated bacteria. The immunity could be transferred to normal

guinea pigs with blood from the immune guinea pigs; that is, antibody was required.

2. Heated serum from immune animals, tested in vitro, was devoid of bactericidal power, but fresh serum was lethal to the cholera bacilli.

3. Heated immune serum would transfer the immunity between animals, and the cholera vibrios were lysed in the passively immunized animal.

It was concluded that heat-stable antibodies in blood could transfer cholera immunity to a living animal and that these antibodies cooperated with a heat-labile substance present in normal animals to create the immunity. When this substance in immune sera was destroyed by heating it at 56° C, antibody alone could not destroy the cholera organisms in vitro. Buchner had earlier described a heat-labile protective activity of blood and had named it alexin.

In 1898 Bordet confirmed Pfeiffer's experiments by demonstrating that fresh normal serum contains a heat-sensitive substance which will dissolve bacteria (bacteriolysis) in the presence of specific antibodies in heat-inactivated antiserum. Bordet also described immune hemolysis following the mixture of red blood cells with specific antibody and alexin. Bordet continued his studies of the hemolytic activity of alexin and demonstrated that hemolytic assays were much simpler than bacteriolytic assays for detecting its presence in sera. Because of his many contributions to an understanding of complement and related studies of immunity, Bordet was awarded the Nobel Prize in 1919. At about this time Ehrlich proposed the term *complement* (something that completes or makes perfect) for alexin (to ward off), and this more meaningful term has persisted.

GENERAL PROPERTIES

Before considering the complicated chemistry of complement and its fractions, it is advisable to consider some of the general properties of complement that serve to distinguish it from immunoglobulins and other serum proteins.

1. Complement is required for the cytolytic destruction of cellular antigens by specific antibodies. Not all cellular antigens are susceptible to dissolution by complement and immunoglobulins. Yeasts, molds, many gram-positive bacteria, most plant

cells, and even most mammalian cells resist complement-mediated cytolysis. The cells that are naturally most fragile—white blood cells of all types, erythrocytes, thrombocytes, and gram-negative bacteria—are the most susceptible to immune cytolysis.

2. The lytic activity of complement in antigen-antibody reactions is destroyed by heating sera at 56° C for 30 minutes. The conditions traditionally used for the heat inactivation of complement do not affect the immunoglobulins that participate in serologic reactions with complement, although IgD and IgE are partially inactivated by these conditions.

3. Only immunoglobulins of the IgM and IgG classes react with complement, and the IgG subclasses are not equally potent in this regard. IgG4 is incapable of activating the complement system, and of the remaining IgG subclasses, IgG3 is the most active. IgA, IgD, and IgE are incapable of functioning with complement. Immunoglobulins activate the classic complement pathway.

4. Complement is bound into all antigen-antibody reactions, provided the immunoglobulin is of the proper class. This fixation of complement occurs even if complement is not required to display the serologic reaction being studied (for example, precipitation and agglutination). It is this characteristic of complement which allowed Bordet and Gengou to develop the complement fixation test in 1901. Binding or fixation of complement by complexes of antigen and antibody initiates the classic activation pathway of complement.

5. Complement activation by nonserologic reactions is possible. The best known of these alternate pathways of complement activation is known as the properdin pathway. The alternate pathways are initiated by complex polysaccharides or enzymes.

6. Complement is a nonspecific serologic reagent in the sense that complement from one species of animal usually will react with immunoglobulins of another species from the same taxonomic order. The more distant the taxonomic position of the two species, the less interaction occurs. Avian complement or fish complement does not react as well with mammalian antibodies as does mammalian complement.

7. Portions of the complement system contribute importantly to chemotaxis, opsonization, immune

adherence, anaphylatoxin formation, virus neutralization, and other physiologic functions.

8. Complement is present in all normal mammalian sera and the sera of most lower animals, including birds, fish, amphibia, and sharks. The complement content of sera, which comprises about 10% of the total globulins, does not increase as a result of immunization.

9. Complement is not a single substance but a complex of nine major proteins that act in consort with one another. All nine are required for cytolytic reactions resulting from the classic pathway. In the properdin activation pathway the first three components of the classic pathway are not required.

The use of several different expressions to denote the participation of complement in a certain activity may lead to confusion until it is recognized that all the terms refer to essentially the same thing. "Complement binding" or "complement fixation" refers to the union of complement or one of its fractions with a substance, usually an immunoglobulin or antigen. Often this results in the expression of a new biologic activity and a change in that component of complement, known as "complement activation." Measurement of the residual complement activity in a serum after complement activation will determine that the complement level has been decreased. This is expressed as "complement consumption" or "complement inactivation," the latter of which is grammatically the exact opposite of complement activation, although the terms refer to basically the same reaction.

CHEMISTRY OF THE COMPLEMENT COMPONENTS
Nomenclature

The components in the classic complement activation sequence, as stated previously, are nine in number. These molecules are numbered sequentially C1 through C9. The individual peptide chains of these proteins are designated by Greek letters, in keeping with the biochemical system for identifying the subunit peptides of proteins that have a quaternary structure. Thus, there is C3α, C3β, C4β, C4γ, and so on.

When a peptide chain is fragmented by proteolysis, the cleavage peptides are denoted by lower case Arabic letters, as in C3a and C3b. It is important to avoid confusion of the Greek and Arabic lettering systems; fragments C3a and C3b arise from C3α. If the fragment loses activity as the result of further proteolysis, the letter i is added as a prefix to indicate inactivation (for example, iC3b).

When a complement protein acquires an enzymatic activity or is otherwise activated, a horizontal bar over the designation for the protein may be used, but this is a less common practice than previously. C1 becomes C$\overline{1}$ when it acquires its esterase activity. When it is desirable to identify the specific peptide fragments, then the appropriate letter designations are used, as in C$\overline{1s}$ or C$\overline{4b,2a}$.

Studies of the alternate pathway have uncovered several additional serum proteins which function with the late-acting components of complement (those which follow C3 in the classic system). At least four additional proteins participate in the properdin alternate pathway. These are properdin, factor B (formerly known as C3 proactivator), factor D (formerly C3 proactivator convertase), and C3b,Bb (the C3 activator). This raises the number of proteins in the complement system to 13—nine classic pathway molecules plus four alternate pathway molecules.

To these 13 molecules, all of which are present in normal serum, additional serum proteins that modulate complement-derived activities must be added. The best characterized complement moderators are C1s INH (inhibitor), Factor I, Factor H, and Ana INH (anaphylatoxin inhibitor) but additional inhibitors are known.

Components of the classic activation pathway

The nine originally described molecules of the complement series, C1 through C9, act in consort with one another when the C1 molecule is activated by certain antigen-antibody reactions. Since C1 is the first component to participate in the reaction, it is referred to as the recognition unit. When this recognition unit becomes activated, the next three components to participate are C4, C2, and C3, in that order rather than in a straight numeric sequence. These three molecules compose the activation unit, so named because important enzyme activities appear during their participation in the sequence. The remaining molecules, C5 through C9, are referred to as the membrane attack complex.

The recognition unit: C1

The first component of the complement cascade is a true macromolecule with a molecular weight of approximately 750,000 and a sedimentation coefficient of 18 (Table 10-1). C1, in its associated form, is a trimolecular complex held together by calcium ions. (Since the alternate pathway does not require Ca^{2+}, a loss of complement activity in the presence of buffers that bind Ca^{2+} indicates use of the alternate pathway.) When the calcium is removed by the use of chelating compounds like ethylenediaminetetraacetic acid (EDTA), C1 dissociates into its three subunits. The three subunits of C1 are designated C1q, C1r, and C1s, which, because of differences in their size and chemical properties, can be separated from each other easily by gel filtration (in calcium-free buffers). One unit of C1q, two units of C1r and two of C1s form the C1 complex.

C1q is the largest of the C1 subunits and has a molecular weight of 410,000 and an $S_{20,w}$ value of 11.2. It has the electrophoretic mobility of a γ_2-globulin, which is notable because most components of complement behave as β-globulins. Normal human serum contains 150 $\mu g/ml$ of C1q.

Chemically, C1q is a novel molecule because of its high content of hydroxyproline, hydroxylysine, and glycine at frequencies of nearly 5%, 2%, and 18%, respectively. Since these three amino acids are so common in collagen, C1q can justifiably be described as a collagen-like molecule. However, this description must be tempered somewhat, since both the amino and carboxyl terminal ends of C1q are typically globular in structure. C1q also can be considered a glycoprotein because it contains about 9.8% of its weight in the form of carbohydrate.

C1q is composed of 18 separate polypeptide chains, each with a molecular weight of approximately 23,000. Although these small proteins are similar in amino acid composition and size, they differ in the amount of carbohydrate that they carry and in electrophoretic mobility. Thus, there are six A chains, six B chains, and six C chains. These appear to be associated as six A-B subunits and three C-C subunits, each held together by disulfide bonds but not covalently linked to the other subunits.

The C1q molecule is so large that it can be viewed in the electron microscope, where it gives

TABLE 10-1
Characteristics of the complement components

Component	Serum concentration ($\mu g/ml$)	Sedimentation coefficient ($S_{20,w}$)	Molecular weight	Number of peptide chains	Electrophoretic position
C1q	150	11.2	410,000	18	γ_2
C1r	50	7.5	83,000	2	β
C1s	50	4.5	83,000	1	α
C2	15	4.5	110,000		β_1
C3	1,250	9.5	180,000	2	β_2
C4	400	10.0	206,000	3	β_1
C5	80	8.7	180,000	2	β_1
C6	60	5.5	120,000	1	β_2
C7	55	6.0	110,000	1	β_2
C8	55	8.0	150,000	3	γ_1
C9	60	4.5	71,000	1	α

the appearance of six globes held on slender shafts that fuse into a common base (Fig. 10-1). The globes serve as the recognition unit and bind to the Fc region of the complement-activating IgM and IgG immunoglobulins. This occurs in the C_H4 domain of IgM but in the C_H2 domain of IgG. All subclasses of IgG are not equally effective receptors for C1q. In descending order of effectiveness, they are IgG3, IgG1, IgG2, and IgG4. IgG4 dissociates so readily that it is not described as a complement-activating globulin. For C1q to initiate the complement cascade it must attach to two immunoglobulin molecules. Since these are adjacent in IgM, IgM is described as a better complement-binding antibody than IgG. IgA, IgD, and IgE do not bind C1q and cannot catalyze the complement cascade.

Although it is traditional to describe C1 activation as an immunoglobulin dependent reaction, a large number of other agents also have this property. Among these, dextran, heparin, polynucleotides and other polysaccharide-containing molecules, lipid A

of LPS, RNA retroviruses, mitochondrion membranes, and certain proteases, such as plasmin, can be mentioned.

C1r and C1s are similar molecules, each composed of a single peptide chain approaching 83,000 mol wt. Each contains about 7% to 9% of its weight in polysaccharide. In their native state C1r and C1s exist as proteolytic zymogens, or proenzymes.

Two moles of C1r and C1s are present in the C1 complex. Activation of the complex occurs first at the C1r level with its conversion to an enzyme with a trypsinlike specificity. The C1s proenzyme is the only known substrate for the C1r enzyme. The attack of C1r on C1s then unmasks the C1s enzyme. The biochemical basis for these alterations is not known. It is assumed that the small activation peptides released, as in other proenzyme-enzyme conversions, is the key alteration. Amino acid sequencing of active C1r and C1s has identified a close homology with other serine-containing proteo-esterases with which they are now classified.

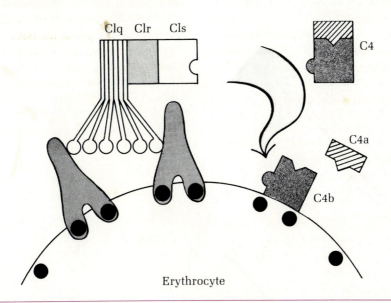

FIG. 10-1

The C1 triad of C1q, C1r, and C1s is held together by calcium ions. When the C1q receptors for the Fc region of complement-activating immunoglobulins bridge two Fc units, its C1s portion becomes activated so that it can cleave C4. The C4b product attaches to the antigen surface, and the C4a peptide is left free.

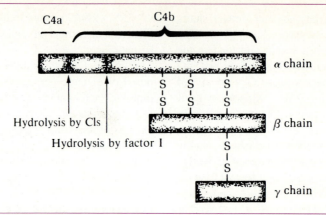

FIG. 10-2

C4 consists of three peptide chains. Hydrolysis of the α-chain by C$\overline{1}$s activates the C4 molecule by releasing the C4a peptide.

The activation unit: C4

The next molecule to participate in the complement sequence is C4 (Table 10-1). C4 has a molecular weight of 206,000 and an $S_{20,w}$ value of 10. It originates from a pro C4 (210,000 mol wt), synthesized by macrophages. It positions itself electrophoretically with the β-globulins. Its concentration in human serum is 400 μg/ml, which makes it second only to C3 in serum concentration. C4 consists of three peptide chains, C4α, C4β, and C4γ, with molecular weights of 95,000, 78,000, and 33,000, respectively. These three chains are joined by disulfide bonds (Fig. 10-2). The attack of C$\overline{1}$s on C4 takes place in the α-chain and releases C4a, which has a molecular weight of about 9,000. The remainder of the molecule, known as C4b, has a molecular weight of about 198,000.

C4b will attach to erythrocyte surfaces, bacterial cell membranes, and other antigens. It does not normally attach to C1. The ability of C4b to attach rather indiscriminantly to proteins is due to the presence of an internal thioester bond involving cysteine and the γ carboxyl group of glutamic acid (Fig. 10-3). The natural instability of this linkage after the removal of C4a permits it to open and then reclose with amino acids on the antigen surface. Free C4b can be removed from the complement cascade by binding to Factor H, formerly known as the

C3b·C4b INAC accelerator. When joined with Factor H, C4b can be converted to iC4b by Factor I, the C3b·C4b inactivator. Cleavage of C4b produces C4c (150,000 mol wt) and C4d (49,000 mol wt).

The C4a molecule consists of 77 amino acids and does not possess any carbohydrate side chains. This small molecule now has been recognized as an anaphylatoxin. Anaphylatoxins are able to bind to mast cells and basophils and cause them to discharge their cytoplasmic granules. (See Chapter 17.) When freed from these cells, the contents of these granules contract smooth muscles, causing edema and shortness of breath.

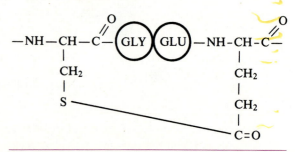

FIG. 10-3

The internal thioester bond in C3 and C4 between cysteine and glutamic acid.

The activation unit: C2

Fraction C2 of complement is a β_1-globulin, with a molecular weight of 110,000 and $S_{20,w}$ of 4.5. It is rather scant in serum, with 15 µg/ml being recorded as the average level. The amino acid composition of C2 is nearly identical to that of factor B of the alternate pathway. The activity of C2 is destroyed when it is combined with *p*-chloromercuribenzoate or iodoacetamide in a molar ratio of 1:2. This indicates that C2 possesses two sulfhydryl groups necessary for its activity. It is not essential for these —SH moieties to be in the reduced condition to measure C2 activity. In fact the treatment of C2 with iodine, which oxidizes the —SH groups to the disulfide or —S—S— forms, results in a ten to twentyfold increase in C2 activity.

The alteration of C2 during the complement sequence has been analyzed, with the discovery that it binds to C4b (Fig. 10-4) and is cleaved by C$\overline{1}$s into C2a and C2b. These proteins have molecular weights of 70,000 and 30,000, respectively. The role of C2b is unclear at this time, but C2a functions with C4b to activate C3 and C5 and may be the critical catalytic portion of the enzyme known as C3 convertase, which is written C$\overline{4b,2a}$.

The activation unit: C3

The substrate for C3 convertase, or C$\overline{4b,2a}$, is C3, that protein of the complement system which is the most abundant in serum, at 1,250 µg/ml (Table 10-1). C3 is a β_2-globulin with an $S_{20,w}$ of 9.5 and a molecular weight of 180,000; it originates from a pro C3 secreted by macrophages. C3 consist of an α-chain with a molecular weight of 105,000 and a β-chain with a molecular weight of 75,000 joined by disulfide bonds (Fig. 10-5). C3 convertase hydrolyzes a peptide bond at positions 77 and 78 in the α-chain to produce C3a, a peptide with a molecular weight of 8,900, which is an anaphylatoxin. The remainder of the molecule is known as C3b, and it attaches to C$\overline{4b,2a}$. C3b is enabled to do this, because, like C4b, it contains an internal thioester bond. The new complex C$\overline{4b,2a,3b}$ is known as C5 convertase, which, like the C3 convertase, relies heavily on C2a for its enzymatic activity.

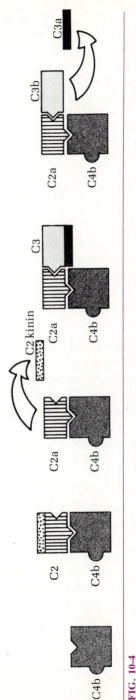

FIG. 10-4

After C4b is produced and attaches to the antigen surface, it is able to combine with C2. C2 kinin is released, leaving the C4b, C2a complex, which is now able to receive C3. C3 then is degraded to release the anaphylatoxin C3a, and its residue remains attached to the C4b, 2a complex.

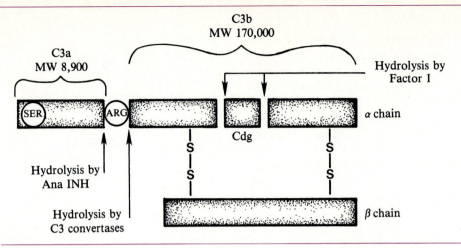

FIG. 10-5

The peptide structure of C3 is similar to that of C5 (Fig. 10-6). Activation of C3 follows a peptide bond cleavage at the carboxyl side of the arginine at residue 77 by C3 convertases of either the classic or alternate pathway. Anaphylatoxic C3a is inactivated upon removal of its terminal arginine by Ana INH. C3b is converted to the inactive iC3b upon hydrolysis by Factor I which is believed to be responsible for producing fragment Cdg.

When C3b is hydrolyzed by Factor I, it is inactivated and referred to as iC3b. Factor I is now believed to split two peptide bonds in C3b rather than one as previously proposed. The peptide released by this action has a molecular weight of only 3000. If cellbound iC3b is degraded by plasma enzymes, the product C3dg is produced. C3dg is subject to further degradation by other enzymes.

The membrane attack complex: C5

The remaining molecules, sometimes referred to as the late acting components, but more frequently as the membrane attack complex, are less well characterized than the aforementioned molecules. This is due to several factors, the foremost of which is their hydrophobic nature and tendency to associate intimately with each other. Polymeric forms of the individual molecules, particularly C9, have hindered molecular studies of the monomeric form of these proteins.

In several respects C5 is much like C3 (Table 10-1). C5 is a β_1-globulin; its molecular weight is 180,000, and its $S_{20,w}$ value is 8.7. These figures are similar to those for C3. Like C3, C5 also is derived from a precursor molecule, in this case pro C5 from macrophages, which has a molecular weight of 220,000. Structurally C5 is also like C3, being composed of two peptide chains, C5α, and C5β, linked by disulfide bonds (Fig. 10-6). C5α has a molecular weight of 105,000 and C5β, 75,000. In parallel with C3a, a C5 convertase, composed of C4b, 2a, and 3b, removes a fragment C5a with a molecular weight of about 16,000 from the α-chain of C5. C5a is an anaphylatoxin and a chemotaxin for granulocytes. It is larger than C3a, partially because of its polysaccharide content. C5b, which remains after the removal of C5a does not contain an internal thioester bond. It can be further degraded to C5c and C5d. The biologic roles of C5c and C5d are not known, but intact C5b, which attaches to the earlier complement components, serves as the receptor for C6 and C7 and is the first element of the membrane attack complex.

The membrane attack complex: C6 and C7

Very little is known about C6 and C7 except that both are β_2-globulins with molecular weights near 125,000 (Table 10-1). C6 is reported to have a molecular weight of 120,000 and C7 one of 110,000. The $S_{20,w}$ values for C6 and C7 are 5.5 and 6, re-

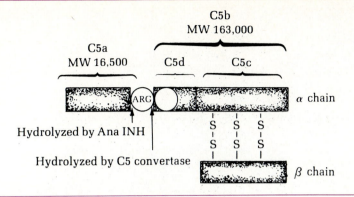

FIG. 10-6
The peptide structure of C5 is reminiscent of that of C3 (Fig. 10-5). C5 convertase cleaves the α-chain next to an arginine residue in C5a. Removal of this arginine by Ana INH inactivates the C5a and C3a anaphylatoxins.

spectively. C6 is available in human serum at a level of 60 μg/ml and C7 at 55 μg/ml. The C5b, C6 union with C3b is very loose and easily dissociated until stabilized by the addition of C7. The participation of C6 and C7 is not accompanied by the appearance of new enzyme activities as noted with the earlier complement components.

The membrane attack complex: C8 and C9

The next molecule to combine in the complement sequence is C8, an unusual molecule consisting of three peptide chains, two of which are covalently linked to each other and a third that is not covalently joined to the other two (Table 10-1). After treatment of C8 with detergents and reducing agents three peptide chains, C8α (69,000 mol wt), C8β (64,000 mol wt), and C8γ (22,000 mol wt), can be isolated. C8γ and C8α are linked by disulfide bonds, and C8β is noncovalently joined to them.

These figures indicate that C8 has a total weight of 150,000. C8 is a γ_2-globulin with an $S_{20,w}$ of 8 and is present in human serum at concentrations of 55 μg/ml.

It is uncertain if C7 or C5b is the attachment site for C8, but it is thought to involve the β chain of the latter. At this point in the cascade a high-affinity phospholipid binding site is generated and the C5b, 6, 7, 8 complex leaves C3b and partially embeds itself in lipid bilayers. At this time the target cells become "leaky" but are not lysed.

The last of the complement molecules to interact is C9 (Table 10-1), an α-globulin like C1s, which is identical to it in $S_{20,w}$ value of 4.5 and similar in molecular weight (71,000 versus 83,000 for C1s). The level of C9 in human serum is 60 μg/ml.

It is uncertain if C9 binds to the γ or β chain of C8 but it is known that from 1 to 18 (average 15) C9 molecules join the complex. The hydrophobic portions of this complex form the outer wall of a cylinder which has a diameter that varies according to the number of C9 molecules incorporated into it. The largest tubules are cone-shaped with an inner diameter of 110 A° and an outer diameter of 210 A° (Fig. 10-7). The hydrophilic core of this transmembrane channel is the tunnel through which the target cells' contents escape in a cytolytic reaction.

Components of the alternate pathway

The original description of an alternate complement pathway was made in 1954 by Pillemer and his associates, who found that cell wall preparations from yeast (zymosan), would activate complement. This activation was related to a newly discovered serum globulin, properdin, and became known as the properdin pathway. Since then, it has been found that many complex polysaccharides will activate this

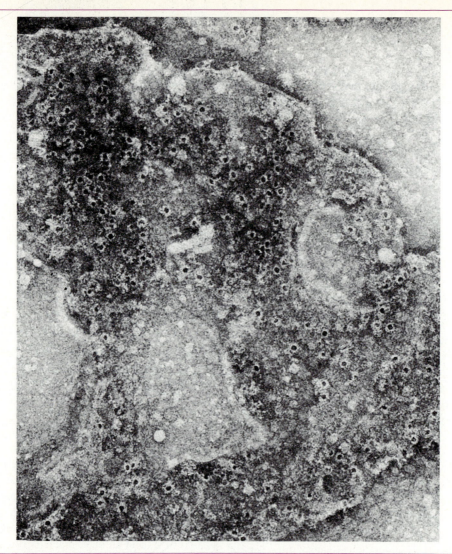

FIG. 10-7
The "holes" in these erythrocytes caused by the erythrocyte-antierythrocyte-complement interaction do not penetrate entirely through the cell membrane. All the holes are about 80 to 100 μm in diameter. (Courtesy R. Dourmashkin and J. Humphrey.)

pathway. Among these are LPS, bacterial capsules, teichoic acids from bacterial cell walls, inulin, dextran, fungal cell walls, and aggregated globulins which are high in carbohydrate content. At least four serum proteins function in the alternate pathway of complement activation that do not contribute to the classic pathway: factor B, factor D, C3b,Bb, and properdin (factor P) (Table 10-2).

An initiating factor for the properdin pathway has not yet been clearly identified, but it is not properdin, as was earlier believed. It is probably the combination of one of the aforementioned polysaccharides

TABLE 10-2

Characteristics of proteins in the alternate complement activation pathway

Component	Abbreviation	Serum concentration (μg/ml)	Sedimentation coefficient ($S_{20,w}$)	Molecular weight	Electrophoretic position	Comment
Properdin	P	25	5.4	184,000	γ_2	Exists as tetramer
C3	C3	1,250	9.5	180,000	β_2	Also intermediate in classic pathway
Factor D	D	2	3	24,000	α	C3 proactivator convertase
Factor B	B	200	5 to 6	93,000	β	C3 proactivator
C3 convertase	C3b,Bb	Unknown	4	63,000	γ	Cleaves C3 at Arg 77-Ser 78
Cobra venom factor	CVF	Not found in serum	6.7	144,000		May be cobra C3b

with C3b, thus protecting it from degradation by Factors H and I, that initiates the alternate pathway.

The question usually posed is, "Where does the C3b originate that is needed for this pathway of complement activation?" It generally is assumed that there is an endogenous generation of C3b from the classic pathway (Fig. 10-8). The actual amount of C3b needed for alternate pathway activation may be trivial. This may arise from non-serologic activation of C1 or trivial serologic reactions that are insufficient in magnitude to be noticed by the host. This C3b, whatever its sources, combines with factor B.

Factor B

Factor B, the C3 proactivator, is a normal serum protein with a molecular weight of 93,000. As such, it has an $S_{20,w}$ of about 6. It is a β-globulin found at a level of 200 μg/ml of serum. Factor B shares several features with C2, such as size, sedimentation rate, single peptide structure, and proenzyme nature. The enzyme nature of factor B is not released until it is bound to C3b and acted on by a protease. This protease is factor D.

Factor D

Factor B in the C3b,B complex (possibly in association with some polysaccharide factor that could generate or stabilize C3b) becomes the substrate for factor D. Factor D is more descriptively referred to as C3 proactivator convertase, since it enzymatically converts the C3 proactivator (factor B) to a state where it too can express an enzymatic activity as the C3 activator. This cleavage of factor B at a single Arg-Lys bond generates two fragments: Ba, an α-globulin with a molecular weight near 33,000 and Bb, a γ-globulin of 60,000 mol wt. Ba is released, but Bb remains bound to C3b. The complex of C3b,Bb now displays the typical features of a serine esterase and is able to hydrolyze C3, e.g. is the C3 convertase of the alternate pathway.

It hydrolyzes C3 at the same peptide bond cleaved by the C4b,2a enzyme of the classic pathway. However, the alternate pathway C3 convertase is labile and decays rapidly. It is stabilized by the addition of properdin. The addition of more C3b to C3b,Bb generates a labile C5 convertase C3b$_n$,Bb, which also is unstable but also becomes stabilized by the addition of properdin. Thus properdin, once thought to be the initial compound of the alternate pathway, now is believed to be its terminal component and to function as a stabilizer for the labile C3 and C5 activating enzymes.

Properdin

Properdin, with an $S_{20,w}$ value of 5.4, is a γ_2-globulin with a molecular weight of 184,000. Pro-

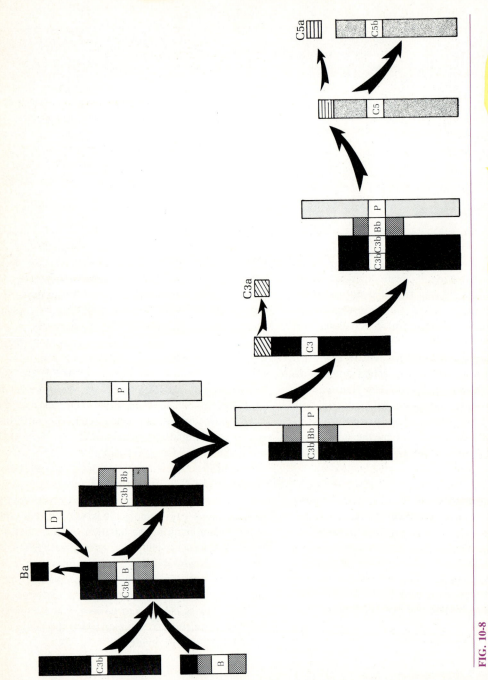

FIG. 10-8

In the alternate activation pathway of complement, C3b formed endogenously complexes with factor B. This renders factor B susceptible to cleavage by factor D. The newly formed C3b,Bb is labile but can hydrolyze C3. C3b,Bb becomes a stable C3 activator when it adds properdin. When more C3b is added to C3b,Bb, it acquires a labile C5 activator role, which is stabilized by the addition of properdin.

perdin contains about 9.8% polysaccharide. Its concentration in normal human serum is 25 µg/ml. Properdin is composed of four peptide subunits, each with a molecular weight of 46,000, held together by hydrogen and ionic bonds. These subunits separate from each other in high-molarity solutions of urea or guanidine. When the dissociating reagents are removed, dimers of the subunits form, which regain about 50% of the activity of intact properdin.

With the generation of stable C3 and C5 convertases the remainder of the pathway from C6 through C9 is ensured. Since the alternate pathway usually occurs in solution rather than on a cell surface, cell lysis is not thought of as a part of this system. Only when the neighboring cell density is high will the C5-C9 complex associate with cells in so-called bystander cell lysis.

Cobra venom factor

Cobra venom factor (or CVF) is a protein found in cobra venom that is capable of combining with factor B to form a complex which can activate C3 via Bb. For complete activation of C3, factor D also is required. Cobra venom factor behaves as cobra C3b. CVF is similar to human C3 in amino acid composition, amino terminal sequence, and pI value and the two molecules are serologically cross reactive.

Complement-derived peptides

At several of the early stages in the complement sequence the activation of the component is associated with limited proteolysis. This generally results in the expression of an enzymatic activity previously masked in a proenzyme. This activation releases low molecular weight peptides of great biologic importance.

C4a

When $C\overline{1}s$ attacks C4, a low molecular weight peptide, C4a, is liberated (Table 10-3). C4a has a molecular weight of only 9,000 and has been identified as an anaphylatoxin.

Anaphylatoxic activity of a molecule refers to its ability to release histamine and basic peptides from mast cells. Since histamine contracts smooth muscle and causes an edema and wheal reaction in skin, these techniques are used to measure anaphylatoxins. C4a contains 77 amino acids, which have a 30% homology with the sequence of C3a and a 39% homology with that of C5a. These three peptides are not serologically cross-reactive.

C2b

$C\overline{1}s$ also cleaves C2 into two unequal halves: C2a of 70,000 mol wt and C2b of 30,000 mol wt. C2a binds with C4b to create C3 convertase or $C4b,\overline{2a}$ and is probably the catalytically active portion of that complex. The biologic significance of C2b is unknown.

C3a

To release C3a, $C\overline{4b,2a}$ hydrolyzes C3 between residues 77 and 78 of its α-chain. This is the same bond ruptured by the C3 convertase formed by the alternate complement pathway, yet the enzymes themselves are clearly separate. Amino acid 77 is an arginine, and this is the carboxyl terminus of C3a. C3a thus consists of 77 amino acids and has a molecular weight of 8,900 (Table 10-3).

C3a is anaphylatoxic. At concentrations as low as 10^{-8}M, C3a is still effective in producing these responses. Removal of the carboxyl terminal arginine by serum carboxypeptidase B, also known as

TABLE 10-3
Properties of the complement-derived peptides

Protein	Source	Molecular weight	Biologic activity	Released by
C2b	C2	37,000	Unknown	$C\overline{1}s$
C3a	α-Chain of C3	8,900	Anaphylatoxic	C3 convertase and C3 activator
C4a	α-Chain of C4	9,000	Anaphylatoxic	$C\overline{1}s$
C5a	α-Chain of C5	16,000	Anaphylatoxic and chemotactic	C5 convertase

anaphylatoxin inhibitor (Ana INH), completely destroys the anaphylatoxic activity of C3a, C4a and C5a.

C5a

C5 convertase, the C4b,2a,3b complex, like C3 convertase, is peptolytic for a single bond in the amino end of the α-chain of C5 and produces C5a (16,000 mol wt) and C5b (163,000 mol wt). C5a also has an arginine as a carboxyl terminal amino acid, and is anaphylatoxic at levels approaching 10^{-10}M. C5a is also chemotaxic for granulocytes. Although des Arg C3a, des Arg C4a and des Arg C5a are no longer anaphylatoxic, des Arg C5a is still chemotactic.

IMMUNOLOGIC AND BIOLOGIC ACTIVITIES OF COMPLEMENT

The vast number of proteins involved in the complement system and the complexities of their interaction, plus the fact that two separate mechanisms have evolved for the activation of the complement system, almost dictate that several important biologic activities would originate from this system. Although all these activities may not be known yet, a rather large number of them are known (Fig. 10-9). Those activities arising from C1, C4, and C2 are expressed only when complement is activated through the classic pathway; those arising from C3 through C9 are expressed after either the classic or alternate pathway activation.

Cytolysis

The classic pathway of complement activation is opened by a serologic reaction between an antigen and immunoglobulin of the IgM or IgG isotypes, and only IgG3, 1, and 2 (in order of activity) of the latter.

There seems to be very little restriction on the na-

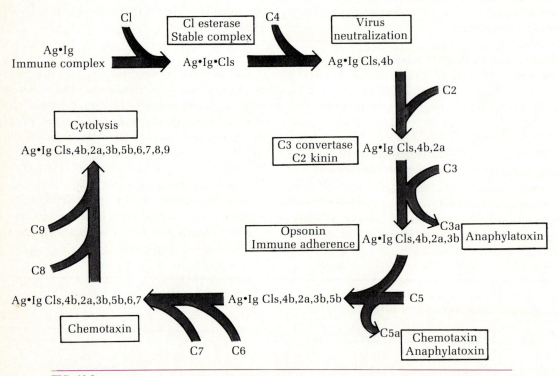

FIG. 10-9

In the classic pathway of complement activation a new biologic activity appears (in *blocks*) at virtually every step of the pathway.

ture of the antigens that will inaugurate (with antibody) the complement sequence. Proteins, polysaccharides, protein or polysaccharide complexes, and hapten-antigen conjugates are all effective, although an occasional antigen that fails to activate complement can be found in any biochemical class. Haptens alone do not initiate the complement cascade, presumably because there is no locus for C4b attachment.

Aggregation of the membrane attack components C5 through C9 on the surface of sensitive cellular antigens, even though the earlier acting components may be dissociated from the cell, will still provoke cytolysis. The number of antibody molecules required for this differs with the immunoglobulin class. By a mathematic correlation of the number of lesions produced in the cell membrane and the number of antibody molecules bound, it was estimated that one IgM molecule and 2,000 to 3,000 IgG molecules were needed to produce a lesion. Two Fc fragments must be bridged by C1 for lysis to ensue. A requirement for multiple molecules of IgM is not necessary, because it has within its own pentameric structure an abundance of complement fixation sites.

Enzyme formation

In the classic complement activation pathway, three new enzyme activities appear. These are C1s esterase and the C3 and C5 convertases. Several enzyme stages exist in the alternate pathway.

C1s esterase is derived from its catalytically inert proenzyme precursor on fixation of the C1 complex to the antigen-antibody pair. C3 convertase activity develops after attachment of C2a and C4b to activated C1. Because this activity does not appear until C2a is bound, C2a is believed to play a critical role in the enzyme. This may be the case with C5 convertase also, since no new enzyme activity has been associated with C3. Moreover, the cleavages of C3 and C5 have so many parallels (for example, substrate size and nature of the peptide bond split) that it is likely that C3 convertase and C5 convertase activities reside in the same portion of the C4b,2a and C4b,2a,3b complexes, respectively.

Factor D is a serine protease normally present in serum. It converts factor B complexed with C3b to an enzyme that then behaves as a C3 or C5 convertase, depending upon the amount of C3b in the complex.

Anaphylatoxins

An anaphylatoxin is any low molecular weight substance of natural origin which will generate a permeability-increasing factor that is inhibited by antihistamines. This is essentially synonymous with a definition of anaphylatoxin as any substance that degranulates mast cells and/or basophils because these cells are the primary source of histamine, which is stored in intracellular granules. Because of the generality of this definition, many substances can be considered as anaphylatoxic. The three known anaphylatoxins generated from complement are C4a (9,000 mol wt), C3a (8,900 mol wt), and C5a (16,000 mol wt). Of these, C4a is the least active. A synthetic octapeptide representing residues 70 through 77 of C3a mimics the complete molecule. A pentapeptide (amino acids 73 through 77) of C4a mimics it. When arginine 77 is removed from either of these, they are no longer anaphylatoxic, whereas C5a loses its anaphylatoxic but retains its chemotactic activity even when the last arginine is removed. A kinin is liberated from C2, but this is apparently different from the vasoactive peptides (kinins) released by anaphylatoxins. (See Chapter 17.)

Chemotaxins

Chemotaxins are substances that induce the migration of leukocytes from an area of lesser concentration to an area of higher concentration of the agent. Chemotaxigens are substances that create chemotaxins from chemotactically inert precursors. In the sense of these definitions C5a is a chemotaxin, and C5 convertase is a chemotaxigen. Another chemotaxin less directly related to the complement cascade is ECF-A. ECF-A originates from mast cell granules where the anaphylatoxic property of C3a, C4a, and C5a would ensure its release.

C3a once was described as a chemotaxin, but this was an error and has been identified as resulting from trace contamination of C3a preparations with C5a.

Opsonization

To detect the direct sensitization of a particle for phagocytic engulfment, it is necessary to have an excess of phagocytic cells in the proximity of the subject particle. Otherwise one might measure the combined action of chemotaxins and opsonins and falsely attribute increased phagocytosis to the latter alone. Opsonins are described in Chapter 5.

Attachment of the C3b to antigen-immunoglobulin complexes improves phagocytosis. Receptors for C3b are found on phagocytic cells, and it is by binding the complex to these receptors that C3b behaves as an opsonin.

Immune adherence

In the traditional serologic agglutination reaction extraneous cells or particulate matter usually are avoided. However, when such particles are present, they are included in the agglutinate in a reaction known as immune adherence or serologic adhesion. This reaction was first described by Levaditi in 1901, who noted bacterial adhesion to platelets in the presence of antibacterial sera. The reaction has been rediscovered and renamed several times since then.

Immune adherence is visually detectable when a particulate antigen, homologous antibody, complement, and indicator particle are present. The indicator particle may be a platelet, erythrocyte, leukocyte, yeast, heterologous bacterium, starch granule, or other. In the course of the reaction the antigen-antibody-complement complex is extended to include the heterologous particle. Analyses with functionally purified components of complement affirm that C3 is the last in the complement series needed for immune adherence. When 50 to 100 C3 molecules are attached to the erythrocyte antigen, adhesion of the indicator particle is just detectable. A maximal reaction requires the fixation of about 1,000 C3 molecules per erythrocyte. Since 10,000 or more C3 molecules per erythrocyte are needed for hemolysis, it is clear that immune adherence is the more sensitive measure of C3. The part of C3 responsible for this activity is C3b.

Immune adherence occurs indiscriminately on any surface. This includes the in vivo attachment of particles to blood vessel walls, which makes them easier prey for phagocytes and must be considered as a protective influence of antibody and complement.

Immunoconglutinins

Lachmann has defined immunoconglutinins as antibodies that display a specificity toward antigenic determinants that are exposed by fixed complement but which are unavailable in free complement. Immunoconglutinin is produced by an animal against its own complement, that is, it is an autoantibody, and arises during ordinary immunization or infections. In the course of the complement fixation the new antigenic determinants are exposed. These new sites appear to be in C3b, although some experiments have suggested that they appear in C4b.

MODULATION OF COMPLEMENT-MEDIATED FUNCTIONS

As described in the preceding section, a multitude of biologic functions are associated with complement and complement-derived peptides. Obviously, biologic control devices have evolved to regulate these activities; otherwise, once initiated, they would continue until the complement system was exhausted. Two principal control systems are known: inactivators, mostly enzymes that destroy the primary structure of the complement protein thus rendering it inactive, and inhibitors, compounds that combine with the complement molecule to halt its further function (Table 10-4).

Complement inactivators

Factor I

A β globulin normally found in serum that cleaves C3b and C4b, and formerly known as KAF and C3b·C4b INAC has now been designated as Factor I. This protein has a molecular weight of 93,000 and is found in serum at a level of 25 μg/ml. Factor I cleaves C3b or C4b only when they are complexed with other proteins, such as the C4 binding protein or Factor H. The α chain of C3b is hydrolyzed at two sites to remove a small peptide of 3000 molecular weight and produce iC3b.

TABLE 10-4

Modulators of the complement system

Modulator	Molecular weight	Electrophoretic mobility	Concentration (μg/ml serum)	Comment
C1s INH	90,000	α_2	100	α_2-Neuraminoglycoprotein
Factor I	90,000	β	25	Synonym of KAF, and C3b·C4b INAC
Factor H	150,000	β	500	Synonym of βIH and C3b·C4b INAC accelerator
Ana INH	300,000	α	35	Carboxypeptidase; acts on C3a, C4a, and C5a
C4 binding protein	60,000	β	Unknown	Complexes with C4
C6 INAC	Unknown	β	Unknown	$S_{20,w}$ is 6.6
S	83,000		500	Binds membrane lipids

In its role as conglutinin activating factor or KAF, C3b in antigen-antibody complexes is altered so that the activity of conglutinin can be expressed. Conglutinin is a β globulin with a molecular weight of 750,000, found at a level of 50 μg/ml of bovine serum. Conglutinin combines with the hemolytically inactive iC3b to cause hemagglutination of erythrocytes that have combined with nonagglutinating quantities of antibody. This conglutinin-complement fixation test is a sensitive indicator of a serologic reaction.

Factor H

Another complement inactivator that has had several name changes is Factor H. Formerly it was known simply as serum β IH to indicate its position in serum electropherograms. Later, it was found to cooperate with Factor I and was labeled as the C3b·C4b INAC accelerator. Factor H is found in human serum at a concentration of 500 μg/ml, as a β globulin with a molecular weight of 150,000. It binds to C3b to retard binding with factor B and accelerates the dissociation of C3b-Factor B complexes. As stated above, it cooperates with Factor I to produce iC3b from C3.

Ana INH

A single enzyme that removes the carboxyl terminal arginine from C4a, C3a, and C5a is inappropri-ately referred to as an inhibitor. In keeping with a system in which enzymes are called inactivators, it really should be termed Ana INAC rather than Ana INH, since it is a carboxypeptidase. Ana INH is a macroglobulin normally present in serum. It is an α-globulin and has a molecular weight of 300,000.

C4 binding protein

Both human and mouse sera contain a β-globulin of 60,000 mol wt that binds to C4, thereby preventing its participation in the complement cascade.

C6 INAC

An inactivator of C6, C6 INAC, is not yet well characterized. It is a β-globulin with an $S_{20,w}$ value of 6.6 and acts on bound, but not on free, C6.

Complement inhibitors
C1s INH

The first molecule described with a known complement-modulating activity was C1s INH, a normal component of the α_2-globulin fraction of human serum. The normal level of C1s INH in human blood is 180 μg/ml. C1s INH is an acid-labile, heat-labile α_2-neuraminoglycoprotein, which is inactivated below pH 6 and above 60° C. Of its molecular weight of 90,000, 17% is in the form of neuraminic acid, and 14% is represented by other carbohydrates.

≡ SITUATION

HANE

Barbara, a 16-year-old white girl, was admitted to the hospital because of repeated attacks of abdominal pain that she had experienced since early childhood. Although early childhood recurrences seldom exceeded 2 or 3 per year, since puberty the attacks had become more frequent and seemed to coincide with the menses. She also complained that severe facial edema, especially of the lips and eyelids, was interfering with her social life. The symptoms usually persisted for 2 or 3 days and then were repeated a month later. Intervening bouts seemed to be associated with mild physical exercise; she had given up guitar lessons because they caused her fingers to swell.

Questions

1. How is the immunologic and clinical diagnosis of HANE established?
2. How does C1s INH regulate this disease?
3. In what way is the complement cascade regulated by current therapeutic programs?

Solution

A definitive diagnosis of $\overline{\text{C1s}}$ INH deficiency on immunologic grounds cannot be made in the usual hospital or clinic. Assays for $\overline{\text{C1s}}$ INH depend on the activity of the patient's serum in neutralizing the action of C1 esterase on synthetic substrates. Traditionally N-acetyl-L-tyrosine ethyl ester (ATEE) is used as the substrate for C1 esterase, which removes the ethyl ester group, liberating the carboxyl group of tyrosine that is titrated with dilute alkali. The C1 esterase inhibitor, incubated with a sample of the esterase, would depress hydrolysis of the substrate. Neither this test nor immunodiffusion tests for the inhibitor are performed in the routine laboratory. This means that the diagnosis is established on indirect laboratory evidence and clinical grounds. The former depends on low complement activity in diluted sera of patients with HANE compared with those of normal persons. Diagnostic features include familial distribution of the disease, anatomic distribution, frequency of the episodes, and response to therapy.

Transfusion of normal plasma to reconstitute the patient's level of $\overline{\text{C1s}}$ INH is one of the most direct means of therapy. It may be the content of plasmin inhibitors in transfused plasma, more than its content of $\overline{\text{C1s}}$ INH, that is therapeutic. Angioneurotic edema frequently is treated just as any acute urticarial condition—with epinephrine and antihistamines. ϵ-Aminocaproic acid is a more specific drug because it is a specific esterase inhibitor. Androgen analogs provide the best therapy since it will correct HANE arising from a total lack of $\overline{\text{C1s}}$ INH or from nonfunctional $\overline{\text{C1s}}$ INH.

Other glycoproteins, including those from egg white, soybean, pancreas, and blood, are also $\overline{\text{C1s}}$ inhibitors. $\overline{\text{C1s}}$ INH will not combine with C1, only $\overline{\text{C1s}}$, and inhibition is achieved at unit stoichiometry, that is, a 1:1 molar ratio. Deficiency of $\overline{\text{C1s}}$ INH results in hereditary angioneurotic edema (HANE), a disease characterized by episodic bouts of edema.

S protein

The S protein is a serum protein that can inhibit the complement system when membrane lipids of an antigen are involved. This specificity of the S protein, a natural protein of serum, is due to its ability to bind surface lipids and interfere with the attachment of C5 and the remaining components of the membrane attack complex.

Complement receptors

Cell receptors for molecules of the complement system participate in phagocytosis, moderate the immune response, serve as cell receptors for viruses, and are important surface markers. Other physiologic roles may be recognized in the future, since there is an increased interest in cell receptors in all fields of science.

Complement receptor type 1, CR1, binds to C3b, iC3b, C4b and C5b. The receptor is a glycoprotein that exists in four major polymorphic forms with molecular weights of 160,000; 190,000; 220,000; and 250,000. This size distribution appears not to be related to the extent of glycosylation, but rather to differences in the peptide itself. The two intermediate-sized molecules are found in an incidence of approximately 99%. Since CR1 is found on a variety of cells including erythrocytes, neutrophils, monocytes; macrophages, B cells and T cells, a variety of physiological roles have been suggested. On neutrophils and cells of the mononuclear system that contain 30,000 CR1/cell, a major role in phagocytosis is accepted. Erythrocyte CR1 (about 500 receptors/cell) is believed to bind to C3b present in soluble immune complexes and to promote their clearance from the circulation. B lymphocyte CR1 may be important in converting these cells into antibody secretors. CR1 may function in its soluble form as a cofactor for C3b·C4b INAC (Factor I).

CR2 binds to C3b, C3d and C3d-g. Thus far, it has been found only on B cells as a 72,000 molecular weight glycoprotein. Until its recent description as the receptor for the Epstein-Barr virus, no function for CR2 had been described.

Type 3 complement receptors (CR3), like CR1, have a wide cell distribution that includes macrophages, LGL, neutrophils and erythrocytes. It binds to the g region of C3d-g and, of course, to C3g. CR3 consists of an α chain of 165,000 molecular weight and a β chain of 95,000 molecular weight, and is part of a family of molecules with identical β chains (see Chapter 5, page 91). On macrophages, CR3 is the Mac 1 antigen.

Other cell surface molecules that interact with proteins of the complement system include those for C1q, factor H, C3a, C4a and C5a. Only a few details are available about these molecules. C1q receptor is unreactive with native C1 because C1r and C1s occupy the collagen region where the receptor binds. After the C1s INH displaces C1r and C1s, then C1q can bind its receptor found on neutrophils, monocytes and a subset of B cells. The receptor for factor H is present on these same cells. The receptor for the anaphylatoxins is discussed in Chapter 17.

Complement phylogeny and ontogeny

Comparative studies on the distribution of the complement components in the sera of animals at several levels of the animal kingdom now have been performed. Invertebrates do not have a classic complement system. Lampreys, which are capable of antibody formation, do not produce complement. All higher life forms have a complement system: elasmobranchs, fishes, amphibia, avians, and mammals. All nine components have been identified only in mammals, however.

All complement components are synthesized early in fetal development, considerably before the appearance of immunoglobulins. C1 has been identified in human fetal intestinal tissue by the nineteenth week of gestation. Tissue cultures of cells taken from human fetal liver at 8 weeks of gestation will synthesize both C4 and C2. Fetal liver, lung, and peritoneal cells taken from fetuses at 14 weeks can be stained successfully with fluorescent anti-C4 and anti-C3. Circulating C4 can be recovered from all fetuses older than 18 weeks and C3 from all those older than 15 weeks.

Determinations of hemolytic complement titers of 44 pairs of maternal and cord sera have revealed that maternal blood contains approximately twice as much complement as cord blood. The complement level of the newborn child reaches the adult level within 3 to 6 months after birth, and the bulk of this recovery occurs within the first 1 or 2 weeks of life. The amount of each individual component of complement in the blood of newborn infants has not been determined, but analyses of C3, C4, and C5 have been accomplished; cord blood contains 38%, 60%, 50%, respectively, of the maternal level of these three components. Maternal C1q titers average about four times those of the newborn infant. Newborn lambs, calves, and pigs are also deficient in complement but repair this defect within the first few weeks of life.

The sources of the complement components in human tissues have been identified. It might be expected that since there are nine major proteins to be considered, several different organs might be involved in the synthesis of these molecules, each organ or tissue being specific for a certain component, but this is not the case.

Tissues of the small and large intestine are the source of all three components of C1. The major intestinal source is the columnar epithelial cell. Monocytes and fibroblasts are also sources of C1q, and C1r and C1s are produced by cultured cells from several organs. Biosynthesis of C2 can be detected in several organs, and eventually cells of the monocyte-macrophage lineage were identified as the cell source. Macrophages are also the source of other components of the classic activation pathway, including C4 and C5, for which the evidence is quite good, and of C6, C7, and C8, where the evidence is less satisfactory. Both C3 and C9 arise from parenchymal cells of the liver.

It should be remembered that C3, C4, and C5 all are derived from precursor molecules that are slightly larger than the active complement component.

Macrophages are the source of factor B, factor D, and properdin.

Complement polymorphism

All complement molecules are not identical in the different species nor within a single species. Indeed allotypic variations already have been described for human C4, 2, 3, 6, 7, 8, and factors B and D. A dozen polymorphic forms of C3 have been identified by simple electrophoresis in agarose or starch gels, in which C3 can be detected easily because of its relatively high concentration in sera. In agarose gels three variants were found in C3. One was an electrophoretically slow (S) variant, and the other two were fast (F) variants, all detected in company with normal C3. Phenotypically a person may be FF, FS, or SS. No significant differences in antigenicity, sedimentation properties, or hemolytic activities have been detected yet in these C3 allotypes.

Polymorphism of human C4 has been noted, with at least 10 different patterns being detected in the immunodiffusion test. Two of these bind to erythrocytes and were erroneously believed to be red blood cell antigens. The human blood groups Chido and Rogers were created as a result of this confusion. Two relatively frequent allotypes and several less common variants of C6 are known. A double pattern of C2 bands has been observed on electrophoresis, and one variant of C7 is known. Both factors B and D of the alternate complement pathway have several electrophoretic variants, which probably are allotypic variants.

Complement genetics

In 1963 serologic studies with a rabbit antiserum to mouse serum globulins distinguished several mouse strains by the ability of the serum from only a few of the strains to precipitate with the antiserum. The variation was designated as due to differences in the quantity of Ss (serum serologic variant) protein in their blood. The gene that regulates Ss formation is situated between the Ir and H-2D regions of the MHC on mouse chromosome 6. Ss is probably a form of murine C4. The structural genes for human C4 also map to the MHC. Another mouse protein originally believed to be present only in the sera of males and thus tagged Slp (sex-linked protein) was found in the high producers of Ss. Slp is the product of a second murine C4 gene, but is functionally inactive. Two human C4 genes are also known. The gene for factor B is also a part of the MHC.

Complement fixation tests
Standard complement fixation test

The complement fixation test takes advantage of two of the properties of complement: its combination in all antigen-antibody reactions, whether or not it is required for that reaction, and the requirement of complement in immunolytic reactions. The complement fixation test is divided into the test system and the indicator system (Fig. 10-10). The test system contains an antigen and a serum believed to contain antibody to that antigen. This serum is heat treated prior to the test to destroy its complement. To these two is added a measured amount of complement in the form of normal guinea pig serum, and an incubation period is allowed. Following this incubation the indicator system, consisting of sheep red blood cells and hemolysin (antibody against sheep red blood cells), is added, and another incubation period is allowed. Hemolysin is identical to hemagglutinin, but has been renamed to more aptly describe its activity in the presence of serum complement.

Interpretation of the complement fixation test is based on the presence or absence of hemolysis in the indicator system. When there is antibody present in the test serum, it combines with the antigen, and complement is fixed into the test system. No erythrocyte lysis occurs. This is referred to as a positive complement fixation test. When there is no antibody in the test serum, complement remains free to be bound later in the indicator system. Erythrocyte lysis is then observed; this is a negative complement fixa-

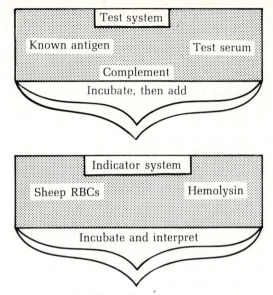

Hemolysis = C fixed in indicator system = negative test
No hemolysis = C fixed in test system = positive test

FIG. 10-10

In the standard complement (C) fixation test the known antigen and test serum are incubated with complement. Then sheep red blood cells and hemolysin are added. If complement was bound in the test serum, the hemolysin cannot lyse the erythrocytes.

tion test. Complement is always fixed in the complement fixation test, either in the test system or in the indicator system. Where it is fixed determines whether the test is positive or negative.

Hemagglutination is not observed in the complement fixation test for the following reason: the antibody to sheep red blood cells is active in a much greater dilution in hemolytic tests than in hemagglutination tests. The amount of antibody required to produce hemagglutination is about 0.01 μg of antibody nitrogen per milliliter of antiserum; only about 0.001 μg of antibody nitrogen per milliliter of antiserum is required for hemolysis. The quantity of hemolysin used for complement fixation is simply too little to cause hemagglutination. The dilution of hemolysin used is so great that it is hardly necessary to heat inactivate it before use, since its complement activity at that dilution is negligible.

The complement fixation test is a delicate test, depending as it does on several serologic reagents, one of which is heat labile. For this reason the quantity of each reagent must be carefully titrated just prior to use, and adequate controls must be applied. For example, the quantity of hemolysin used is determined first by a hemolysin titration. This is performed by making a dilution series of hemolysin in buffer, adding a constant, excess amount of guinea pig complement to each tube, and observing for hemolysis after a suitable incubation period. The hemolysin dilution series should be carried out until dilutions of several thousand are achieved. The extent of hemolysis is either estimated visually, based on an end point of 100% hemolysis, or measured in a colorimeter for an exact reading of the 50% hemolytic end point. From this assay the exact amount of hemolysin needed to produce lysis of 50% of the erythrocytes is determined, and in the complement titration test a multiple of two to five times this amount is used to ensure sufficient reagent in that titration.

To determine the hemolytic activity of complement, different quantities of fresh complement are added to tubes containing sheep red blood cells and hemolysin. After incubation the degree of lysis is read colorimetrically, and the amount of complement required for 50% hemolysis is determined. This is referred to as the CH50 unit, and in the complete complement fixation test two CH50 units of complement are the minimum amount employed. Four to five CH50 units of complement may be used. This means that in a positive complement fixation test as many as five CH50 units of complement must be fixed in the test system; otherwise some complement will be left free to interact in the indicator system.

Separate anticomplementary controls on the antigen are necessary. This includes antigen, complement, sheep red blood cells, and hemolysin (the latter two sometimes premixed and referred to as sensitized erythrocytes). If this tube does not exhibit lysis, it is because of an anticomplementary activity of the antigen. A separate anticomplementary control of the serum also is performed as proof that the serum did not contain nonspecific complement-inactivating substances. If the antigen or serum were anticomplementary and such controls were not included, false positive complement fixation test results of a serious nature could be reported. Since complement is heat labile, a positive lytic control containing only complement and sensitized red blood cells also is included.

The titer of a complement-fixing antiserum is determined in the same way as the titer in most other serologic tests, that is, by testing dilutions of the antiserum.

The complement fixation test can be applied to virtually any antigen-antibody system. It is especially useful when only small quantities of antigen or antibody are available because it is a very sensitive serologic procedure. Moreover certain serologic tests are difficult to demonstrate by other means. For example, antibodies to viruses can be identified much more quickly and less expensively by complement fixation than by animal neutralization tests. If one has a known antiserum, it can be used in complement fixation assays for the antigen. Thus the complement fixation test can be used to determine either antigen or antibody.

The complement fixation test has been used to detect and quantitate antibodies of patients infected with viruses of poliomyelitis, mumps, smallpox, influenza, St. Louis encephalitis, measles, herpes, and adenovirus; bacteria such as *Treponema, Mycobacterium, Neisseria,* and *Hemophilus* organisms; fungi such as *Histoplasma, Blastomyces,* and *Coccidioides* organisms; and many others. Antigens of all varieties have been used in complement fixation tests: enzymes, serum proteins, those of viral, bacterial, rickettsial, and fungal origin, thyroid tissue, blood group substances, etc. Theoretically there is no limit to the antigens or antisera that can be used in this test; this is what has made the complement fixation test so widely appreciated.

The Wassermann test

The most extensive use of the complement fixation test has been in the serologic diagnosis of syphilis by the Wassermann test and its variations. In this test, as originally designed, extracts of the liver of fetuses, stillborn because of syphilis and teeming with *Treponema pallidum,* were used as the antigen. The antibody in a patient's serum, combining with this antigen and fixing complement in the test system, was thought to be a specific antitreponemal antibody. It subsequently was discovered that this antibody would fix complement when alcoholic extracts of normal human or animal tissues were used as the antigen. The antigen now used is a purified alcoholic extract of beef heart to which lecithin and cholesterol have been added. This is known as cardiolipin. The lecithin is added to reduce the anticomplementary activity of the antigen and to replace the lecithin that is removed in the purification procedure. The antigen will not fix complement if cholesterol is omitted.

Since the Wassermann antibody reacts with nonspecific antigen, it is clear that it is not an antibody of the usual type. This view is fortified by the rapid disappearance of this antibody during successful therapy. For these reasons the terms *syphilitic reagin* or *Wassermann reagin* have been applied to this antibody. Caution must be taken not to confuse this with allergic reagin, now known as IgE. Syphilitic reagin may be an unusual autoantibody that reacts with tissue. This "antibody" could be formed originally against treponemal altered autoantigens.

Truly specific serologic tests for syphilis have

been developed using antigens prepared from *T. pallidum* spirochetes taken from experimental lesions in rabbits or cultured in vitro. These procedures have replaced the Wassermann test as a diagnostic device for syphilis. In these instances immunologically specific antibody is measured; the titer of this antibody remains high during and after successful therapy.

REFERENCES

Asghar, S.S.: Pharmacological manipulation of complement system, Pharmacol. Rev. **36:**223, 1984.

Bhakdi, S., and Tranum Jenen, J.: Membrane damage by complement, Biochim. Biophys. Acta **737:**343, 1983.

Colten, H.R.: Biosynthesis of the MHC-linked complement proteins (C2, C4, and factor B) by mononuclear phagocytes, Molec. Immunol. **19:**1279, 1982.

Colten, H.R.: Molecular basis of complement deficiency syndromes, Lab. Invest. **52:**468, 1985.

Colten, H.R.: Molecular genetics of the major histocompatibility linked complement genes, Springer Semin. Immunopathol. **6:**149, 1983.

Cooper, N.R.: The classical complement pathway: activation and regulation of the first complement component, Adv. Immunol. **37:**151, 1985.

Fey, G., Domedy, H., Wiebauer, K., Whitehead, A.S., and Odink, K.: Structure and expression of the C3 gene, Springer Semin. Immunopathol. **6:**119, 1983.

Guenther, L.C.: Inherited disorders of complement, J. Amer. Acad. Dermatol. **9:**815, 1983.

Hartung, H.P., and Hadding, U.: Complement components in relation to macrophage function, Agents Actions **13:**415, 1983.

Hugli, T.E.: Structure and function of the anaphylaxtoxins, Springer Semin. Immunopathol. **7:**193, 1984.

Kazatchkine, M.D., and Nydegger, U.E.: The human alternative complement pathway: biology and immunopathology of activation and regulation, Prog. Allergy **30:**193, 1982.

Lachman, P.J., and Hughes-Jones, N.C.: Initiation of complement activation, Springer Semin. Immunopathol. **7:**143, 1984.

Loos, M.: The classical complement pathway: mechanism of activation of the first component by antigen-antibody complexes, Prog. Allergy **30:**135, 1982.

McPhaden, A.R., Lappin, D., and Whaley, K.: Biosynthesis of complement components, J. Clin. Lab. Immunol. **8:**1, 1982.

Muller-Eberhard, H.J.: The membrane attack complex, Springer Semin. Immunopathol. **7:**93, 1984.

Muller-Eberhard, H.J.: The membrane attack complex of complement, Ann. Rev. Immunol. **4:**503, 1986.

Perez, H.D., and Goldstein, I.M.: Regulation of the biologic activity of C5-derived peptides, Adv. Inflamm. Res. **2:**1, 1981.

Porter, R.R.: The complement components of the major histocompatibility locus, CRC Crit. Rev. Biochem. **16:**1, 1984.

Ratnoff, W.D., Fearon, D.T., and Austen, K.F.: The role of antibody in the activation of the alternative pathway, Springer Semin. Immunopathol. **6:**361, 1983.

Schreiber, R.D.: The chemistry and biology of complement receptors, Springer Semin. Immunopathol. **7:**221, 1984.

Volanakis, J.E.: The complement system: 1983, Surv. Immunol. Res. **3:**202, 1984.

Wright, S.D., and Griffin, F.M., Jr.: Activation of phagocytic cells C3 receptors for phagocytosis, J. Leuk. Biol. **38:**327, 1985.

Ziccardi, R.J.: The first component of human complement (C1): activation and control, Springer Semin. Immunopathol. **6:**213, 1983.

See related **Reading 5,** page 424.

SEROLOGY

Serology with labeled antibodies

≡ GLOSSARY

antiglobulin test A test to determine the presence of one globulin (antibody) by using a second globulin (antibody) with a serologic specificity for the first.

avidin/streptavidin Proteins from egg white and streptomyces, respectively, that bind firmly to biotin.

double antibody technique Often an antiglobulin procedure, but sometimes varied so that two antibodies react with the same antigen.

ELISA Enzyme linked immunosorbent assay.

enzyme linked immunosorbent assay A serologic test that utilizes an enzyme labeled reagent.

equivalence point That dilution in a serologic titration in which all the antigen has combined with all the antibody.

FAB Fluorescent antibody.

fluorescent antibody An immunoglobulin conjugated to a fluorescent dye for use in ultraviolet microscopy.

heterobifunctional cross-linker A chemical with two reactive groups capable of covalently joining two proteins.

optimal proportions That dilution in a serologic titration that becomes positive in the shortest time.

postzone Failure of a serologic reaction to occur in extreme dilutions of antibody.

protein A A protein on the surface of *Staphylococcus aureus* that binds IgG.

prozone Failure of a serologic reaction to occur in a high concentration of antibody.

radioimmunoassay A serologic test in which one of the reagents is labeled with a radioisotope.

RIA Radioimmunoassay.

solid phase radioimmunoassay A radioimmunoassay in which one of the reactants is bound to a surface.

titer The greatest dilution of antigen or antibody that will produce the desired result in a serologic test.

. . .

The presence of antibodies in an antiserum is demonstrated by performing a serologic reaction. The end result of the reaction may be a clumping or agglutination of particulate antigens, a precipitation of fluid antigens, a binding of the antigen without any outward evidence of the reaction, or some other type of reaction, depending on the physical nature of the antigen and the conditions imposed on it.

SEROLOGIC TESTING

In the usual serologic test a dilution series of the antiserum is prepared, and to this an appropriate quantity of antigen is added. Additional tubes lacking antigen or antiserum are prepared as controls for the stability of the two serologic reagents. After a suitable incubation time at a specified temperature the test is examined for the evidence of a serologic reaction. The dilution of the serum in the last tube to exhibit a positive test is the titer of the antiserum.

In such a dilution series, several zones of the serologic reaction may be noted. In the first few tubes, where the antiserum concentration is greatest, a positive test may not be apparent; this is the prozone. In the last tubes in the dilution series, a negative result always should be observed; otherwise, the final titer cannot be determined. This obviously is caused by dilution of the antiserum to the point at which there are too few antibody molecules present to produce a positive test. The dilution of optimal proportions is that dilution in which the serologic reaction is visible in the shortest time. When different preparations of antisera are used and the optimal proportion for each is calculated, it is observed that the ratio of antigen to antibody is nearly constant. The equivalence zone or tube is that in which all of the antigen has combined with all of the antibody, so that no excess of either molecule remains.

MECHANISM OF THE SEROLOGIC REACTION

Bordet proposed that the serologic reaction takes place in two phases. In the first phase combination of the reactants occurs; this is followed by the second phase, aggregation. The first stage takes place almost instantaneously, although there is no external evidence that combination has occurred. Proof that combination takes only a few moments is seen in the experiment in which bacteria and specific antibody are mixed and immediately pelleted in a centrifuge. Examination of the supernatant fluid will reveal that it is now devoid of specific immunoglobulin. Antigen and antibody can combine in the absence of electrolytes. Combination is the portion of the reaction wherein the major change in free energy occurs.

In the second stage of the reaction, aggregation of antigen-immunoglobulin complexes occurs. This phase takes time, requires electrolytes, and involves very little change in free energy. This phase does not occur when monovalent antibodies or monovalent haptens are involved in the reaction.

Marrack developed a theory of serologic reactions on the assumption that antigen and antibody molecules unite through their specific determinant groups and that these groups have a special affinity for each other. This union of antigen with antibody is assumed to be a firm but dissociable combination. Aggregate formation consists of the dissociation and recombination of these molecules with each other until a reasonably stable network of alternating antigen and antibody molecules is formed. At the equivalence point all the antigen and all the antibody mol-

ecules are consumed in lattice formation. It should be noted that lattice formation with simple antigens, which do not contain more than 1 mole of a specific antigenic determinant per molecule, requires the presence of two different species of antibody in the antiserum, each directed against different antigenic sites (Fig. 11-1). When there is an excess of antibody (prozone), aggregation is not observed because, as an antibody dissociates from the antigen, there is a better chance for one of the free antibody molecules than for an antibody that already is attached to an antigen to combine with the original molecule of antigen (Fig. 11-2). Essentially the reverse situation occurs in postzone, where too little antibody is present to produce a complete reaction (Fig. 11-3).

In Marrack's hypothesis one can visualize how antigen-antibody complexes of unequal composition (varying proportion or multiple proportion) could occur, since aggregation of a multivalent antigen molecule would be possible when only two or three of its valence sites are combined with antibody. The inability of monovalent haptens or antibodies to produce aggregation is also self-evident. Furthermore, if antibody is reacted with an excess of hapten so that all combining sites are saturated, there is no possibility for a hapten-conjugated antigen to combine and form a lattice with the antibody. This is the basis for the hapten inhibition reaction.

Although the combination of antigen or hapten with antibody may be firm, it is still dissociable and reversible. This is true of essentially all chemical reactions, but it is sometimes difficult to demonstrate for a specific chemical reaction in which the equilibrium constant is in favor of product formation. This is not true of serologic reactions, in which dissociation and recombination are fairly easy to demonstrate.

A modern illustration of the reversibility of serologic reactions involves the addition of sheep red blood cells to hemolysin in proportions that bind all the hemolytic antibody. Complement, required for lysis of the erythrocytes by hemolysin, must be absent. Then ^{51}Cr-labeled sheep red blood cells are added, and incubation is continued. Complement then is added to initiate the lytic reaction. Only those cells coated with antibody will rupture. The unlysed

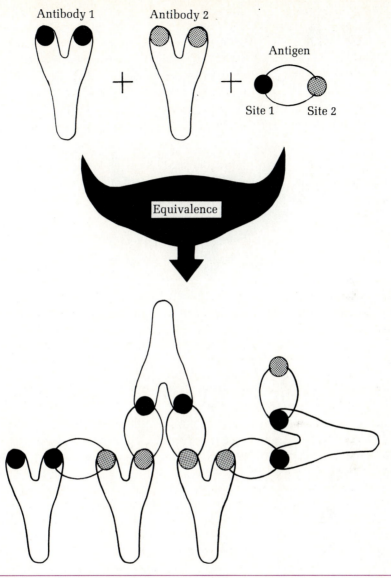

FIG. 11-1

The combination of antigen with antibody at equivalence. Notice that all molecules of both reactants are combined in the lattice and that when an antigenic determinant occurs only once on an antigen molecule, two species of antibody are required for the reaction.

cells are sedimented by centrifugation, and ^{51}Cr in the supernatant fluid is measured. This is evidence of the antibody shift to the labeled red cells added after all antibody had been bound initially to the unlabeled cells.

RELATIVE SENSITIVITY OF SEROLOGIC REACTIONS

Several in vitro and in vivo serologic reactions are available and useful in identifying antigens or antibodies. These reactions differ in their physical con-

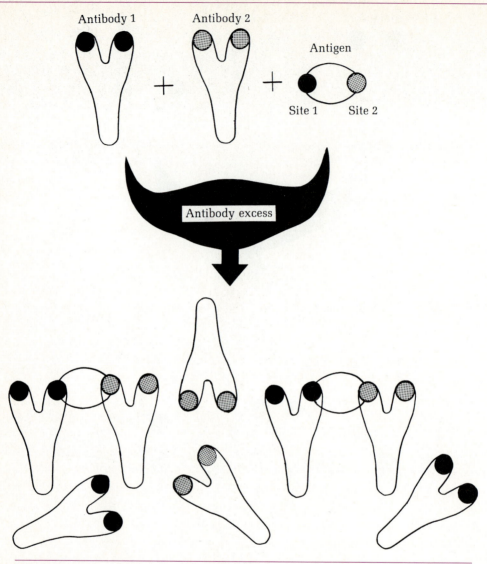

FIG. 11-2
Excess of antibody molecules in prozone with little or no lattice formation.

ditions and in their requirement for external reagents such as white blood cells, serum complement, conglutinin, and test animals. Furthermore these tests may measure different molecular species of antibodies. Thus, it is not surprising that these tests should differ significantly in their sensitivity for detecting antibody (Table 11-1).

One of the least sensitive tests is precipitation, and the fluid and gel tests are of approximately the same insensitivity. For a positive precipitation reaction, 3 to 15 μg of antibody nitrogen per milliliter of serum is usually necessary, but some tests may require more. Several tests require only 0.01 to 1.0 μg of antibody nitrogen per milliliter; these include

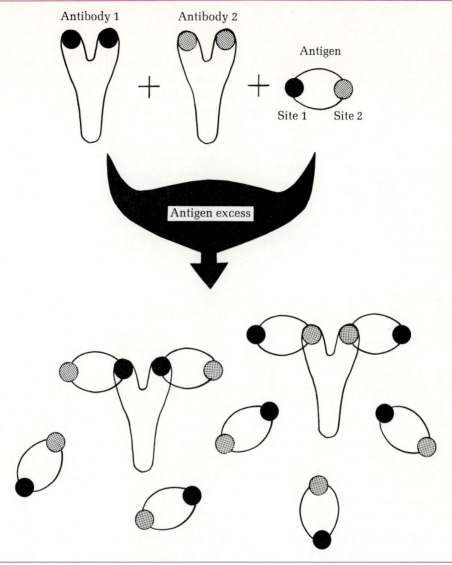

FIG. 11-3

Excess of antigen in postzone with little or no lattice formation.

bacterial agglutination, toxin neutralization, complement fixation, passive cutaneous anaphylaxis, Schultz-Dale reaction, Prausnitz-Küstner (P-K) reaction, and flocculation tests for syphilis. Tests that require only 0.001 to 0.01 μg of antibody nitrogen per milliliter include hemolysis, RIA, enzyme immunoassay, conglutinating complement adsorption, bacteriolysis, and passive hemagglutination. Of these, passive hemagglutination, RIA, enzyme immunoassay, virus neutralization, hemolytic, and bacteriolytic tests are cited as the most delicate. Naturally, there is much variation with the exact procedure used, but under the most optimal conditions as little as 0.00001 μg of antibody nitrogen in 1 ml of antiserum may suffice to produce a positive reaction in these tests.

TABLE 11-1

Comparative sensitivity of serologic tests

Serologic test	Positive test requires
Fluid precipitation	
Interfacial (ring) test	20 to 30 μg antibody nitrogen/ml
Quantitative, colorimetric	3 to 10
Quantitative, nephelometric	0.5 to 3
Gel precipitation	
Double diffusion (Ouchterlony)	3 to 15
Single diffusion (Oudin)	12 to 110
Radial diffusion (Mancini)	3 to 10
Immunoelectrophoresis	50 to 200
Bacterial agglutination	0.01
Hemagglutination	
Direct	0.5 to 1.0
Passive (indirect)	0.001 to 0.03
Hemolysis	0.001 to 0.003
Complement fixation	0.01 to 0.1
Toxin neutralization (diphtheria)	0.01
Anaphylaxis, passive cutaneous	0.01 to 0.03
RIA, enzyme immunoassay	0.001 or less
Bacteriophage or virus neutralization	1 molecule of antibody
Immunocyte adherence	1 antibody-producing cell
Fluorescent antibody	1 antibody-producing cell
Jerne PFC	1 antibody-producing cell

In certain systems the serologic reaction cannot proceed to its second, or aggregative phase. Haptens by definition consist of but a single antigenic determinant and, since they lack a multivalent character, are unable to form a serologic lattice work. On the other hand, some antisera contain high levels of antibodies, referred to as monovalent, incomplete, or blocking antibodies, which fail to aggregate with antigen, and this is typical of normal IgE molecules. It is a known property of IgE to combine with antigens or haptens in vitro, but be unable to continue into agglutination, precipitation, complement fixation, and other processes. The presence of high levels of

IgE or IgE-like immunoglobulins in a serum does much to explain the prozone phenomenon and the blocking antibody effect. Blocking antibodies are those which, by binding to an antigen, block the attachment of other antibodies or cells with the antigen receptors. Blocking antibody used in this sense is unable to aggregate the antigen.

Under certain circumstances, deliberate efforts to prevent development of the aggregative portion of the serologic reaction can be rewarding. When expensive reagents are used, it is obviously economic to use the reactants at the greatest dilution possible. When this is the case, the reaction is rarely detectable with the unaided eye. Reliance must be placed on sophisticated instrumentation or serologic procedures to note that the reaction has occurred. Frequently this involves the use of labeled haptens, antigens, or antibodies.

TRADITIONAL HAPTEN REACTIONS

Since the reaction of a hapten with its antibody cannot progress through the aggregation phase and become directly visible, serologic tests for hapten-antibody interaction are dependent entirely on changes that occur in the first, or combination, phase of the serologic reaction. Historically this has been done by measuring the influence the hapten may have on the aggregation of the antihapten with the hapten-antigen conjugate; that is, the hapten inhibition test. The hapten inhibition test has been superceded by numerous, more sensitive tests.

In the hapten inhibition test increasing quantities of hapten are mixed with an appropriate (constant) amount of antibody or antiserum specific for the hapten and incubated prior to the addition of a fixed amount of hapten-antigen conjugate. After a second incubation the extent of the inhibition by hapten of the expected complete reaction with the hapten-antigen conjugate can be calculated. This technique permitted Landsteiner and others to originate many ideas about hapten-immunoglobulin interactions that are still valid today.

An alternative reaction to hapten inhibition is equilibrium dialysis, from which the equilibrium constant of the hapten-antibody system can be determined. The experimental arrangement for equilibrium dialysis requires the placement of the antibody (antiserum or its globulin fraction) within a dialysis membrane. This dialysis bag is placed in a container filled with a solution of the hapten. The concentration of the hapten in this solution must be known. During the incubation that follows, the hapten is able to diffuse freely across the dialysis membrane, but the antibody, because of its larger size, cannot. When equilibrium has been reached, the concentration of hapten inside and outside the dialysis bag is determined. These measurements are corrected for nonspecific binding by the dialysis membrane and normal γ-globulin solutions in appropriate controls. The increase in the concentration of hapten inside the dialysis tube, compared with its concentration outside the tube, is a measure of the hapten actually bound by the antibody and held inside the dialysis membrane. Relatively simple calculations allow this information to be converted into the average dissociation constant as well as providing direct proof that a hapten-antibody reaction has occurred.

A simpler and more rapid procedure that yields the same information is the fluorescence-quenching technique. Nearly all proteins fluoresce when activated by ultraviolet light at or near the absorption maximum of phenylalanine, tyrosine, and tryptophan—between 280 and 350 nm. However, the fluorescent light emitted is at 350 nm; so the preferred choice of excitation light is in the lower wavelength range. When an antibody molecule combines with a hapten, its fluorescence is quenched, presumably by a transfer of its excitation energy to the hapten rather than into light energy. This quenching of fluorescence is easily quantitated in a spectrofluorometer. The extent of this quenching is mathematically relatable to the quantity of hapten bound, and thus can be treated to derive an association constant of the antibody. One distinct limitation to this method is the requirement for purified antibody solutions. Certain haptens do not absorb the excitation energy very easily and thus are poor quenchers.

RADIOIMMUNOASSAY (RIA)

The impetus for the development of RIAs stemmed from the pioneer work of Berson and Yalow in the middle 1950s. These investigators were interested in diabetes and believed that diabetic individuals might eliminate insulin too rapidly from their bodies, thus creating a hormonal insufficiency. To test this, they injected radiolabeled insulin into normal and diabetic subjects. Contrary to their hypothesis, they observed that the insulin was retained longer in the blood of diabetics. Further studies revealed that this was caused by the presence of insulin antibodies in diabetics. When a combination of radiolabeled and unlabeled insulin was injected, it was noted that the unlabeled hormone competitively inhibited antibody binding by the labeled hormone. When this information was translated from those in vivo experiments to in vitro conditions, the basis for the development of RIA tests for many antigens and haptens was founded.

One arrangement for RIAs establishes a competition of a known amount of radiolabeled antigen (or hapten) and an unknown amount of the same unlabeled antigen with a limited, standard amount of antibody. The amount of antibody used is determined by an earlier titration with labeled antigen and is usually the amount of antibody or antiserum that will bind 70% of the antigen; however, a simpler mathematic explanation of the reaction based on 100% binding is used here. If it is assumed that only the IgG class of antibody is involved in the reaction, then 100 molecules of immunoglobulin will bind 200 molecules of antigen (hapten), since each IgG molecule has two binding sites. If a mixture of 200 molecules of radiolabeled antigen and 200 molecules of unlabeled antigen is incubated with the 100 molecules of IgG, it is obvious that half the radiolabeled antigen will be displaced from the antibody, creating a bound-free ratio of 1:1 (Fig. 11-4). Thus in any experimental determination that results in a 50% diminution in binding of the radiolabeled antigen, the concentration of the unknown sample is exactly the same as that of the known. It follows logically that other bound-versus-free ratios of antigen could be used to determine other concentrations of the unknown antigen.

A critical part of any RIA is clearly the problem of distinguishing between the bound and free portions of the labeled antigen (hapten). If the antigen precipitates with the antibody, the unbound mole-

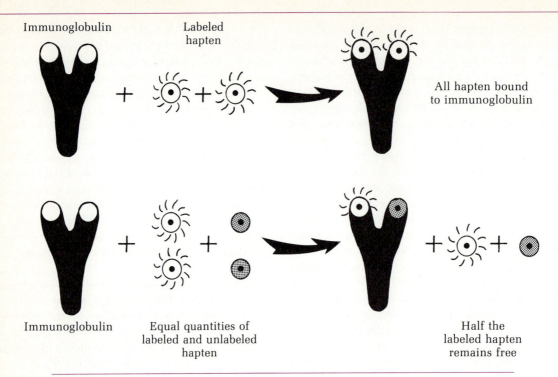

FIG. 11-4

In a preliminary titration prior to the RIA test the amount of radiolabeled hapten (or antigen) that will react with a standard amount of antibody is determined. In this example two parts of hapten saturate one part of immunoglobulin. To determine the amount of hapten in a solution of unknown concentration, it is added to two parts of labeled hapten and one part of immunoglobulin. After the reaction is complete, if one finds that half the labeled hapten is bound to the antibody and half is free, then the unknown solution contained two parts of hapten.

cules can be removed simply by washing the precipitate. The difference in the amount of radiolabel added and that recovered in the precipitate is then the amount of free antigen. As a matter of practical application, RIA tests of this type usually are not performed. RIA tests are conducted more frequently with nonprecipitating haptens, or, for reasons of economy, with antigen or antibody solutions diluted beyond their capacity to form a visible reaction. Under these conditions some physicochemical method must be used to separate the bound and free haptens.

When the antigen is of low molecular weight, or when a hapten is used, advantage can be taken of the insolubility of immunoglobulins in 50% saturated ammonium sulfate to separate the free from the immunoglobulin-bound hapten. After the reaction is

complete, the mixture is adjusted to 50% saturation with ammonium sulfate. This precipitates the antibody and its bound antigen but leaves the unbound antigen in solution. Counting the radioisotope content of the precipitate and subtracting this from the amount of isotope added indicates how much labeled antigen was displaced, which is the amount of unlabeled antigen present in the unknown. Alternately, the calculation can be based on how much radiolabeled antigen remained unprecipitated. Precipitants other than ammonium sulfate may be used. The only restriction is that they must not precipitate the free antigen nor affect any dissociation of the bound antigen from the antibody.

A second method of precipitating soluble antibody-antigen complexes is by the double antibody procedure, or antiglobulin method, sometimes referred to as an "immunologic sandwich." In this form of RIA testing it is necessary to know the species origin of the primary antibody being used in the assay and to have a secondary antibody that will precipitate that species of γ-globulin. If the competitive binding portion of the assay uses a rabbit antibody, the experimenter needs an antibody against rabbit γ-globulin to complete the test. If the original antiserum is of goat origin, then an antibody against goat γ-globulin is needed. The primary antibody and its bound antigen are precipitated by the antiglobulin. The primary immunoglobulin serves both as an antibody and as an antigen and is the "meat" of the sandwich. Unbound antigen is not affected by the secondary antibody and remains in solution.

There is nothing mysterious about the ability of a γ-globulin to serve as an antigen. It meets all the criteria of an antigen when injected into a foreign species. γ-Globulins contain allotypic determinants in their Fab and Fc portions, and the combination of the Fab portions with an antigen does not sterically block the attachment of antibodies to the Fc determinants.

An innovative approach to the harvesting of soluble antigen-antibody complexes has been the use of protein A. This protein is present on the surface of certain strains of *Staphylococcus aureus,* where it is covalently linked with the peptidoglycan support structure of the cell wall. Protein A has been isolated from lysed preparations of *S. aureus* and identified as a single peptide of 42,000 mol wt. Protein A has four binding sites for the Fc domain of IgG, enabling it to combine with IgG that has already bound to antigen. The human IgG subclasses 1, 2, and 4, but not 3, react with protein A. Since protein A does not bind with free antigens, soluble protein A, protein A attached to insoluble particles, or even intact *S. aureus* can be used to insolubilize antigen-antibody complexes as a substitute for an antiglobulin technique.

A third method of RIA is referred to as a solid phase RIA. In this variation the antibody already is provided or converted to an insoluble form. In one form of the test, the antibody is allowed to attach by physical adsorption to the inner surface of polystyrene assay tubes or wells in a plate. A known amount of the labeled antigen and an unknown quantity of unlabeled antigen are added. After an incubation period the unreacted reagents are rinsed from the wells, and the amount of isotope bound to the well is determined. Any decrease from the amount added is an index of the quantity of antigen in the unknown. Titrations with known quantities of the competing unlabeled antigen should be conducted to establish a standard curve and simplify subsequent calculations.

It is not always necessary to use competitive inhibition procedures to measure the amount of antigen in an unknown solution. One can adsorb a primary antibody to the polystyrene wells, add antigen, and then add radiolabeled antibody. The amount of radioisotope that is retained in this immunologic sandwich is an index of the amount of antigen.

In those RIA procedures that rely on spontaneous adsorption of proteins to wells in plastic trays, a blocking step is needed. In the preceeding paragraph, for example, it is necessary to prevent nonspecific adsorption of the antigen by interposing a rinse with a solution of gelatin, bovine serum albumin, or other non-interfering protein between the additions of the primary antibody and antigen. Alternatives include coupling the antibody to cellulose, Sepharose, or Sephadex or embedding it in porous glass beads or polyacrylamide particles as the solid phase support. The cross-linked dextrans (Sephadex or Sepharose) and porous glass entrap the large antibody molecules within their matrix yet still permit the entry and exit of smaller molecules by simple diffusion. After equilibrium is reached, centrifugation separates the bound antigen from the free.

Regardless of the exact RIA procedure used, the great advantage of all RIAs is their sensitivity. Commercially available RIA kits may detect as little as one nanogram (a billionth of a gram) or a picogram (10^{-12} gram, or a trillionth of a gram) of antigen. This is obviously of great significance in monitoring or determining the blood level of certain hormones or therapeutic agents that seldom exceed a few micrograms per milliliter. RIA procedures have the disadvantage of relatively great expense in terms of both the reagents and radioisotope-counting equipment and the unavoidable hazards associated with radioisotopes. These features obviously have not been a serious handicap to the clinical application of RIA. RIA procedures are currently in use for monitoring cardiovascular function, reproductive functions, hematopoietic function, and various other metabolic functions and are available for the quantitation of opiates, barbiturates, amphetamines, and other abused drugs (Table 11-2). Detection of hepatitis-associated antigen is another important application of RIA.

For RIA tests not all radioisotopes are of equal utility. Many isotopes have a half-life of only a few days, and any serologic reagent incorporating them would have too brief a shelf life to be of much use. Isotopes of iodine—^{125}I (half-life, 57.5 days) and ^{131}I (half-life, 8 days)—are the two most frequently used isotopes in immunology. Advantages of their use include the ease of in vitro labeling, which allows for labeling of a predetermined activity, and, in the case of ^{131}I, the emission of γ-rays of relatively high energy.

ENZYME-LINKED IMMUNOSORBENT ASSAYS (ELISA)

The expense, intrinsic hazards, and instability of the reagents used in RIAs spurred a search for other labels that could be used with serologic reagents—haptens, antigens, and antibodies. Several nonisotopic labels have been employed, including fluorescent dyes and enzymes. The advantages offered by enzyme-linked immunosorbent assays (ELISA) are those of most antibody-labeled reactions, and include specificity, sensitivity, rapidity, inexpensiveness, and safety.

Since the enzyme label is the critical portion of enzyme immunoassay methods, its selection is very important. The primary criteria are that the enzyme be stable under the conditions used for storage, cross-linking, and assay, have a high specific activity or substrate turnover number, and be inexpensive. Equally important is that the enzyme must be absent from the antigen or antiserum preparation to be used in the serologic tests; otherwise false positive tests would result. False negative results could stem from the presence of enzyme inhibitors or inac-

TABLE 11-2

A partial list of biologically important substances measured by RIA

Follicle-stimulating hormone (FSH)	Digoxin
Adrenocorticotropic hormone (ACTH)	Digitoxin
Human chorionic gonadotropin (HCG)	Renin
Pituitary human growth hormone (HGH)	Vitamin A
Luteinizing hormone (LH)	Folic acid
Luteinizing hormone release factor (LHRF)	Hageman factor
Thyroid-stimulating hormone (TSH)	cAMP
Human placental lactogen (HPL)	cGMP
Melanocyte-stimulating hormone (MSH)	Plasmin
Parathyroid hormone (PTH)	Trypsin
Calcitonin (CT)	Chymotrypsin
Insulin	Carboxypeptidase
Glucagon	Elastase
Oxytocin	Hepatitis virus
Vasopressin	Mouse leukemia virus
Prolactin	CEA
Gastrin	AFP
Secretin	AHP
Bradykinin	Properdin
Cholecystokinin (CCK)	C1 esterase
Thyroxine (T_4)	C1q
Triiodothyronine (T_3)	Fibrinogen
Corticosteroids	IgG
Estrogens	IgE
Androgens	Myelin basic protein (MBP)
Prostaglandin	Cholera toxin

tivators in the serologic reagents. Appropriate controls must be incorporated into the tests to identify these potential problems in ELISA.

At least nine different enzymes have been used in ELISA (Table 11-3). These are horseradish peroxidase, alkaline phosphatase from *Escherichia coli* or calf intestinal mucosa, glucose oxidase and glu-

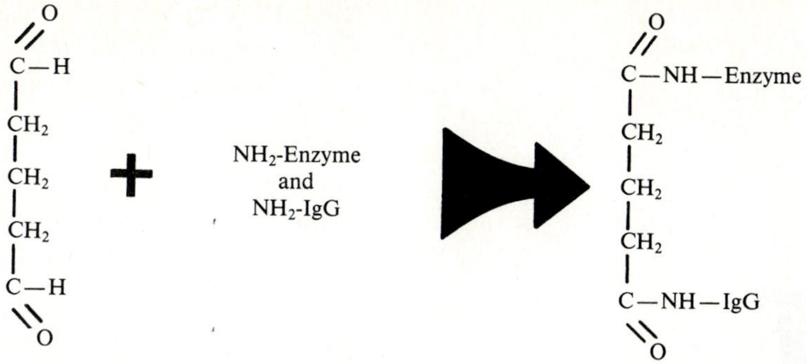

FIG. 11-5

Glutaraldehyde has two aldehyde groups and by proper adjustment of reagent proportions will bind to two separate proteins.

TABLE 11-3

Enzymes employed in enzyme immunoassay

Enzyme	Source	Molecular weight
Peroxidase	Horseradish	40,000
Alkaline phosphatase	*Escherichia coli*	80,000
Glucose oxidase	*Aspergillis niger*	160,000
Lysozyme	Egg white	14,400
Malate dehydrogenase	Pig heart	70,000
β-Galactosidase	*Escherichia coli*	540,000
G6PD	*Leuconostoc mesenteroides*	104,000
Acetylcholinesterase	*Electrophorus electricus* (electric eel)	260,000

coamylase from fungal sources, egg white lysozyme, malate dehydrogenase from pig heart mitochondria, β-galactosidase from *E. coli,* glucose-6-phosphate dehydrogenase (G6PD) from *Leuconostoc mesenteroides,* and acetylcholinesterase from the electric eel. Peroxidase and alkaline phosphatase have been the most widely used, but lysozyme and G6PD are available in commercial preparations. One advantage of lysozyme, in addition to its stability, is its low molecular weight (14,400), so several molecules can be attached to each immunoglobulin molecule without fear of problems related to steric hindrance. This also minimizes steric hindrance of the antigen-antibody reaction by enzyme, since its size is small compared with that of the antibody molecule.

Glutaraldehyde is a bifunctional cross-linker used to join the enzyme to the antigen or antibody. The reaction proceeds through the dialdehyde portion of the molecule and amino groups on the reactants. A unique and valuable aspect of the glutaraldehyde-peroxidase reaction is that only one aldehyde group attaches to the enzyme so that peroxidase-peroxidase dimers are rarely formed (Fig. 11-5). Substituted maleimides are also useful in linking two proteins especially when one contains free thiol groups or can be thiolated (Fig. 11-6). Other bifunctional reagents used in the past include toluene 2,4-diisocyanate, tetrazotized *o*-dianisidine, difluorodinitrophenyl derivatives, and substituted carbodiimides (Fig. 11-7). Several enzyme conjugates have proved stable for more than a year. Here it must be remembered that the half-life of ^{131}I is only 8 days.

A recently popularized system for binding radioisotopes or enzymes into serologic reactions utilizes

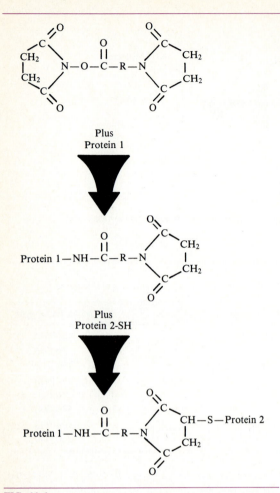

FIG. 11-6

Maleimide derivatives can bind to two separate proteins, one through an amide bond (Step 1) and the other through a thioether bond (Step 2).

the avidin or streptavidin/biotin catch systems. Avidin is an egg-white glycoprotein with a molecular weight of 66,000 that is capable of binding to four equivalents of biotin. This union is not easily dissociated, but because of its isoelectric point near pH 10, avidin tends to bind ionically to many substances. Nonspecific adsorption of this type has limited the usefulness of the avidin-biotin system in immunologic reagents. Streptavidin (mol wt 60,000), from *Streptomyces avidinii* is much like avidin but has an isoelectric point near pH 5. In physiologic so-

lutions, it is less apt than avidin to bind to other reagents nonspecifically, and thus is a superior detector of biotin and of any immunological reagent to which biotin is bound.

In Fig. 11-8, an illustration of the avidin/biotin system is depicted in which an antibody is attached to an antigen on a cell's surface. A biotinylated antiglobulin with a serologic specificity for the first antibody reacts with it. Thereafter, a labeled avidin (or streptavidin molecule) is added. Signals from the enzyme or isotope label are used to quantitate the extent of the first serologic reaction. In the avidin/biotin system, it is also possible to use biotin as the immunoglobulin marker and avidin as the enzyme carrier.

The conjugate of enzyme with antigen or of enzyme with antibody must be separated from unreacted molecules or from the homodimers formed during the cross-linking step. This depends almost entirely on size differences among the reaction products and is accomplished by filtration through membranes of selected pore size or by molecular sieving chromatography. For example, lysozyme labeling of a purified immunoglobulin preparation would produce free lysozyme, lysozyme-lysozyme, lysozyme-immunoglobulin, immunoglobulin-immunoglobulin, and free immunoglobulin as the hypothetical end products. The use of an excess of lysozyme and cross-linking reagents would be expected to reduce the amount of immunoglobulin left unreacted. Filtration through a membrane with a pore size of 50,000 would allow the excess lysozyme and lysozyme-lysozyme dimers to pass but would retain the larger molecules. Then a filter with a pore size near 200,000 could be used to allow the desired conjugate to pass and to retain the immunoglobulin-immunoglobulin dimers. By collecting those fractions with enzyme activity which are eluted from a molecular sieving column, and selecting only that one with antibody activity, one can separate the enzyme-linked antibody from the unwanted molecules.

Enzyme activity generally is determined spectrophotometrically. Alkaline phosphatase is easily determined by the color change associated with cleavage of *p*-nitrophenylphosphate as the substrate. The oxidizing activity of the H_2O_2 formed by glucose

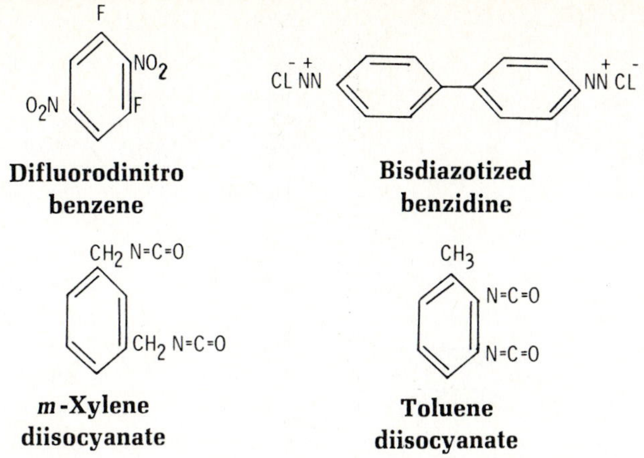

FIG. 11-7

Divalent coupling reagents used for ELISA and ferritin-labeled antibody procedures. Under ideal conditions one molecule of coupling reagent is simultaneously attached to one molecule of enzyme or ferritin and one molecule of antibody.

oxidase is its measure of concentration. Peroxidase is measured by its ability to change the color of *o*-dianisidine. Other enzymes have equally simple colorimetric or spectrophotometric quantitation methods. Thus, if an enzyme-labeled antibody is bound serologically to a solid phase antigen contained in a tube, it is only necessary to add the enzyme substrate in a suitable buffer and follow spectrophotometrically the appearance of the enzyme end product within a specific time period. This quantitates the amount of enzyme present and the amount of antigen. A decrease in the amount of bound enzyme activity created by preincubation of free antigen with the labeled antibody is then a reflection of the amount of free antigen in an unknown solution.

ELISA methods may be even more sensitive than RIA methods (Table 11-4). In the latter, when the radionuclide emits the γ or β particle, it is then less radioactive or inactive and cannot be measured again as a radioisotope. In ELISA, the enzyme catalyzes a change in a substrate molecule, but the enzyme itself is not consumed in this process. The enzyme molecule continues to act on more substrate molecules and in the form of the end products produced can give off literally thousands of signals of its presence.

Four forms of enzyme immunoassay have been developed: the competitive binding test, the immu-

noenzymometric test, the sandwich method for antigen or antibody, and the homogeneous enzyme immunoassay. Only the competitive binding test is properly referred to as the ELISA procedure. The ELISA test was the first to be developed and is patterned exactly after the standard competitive RIA procedure. Labeled and unlabeled antigens compete for attachment to a limited quantity of solid phase antibody. The enzyme label that is displaced is quantitated, and the calculations that follow are essentially the same as in RIA procedures. Again, in ELISA tests in which the solid phase relies on a nonspecific binding of an immunoglobulin or antigen to a plastic surface, blockade of nonspecific binding sites with gelatin or bovine albumin is required. Then the subsequent binding of any reagent can only be due to immunological specificity.

In the immunoenzymometric procedure an unknown quantity of antigen is reacted with an excess of labeled antibody, and then solid phase antigen is added. Centrifugation removes the unreacted enzyme-linked antibody molecules. Then enzyme activity associated with the soluble phase is measured, and this is an expression of the antigen concentration in the unknown sample.

The sandwich technique relies on the multivalence of antigen and its capacity to bind simulta-

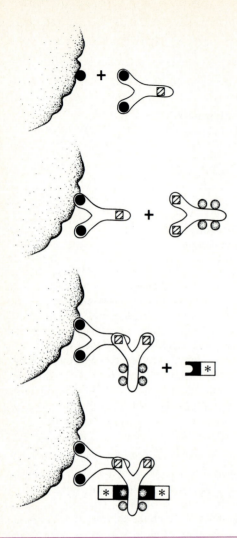

FIG. 11-8

In this illustration of the avidin-biotin labeling system, the primary antibody is bound to an antigen on the surface of a cell. A biotinylated second antibody reacts with the primary antibody. Avidin, labeled with enzyme or isotope, reacts with biotin on the second antibody. In this way, the presence and the quantity of the original antigen can be determined.

neously with two molecules of antibody. The first antibody molecule, used in excess, is a solid phase reactant. Nonspecific protein binding sites are then blocked with gelatin and antigen is added. After this reaction is completed, an enzyme-labeled antibody is

TABLE 11-4

A partial list of biologically important substances measured by enzyme immunoassay

Antigen or hapten	Enzyme label
Human serum albumin	Glucose oxidase
CEA	Alkaline phosphatase
AFP	Alkaline phosphatase, glucose oxidase, peroxidase
Haptoglobin	Alkaline phosphatase
IgE	Alkaline phosphatase
IgG	Alkaline phosphatase, glucose oxidase, peroxidase, β-galactosidase
Insulin	Alkaline phosphatase, peroxidase, β-galactosidase
Human placental lactogen	Peroxidase
Estrogens	Peroxidase
Chorionic gonadotropin	Peroxidase, acetylcholinesterase
Progesterone	β-Galactosidase
Digoxin	G6PD
Morphine	Lysozyme, malate dehydrogenase
Thyrotropin	Alkaline phosphatase
α_2-Globulins	Peroxidase
Cortisol	β-Galactosidase
Cholera toxin	Alkaline phosphatase
Streptolysin O	Glucose oxidase
Hepatitis B virus	Peroxidase
κ or γ L chains	Alkaline phosphatase
Hog cholera virus	Peroxidase
Rubella virus	Alkaline phosphatase
Malarial parasites	Alkaline phosphatase
Amphetamine	Lysozyme
Phenobarbital	G6PD
Methadone	Lysozyme

added and incubated with the complex resulting from the first phase. The labeled antibody now combines with the available determinants on the antigen. Excess antibody is removed by washing, and enzyme activity is determined. As before, the amount of enzyme bound to the complex is an indirect expression of the amount of antigen in the sample. This procedure is also commonly described as an ELISA technique.

c

≣ SITUATION

THE GRAD STUDENT MIXER

As the Graduate Student Association mixer was about to break up, a fellow you recognized as a student in the biochem. department approached you. He introduced himself and asked, "Can I pick your brain for the price of a beer?"

"Sure, as long as it's a mug!"

"Good, I need help from an immunologist. I've got a problem."

With that introduction he briefly outlined his doctoral research project. His advisor had been carrying a cell culture line for several years that was capable of producing nanogram quantities per milliliter of an exciting new hormone. All efforts to increase the yield of hormone by manipulating the composition of the growth medium had failed. This also was hampered by the fact that the biologic assay for the hormone, a molecule of only 17,500 mol wt, was expensive, time consuming, and subject to excessive variability. Now the possibility of selecting mutant cells with a greater hormone-synthesizing capacity was under consideration. Would it be possible to develop an immunoassay for tiny quantities of hormone that could be used to recognize the desired mutant cells and to more satisfactorily quantitate the hormone in culture fluids?

Questions

1. What are the antigen and immunization demands in problems such as the one just outlined?
2. What serologic procedures are sufficiently sensitive to quantitate nanogram amounts of an antigen or hapten?
3. Which serologic procedures are applicable to the recognition of specific antigens in or on cells?
4. Are the procedures meeting the demands of questions 1, 2, and 3 practical in terms of expense, time to develop (as for a Ph.D. dissertation), reproducibility, etc.?

Solution

To recognize and quantitate an antigen, it is necessary to produce a high-titer, specific anti-serum. This is an aspect of research problems like the one being considered here which is often more troublesome than it first appears. The primary requirement, of course, is to have an adequate supply of a highly purified preparation of the antigen. "An adequate supply" was a deliberately chosen vaguely stated phase. The immunologist would like to have several milligrams to enable the immunization of several rabbits or other species. Low molecular weight antigens are not as potent as those of larger size. Thus a large group of animals usually is selected for immunization with these antigens. This would make a larger demand on the ideal amount of antigen needed. Clearly the use of adjuvants is important in problems in which antigen supply is limited. Fortunately several good adjuvants are available. One method—an adjuvant-based method combined with antigen purification—might apply here. It is possible to identify an antigen in polyacrylamide gels where it has been electrophoretically separated from other antigens and use the antigen-gel mixture directly in the immunization. The matrix of the gel slows the release of antigen into the true physiologic milieu of the immunized animal and thus behaves as a depository adjuvant.

It is undoubtedly important to attempt the development of hybridomas in this instance. Hybridoma cells may even be detected that are specific for the hormone-active determinants, a feature that would be far superior to biological assays for the hormone.

The most sensitive serologic procedures are the antigen- (or hapten-) binding reactions that economize on the amount of antigen used by eliminating the large amount of reactants needed to produce a second phase in the serologic reaction. The sensitivity of these tests almost always is related to the ability of a modified form of the antigen or antibody to display an easily detectable recognition signal. This may be done through the agency of fluorescent dyes, radioisotope or enzyme labels, or other alterations of the chemistry of the antigen or antibody.

The methods most adaptable to quantitating tiny amounts of antigen in solution would be RIA or enzyme-linked immunoassay. As described in this chapter, nanogram or picogram quantities per milliliter, or in some instances even per deciliter or liter, can be accurately determined by these techniques under ideal assay conditions. Preference for one or the other of these two methods would be based on criteria such as availability of radioisotope-counting equipment and general experience with radioisotopic or enzymatic techniques and related subjects, since the methods are very similar in sensitivity and in technical performance.

Immunohistochemical localization of antigens on cell surfaces is possible through techniques such as the horseradish peroxidase or ferritin antibody methods used in electron microscopy. Since there is no apparent need to involve electron microscopy in this problem, fluorescent or enzyme-linked methods would be preferred. Indirect methods are more sensitive than direct methods and would be recommended here. The limits of antigen detection by immunocytochemical methods are uncertain, but there is no reason to suspect other than success in their application here.

The practicality of the procedures outlined needs no further testimony than the abundance of such methods already available for problems with demands similar to those presented here. As with any research problem, a prediction as to time and cost must be tempered by the intangible: luck. Ordinarily the development of a completely satisfactory solution to the problems presented here would be more than an average Ph.D. candidate could accomplish in the time usually needed to complete degree requirements.

The homogeneous enzyme immunoassay system does not require a solid phase reactant. It relies on an inhibition of enzyme activity by combination of antibody with an enzyme-labeled antigen or hapten. This does not occur with all systems but can be a valuable serologic method for measuring haptens. Enzyme inhibition is presumed to occur because of steric effects. When the hapten is surrounded by the immunoglobulin, the enzyme is masked from its substrate.

The parallels between ELISA and RIA are apparent, and the simplicity and economy of the former are two reasons why many RIA tests have been replaced by their ELISA counterparts.

Although immunoblotting is perhaps as much a variation of precipitation testing as immunobinding, the amplification of immunoblotting reactions by enzyme techniques makes it an appropriate continuation of ELISA methodology. Immunoblotting is a form of solid phase ELISA whose development was hinged to the formulation of activated cellulose papers or membranes. Nitrocellulose papers can be ionically or covalently bonded to proteins that are applied directly to the paper or transferred to it by placing the paper on protein-containing gels. Alternatively, bifunctional cross-linkers can be used to insure covalent attachment of antigen to the cellulose. Such papers can then be used as a source of solid-phase antigen. After protein fixation to the cellulose, it is blocked with gelatin and the subsequent application of an enzyme linked antibody will detect the location and quantity of antigen as in ordinary ELISA tests.

FLUORESCENT ANTIBODY METHODS

Fluorescent antibodies (FAB) are antibody preparations that are chemically coupled to a fluorescent dye. The conjugation of the reactants is performed so that the serologic activity and specificity of the γ-globulin and the fluorescent character of the dyes are preserved in a single molecule. Efforts to label antibodies with visually detectable carriers date back more than 50 years. No true success was achieved until the early 1940s, when Coons developed the fluorescent antibody method.

The fluorescent technique makes use of special dyes referred to as fluors or fluorochromes. Fluors are chemical substances that are capable of absorbing a short wavelength of light and instantaneously emitting a longer wavelength light. The dyes used for fluorescent antibody absorb in the ultraviolet and short blue range (200 to 400 nm) and emit a visible light. The exact absorption spectrum of the fluor and that of its emitted light are characteristic for each fluor. The color of the emitted light is not a characteristic of the excitation light.

The fluorochromes usually chosen are fluorescein, a rhodamine such as lissamine rhodamine B, and 1-dimethylaminonaphthalene-5 sulfonic acid (DANSYL) (Fig. 11-9). Fluorescein and DANSYL give off a green or yellow-green light, and rhodamine gives off an orange-red hue. Texas red is another label that emits an orange-red fluorescence. All three are easily bonded to the free amino groups of the antibody molecule. Fluorescein ordinarily is purchased in the form of fluorescein isothiocyanate, which forms a thiocarbamido linkage with amino

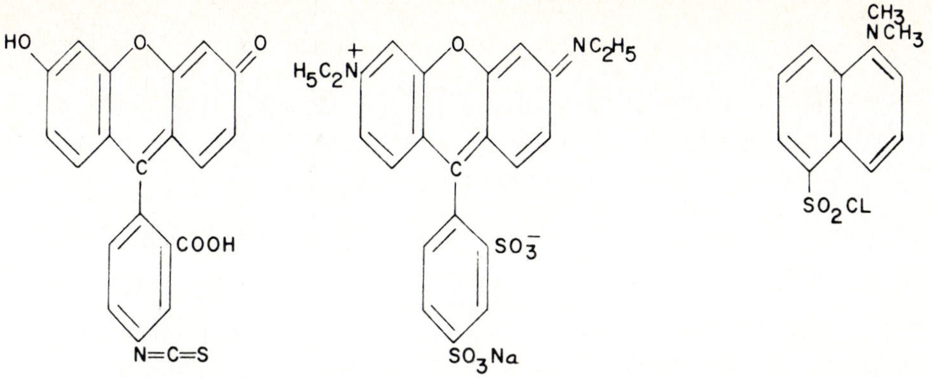

**Fluorescein
isothiocyanate**

**Lissamine
rhodamine B**

**1-Dimethylamino-
naphthalene-
5-sulfonyl
chloride
(DANSYL)**

FIG. 11-9

Three fluorochromes often used in fluorescent labeling of antibodies. All three of these compounds couple to the amino groups of proteins. Under ultraviolet illumination fluorescein and DANSYL emit a green or yellow-green light and rhodamine a red-orange light.

groups of protein. Rhodamines and DANSYL more often are prepared as sulfonyl chlorides, which form sulfonamido bonds with proteins. Since free amino groups of lysine are not especially critical to the activity of the antibody, the covalent bonding of these ligands does not destroy the antibody activity unless carried to excess.

The antibody preparation to be labeled should be a purified γ-globulin preparation, since most fluors will label albumin and even α- and β-globulins much better than γ-globulins. Unless these serum proteins are excluded, the fluorescent antibody preparation will suffer from the dual handicap of low fluorescence and nonspecific staining by the other labeled serum proteins. Specific labeling directions will differ slightly for different fluors and generally are based on specific dye/protein ratios. Careful adherence to the directions is necessary to avoid losses of antibody activity and nonspecific staining caused by overlabeling. Unreacted fluor can be removed by gel filtration or dialysis. Dilutions of the labeled antibody then should be tested on known preparations

to determine its activity and nonspecificity. Fluorescent antibody preparations with a high nonspecific background staining may be absorbed repeatedly with dried acetone powders of animal tissues to improve their quality. Background staining of tissue preparations with labeled albumin or simple dyes such as Evans blue or Congo red will quench nonspecific staining and improve contrast.

Fluorescence microscopy is more demanding than ordinary light microscopy, since objects are always much dimmer. A conventional microscope of good quality can be used. There is no need for quartz optics, even though an ultraviolet light source is used. The usual physical arrangement is depicted in Fig. 11-10. A high-pressure lamp emitting ultraviolet and short blue light is needed. The light is filtered by the primary filter to remove light longer than 450 to 500 nm. Heat filters usually are required because of the intensity of the mercury lamp. A front-surfaced mirror diverts the light into the condensor. A darkfield condensor is preferred, because it is easier to see a point of colored light on a black field than against a

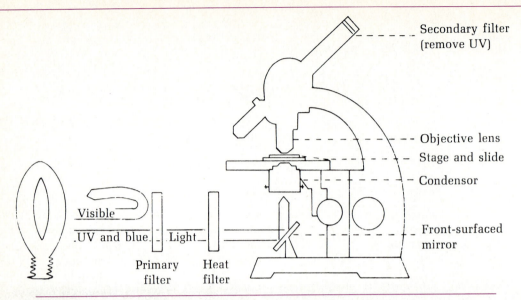

Secondary filter
(remove UV)

Objective lens

Stage and slide

Condensor

Front-surfaced
mirror

Visible

UV and blue   Light

Primary
filter

Heat
filter

FIG. 11-10

Physical arrangement for fluorescent antibody microscopy. The primary filter transmits only ultraviolet *(UV)* and blue light. Heat rays are removed by the heat filter, and the light is diverted into the darkfield condensor by a front-surfaced mirror. Visible light emitted by fluorescent-labeled materials passes through the tube of the microscope, where a secondary filter removes stray ultraviolet light rays. Quartz optics are not required.

bright white background. When the light coming through the condensor strikes the fluorescent antibody on the specimen slide, the fluor emits a visible light. This visible light, mixed with some ultraviolet light rays, progresses up the tube of the microscope to the observer. A secondary filter is used to remove the damaging ultraviolet light. Since the objects are often only faintly visible, this technique should be performed in a darkened room. For the same reason a monocular microscope may be preferred on some occasions.

Fluorescent antibodies are specific histochemical reagents capable of reacting with and identifying specific antigens. The antigen is fixed to an ordinary microscope slide. Impression smears, thin tissue sections, or alcohol-fixed bacterial smears may be used. In the direct fluorescent antibody procedure the labeled antibody is flooded onto the slide and allowed to react with the antigen. Gentle washing will remove the uncombined antibody. The slide is placed under the microscope. Wherever fluorescence is not-

ed, one can be confident that the antigen is present, provided appropriate controls have been applied. The most suitable control is the blocking test. In the blocking test the antigen preparation first is reacted with an unlabeled portion of antiserum. Combination of this antiserum with the antigen will prevent the combination of the subsequently applied fluorescent antibody.

The blocking reaction is important from two aspects: it provides the most useful control for the direct test, and it provides a method of demonstrating antibody in a serum without the effort, time, and expense of attaching a fluor to each serum specimen. Thus the blocking test itself becomes a useful tool for identifying unknown sera.

The indirect fluorescent antibody method is based on the antiglobulin, or immunologic sandwich, procedure. Two steps are required; the first uses the antigen and an unlabeled antibody derived from some known species, possibly a rabbit, and is to this point the same as the first stage of the blocking test. After

Direct FAB

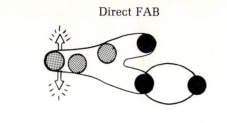

Indirect FAB

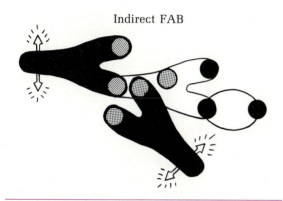

FIG. 11-11

Direct and indirect fluorescent antibody *(FAB)* procedures. In the direct procedure the antibody specific for the antigen is labeled. In the indirect procedure the antigen is reacted with its antibody, in this case of rabbit origin, and then with a fluorescent antibody versus rabbit γ-globulin. This diagram indicates why the indirect reaction produces a more brilliant fluorescence and a more sensitive test.

the uncombined antibody is washed away, the preparation is exposed to a fluorescent antirabbit globulin. This attaches to the rabbit globulin, which in turn is attached to the antigen (Fig. 11-11); thus the antigen is indirectly rendered fluorescent. A blocking control also can be applied to the indirect method.

The indirect method has certain advantages over the direct method: (1) it is more sensitive, since the unlabeled antibody, while serving as an antigen for the labeled antibody, provides many more combining sites than the original antigen itself; (2) it is more easily controlled, since more reagents are used and their concentrations are easily adjusted; and (3) it

may conserve the number of fluorescent antibodies that must be prepared. In the identification of a wide variety of antigens for which rabbit antisera are available, the only fluorescent reagent required is the labeled antirabbit globulin. Even this is not required if one prefers to use a fluoresceinated protein A as the second reagent. However, the indirect procedure does have the disadvantages of requiring more time and more reagents and being less specific.

The two procedures just described illustrate the two basic applications of the fluorescent antibody method: the identification of antigens with labeled antibody, as in the direct method, and the identification of antibody by either the blocking test or the indirect method. Antibody also can be localized by using fluorescent antigens. These methods are adaptable to widely varying serologic problems.

Phycobiliproteins, highly pigmented proteins that algae use in photosynthesis, are a recent addition to fluorescent microscopy. Phycoerythrin, one of these proteins, has a molecular weight of 240,000 and an emission maximum near 576 nm, different from the conventional fluors used in FAB assays. Its absorbance maximum is also quite different from fluorescein, so that the two dyes can be used in conjunction with each other. Phycobiliproteins may become useful antibody labels, because they fluoresce 10 to 30 times the intensity of fluorescein.

A frequently used alternative to fluorescent labels is the peroxidase-antiperoxidase system. In the direct method, an antibody labeled with horseradish peroxidase is reacted with the antigen. Then 3,5 diaminobenzidine, the peroxidase substrate, is added in order to quantitate the reaction. In the indirect method, a second antibody labeled with peroxidase and having a serologic specificity for the primary antibody is allowed to react with it. When enzyme substrate is added, the reaction can be quantitated. In a third variation—the peroxidase-antiperoxidase or PAP technique—the second antibody is not labeled, but a labeled third reagent is used. In the PAP procedure, the primary rabbit antibody combines with antigen. A goat anti-rabbit globulin reacts next. Then a soluble immune complex of rabbit antiperoxidase combined with the enzyme peroxidase is added. The goat anti-rabbit globulin already bound to the primary rabbit antibody also binds the complex, thus incorporating peroxidase into the system. Since the antiperoxidase does not totally inhibit the peroxidase, once again addition of the enzyme substrate will detect the enzyme's location. This is possible because the enzyme product is insoluble and remains at the location of the original antigen. The PAP method is still considered one of the most useful immunohistochemical procedures available.

The procedure used in the past for the diagnosis of animal rabies, when time is often of the essence, may require 3 weeks. With fluorescent antibody, the time can be shortened to a few hours or a few days. Often when a person is bitten by a presumably rabid dog, the dog is killed. (This is absolutely the wrong thing to do, but in moments of panic the best judgment is seldom used.) The dog brain is then stained by Seller's method to identify the pathognomonic rabies inclusion bodies. If the brain has been severely damaged, or if the dog had only recently acquired rabies, these bodies may not be seen. If they are not, an emulsion of the brain is injected into mice. An incubation period of 3 weeks is allowed before the mice are examined to see if they have acquired rabies. In the meantime, a decision has to be made as to the advisability of administering rabies vaccine to the bitten person. The Pasteur method of rabies vaccination has the inherent danger of initiating autoimmune encephalitis, so this vaccination procedure is not practiced recklessly. The application of fluorescent antibody to sections of the dog brain can obviate much of this problem. Such an antibody will specifically identify rabies virus in tissue, even in badly damaged tissue where the typical Negri inclusion bodies are absent by ordinary procedures. Within hours the decision becomes self-evident as to whether rabies immunization is needed.

A second major area of application of the fluorescent antibody method has been in the study of immunology itself—the site of antibody formation (Fig. 11-12), the nature of serum sickness, the autoimmune diseases, and other topics. Several approaches for locating the site of antibody formation have been employed. Tissue sections of an immune animal are flooded with antigen first and then with fluorescent antibody. Only in this way is there an immunologically specific localization of tissue or cellular antibody. By using two differently labeled fluorescent antibodies in doubly immunized animals it has been found that each plasma cell makes antibody to only one antigen.

APPLICATIONS TO ELECTRON MICROSCOPY

Ferritin is a protein of 465,000 mol wt whose biologic function is the transportation of iron. Nearly 23% of the molecule is iron, in the form of ferric hydroxide-phosphate salt. The complexed iron is situated in four discrete micelles about 55 Å in diameter. The iron micelles are electron opaque.

Antibodies can be joined to ferritin (or other proteins) by divalent ligands. The compounds used for this purpose are difluorodinitro benzene, bisdiazobenzidine, toluene diisocyanate (or diisothiocyanate), *m*-xylene diisocyanate, carbodiimides, and others (Figs. 11-5, 11-6, and 11-7). As mentioned earlier a complication arises from the use of these compounds with two proteins in that it is just as likely that two antibody molecules or two ferritin molecules will be joined as one antibody to one ferritin. Since two ferritins are much larger and two

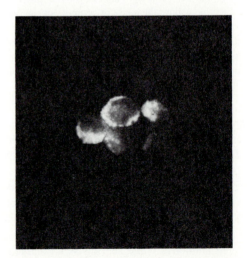

FIG. 11-12

A fluorescent antibody stain of a cluster of lymphocytes that are producing immunoglobulins. The antibody was specific for κ-chains. (Courtesy Dr. R. Lynch.)

Möller G.

Demonstration of mouse isoantigens at the cellular level by the fluorescent antibody technique.

J. Exp. Med. **114**:415-34, 1961.   [Institute for Tumor Biology, Karolinska Institutet Medical School, Stockholm, Sweden]

The fluorescent antibody method applied to living cells in suspension demonstrated that H-2 and non-H-2 histocompatibility antigens were localized to the cell membrane. A proportion of lymphocytes but not other cells, treated with only anti-immunoglobulin antisera exhibited staining of part of the membrane, giving rise to fluorescent crescents. This staining revealed surface bound immunoglobulin produced by the lymphocytes themselves. (The SCI® indicates that this paper has been cited in over 535 publications since 1961.)

Year

'61	'62	'63	'64	'65	'66	'67	'68
0	7	11	8	17	12	24	34

Citations

Göran Möller
Department of Immunobiology
Karolinska Institute
Wallenberglaboratory
104 05 Stockholm
Sweden

May 16, 1984

"This was my second scientific publication and the result of nearly two years' frustrating work. In 1959, I started to do research in immunology and my first task was to find a suitable research project. I was reading the proceedings of a recent symposium,[1] which was introduced by Peter Medawar. The first paragraph of his paper listed a number of unsolved problems in the form of questions. This was excellent for me and I selected two questions from his list and made them into my research projects. The first was to determine the intracellular and histological localization of H-2 transplantation antigens and the second to study their phenotypic expression during ontogeny. I thought it would be easy to show the intracellular localization of the antigens by the fluorescent antibody method, which at that time was used only with tissue sections. After labelling antibodies with fluorescein—not so easy at a time when you had to start to prepare the fluoresceinisothiocyanate yourself—I applied them to tissue sections, but only obtained a diffuse nonspecific staining.

"My other Medawar-inspired project progressed better, and for various reasons I became interested in pinocytosis of cells during ontogeny. I used fluorescein labelled albumin to study pinocytosis and then observed that the great majority of cells did not take up the fluorescein and, after washing, they remained totally unstained in contrast to the tissue sections. It occurred to me that the use of living cells instead of tissue sections could solve the problem with the nonspecific staining. The first experiment with living cells worked well: all cells in the experimental group exhibited membrane staining and none in the control group. The use of living cells solved a technical problem and clearly demonstrated that H-2 antigens were membrane bound.

"However, a proportion of lymphocytes, in contrast to all other cells, stained when treated only with a fluorescent rabbit antimouse immunoglobulin antiserum. It was also membrane staining, but different from the ring staining seen with anti-H-2 sera. The antibodies were localized in one part of the lymphocytes only, making them look like the crescent of the moon. I showed that the stained structures were membrane bound immunoglobulin and that the immunoglobulin was produced by the lymphocytes and not passively picked up. I also found that they were absent in lymphocytes from embryos and appeared shortly after birth. This was the first demonstration of immunoglobulin receptors on the surface of B lymphocytes, although T and B cells had not yet been discovered.

"I am slightly surprised that the paper has been cited often for two reasons. First, it had little impact after its publication. It took seven years for the first confirmation of the membrane localization of H-2 antigens[2] and nine years before membrane immunoglobulin receptors were rediscovered and crescent formation renamed cap formation.[3]

"The second reason is that the fluorescent antibody method applied to living cells is now a routine method and I would not expect most immunologists to care about the original discovery. The same applies to the existence of membrane bound immunoglobulins. It is part of the common knowledge in immunology and reference to the original work done 23 years ago is not necessary."

1. Albert F & Medawar P B, eds. *Biological problems of grafting.* Oxford Blackwell, 1959. 453 p.
2. Cerossini J C & Brunner K T. Localization of mouse isoantigens on the cell surface as revealed by immunofluorescence. *Immunology* **13**:395-405, 1967. (Cited 130 times).
3. Raff M C, Sternberg M & Taylor R B. Immunoglobulin determinants on the surface of mouse lymphoid cells. *Nature* **225**:553-4, 1970. (Cited 470 times.)

then is measured with radiolabeled antihuman globulin. Immune complexes that are not yet fully saturated with complement will bind additional complement in a modified form of the complement fixation test.

REFERENCES

Albertini, A., and Ekins, R., editors: Monoclonal antibodies and developments in immunoassay, Amsterdam, 1981, Elsevier/North-Holland, Biomedical Press.

Aloisi, R.M., and Hynn J., editors: Immunodiagnostics, New York, 1983, Alan R. Liss, Inc.

Avrameas, S.: Enzyme immunoassays and related techniques: development and limitations, Curr. Top. Microbiol. Immunol. **104**:93, 1983.

Avrameas, S., Druet, P., Masseyeff, R., and Feldman, G., editors: Immunoenzymatic techniques, Amsterdam, 1983, Elsevier Science Publishers.

Beutner, E.H., Nisengard, R.J., and Allini, B., editors: Defined immunofluorescence and related cytochemical methods, Ann. N.Y. Acad. Sci. **420**:1, 1983.

Boguslaski, R.C., Maggio, E.T., and Nakamura, R.M., editors: Clinical immunochemistry: principles of methods and applications, Boston, 1984, Little Brown and Company.

Bullock, G., editor: Techniques in immunocytochemistry, Orlando, 1984, Academic Press, Inc.

Collins, W.P., editor: Alternative immunoassays, Chichester, 1985, John Wiley and Sons, Ltd.

Cuello, A.C., editor: Immunohistochemistry, Chichester, 1983, John Wiley and Sons, Ltd.

DeLellis, R.A., editor: Diagnostic immunohistochemistry, New York, 1981, Masson Publishing USA, Inc.

DeLellis, R.A., editor: Advances in immunohistochemistry, New York, 1984, Masson Publishing USA, Inc.

Grieco, M.H., and Meriney, D.K.: Immunodiagnosis for clinicians, Chicago, 1983, Year Book Medical Publishers, Inc.

Hunter, W.M., and Corrie, J.E.T., editors: Immunoassays for clinical chemistry, ed. 2, Edinburgh, 1983, Churchill Livingstone.

Jaffe, F., and Behrman, H.R., editors: Methods of hormone radioimmunoassay, ed. 2, Orlando, 1979, Academic Press, Inc.

Langone, J.J.: Use of labeled protein A in quantitative immunochemical analysis of antigens and antibodies, Jour. Immunol. Methods **51**:3, 1982.

Lefkovits, I., and Pernis, B., editors: Immunological methods, vol. 3, Orlando, 1985, Academic Press, Inc.

Mayer, R., and Walker, J.: Immunochemical methods in the biological sciences, Orlando, 1980, Academic Press, Inc.

Nakamura, R.M., Dito, W.R., and Tucker, E.S., III: Immunologic analysis, New York, 1982, Masson Publishing USA, Inc.

Ngo, T.T., and Lenhoff, H.M., editors: Enzyme-mediated immunoassay, New York, 1985, Plenum Press.

Polak, J.M., and VanNoorden, S., editors: Immunocytochemistry, Bristol, 1983, John Wright and Sons Ltd.

Polak, J.M., and Varndell, I.M., editors: Immunolabelling for electron microscopy, Amsterdam, 1984, Elsevier Science Publishers B.V.

Sternberger, L.A.: Immunocytochemistry, ed. 3, New York, 1986, John Wiley and Sons, Inc.

Thorell, J.I., editor: Radioimmunoassay design and quality control, Oxford, 1983, Pergamon Press Ltd.

Towbin, H., and Gordon, J.: Immunoblotting and dot immunobinding—current status and outlook, Jour. Immunol. Methods **72**:313, 1984.

Wordinger, R.J., Miller, G.W., and Nicodemus, D.S.: Manual of immunoperoxidase techniques, Chicago, 1983, American Society of Clinical Pathologists.

See related **Reading 6,** page 428.

particles impedes penetration of these reagents into thick tissue sections; thus, their primary use is in surface labeling.

IMMUNE COMPLEXES

The ability to detect free antibody or free antigen in serum, spinal fluid, or other specimens represents an ideal condition in which one of the two reagents needed for a serologic reaction is present in excess. In the past few years it has been recognized that this is not always the case and that the antigen and antibody may already have combined in vivo. This makes it difficult, if not impossible, to detect either of them by standard serologic reactions. The complexes that contain an excess of antibody often are cleared rapidly by the phagocytic system. When the opposite is the case and antigen is in excess, the complex may circulate for 24 to 36 hours, during which time gradual deposition on target tissues occurs. Particularly when complement is bound into the matrix, the possibility of tissue damage and inflammation exists. For this reason it is important to recognize the presence of circulating immune complexes before tissue deposition creates tissue damage.

Immune complexes have been recognized in the blood of patients with malaria, leprosy, viral hepatitis, group A streptococcal infections, subacute bacterial endocarditis, dengue, schistosomiasis, and other infections. Indeed a transient "complexemia" can be anticipated in many infectious diseases. One whole subdivision of allergy is referred to as immune complex allergy. (See Chapter 18.) This includes conditions such as serum sickness, allergic pneumonitis, and the Arthus reaction. Several autoimmune diseases have an important component with the formation or deposition of immune complexes. Among these, rheumatoid arthritis, systemic lupus erythematosus (SLE), poststreptococcal glomerulonephritis, and rheumatic fever, pemphigus vulgaris, bullous pemphigoid, and myasthenia gravis (MG) are discussed in Chapter 19.

At present the techniques designed to detect immune complexes deposited in or on tissues are superior to the procedures used to recognize them in body fluids. Immune complexes in tissues are easily

detected by fluorescent antibody methods using labeled antibodies specific for complement or a specific immunoglobulin. Fluorescein-labeled protein A will identify IgG in tissues. Among the currently employed techniques are those which rely on the presence of immunoglobulin in molecular aggregates larger than their expected size (150,000 to 900,000 mol wt). "Abnormal" sizes of antibody can be measured by ultrafiltration, gel filtration, gradient density centrifugation, etc., and when detected, they indicate the presence of antibody in association with other (antigen) molecules. Immune complexes frequently have different solubility properties than normal globulins, and this can be detected by precipitation in the cold (cryoglobulins are often antigen-complexed globulins) or with PEG. Antigen-complexed antibody can be recognized by antiglobulin methods either while held in the complex or after dissociation of the antibody from the complex. For example, an antibody to human γ-globulin, known as RF, can be adsorbed onto latex particles and used in passive agglutination tests to detect human IgG. If this reagent agglutinates in a fraction of human serum known to contain molecules greater than 150,000 mol wt, this indicates the presence of immune complexes in that fraction. Cryoglobulin precipitates formed in the cold can be dissolved at 37° C and tested with the reagent. Protein A has been adsorbed onto insoluble carriers and used as an immunosorbent for purifying IgG, and this technique is adaptable to measuring IgG in unusual size ranges typical of immune complexes.

The Fc region of the immunoglobulin in complexes usually remains exposed, even though the Fab portions are bound to the antigen. Many types of cells have receptors for the Fc region of immunoglobulins and respond differently on exposure to these complexes, depending on the nature of the cell. Platelets are aggregated by Fc domains in immunoglobulins, and it may be possible to capitalize on this so that only complexes and not free globulin will agglutinate platelets. Macrophages, neutrophils, B lymphocytes, Raji's cells, and K cells all have Fc receptors, and all but K cells have receptors for complement component C3b. When immune complexes are bound to Raji's cells, the globulin in the complex then is measured with radiolabeled antihuman globulin. Immune complexes that are not yet fully saturated with complement will bind additional complement in a modified form of the complement fixation test.

REFERENCES

Albertini, A., and Ekins, R., editors: Monoclonal antibodies and developments in immunoassay, Amsterdam, 1981, Elsevier/North-Holland, Biomedical Press.

Aloisi, R.M., and Hynn J., editors: Immunodiagnostics, New York, 1983, Alan R. Liss, Inc.

Avrameas, S.: Enzyme immunoassays and related techniques: development and limitations, Curr. Top. Microbiol. Immunol. **104**:93, 1983.

Avrameas, S., Druet, P., Masseyeff, R., and Feldman, G., editors: Immunoenzymatic techniques, Amsterdam, 1983, Elsevier Science Publishers.

Beutner, E.H., Nisengard, R.J., and Allini, B., editors: Defined immunofluorescence and related cytochemical methods, Ann. N. Y. Acad. Sci. **420**:1, 1983.

Boguslaski, R.C., Maggio, E.T., and Nakamura, R.M., editors: Clinical immunochemistry: principles of methods and applications, Boston, 1984, Little Brown and Company.

Bullock, G., editor: Techniques in immunocytochemistry, Orlando, 1984, Academic Press, Inc.

Collins, W.P., editor: Alternative immunoassays, Chichester, 1985, John Wiley and Sons, Ltd.

Cuello, A.C., editor: Immunohistochemistry, Chichester, 1983, John Wiley and Sons, Ltd.

DeLellis, R.A., editor: Diagnostic immunohistochemistry, New York, 1981, Masson Publishing USA, Inc.

DeLellis, R.A., editor: Advances in immunohistochemistry, New York, 1984, Masson Publishing USA, Inc.

Grieco, M.H., and Meriney, D.K.: Immunodiagnosis for clinicians, Chicago, 1983, Year Book Medical Publishers, Inc.

Hunter, W.M., and Corrie, J.E.T., editors: Immunoassays for clinical chemistry, ed. 2, Edinburgh, 1983, Churchill Livingstone.

Jaffe, F., and Behrman, H.R., editors: Methods of hormone radioimmunoassay, ed. 2, Orlando, 1979, Academic Press, Inc.

Langone, J.J.: Use of labeled protein A in quantitative immunochemical analysis of antigens and antibodies, Jour. Immunol. Methods **51**:3, 1982.

Lefkovits, I., and Pernis, B., editors: Immunological methods, vol. 3, Orlando, 1985, Academic Press, Inc.

Mayer, R., and Walker, J.: Immunochemical methods in the biological sciences, Orlando, 1980, Academic Press, Inc.

Nakamura, R.M., Dito, W.R., and Tucker, E.S., III: Immunologic analysis, New York, 1982, Masson Publishing USA, Inc.

Ngo, T.T., and Lenhoff, H.M., editors: Enzyme-mediated immunoassay, New York, 1985, Plenum Press.

Polak, J.M., and VanNoorden, S., editors: Immunocytochemistry, Bristol, 1983, John Wright and Sons Ltd.

Polak, J.M., and Varndell, I.M., editors: Immunolabelling for electron microscopy, Amsterdam, 1984, Elsevier Science Publishers B.V.

Sternberger, L.A.: Immunocytochemistry, ed. 3, New York, 1986, John Wiley and Sons, Inc.

Thorell, J.I., editor: Radioimmunoassay design and quality control, Oxford, 1983, Pergamon Press Ltd.

Towbin, H., and Gordon, J.: Immunoblotting and dot immunobinding—current status and outlook, Jour. Immunol. Methods **72**:313, 1984.

Wordinger, R.J., Miller, G.W., and Nicodemus, D.S.: Manual of immunoperoxidase techniques, Chicago, 1983, American Society of Clinical Pathologists.

See related **Reading 6,** page 428.

Möller G.

Demonstration of mouse isoantigens at the cellular level by the fluorescent antibody technique.

J. Exp. Med. **114**:415-34, 1961.   [Institute for Tumor Biology, Karolinska Institutet Medical School, Stockholm, Sweden]

The fluorescent antibody method applied to living cells in suspension demonstrated that H-2 and non-H-2 histocompatibility antigens were localized to the cell membrane. A proportion of lymphocytes but not other cells, treated with only anti-immunoglobulin antisera exhibited staining of part of the membrane, giving rise to fluorescent crescents. This staining revealed surface bound immunoglobulin produced by the lymphocytes themselves. (The SCI® indicates that this paper has been cited in over 535 publications since 1961.)

Year

'61	'62	'63	'64	'65	'66	'67	'68
0	7	11	8	17	12	24	34

Citations

Göran Möller
Department of Immunobiology
Karolinska Institute
Wallenberglaboratory
104 05 Stockholm
Sweden

May 16, 1984

"This was my second scientific publication and the result of nearly two years' frustrating work. In 1959, I started to do research in immunology and my first task was to find a suitable research project. I was reading the proceedings of a recent symposium,[1] which was introduced by Peter Medawar. The first paragraph of his paper listed a number of unsolved problems in the form of questions. This was excellent for me and I selected two questions from his list and made them into my research projects. The first was to determine the intracellular and histological localization of H-2 transplantation antigens and the second to study their phenotypic expression during ontogeny. I thought it would be easy to show the intracellular localization of the antigens by the fluorescent antibody method, which at that time was used only with tissue sections. After labelling antibodies with fluorescein—not so easy at a time when you had to start to prepare the fluoresceinisothiocyanate yourself—I applied them to tissue sections, but only obtained a diffuse nonspecific staining.

"My other Medawar-inspired project progressed better, and for various reasons I became interested in pinocytosis of cells during ontogeny. I used fluorescein labelled albumin to study pinocytosis and then observed that the great majority of cells did not take up the fluorescein and, after washing, they remained totally unstained in contrast to the tissue sections. It occurred to me that the use of living cells instead of tissue sections could solve the problem with the nonspecific staining. The first experiment with living cells worked well: all cells in the experimental group exhibited membrane staining and none in the control group. The use of living cells solved a technical problem and clearly demonstrated that H-2 antigens were membrane bound.

"However, a proportion of lymphocytes, in contrast to all other cells, stained when treated only with a fluorescent rabbit antimouse immunoglobulin antiserum. It was also membrane staining, but different from the ring staining seen with anti-H-2 sera. The antibodies were localized in one part of the lymphocytes only, making them look like the crescent of the moon. I showed that the stained structures were membrane bound immunoglobulin and that the immunoglobulin was produced by the lymphocytes and not passively picked up. I also found that they were absent in lymphocytes from embryos and appeared shortly after birth. This was the first demonstration of immunoglobulin receptors on the surface of B lymphocytes, although T and B cells had not yet been discovered.

"I am slightly surprised that the paper has been cited often for two reasons. First, it had little impact after its publication. It took seven years for the first confirmation of the membrane localization of H-2 antigens[2] and nine years before membrane immunoglobulin receptors were rediscovered and crescent formation renamed cap formation.[3]

"The second reason is that the fluorescent antibody method applied to living cells is now a routine method and I would not expect most immunologists to care about the original discovery. The same applies to the existence of membrane bound immunoglobulins. It is part of the common knowledge in immunology and reference to the original work done 23 years ago is not necessary."

1. Albert F & Medawar P B, eds. *Biological problems of grafting.* Oxford Blackwell, 1959. 453 p.
2. Cerossini J C & Brunner K T. Localization of mouse isoantigens on the cell surface as revealed by immunofluorescence. *Immunology* **13**:395-405, 1967. (Cited 130 times).
3. Raff M C, Sternberg M & Taylor R B. Immunoglobulin determinants on the surface of mouse lymphoid cells. *Nature* **225**:553-4, 1970. (Cited 470 times.)

antibodies substantially smaller than one of each, the three forms of coupled protein molecules can be separated by gel filtration. The desired product can be used in the direct or indirect procedure to histochemically localize antigens or antibodies by electron microscopy (Fig. 11-13).

Two different enzymes, horseradish peroxidase and alkaline phosphatase, have been used as histologic reagents in electron microscopy. Horseradish peroxidase has a molecular weight of 40,000 and alkaline phosphatase a molecular weight of 80,000. Both these molecules are appreciably smaller than ferritin, so there is much less steric hindrance of immunoglobulin molecules bearing these enzymes than if they were labeled with ferritin. Because of this,

several enzyme-labeled antibodies may attach to a single molecule of antigen that would have space for only one ferritin-labeled antibody. A second advantage of the enzyme-bound antibodies, as mentioned earlier in regard to ELISA tests, is that the enzymes are catalytic reagents which will convert many molecules of substrate to an electron-dense end product. These many molecules of product are much easier to detect than a single molecule of ferritin-labeled antibody. Thus, the enzyme-labeled antibodies are more sensitive reagents.

Antibodies conjugated to colloidal gold have been used as histologic reagents for light microscopy, and, because of their opacity to electrons, in electron microscopy as well. The size of the colloidal gold

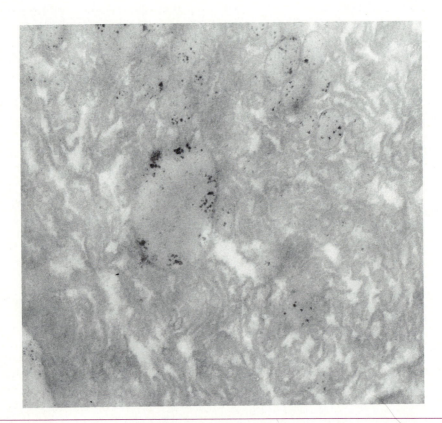

FIG. 11-13
Ferritin labeling of colloid vesicles of a thyroid gland with ferritin-labeled antithyro-globulin. The dark granules of ferritin are localized only in the homogeneously staining colloid. (Courtesy Drs. D. Senhauser and E. Adelstein.)

Precipitation

≡ GLOSSARY

CIEP Counterimmunoelectrophoresis.

counterimmunoelectrophoresis Electrophoresis of antigen and antibody toward each other through a gel.

crossed immunoelectrophoresis Electrophoresis of antigens through a neutral gel followed by electrophoresis at 90° to the first axis and into an antibody-containing gel.

Elek test A double immunodiffusion test similar to the Ouchterlony test.

flocculation 1. A specific type of precipitation that occurs over a narrow range of antigen concentration. 2. Aggregation of colloidal particles in a serologic reaction, as in syphilis serology.

immunodiffusion The diffusion of soluble antigens and/or antibodies toward each other and their precipitation in gel.

immunoelectrophoresis An electrophoretic displacement of antigen(s) or antibodies followed by immunodiffusion.

incomplete antibody An antibody that does not continue into the aggregative phase of the reaction with antigen.

Mancini's test A radial immunodiffusion test, usually based on diffusion of antigen through a gel containing antibody.

monovalent antibody An incomplete antibody.

Ouchterlony test An immunodiffusion test based on diffusion of both antigen and antibody through gels.

precipitation Formation of an insoluble complex of antibody with soluble antigen.

Quellung reaction Precipitation of specific antibody on the capsule of an organism, producing the appearance of capsular swelling.

radial immunodiffusion The Mancini test.

rocket immunoelectrophoresis The electrophoresis of an antigen into a gel containing antibody to form precipitates that are spear shaped.

■   ■   ■

The precipitation of antibodies by fluid antigens is one of the most useful of all serologic tests, partially because most antigens, if they are not already fluids, can be converted to fluid form by simple solubilization procedures. Another reason precipitation tests are so useful is that they can be varied in so many purposeful ways. Precipitation can be studied in either fluid or gelled media. Precipitation tests can be converted to one of the most sensitive forms of the serologic reaction: the passive hemagglutination test. Even when precipitation does not normally occur—

as with the combinations of haptens and antibody—double antibody procedures can be used to develop the reaction as a precipitation test.

FLUID PRECIPITATION
Procedures

The phenomenon of serologic precipitation in a fluid medium was discovered in 1897 by Kraus, who found that culture filtrates of enteric bacteria would precipitate when mixed with homologous antisera but not with heterologous antisera. In 1902 Ascoli modified the precipitation test to an interfacial, or ring type test. In this form of precipitation small tubes partially filled with antiserum, which is usually the most dense of the reactants, are carefully overlaid with dilutions of the antigen. As the reactants diffuse into each other, precipitation occurs at their interface. The plane of precipitate gives the illusion of a ring when seen from the side (Fig. 12-1).

Lancefield, when serologically typing the streptococci, adapted the Kraus method to a capillary precipitation technique. In this instance very small quantities of premixed antigen and antibody are drawn into capillary tubes that have an inside diameter of only 1.5 to 2 mm. Except for the quantity of reagents used, the capillary precipitation test is the same as that described by Kraus. In each of these methods incubation at room temperature for periods of a few minutes to 24 hours is allowed before the results of the test are recorded.

The exact physical form of the test is largely a matter of individual choice. Interfacial tests become positive rather quickly and tend to avoid prozone phenomena. The capillary test has two advantages: it conserves the serologic reagents, and it permits a rough quantitation of the reaction because the precipitate falls out of solution and accumulates at the bottom of the fluid column (Fig. 12-2). The height of this precipitate can be measured and used as an esti-

mate of the amount of antibody present and the equivalence zone.

Since precipitation tests involve two reagents, both of which are in a fluid condition, two inherently different methods of procedure are possible. The method described by Ramon in 1922 specifies that dilutions of antibody should be mixed with a constant amount of antigen. In the second form of the test, advanced by Dean and Webb in 1926, the antibody concentration is held constant and is mixed with different dilutions of the antigen.

The Dean and Webb method (the α procedure) is in reality a measure of the least amount of antigen that will coprecipitate with antibody, whereas the β procedure (Ramon's procedure) is a measure of the least amount of antibody that will react with a certain concentration of antigen. Despite the fact that, from a theoretic standpoint, the Ramon procedure is more satisfying (it is actually measuring antibody), the α procedure has been more widely used. The reason for this is that the antigen can be diluted over a wide range, perhaps several hundredfold if one begins with a 1% antigen solution, and still yield a positive test with a high-titer antiserum. In this way, antisera of different precipitating titers are distributed over a broad scale, and comparisons of sera with each other are easily made. In the Ramon method, with a 1% antigen solution, the antibody titers fall within a very narrow range. The comparison of antiserum potency by titer is not meaningful unless the exact conditions of the test are described. Antiserum potency is best determined by the quantitative precipitation method.

In capillary precipitation tests the usual prozone and postzone are easily detected (Fig. 12-2). In this titration of bovine serum albumin versus its rabbit antiserum, a partial prozone in the first two capillary tubes is evident. Following the region of prozone, the tubes reveal a gradual increase in the amount of precipitate as the equivalence point is reached. Thereafter a gradual decrease in the amount of precipitate is evident as antigen dilution places the system gradually into the postzone area.

Antigens and antibodies

The precipitation test places virtually no restriction on the type of antigen employed, except that it

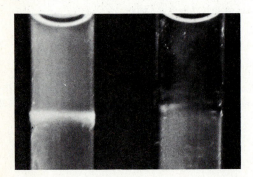

FIG. 12-1
Interfacial (ring precipitin) test. Antiserum to bovine serum albumin is seen in bottom of each tube. The left tube (positive) has been overlayered with bovine serum albumin and the right tube (negative) with human serum albumin. (Courtesy William Krass.)

must be in a fluid condition. The respective efficiency of IgG, IgM, and IgA in precipitation decreases in that order. The maximum sensitivity of qualitative precipitation tests is in the range of 3 to 15 μg of antibody nitrogen per milliliter of serum. This is equivalent to approximately 25 μg of antibody protein.

Applications

Precipitation tests have been adapted to a great variety of purposes, so only two examples will be described here.

In forensic medicine it is sometimes necessary to determine if bloodstains are of human or lower animal origin; for example, in cases of suspected homicide. Cloth bearing the bloodstain is extracted with saline and is treated as antigen in precipitation tests. The antisera required are those against human and other species of serum proteins. A precipitation test is arranged with each antiserum and the stain extract. Precipitate formation with one of the antisera will identify the animal source of the bloodstain. Bloodstains can be identified not only as to their species origin but also as to their exact blood type by the use of specific antisera against the blood group antigens. Such information is obviously useful in criminal proceedings.

Fluid precipitation tests also are used to detect adulteration of beef with meat of a lower quality or with soybean protein. If hamburger is extracted with saline and is centrifuged, the supernatant can be considered as the antigen. Precipitation tests conducted with antisera to several domestic and wild animals and to soy protein will determine if the hamburger contains only beef or has been adulterated with "foreign" proteins.

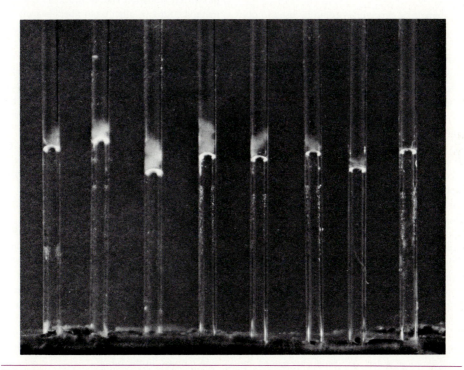

FIG. 12-2

A capillary precipitin test with dilutions of antigen (bovine serum albumin) premixed with the specific antiserum before being drawn into capillary tubes. Note the slight prozone because of antigen excess in the first two tubes and the postzone in the last tubes at right. The final tube contained no antigen and is a negative control. (Courtesy William Krass.)

≡ SITUATION 1

A PIG IN A POKE

Dwight V., a 58-year-old businessman, left a meeting late at night in a city 25 miles from his home just as a heavy snowstorm struck. When he was still nearly 10 miles from home, a heavy flurry completely blinded him. Just then he felt his car strike a solid object. He pulled to the shoulder of the road as soon as he could see, stopped his car, got out, and with aid of a flashlight examined the roadway and car. Seeing nothing unusual, he proceeded homeward.

The next morning the newspaper lead story described a hit-and-run death in the snowstorm on the highway Dwight V. had taken and at about the distance from town where his own incident had occurred the night before. Clearly shaken, he went to the garage and looked at his car. Some blood and a small piece of flesh clung to the right front wheel suspension below the bumper.

Questions

1. What immunologic procedures could be used to determine if the blood and tissue are of human origin?
2. Are precipitin tests the only serologic means of identifying bloodstains?
3. If tests prove the human nature of the blood and tissue specimens, what tests could be conducted to further identify the individual source of these materials?

Solution

The time-proved method for identifying the origin of tissue is the precipitation test, customarily performed by the interfacial, or ring, technique. The test can be performed simply, inexpensively, and with known limits to its sensitivity. Basically the test depends on the extraction of protein and polysaccharide antigens from the unknown tissue, blood, or seminal stain with isotonic saline. In the case of solid tissue this will require grinding or homogenization of the sample in a small blender. The extract is clarified by centrifugation and layered over antisera of known specificity, such as antihuman albumin, antihuman serum, antidog serum, or antichicken serum. The development of positive tests identified the species origin of the sample.

The precipitation test has not been superceded by other methods, but other methods have been developed for identifying the species and blood group status of unknown samples and are proving satisfactory. In the realm of precipitation tests double immunodiffusion methods are useful substitutes for the interfacial test. In this method it is not always necessary to clarify the extract, since this is accomplished to some degree as the antigen-containing preparation diffuses through the agar. The test is more time consuming and less sensitive than interfacial precipitation tests. Counterimmunoelectrophoresis appears to combine the rapidity and sensitivity of the fluid precipitation test with the advantages of immunodiffusion. The principal antigens detected are albumin and the α-globulins, since they are the most electronegative.

For further identification of dried bloodstains the testing of extracts against anti-A, anti-B, and even anti-H(O) sera in precipitation tests remains the standard method. Other methods that may be used include mixed agglutination and absorption-elution. In the first method cotton or other cloth fibers bearing the stain are used directly, since the red cell debris is firmly adsorbed to the fibers. The fibers are incubated separately with anti-A and anti-B sera. Then A cells are added to the first mixture and B cells to the second. If A antigens are present on the fibers, the corresponding antibody will attach to the fibers and then to the indicator cells used in the second incubation. In negative tests the indicator cells are easily washed free from the fibers. The absorption-elution method is similar except the absorbed antibody is eluted from the fibers with heat and tested for its capacity to agglutinate indicator cells in a separate test.

Serologic methods are also available to identify proteins in which allotypic variations occur, such as the variants of hemoglobin, transferrin, double albumin, and haptoglobin. These markers are very helpful in the identification of specific individuals. For several enzymes in which electrophoretic variants are known, simple electrophoresis is useful in identifying the source of the bloodstain. Phosphoglucomutase and serum cholinesterase are examples. Methods to identify HLAs also are being developed but are not used frequently in forensic medicine. However, they definitely will be used in the future.

QUANTITATIVE PRECIPITATION

Undoubtedly one of the most important advances in serologic technique occurred in 1932 when Heidelberger and Kendall developed the quantitative precipitation technique. This was soon followed by the application of quantitative chemical procedures to other serologic tests. Several kinds of information can be derived from quantitative serology; concerning precipitation this information includes the following points:

1. An exact expression of the amount of precipitating antibody in an antiserum (This is extremely important when comparing the potency of different lots of antisera.)
2. Proof of the antigen-antibody reaction in varying proportions
3. The functional valence of the antigen
4. An estimation of the relative heterogeneity of the antigen-antibody system
5. The distinction of precipitating and flocculating antisera
6. A measure of the contribution of serum complement to the serologic reaction
7. A quantitative expression of the amount of nonprecipitating antibody present

To perform the quantitative precipitation test, dilutions of antigen are mixed with a constant amount of heat-inactivated antiserum in a volume of 1 ml. (A smaller final volume may be used if microchemical techniques will be employed later.) Both the antigen and antibody solutions should be clarified by vigorous centrifugation if necessary. Controls containing the greatest concentration of antigen used and undiluted controls of antiserum adjusted to volume with buffer also are prepared. After proper mixing all tubes are stoppered and incubated, first for 30 minutes at 37° C and then for an additional 2 days at 4° C. The precipitates should be resuspended after the first day in the refrigerator. After the second day the tubes should be centrifuged in the cold and the supernatant fluids used to determine the zones of equivalence, antigen excess, and antibody excess. The precipitates are washed with cold buffer three times and after the final wash are dissolved so that chemical analyses for protein content can be made. A plot of the amount of antigen added versus the amount of total precipitate is prepared.

The results of a hypothetical quantitative precipitin test are presented in Table 12-1 and Fig. 12-3.

Table 12-1 shows that the amount of precipitate formed in each tube increased as more antigen was added only until the sixth tube, after which the quan-

---

TABLE 12-1

Data from quantitative precipitation test

Tube	Antigen added (mg nitrogen)	Total precipitate (mg nitrogen)	Excess reagent*	Antigen precipitated (mg nitrogen)	Antibody (mg nitrogen)	Antibody nitrogen/antigen nitrogen
1	0.003	0.093	ABY	0.003	0.090	30.0
2	0.005	0.145	ABY	0.005	0.140	28.0
3	0.011	0.249	ABY	0.011	0.238	21.7
4	0.021	0.422	ABY	0.021	0.401	19.1
5	0.032	0.571	ABY	0.032	0.539	16.8
6	0.043	0.734	—	0.043	0.691	16.1
7	0.064	0.720	Ag	—	—	—
8	0.085	0.601	Ag	—	—	—
9	0.171	0.464	Ag	—	—	—
10	0.341	0.386	Ag	—	—	—
11	0.525	0.314	Ag	—	—	—
12	0.683	0.241	Ag	—	—	—

*ABY, Antibody; Ag, antigen.

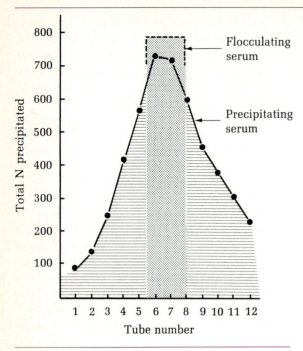

FIG. 12-3

A quantitative precipitin curve plotted from the data in Table 12-1 is seen in the solid line. Both the prozone and postzone effects (diminished amount of precipitate in the presence of excess antigen or antiserum) are apparent. A flocculating serum would precipitate over a narrow range of antigen concentration, as indicated by the broken line.

tity of precipitate decreased. Tests of the supernatant fluids from each tube revealed that tube 6 is the only tube in which all the antigen and all the antibody were precipitated, and it is thus the equivalence point. For this tube the amount of antibody precipitated can be calculated by subtracting the amount of antigen added from the total amount of precipitate $(0.734 - 0.043 = 0.691)$. This gives an exact expression of the amount of antibody in this antiserum.

Since all the antigen is precipitated in tubes 1 through 6, the amount of antibody contributing to the precipitate in each tube is easily determined by difference. When this is done, it is noted that the ratio of antibody to antigen in the precipitate varies. This is proof of the varying proportions of antigen and antibody in the serologic reaction. The proportions in tube 6 are useful in calculating the serologic

valence of the antigen if its molecular weight is known and if it is assumed that IgG is the only species of antibody contributing significantly to the precipitate. The formula used is:

$$\text{Valence} = \frac{\text{Ratio of antibody to antigen} \times \text{Molecular weight of antigen}}{\text{Molecular weight of antibody} \; (150{,}000)}$$

Since these data were derived from the use of bovine serum albumin as the antigen and it has a molecular weight of 36,000, the equation becomes:

$$\text{Valence} = \frac{16.1 \times 36{,}000}{(150{,}000)} = \frac{579{,}000}{150{,}000} = 3.8$$

Naturally a whole integer should be the result, and the answer here would be rounded off to 4. This yields a functional valence of approximately 1 to 10,000 of molecular weight, which is in the expected range. Any great deviation from a whole number may be an indication of a large quantity of nonprecipitating antibody.

Fig. 12-3 shows a reasonably symmetric curve, plotted from the data of Table 12-1, typical of the results when a purified antigen is tested against its antiserum. The experimental curve is also typical of precipitating, or R type, antisera, as compared with H, or flocculating, antisera. R precipitation curves are typical of rabbit and human antisera. The H class, typified by horse antisera, precipitates only in a narrow range of antigen concentration, with soluble complex formation being the rule outside that zone. This is illustrated in Fig. 12-3 for comparative purposes. *Flocculation* is a term with dual meaning in immunology. Its original use was for H precipitation tests, but it also has been used to describe aggregation of lipidlike particles that serve as the antigen in serologic tests for syphilis; flocculation in this sense is more akin to agglutination.

The contribution of serum complement to the system is determined by comparative trials using fresh and heat-inactivated sera. The increased amount of nitrogen precipitated in the former situation results from the contribution by complement.

Nonprecipitating antibody also can be detected by precipitation tests. To perform the double antibody procedure to detect nonprecipitating antibody, one must know its species origin. For example, if rabbit antibody were used, the addition of goat, equine, or other antibody to rabbit γ-globulin would precipitate the monovalent antibody. The rabbit incomplete antibody serves as an antibody with the original antigen, a reaction that takes place exclusively via the Fab portions of the immunoglobulin molecule; but this leaves its Fc portions free to serve as antigen and to combine with the goat antirabbit γ-globulin. This precipitation produced by the antiglobulin can be quantitated exactly as in the usual precipitation test, and the amount of nonprecipitating antibody in a serum can be expressed in exact units of weight.

Laser beam technology has added a modern approach to quantitative serology by improving nephelometry. In nephelometry a light beam is passed through a solution or suspension, and the amount of light scattered from its original path is measured. The quantity of this scattered light is an index of the concentration of the suspension. Heretofore the measurement of immunoprecipitates or immune complexes by nephelometry was unsuitable because of its lack of sensitivity and inability to detect small differences in the amount of precipitate formed under different circumstances. This has been overcome by laser beams with a greater strength than the usual light sources and the ability to measure light that is deflected only slightly from its original path. Consequently immune complexes that produce only a slight haze in a solution can be quantitated, and nephelometric procedures are used in clinical immunology to quantitate several serum proteins. In performing these tests the antiserum and antigen solutions should be free of any contaminating particles.

IMMUNODIFFUSION

Between 1946 and 1948 three separate studies established that precipitation tests performed in gels could provide several advantages over fluid tests. One of the principal advantages of these tests is the ease by which multiple antigen-antibody systems can be identified. The report by Oudin (France) published in 1946 described a single diffusion system. Two years later Elek (England) and Ouchterlony (Sweden) both published their data on a double gel diffusion technique. In 1953 a third technical variation of the gel immunodiffusion test was described, but this was also a double diffusion procedure and had no significant advantage over the Ouchterlony procedure. The three techniques are distinguishable on the basis of the number and dimension of the diffusion. Since only one reagent diffuses in the Oudin test, it is described as a single diffusion–single dimension system. Both the Elek and Ouchterlony procedures are double diffusion–two dimension systems, and the third procedure, devised by Oakley and Fulthorpe, is a double diffusion–single dimension system. Obviously there can be at least one other class, a single diffusion–double dimension system. This often is called radial immunodiffusion and has been very useful in developing quantitative gel precipitation techniques. It was first devised by Feinberg in 1957 and was modified by Mancini in 1963.

Gel immunodiffusion tests are most commonly performed in purified agarose gels. Agar is a mixture of two principal linear polysaccharides: agaropectin, the portion containing the acid residues, and agarose, which is neutral. Agar and agarose form gels that are essentially impermeable to molecules with a molecular weight greater than 200,000. Since most serologic precipitates exceed this molecular weight (one IgG plus two antigen molecules), the precipitates are held in the agarose when extraneous proteins are washed from the agar. Because of this, immunoprecipitates can be stained for protein, lipid, or special enzyme activities, which adds to the information obtainable by gel diffusion analyses.

Single diffusion in one dimension

The Oudin procedure is a single diffusion–single dimension gel precipitation test. An antiserum or purified antibody is added to a 0.7% solution of agarose that has been melted and allowed to cool to about 50° C. Proteins in solution usually do not coagulate at temperatures below 60° to 65° C, and agarose congeals at about 45° C; so the temperature chosen will protect the antibody and allow adequate mixing of the reactants. This fluid agarose–antiserum mixture is placed in a tube of convenient size and is allowed to gel. Care should be taken to avoid depositing any of this mixture on the sides of the tube.

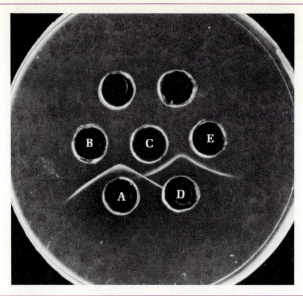

FIG. 12-4

This Ouchterlony immunodiffusion test shows two reactions of serologic identity and a reaction of nonidentity. Well A contains an antiserum to an *Escherichia coli* toxin. The toxin was placed in wells B and C. Well D contains antiserum to human lactoferrin. Lactoferrin was placed in wells C and E. (Courtesy Drs. R. Finkelstein and B. Marchlewicz.)

The fluid antigen is layered over the gelled antiserum. The concentration of the antigen should be considerably greater than the equivalence concentration. If the tube is small enough in diameter to hold the fluid layer in place by surface tension, the tube is placed on its side. This eliminates any effect of hydrostatic pressure on the diffusion of the antigen into the antiserum layer.

As the fluid antigen diffuses into the agarose, it dilutes itself to the proper concentration to precipitate with the antiserum. A disc of precipitate will become visible in the tube when this occurs. The precipitin band that forms will move down the tube according to the time elapsed, the concentration of the antigen in solution, the concentration of antibody in the agarose, the temperature, and the pore space in the agar. Movement of the precipitin band is more apparent than real. As the increasing antigen concentration at the rear face forces the antigen concentration there into a zone of antigen excess, the precipitate dissolves. Simultaneous movement of the antigen at the front of the band forward into a new position

for an equivalence concentration causes precipitation in front of the old precipitin band. Because of the dissolution and reformation of the precipitate, it appears to move down the precipitin tube. This process is repeated continuously until the position of the precipitate stabilizes. At this time the precipitate is observed as a sharp, distinct band with only a very faint fuzziness at its edges. This fuzziness is less likely to exist with "flocculating" sera, which form precipitates only within a restricted zone of antigen concentration, than with R antisera. In the Oudin procedure, only one of the reactants diffuses; this is in a straight line, so the procedure is aptly named a single diffusion–single dimension system.

In immunodiffusion tests a single antigen and its antibody will form only a single precipitin line. A mixture of antigen-antibody systems will present multiple bands, theoretically one band for each system. Exceptions occur when two antigens with equivalent diffusion rates diffuse into an antiserum that contains their respective antibodies in equal concentration. In such a case the equivalence concentra-

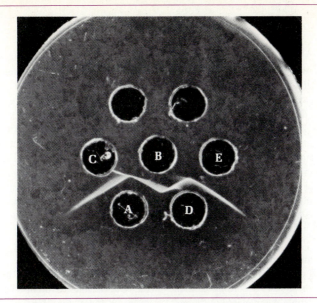

FIG. 12-5

In immunodiffusion reactions of partial identity spurred precipitation lines are seen. Well A contains an antiserum to a toxin from a human strain of *Escherichia coli*. This toxin was placed in well B. Toxin from a porcine strain of *E. coli* was placed in well C. Antiserum to the toxin of a porcine strain of *E. coli* was placed in well D and its corresponding antigen in well E. (Courtesy Drs. R. Finkelstein and B. Marchlewicz.)

tions in the two systems would occur in a single plane. The two precipitates thus would be superimposable and recorded as a single precipitate. Therefore in gel diffusion precipitation tests the number of precipitation bands observed will represent the minimal number of possible antigen-antibody systems functioning.

Double diffusion in one dimension

In the double diffusion–single dimension gel precipitation tests, a zone of neutral agar is placed between the fluid antigen and fluid antiserum in a tube. The principles of the Oudin technique apply, the only variation being that both reagents are diffusable.

Double diffusion in two dimensions (Ouchterlony technique)

To perform the double diffusion–double dimension test, better known as the Ouchterlony test, reservoirs are cut or molded into agarose on a flat sur-

face. The exact number, position, and shape of the wells are mostly matters of choice. The wells are filled with appropriate solutions of antigens and antiserum, covered to prevent evaporation, and observed periodically for several days. Precipitin bands may become visible in a few hours if concentrated reagents and/or a micromethod is used. The same general rules observed for the other gel diffusion tests concerning the number and position of the developing precipitin lines apply here as well.

If two wells for antigen are placed in opposition to a well containing antiserum, three principal types of reaction may be detected (Figs. 12-4 and 12-5). These differ physically in the way the two precipitation arcs from the separate antigen wells merge. In a reaction of serologic identity the intercepts of the two precipitation lines merge into a single arc; this means that the antiserum cannot distinguish one antigen from the other. In reactions of nonidentity the lines cross completely; this is evidence that the two antigens are reacting with two entirely different anti-

☰ SITUATION 2

THE IMMUNOLOGY LABORATORY

Your advisor was called away from the university on Friday because of a death in his family. He expected to be absent until late Monday night. In a brief note he asked you to arrange for the Tuesday meeting of his immunology laboratory course. He informed you of the location of his stock antigens and antisera and specifically informed you his class should perform an experiment designed to display the multiplicity of antigens in a solution. He insisted that you pretest the experiment so that the proper concentrations of the reagents could be prepared by him Tuesday morning before his class.

Questions

1. What serologic tests are available to demonstrate that a solution contains more than one antigen?
2. How would you rank these tests according to their ability to reveal the multiple components in the antigen mixture?
3. Which of the tests would require the least amount of reagents?
4. In terms of reagent costs, equipment needs, and time of performance, which of these tests could you most conveniently pretest and then have a class perform in a 2-hour laboratory period?

Solution

There are, in fact, many serologic reactions which can be used to prove that a solution contains more than one antigen, including RIA, complement fixation, and quantitative fluid precipitation tests. With fluid antigen solutions it is possible to establish a dilution series of the antigen and test these dilutions with a constant amount of antiserum. When a bimodal response is observed, then one can be certain that two or more antigens are present in the antigen solution. The bimodal response is seen because the two antigens and their corresponding antibodies are rarely at equivalence at the same dilution. Thus, when one of the antigen-antibody systems is at equivalence, the other is in prozone or postzone. When the second system reaches equivalence, then the first is in antigen postzone. As more and more antigen-antibody systems participate, the response curve shifts from a simple bimodal to a trimodal form to a broad plateau, since one or more of the systems is in or near equivalence at every point in the antigen dilution series. For this reason quantitative fluid

precipitation, RIA, complement fixation tests, etc. are not ideally suited for a situation such as that presented in this case.

Using antibodies, each bearing a different colored fluorochrome, radioisotope, enzyme, or other label, to different antigens in the mixture, it is possible to measure the simultaneous function of different antigen-antibody systems in a mixture. These methods usually are applied to particulate antigens and histochemical procedures but can be adapted to soluble antigens rendered insoluble or attached to particulate carriers.

The student in this situation should quickly recognize the advantage of immunodiffusion techniques to solve the problem. The two major varieties of immunodiffusion are unaided, or simple, immunodiffusion and immunoelectrophoresis. In the first category are included the Ouchterlony, Oudin, and Mancini gel diffusion tests. Of these, the Mancini and Ouchterlony tests are easiest to arrange and to interpret and are consequently the most popular. The Mancini test is particularly suited to the quantitation of antigens but can be used for their enumeration as well, each antigen producing a separate ring of precipitate. The Ouchterlony test is more suited to the enumeration of antigens and can be used to identify an antigen in a mixture with a known antigen. Both tests suffer to some extent from delays in reading the results until diffusion is nearly halted, and the final results may not be available until several days after the tests were begun. This does not prevent recording data earlier as long as it is understood that the results may change slightly in the ensuing days. Depending on the physical circumstances of the test, as little as 3 μg of antigen per milliliter can be detected.

Because the diffusion rates of two antigens through a gel may be nearly identical, two antigen-antibody systems may precipitate at essentially the same location. This prospect is minimized if an electric potential is used to move the antigens, since the antigens will very likely have different isoelectric points. As a consequence, immunoelectrophoretic diffusion tests are more likely to display the multiplicity of antigen-antibody systems in a mixture of precipitating systems than is simple immunodiffusion. Of the available methods, ordinary immunoelectrophoresis and counterimmunoelectrophoresis are the simplest to arrange, although the restricted diffusion distance in the latter test may mask the true number of precipitating systems. Crossed immunoelectrophoresis, since it relies on antibody in an agarose slab, is unlike the previous two tests in that it is subject to prozone phenomena, which may prevent the formation of one or more precipitates. To prevent this, several pretitration runs may be necessary to establish the correct conditions.

Although immunoelectrophoretic diffusion tests are more sensitive in defining the number of antigens in a mixture, they are no more sensitive than simple immunodiffusion tests in measuring small quantities of an antigen, 1 to 3 μg/ml being the usual lower limit. This is true because the immunologic development in both types of tests usually takes place via simple diffusion.

Faced with the handicap of time and inexperience, it would probably be best for this student to prepare for the Ouchterlony immunodiffusion and either regular immunoelectrophoresis or counterimmunoelectrophoresis. If the student is fortunate, the Ouchterlony test might identify two serologic systems and the latter more than two.

All the simple immunodiffusion tests performed as microtechniques can be conducted with as little as 25 μl of antigen or antiserum, but larger volumes are needed if the tests are performed as macrotechniques. This is probably desired for a class exercise even though it may consume five to ten times more of the reagents. Students seldom are able to deposit 25 μl of solution in reservoirs of only 2 mm diameter in Ouchterlony plates without practice. Spilling the reagents on the agarose surface or deforming the reservoir will mar the results of the exercise. Since the Mancini and crossed immunoelectrophoretic procedures rely on antiserum incorporated into an agarose film, 0.1 to 0.5 ml of this reagent may be needed per test. Since the antiserum can be diluted fivefold to 500-fold, this does not stress the supply of antiserum. For immunodiffusion tests the amount of reagents used is seldom a limiting factor.

bodies. Both the second antigen and second antibody pass through the precipitate produced by the first antigen-antibody system. In reactions of partial identity, in which one antigen is cross-reactive with but not serologically identical to the other, a spurred intercept is noted. This is the result of precipitation of one antibody by determinants of the simplest antigen and the movement through that precipitate of antibody molecules with specificity only for determinants found in the more complex antigen. Viewed in another way, the simpler antigen adsorbs out its own antibody, but the antibody that is specific for the additional antigenic determinants of the second antigen passes through that precipitate and reacts with the more complex antigen. Hence the spur points toward the simpler antigen. The ease with which two antigens can be established as serologically identical or different is the prime advantage of the Ouchterlony test over other immunodiffusion assays.

Radial quantitative immunodiffusion

A fourth form of immunodiffusion test first was described by Feinberg in 1957. It is now most widely known as the Mancini test or the radial immunodiffusion test. A major advantage of this technique is that it is a quantitative procedure. Micro-

gram quantities of antigen can be accurately determined by the method.

The Mancini technique is a single diffusion–double dimension system in which the antiserum is incorporated in the agarose gel, which is solidified on a flat surface. Small wells are cut in agarose and filled with antigen. Radial diffusion of the antigen produces a ring of precipitate, the diameter of which is proportional to the concentration of the antigen (Fig. 12-6).

The most intensive use of radial immunodiffusion is in clinical laboratories where it is necessary to determine the exact amount of various protein antigens in serum. Radial immunodiffusion is the best laboratory aid for the diagnosis of hypogammaglobulinemia of IgG, IgM, or IgA, the determination of myelomas of one of these immunoglobulin classes, and the quantitation of complement components C3 and C4, haptoglobin, lysozyme, α_1-antitrypsin, and of other serum proteins.

IMMUNOELECTROPHORESIS

There are two recognized handicaps to ordinary immunodiffusion tests. Incubations of several hours or even days are needed to ensure that equilibration of the system has occurred, and there is the possibil-

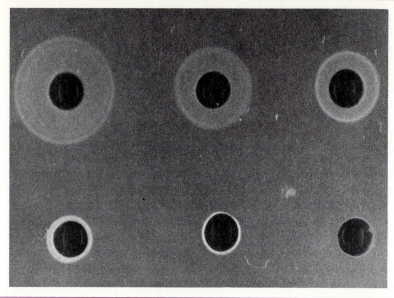

FIG. 12-6

The Mancini (radial immunodiffusion) test. Antigen in the upper wells was at a concentration of 10, 5, and 2.5 µg/ml, reading left to right. In the lower row only the left well received antigen (1.2 µg/ml). (From Barrett, J.T.: Basic immunology and its medical application, ed. 2, St. Louis, 1980, The C.V. Mosby Co.)

ity that two or more precipitation bands may form in the same plane and prevent an accurate enumeration of the antigen-antibody systems involved. Both these objections may be overcome in immunoelectrophoretic procedures. In immunoelectrophoresis a direct electric current is forced through a gel containing antigen and/or antibody. If the antigen is actually a mixture of antigens, the electrophoretic phase of the test generally will displace the antigens from one another. The probability of two molecules having exactly the same electrophoretic mobility is unlikely. Because of this difference in the ionic properties of antigens, each will form a visibly distinct band of precipitate in the second immunodiffusion phase of the procedure.

In standard immunoelectrophoresis the electrophoretic portion of the method is followed by regular immunodiffusion. In a few variations of immunoelectrophoresis both antigen and antibody are set in motion by the electric field. In other instances the antigen is electrophoresed into a slab of antibody.

In both cases the immunoprecipitates are formed quickly and are nearly complete during the electrophoretic phase of the test.

Counterimmunoelectrophoresis

The immunodiffusion technique in which both antigen and antibody are displaced electrophoretically (in opposite directions and toward each other) is the immunoelectrophoretic variant to the double diffusion–single dimension test.

In counterimmunoelectrophoresis, countercurrent immunoelectrophoresis, or immunoosmophoresis, paired wells in an agarose film are charged with antigen and antiserum (or antibody). The agarose is buffered at pH 8.2 and is connected by paper wicks to buffer-filled reservoirs to complete an electric circuit. The electric potential is applied, and the reactants move toward each other if the test has been properly arranged. In the pH range below 8.2 the immunoglobulin molecules will carry a slight positive charge that will cause their movement toward

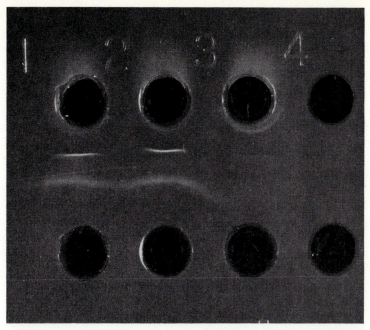

FIG. 12-7

Counterimmunoelectrophoresis of a heat-extracted antigen from *Bacteriodes fragilis* versus its antiserum produced the dual precipitation pattern seen in wells 1 and 2. A dilution of the antigen produced a trace precipitate in well 3. Well 4 was a control system in which normal rabbit serum was used. (Courtesy T. Ellis.) (From Barrett, J.T.: Basic immunology and its medical application, ed. 2, St. Louis, 1980, The C.V. Mosby Co.)

the cathode. At pH 8.2 the immunoglobulins are essentially uncharged but are carried toward the antigen by the fluid through the gel, a process known as electroendosmosis. Antigens having an acidic isoelectric point will bear a negative ionic charge at alkaline pH and will be displaced toward the anode. Thus the serologic reactants will be driven toward each other by the electric potential, and this will accelerate their precipitation (Fig. 12-7).

Counterimmunoelectrophoresis is a time-saving procedure, qualitative rather than quantitative in nature, and most easily performed with electronegative antigens. Fortunately many antigens are negatively charged at an alkaline pH; these include the albumin, β- and α-globulins, many polysaccharides, nucleoproteins, and glycoproteins. This encompasses a wide range of antigens of practical interest: viruses, bacterial polysaccharides, serum proteins, etc. More-

over it is possible to improve the anodic migration of many proteins, including immunoglobulins, by acetylation or carbamylation reactions with their amino groups. Contrariwise, acidic groups (COOH, SO_3H_2) can be added to neutral antigens to provide them the necessary mobility for standard counterimmunoelectrophoresis procedures.

Rocket immunoelectrophoresis

Rocket immunoelectrophoresis is the most used synonym for single crossed immunoelectrophoresis, spike immunoelectrophoresis, the Laurell technique, or electroimmunoassay. This is a quantitative method similar in concept and application to the Mancini test with the added dimension of electrophoresis.

To conduct this test, the antiserum is incorporated into an agarose film adjusted to pH 8.6, the isolectric point of the immunoglobulins at which these proteins are electrophoretically immobile. The antigen specific for the antiserum is placed in small reservoirs along one edge of the antibody-containing slab or in a narrow film of neutral agarose placed against it. The electric potential is applied so that it will draw the antigen into the antibody-agarose layer, that is, with electronegative antigens at pH 8.6 the antigens would move toward the anode. As the antigen molecules contact the antibody molecules, precipitation begins. As the concentration gradient of the antigen changes, dissolution of the precipitate and reprecipitation take place at a steadily increasing distance from the antigen reservoir. At the end of the run the length of the cone-shaped precipitate is directly proportional to the concentration of the anti-

gen (Fig. 12-8). When a series of antigen solutions of known concentration is examined, it is possible to construct a standard curve to determine the concentration of the antigen in an unknown preparation.

Crossed immunoelectrophoresis

This method initially was described by Ressler in 1960 but perfected by Laurell in the years following 1965. The method is also known as double crossed immunoelectrophoresis or two-dimensional immunoelectrophoresis.

This method requires, as its first stage, the simple electrophoresis of an antigen mixture in agarose. Thereafter this agarose strip is transferred to the edge of a second plate and positioned against an agarose slab containing an antiserum. Now the second elec-

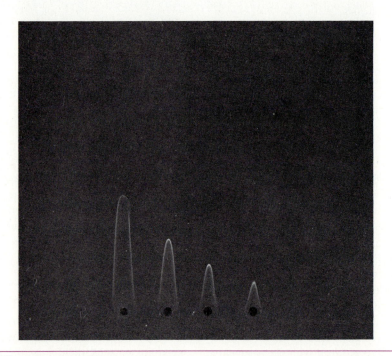

FIG. 12-8
Result of rocket immunoelectrophoresis of four different concentrations of complement component C3 against its monospecific antiserum. A twofold dilution series of the antigen was made beginning at the left and progressing to the right. Notice that the adjacent rocket heights do not differ by twofold, although the peak areas do. The left rocket did not form a perfect spear because of premature termination of the electrophoresis. (From Barrett, J.T.: Basic immunology and its medical application, ed. 2, St. Louis, 1980, The C.V. Mosby Co.)

trophoretic step is applied, only this time the electric field is arranged at right angles to the original separation. This draws the antigens from their original positions in the neutral agarose slab into the antibody-containing film. As in counterimmunoelectrophoresis, the buffer system is adjusted to pH 8.6 to hold the antibody molecules immobile. As the antigens move into the antiserum layer, spears or rockets of precipitation develop (Fig. 12-9). Intercepts of these precipitation arcs will indicate their serologic unrelatedness or partial identity. Reactions of serologic identity are not observed.

Crossed immunoelectrophoresis is primarily a method for the enumeration of antigen-antibody systems in a mixture.

Ordinary immunoelectrophoresis

The original immunoelectrophoretic modification of gel precipitation tests was the immunoelectrophoretic procedure of Grabar and Williams.

The physical arrangement for ordinary immunoelectrophoresis requires that an agarose film on a flat

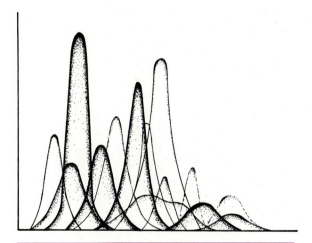

FIG. 12-9

The electrophoretic displacement of a complex mixture of antigens in an agarose gel followed by a subsequent electrophoretic displacement at 90° to the original into an antiserum-containing gel produced this pattern of precipitation. Crossed immunoelectrophoresis is a useful research technique when a complete analysis of a mixture of many antigens is needed.

surface be placed in an electric field after the antigen mixture has been added to a small reservoir cut in the agar. Prior knowledge of the electrophoretic behavior of the antigens at the pH of the buffer used is desirable so that the electric force can be applied in sufficient strength and for a long enough period to permit an adequate separation of the antigens. After the electrophoresis a trough the length of the glass plate or slide is cut from the agarose and is filled with antiserum. Double diffusion in two dimensions begins, and after a suitable period of incubation areas of precipitate will develop just as in the usual Ouchterlony technique (Fig. 12-10).

Although immunoelectrophoresis is very useful in separating antigens and has a very high resolving power, it is somewhat difficult to identify a specific precipitin arc as originating from a known antigen. Parallel immunoelectrophoresis of a purified antigen preparation, even on the other half of the same slide, will not always present a perfect enough mirror image of the band in question to afford exact identification. This is especially difficult when several bands are situated closely together. To circumvent this handicap in antigen identification, the common antigen technique is employed. This involves the preparation of a second antigen trough, placed so that the electrophoretically separated antigens are between the antigen and serum troughs. This second trough is for the purified antigen, which diffuses toward the antiserum and precipitates with it in a straight line, except for that area where the antigen concentration was reinforced by the electrophoretically positioned antigen. In this region an arc is formed that fuses perfectly with the straight line, thus identifying the antigen involved.

CAPSULAR SWELLING (QUELLUNG REACTION)

One of the broader modifications of the precipitation test is the Quellung reaction. In 1902 Neufeld described the apparent swelling of the capsule of a bacterial organism when it was mixed with homologous antiserum. The German word *Quellung* means swelling, and the reaction has become known as the Quellung reaction. There is some disagreement as to whether capsular swelling actually occurs. The reac-

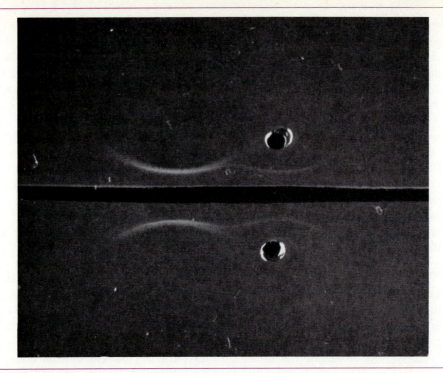

FIG. 12-10

In the immunoelectrophoretic identification of Factor B and Bb a mixture of the two is placed in wells cut in an agarose film. The two proteins have dissimilar electrophoretic mobilities, with Factor B moving further. When the plate is developed by adding anti-Factor B serum to the trough, Factor B forms a heavy precipitation line and Bb a light precipitation line, with the latter nearer the starting point (the well). (From Barrett, J.T.: Basic immunology and its medical application, ed. 2, St. Louis, 1980, The C.V. Mosby Co.)

tion may be viewed as the binding of antibody molecules to the periphery of the bacterial capsule, rendering its outline more visible. This fine precipitate actually may be at a point more distant than the apparent outer margin of the capsule because unstained capsules are very difficult to see under the ordinary light microscope. Thus swelling may be more apparent than real.

ARTHUS REACTION

The precipitin reaction can occur in vivo when sizable quantities of antigen are injected intradermally or subcutaneously into animals with a high antibody titer. The precipitate that develops blocks the local capillary bed and prevents the exchange of the nutrients and wastes from the injection site. This encourages the development of tissue necrosis, which is known as the Arthus reaction. (See Chapter 18.)

REFERENCES

Axelsen, N.H., editor: Handbook of immunoprecipitation-in-gel techniques, Oxford, 1983, Blackwell Scientific Publications.

Bjerrum, O.J., editor: Electroimmunochemical analysis of membrane proteins, Amsterdam, 1983, Elsevier Science Publishers.

Cawley, L.P., Minard, B.J., and Penn, G.M.: Electrophoresis and immunochemical reactions in gels: techniques and interpretation, Chicago, 1978, American Society of Clinical Pathologists.

Emmett, M., and Crowle, A.J.: Crossed immunoelectrophoresis:

qualitative and quantitative considerations, J. Immunol. Meth. **50:**R65, 1982.

Lefkovits, I., and Pernis, B., editors: Immunological methods, vol. I-III, Orlando, 1985, Academic Press, Inc.

Peacock, J.E., and Tomar, R.H.: Manual of laboratory immunology, Philadelphia, 1980, Lea and Febiger.

Rose, N.R., and Friedman, H., editors: Manual of clinical immunology, ed. 3, Washington, 1986, American Society for Microbiology.

Thompson, R.A., editor: Technologies in clinical immunology, ed. 2, Oxford, 1981, Blackwell Scientific Publications.

Towbin, H., and Gordon, J.: Immunoblotting and dot immunobinding—current status and outlook, J. Immunol. Meth. **72:**313, 1984.

Ward, A.M., and Whicher, J.T., editors: Immunochemistry in clinical laboratory medicine, Baltimore, 1979, University Park Press.

Agglutination and hemagglutination

≡ GLOSSARY

ABO antigens   Antigens of the major human blood group system.

agglutination   Aggregation of a cellular or particulate antigen by an antiserum containing antibodies to one or more surface antigens.

agglutinin   An antibody directed toward surface antigens and capable of causing agglutination.

agglutinin adsorption   Removal of some of the antibodies in an antiserum by reacting them with the cellular antigen, which afterward is removed by physical procedures such as filtration or centrifugation.

blood group antigen   Antigens that are genetically determined and which are present on the surface of red blood cells.

Boyden's technique   A procedure for attaching protein antigens to erythrocytes by first treating the cells with tannic acid.

H antigen   The flagellar antigen(s) of bacteria.

H substance   An antigen on the human erythrocyte that is a precursor substance for the A and B antigens.

hemagglutination   The agglutination of erythrocytes, especially by antiserum.

O antigen   Surface somatic antigens of bacteria; not to be confused with ABO antigens of human erythrocytes.

passive hemagglutination   Hemagglutination resulting from antibodies directed toward antigens adsorbed to the erythrocyte surface.

Rh antigens   A system of human blood group antigens shared by the rhesus monkey.

tanned erythrocyte   One treated with tannic acid in preparation for passive hemagglutination tests.

Widal test   A bacterial agglutination test.

Weil-Felix test   An agglutination test used to diagnose certain rickettsial diseases.

■   ■   ■

The initial demonstration of immune hemagglutination was performed in 1900 by Ehrlich and Morgenroth, who immunized goats with the red blood cells of other goats (alloimmunization or isoimmunization). The resulting antisera were capable of distinguishing the red blood cells of different goats from each other, since some were hemagglutinated and some were not. This permitted the creation of the first blood cell groups. Human erythrocyte alloantibodies were described in 1901 by Landsteiner. This is the discovery which opened the way to successful blood transfusion, to a better understanding of erythroblastosis fetalis, and to other hemolytic diseases. In 1930, Landsteiner received the Nobel Prize for his discovery of human blood groups.

ABO(H) BLOOD GROUP SYSTEM

Landsteiner made multiple crosses of erythrocytes and serum from himself and his associates, and originally identified three types of persons, those currently designated A, B, and O. In a subsequent report, the existence of a fourth group, AB, was noted. The relationship of these four groups to one another, recorded in Table 13-1, requires only a

TABLE 13-1

ABO(H) blood group system

Blood group phenotype	Antigen on red blood cells*	Antibody in serum	Genotype	Distribution in United States (percent)
A	A	Anti-B	AA, AO	42
B	B	Anti-A	BB, BO	10
O(H)	Neither A nor B	Both anti-A and anti-B	OO	45
AB	Both A and B	Neither anti-A nor anti-B	AB	3

*Cells of all blood groups contain the H substance.

minimum of additional explanation. Every group A person has an antigen on the erythrocytes, which arbitrarily was designated as A, and has an antibody in serum that reacts with red blood cells bearing the B antigen. The reverse is true of the group B person, whose erythrocytes all contain the B antigen and whose serum contains an antibody to the A antigen. Persons in group O lack both the A and B antigens but have antibodies to both A and B antigens in their sera. The reverse situation is true for AB persons, who have both the A and B antigens on each erythrocyte but lack both A and B antibodies in their sera. It can be noted immediately that an antigen and its corresponding antibody do not coexist in one individual. Coexistence of a common antigen and antibody would be incompatible with life, since in vivo hemagglutination and hemolysis would result. This would block the circulation and destroy that person's red blood cells.

The blood group designations A, B, O, and AB are designations of phenotype. It has been postulated that the blood group antigens are inherited according to simple mendelian genetics involving three allelic genes, A, B, and O. These genes exist as pairs on the two sets of chromosomes present in the nucleus of all except the haploid germ cells (sperm and ovum). If the same characteristic is on both genes, then the person is homozygous. In the blood system this would be exemplified by the group O person, each gene lacking the A and B characteristic. The genotype of such a person would be OO. It is in fact artificial to refer to the O gene as a true gene, since it does not control the production of a specific prod-

uct. This is not the case with the A and B genes, which control the synthesis of definite antigens. An AB person, who produces both antigens, is heterozygous, that is, capable of producing germ cells of which half transmit the A gene and half the B gene to the zygote. In contrast to group O persons, who are restricted to the homozygous state, and to group AB persons, who are restricted to the heterozygous state, persons in groups A and B may be either homozygous (AA, BB) or heterozygous (AO, BO). This is important in solving cases of uncertain parentage or in identifying misplaced infants.

Group O persons are not absolutely devoid of antigens related to the A and B antigens. Group O cells contain an H substance, which is a precursor to the A and B antigens. The H gene regulates the production of the H substance, some of which is converted to the A and B antigens by products of the A and B genes. Some of the H substance remains unconverted and can be detected on A and B cells.

The distribution of the ABO(H) blood groups in the United States is approximately 45% O, 42% A, 10% B, and 3% AB. These values will differ slightly in separate racial or ethnic groups, which represent "isolated" genetic populations because of the tendency to marry within the group. For example, the distribution in blacks is 49% O, 28% A, 20% B, and 3% AB.

About 80% of A and AB blood cells are easily agglutinated by anti-A serum, but the remaining 20% are difficult to clump because of the presence of A_1 and A_2 subgroups within the A group. The A_1 cells have both the A_1 and A_2 antigens, and the A_2

cells have only the A_2 antigen. Since the usual anti-A serum contains both anti-A_1 and anti-A_2, it is a more potent reagent for the A_1 cells than it is for A_2 cells. Incubation of anti-A serum with A_2 cells will remove the A_2 antibody (agglutinin adsorption) and leave an antiserum that is specific for the A_1 antigen. Of the 42% of the population referred to as group A, actually about 34% (42×0.8) are A_1, and 8% are A_2. Likewise, the AB persons are divisible into those who are A_1B (2.5%) and those who are A_2B (0.5%).

Less important subgroups of the A antigen include A_3, A_x, and A_m. Variants of the O and B groups are also known but are quite rare.

ABO(H) antigens

Antigens of the ABO(H) system are present on erythrocytes from fetal life onward and can be found on most other cells as well. In each instance, the antigen exists as an integral part of the cell membrane. Estimates of the number of A sites on a single erythrocyte have varied widely, from as low as 120,000 to as high as 1,170,000. The number of B sites has been estimated to be from 310,000 to 830,000 per cell. A figure of 500,000 for each is probably a satisfactory compromise of these estimates at present.

Information concerning the chemistry of the A, B, and H antigens has come from three major sources: (1) the agglutination of erythrocytes by lectins, (2) the enzymatic and chemical degradation and analysis of the blood group substances from human and lower animal sources, and (3) inhibition of the serologic reaction between red blood cells and antibodies by monosaccharides and oligosaccharides of known structure. The results of these independent approaches have been mutually supportive, and now the structure of the immunodominant portion of these molecules generally is agreed on.

Lectins from *Phaseolus limensis* and *Vicia crassa* are specific agglutinins for group A erthrocytes. These lectins and antisera that are specific for the A antigen are inhibited by N-acetyl-D-galactosamine, and the disaccharide N-acetyl-D-galactosaminyl-β-1,3-D galactose is an even better inhibitor. Chemical studies have identified this structure as the terminal portion of the A antigen. Parallel studies with the B antigen, though hampered by the scarcity of B spe-

cific lectins, have identified D-galactosyl-β-1,3-D galactose as its terminal disaccharide. Each of these arises from separate enzyme transformations of the H substance (Fig. 13-1).

ABO(H) antibodies

One of the great mysteries of the ABO(H) blood group system is that the alloantibodies are naturally present in the sera of all but group AB persons. The antibodies are barely detectable in the sera of newborn infants, but in the first few months after birth these agglutinins gradually increase in titer. This fact has been used to determine if infants are undergoing a normal maturation of their "bursal dependent," or immunoglobulin-producing, system. The uniform upward progression of ABO agglutinin titers in infancy and early childhood has been cited as evidence that an immunizing experience, occurring during these early months of life, is responsible for their production. It is known that during this same period enteric bacteria of several types begin to colonize the intestinal tract. Some of these bacteria are noted for their polysaccharide antigens, which are described in chemical terms later in this chapter. Exposure of this sort to an organism with an antigen that is structurally related and cross-reactive with the ABO antigens may be the source of the alloantibodies.

This hypothesis for human A and B isohemagglutinin formation has been supported by experiments in germ-free chickens. Chickens reared in the usual fashion have anti-human B in their sera, but germ-free chickens do not. If these germ-free chickens are deliberately contaminated with *Escherichia coli*, which synthesizes a B-like antigen, anti-B appears in the chicken sera. A- and B-like antigens are also present in *Shigella, Salmonella,* and other coliform bacteria. The reason that group A persons produce only anti-B is that their own A antigens produced early in fetal life have rendered them immunotolerant to the A antigen.

Hemagglutination testing

Hemagglutination relies on the bridging of red blood cells with antibody molecules. Most of the naturally occurring allohemagglutinins are antibodies of the IgM class. Partially because of their high se-

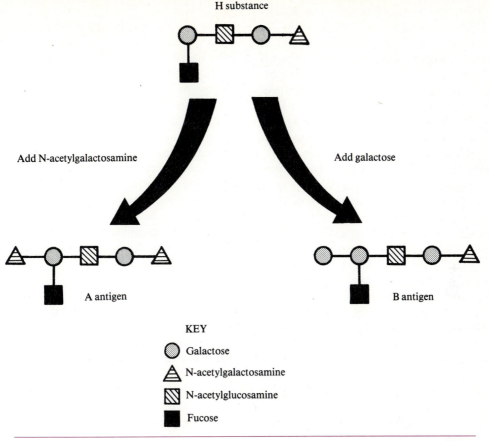

H substance

Add N-acetylgalactosamine

Add galactose

A antigen

B antigen

KEY

◯ Galactose

△ N-acetylgalactosamine

▨ N-acetylglucosamine

■ Fucose

FIG. 13-1

The H substance, which has a fucose attached to its terminal galactose, is modified by the addition of N-acetylgalactosamine to become the A antigen or the addition of galactose to become the B antigen.

rologic valence, these immunoglobulins are very efficient hemagglutinins. They function well in the ordinary hemagglutination tests in physiologic saline diluent and are by definition "complete" antibodies. Many of these IgM hemagglutinins are known as cold agglutinins because of their unique thermal amplitude, functioning much better at 25° or even 4° C than at 37° C, at which they are essentially inactive. When hemagglutination tests that are positive at 4° C are warmed to 37° C, the clumped cells redisperse, and the test becomes negative. Antibodies that function best at 37° C such as the IgG agglutinins are known as warm agglutinins.

Possibly because of their smaller size or lower serologic valence, the IgG antibodies are less efficient hemagglutinins than the IgM antibodies, and some may fail to clump erythrocytes in standard physiologic saline. By definition, then, these are "incomplete" antibodies. There is as yet no evidence that incomplete antibodies are structurally different from complete IgG antibodies. Cells coated with incomplete antibodies can be agglutinated with Coombs' reagent (antihuman globulin).

Hemagglutination tests are interpreted by two different methods. In the standard tube test, dilutions of the antiserum are incubated with a volume of red blood cells, usually 1 or 2 ml at a concentration of about 2%, and then observed macroscopically for clumping. In the case of weak agglutination, or when time is important and the incubation period must be abbreviated, light centrifugation of the tubes is helpful. After centrifugation the tubes are tapped gently with the finger to resuspend the cells. Cells that do not disperse evenly are agglutinated; agglutinated cells usually are graded as to heavy, moderate, or weak agglutination.

The cell sedimentation pattern also can be used to interpret hemagglutination, either in tubes or in microtiter trays (Fig. 13-2). For this test more dilute erythrocyte suspensions are used and are mixed with antiserum and incubated as usual. Centrifugation may be employed if needed. The settling pattern in the bottom of the wells is examined; when the cells form a dark red central button, the test is recorded as negative. Agglutinated cells are spread evenly over the bottom of the well, except in instances of very heavy agglutination, when ragged or "torn" edges of the cell pattern are typical.

Hemagglutination tests usually require antisera with an antibody content of only 0.001 to 0.01 μg/ml. As will be seen in the discussion of passive hemagglutination, less sensitive serologic tests may be converted to hemagglutination tests for improved sensitivity in detecting antibodies.

RH BLOOD GROUP SYSTEM

The Rh factor was described by Landsteiner and Wiener in 1940 as an antigen common to 85% of all human erythrocytes and those of the rhesus monkey. (The symbol for the Rh system has been taken from the first two letters of the word *rhesus*.) This shared antigen was discovered by hemagglutination testing of human red blood cells with antisera prepared in rabbits against rhesus monkey erythrocytes. Natural alloagglutinins against the Rh antigen do not occur; this fact probably accounts for the 40-year gap between the discovery of the ABO and the Rh blood group systems. Since the discovery of the initial Rh antigen it has become clear that more than 30 antigens must be considered as Rh antigens (Table 13-2). For practical reasons only the major Rh antigens are included in this discussion.

Nomenclature

Three independent nomenclature systems have arisen for the Rh antigens, two of which are in widespread use. In the Fisher-Race system capital and lower case letters (C, D, E, c, d, e,) are used to designate the six most commonly detected antigens. Actually only five of these may exist, since it has been impossible to produce antisera to the d antigen. Consequently d may represent only the absence of D. The D antigen is the most potent of these antigens

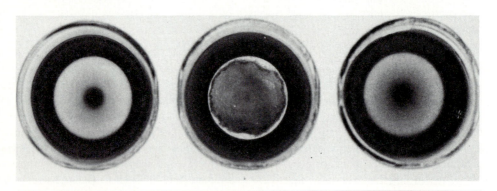

FIG. 13-2

Hemagglutination as seen by the settling patterns of the erythrocytes. A dark center indicates no hemagglutination, whereas a uniform distribution of erythrocytes across the bottom of the tubes is evidence of positive hemagglutination. These tubes would be read as negative, very strongly positive, and questionable or very weakly positive *(left to right)*.

and is synonymous with Rh antigen, as used in the original sense of Landsteiner and Wiener, or the Rh_0 antigen in the Wiener nomenclature system. Thus the 85% of the population who are Rh positive have the D antigen (Rh_0 antigen) on their red blood cells, and the 15% lacking this antigen are referred to as Rh-negative.

According to the interpretation by Fisher and Race the genes that regulate the synthesis of the Rh antigens exist as the allelic pairs Cc, Dd, and Ee, which reside at three separate but neighboring loci. Currently this interpretation is less favored than that of Wiener, but because of its simplicity, the Fisher-Race nomenclature remains a popular system in many laboratories.

The Wiener nomenclature system is more complex than the Fisher-Race system, since the letters Rh are varied between capital and lower case and are

TABLE 13-2

Partial list of human blood group systems

System	Number of antigens	Antigens			
ABO(H)	4	A_1, A_2, B, H plus four interactions with the I system			
Rh	33	Rh1	Rh_0, D	Rh18	Hr
		Rh2	rh', C	Rh19	hr^s
		Rh3	rh'', E	Rh20	VS, e^s
		Rh4	hr', c	Rh21	C^G
		Rh5	hr'', e	Rh22	CE
		Rh6	hr, f, ce	Rh23	D^w (Wiel)
		Rh7	rh_i, Ce	Rh24	E^T
		Rh8	rh^{w1}, C^w	Rh25	LW
		Rh9	rh^x, C^x, ce^s	Rh26	c-like (Deal)
		Rh10	hr^v, V	Rh27	cE
		Rh11	rh^{w2}, E^w	Rh28	hr^H
		Rh12	rh^G, G	Rh29	RH
		Rh13	Rh^A	Rh30	Go^a, C^{Cor}
		Rh14	Rh^B	Rh31	hr^B
		Rh15	Rh^C	Rh32	Troll (Reynolds)
		Rh16	Rh^D	Rh33	Ro^{Har}
		Rh17	Hro		
MN	28	M, N, S, s, U, U^B, M_1, M^A, M^C, M^g, M^V, Tm, Sj, Mi^a, Vu, Mur, Hill, Hu, He, M^e, Vr, St^a, Mt^a, Ri^a, Cl^a, Vr^a, Ny^a, Sul			
P	4	P_1, P_2, p, Tja, plus one interaction each with ABO (Luke) and with I(IP)			
I	5	I, i, i_2, I^t, I^D			
Lutheran	3	Lu^a, Lu^b, Lu^{ab}			
Kell	10	K, k, Kp^a, Kp^b, Js^a, Js^b, Kp^o, K^w, KL, Ul^a			
Lewis	6	Le^a, Le^b, Le^c, Le^x, Le^{ab}, Mag			
Duffy	3	Fy^a, Fy^b, Fy^3			
Kidd	2	Jk^a, Jk^b			
DBG	4	Ho, Ho-like, Ot, DBG			

Low-frequency antigens, not grouped: Be^a, By, Evans, Good, Box, Job, Kam, Lev, Mag, Nij, Or, Rd, Rm, Sf, Spl,Ta^a, Tr^a, Ven, Wb, Zd, and many others

High-frequency antigens not grouped: AT^a, Bra, Co^a, Ge, Kelly, Lan, Sd^a, Yus, and many others modified with subscripts (Rh_0, rh_1) or superscripts (Rh^A) to identify the different antigens. Consequently there is a greater chance for error in bookkeeping and in written records. In the Wiener system rh', Rh_0, and rh'' represent C, D, and E of the Fisher-Race system, and hr' and hr'' are c and e (Table 13-2).

The third nomenclature system is a simple numeric system proposed by Rosenfield in 1962 in which $Rh1 = Rh_0 = D$, etc. (Table 13-2). The numeric system has not yet been widely accepted as a neutral solution for those debating the merits of the Wiener and Fisher-Race systems.

Regardless of the system of nomenclature or the exact modes of inheritance, it is agreed that an allelic system is followed. Thus, an Rh-positive person may be either homozygous or heterozygous, but an Rh-negative person is necessarily homozygous. This is an important consideration when discussing HDN caused by maternal-fetal Rh incompatibility.

Rh antigens and antibodies

The number of Rh_0 (D) antigen sites on human erythrocytes has been variably estimated to be between 2,000 and 33,000 per cell. If we accept 10,000 to 15,000 as an average value, then the number of A or B sites per cell exceeds the number of Rh_0 sites by about fortyfold.

Human immunoglobulins to the Rh antigens differ from the hemagglutinins to the ABO(H) antigens in that the former arise from genuine alloimmunization and do not exist as "natural" antibodies. Thus an Rh-negative person does not axiomatically have antibodies to the Rh_0 antigen. As described earlier, Rh-negative means the absence of Rh_0, or D; so an Rh-positive person cannot make antibodies to an antigen that does not exist. (Notice that this applies only to D and d; a person who is genetically CDE [and Rh-positive] can make antibodies to antigens c and e.) Alloantibodies directed toward the Rh antigens may be of the IgM or IgG class. The route of immunization is from improper transfusion of Rh-positive blood into an Rh-negative recipient or maternal immunization by Rh-positive fetal erythrocytes. Mild or recent antigen exposure will favor IgM, and more intensive immunization will favor IgG.

Hemolytic disease of the newborn

Hemolytic disease of the newborn, sometimes called erythroblastosis, is most commonly the result of the transplacental migration of maternal anti-Rh globulins into the circulatory system of the developing fetus. The ensuing serologic reaction destroys the fetal erythrocytes. This condition is discussed fully in Chaper 18.

MISCELLANEOUS HUMAN BLOOD GROUP SYSTEMS

The second blood group system to be discovered, the MN system, was reported by Landsteiner and Levine in 1927, more than a decade prior to the discovery of the Rh system. These antigens were detected by the use of specific sera produced in rabbits, and the letters *M* and *N* were chosen arbitrarily. The two original antigens of this system are inherited in the same way as the A and B antigens so that three blood groups are possible: MM, MN, and NN. There is no group corresponding to O. The frequency of the M, MN, and N groups in the white population is 29%, 50%, and 21%, respectively. Human anti-M is fairly frequent; anti-N is more rare. Detection of M and N antigens now is accomplished with a lectin of *Iberis amara* for the M antigen and of *Vicia graminea* or *Bauhinia purpura* for the N antigen.

The MN system now has been expanded to include at least 28 different antigens. The best known of these additional antigens are S, s, and U. Nearly 100% of white and 95% of blacks have the U antigen. The S and s antigens are inherited in a four-gene complex with M and N, permitting the combinations MS, Ms, NS, and Ns. Much is yet to be learned about the chemistry of these antigens, but the evidence currently available indicates that M and N are dependent on a complex polysaccharide core modified by *N*-acetylneuraminic acid groups.

Antigens and antibodies of the I blood group system have some interesting relationships to several disease conditions and to human development. The discovery of the I blood group was made in 1956 by Wiener and his associates, who suggested that the cold agglutinin found in patients with hemolytic anemia was directed against a specific antigen. This antigen, the I antigen, is present on virtually 100% of human adult red blood cells and is one of the two major antigens in this group, the other antigen being i. Agglutinins with anti-I activity are thus autoantibodies, and, as indicated, most of these antibodies have a unique thermal amplitude, reacting at 4° C but hardly at all at 37° C. Anti-i exists with a high frequency in patients with infectious mononucleosis, but the basis for this relationship is uncertain.

Fetal erythrocytes and those taken from cord blood or newborn infants do not react with anti-I. During the first months of life these i cells tend to disappear and by the second year of life are replaced by I cells of the adult type. Adult type cells still contain traces of the i antigen; so this i $\rightarrow$ I transition probably is related to an enzymatic "maturation" that converts the i substance to the I antigen. Red blood cells of persons with chronic hemolytic anemia or hypoplastic anemia react strongly with anti-i. Thus immature erythrocytes originating from natural or disease conditions are deficient in I but have the precursor i substance.

New blood cell antigens continuously are being discovered. When it can be shown that the inheritance of two or more antigens is interrelated, then the antigens are placed in a blood group. If the inheritance of these antigens is unrelated to the inheritance of a preexistent group, the creation of a new blood group system is justified. The time required to make these decisions is often considerable, perhaps several years. During this time the presumed new antigen or blood group has to be named in some way so that it is not confused with existing blood group systems. The first red cell antigens to be discovered were assigned capital letters A and B, and then later M and N, and still later C and D of the Rh system. When the suggestion of an alphabetical order was broken in the formation of the MN group, then one or more letters from the name of the first individual known to have the antigen or antibody was used, as in Rh (rhesus), K (Kell), and Le (Lewis). The letters need not come from the first part of the name; the name ending also can be used, as in Fy (Duffy). As additional antigens were discovered within a group, subscripts, superscripts, changes in case, and combinations of these were used to name the new antigens.

In this way A_1, rh', rh'', Rh_0, Le^a, and others were created. Currently there is a tendency to use the first three or more letters of the person's last name for new blood group antigens. The result of this mixture of nomenclature systems is that there is no simple method for learning blood group antigens.

Blood cell antigens often are described as public or private antigens, depending on their incidence. "Public" antigens are those which are unusually common but not a part of a known group; At^a, Co^a, Ge, and Lan are examples. In many instances these antigens later are placed in new or existing groups. "Private," or "family," antigens generally have an incidence of less than 0.25%. Such antigens are especially useful in identifying specific individuals or groups and are valuable genetic tools.

Blood group systems depending on antigenic variations of white blood cells and platelets also have been constructed. Those based on leukocyte antigens are discussed in Chapter 15, where their importance as histocompatibility antigens is explained.

APPLICATIONS OF HEMAGGLUTINATION
Blood transfusions

The practical importance of blood groups and blood grouping in modern medicine is immeasurable. The increasing use of blood transfusions has made hemagglutination the most frequent serologic test performed. In blood transfusions, the ideal goal is that the recipient be given exactly his or her own type of blood. For example, a group A person should not receive group B blood, since the blood would be destroyed by the B alloagglutinins of the group A person. A group A person might be given group O blood, despite the known content of anti-A in the latter. This is often a safe procedure, since in the transfusion the anti-A globulins will be diluted extensively in the recipient, possibly beyond the titer of their activity. It is on this basis that the group O person has been described as the "universal donor" and the group AB person as the "universal recipient." In emergencies this may be an acceptable operating procedure, but in everyday blood banking an exact matching of donor and recipient blood is the goal.

All laboratories formerly performed two tests to

determine the suitability of a transfusion. These are called the major and minor cross matches. The major cross match, called major because it is of greater importance, is performed by mixing the serum of the recipient with the blood cells of the donor. If agglutination occurs, this blood cannot be given to the recipient for the obvious reason that the recipient has antibodies which will destroy the donor cells. In the minor cross match the recipient's cells are mixed with the donor's serum. If agglutination occurs, the blood should not be given because the donor's serum contains antibodies capable of attacking the recipient's cells. It is only during a true emergency that such blood can be given. A positive minor cross match destroys the concept of O blood being the universal donor, since it contains both anti-A and anti-B globulins and only can match with O blood. Similarly, since AB blood is agglutinated by all except group AB sera, an AB person is not a universal recipient.

In actual practice the minor cross match is not used extensively, and the major cross match, now called the compatibility test, is the only test being used. Compatibility testing has the major limitation of not detecting antigens. For example, the Rh antigen would not be detected in a donor's blood by cross matching with a nonimmune Rh-negative person. Transfusion of such blood would actively immunize the recipient and set the stage for a subsequent transfusion reaction if similar Rh-positive blood were given again. Incomplete antibodies can be identified in the compatibility test by performing the Coombs test after the incubation of donor cells and recipient serum.

Personal identification

Because of the large number of blood group antigens that are now known, it is almost possible to identify a specific individual by his or her own special combination of antigens. This fact, coupled with an understanding of genetic principles, has led to a number of forensic applications based on erythrocyte antigens. In paternity suits, certain combinations of blood types in the mother and child will exclude the possibility of certain men being the father. For example, an AB man cannot father a group OO child;

an A woman and an A man cannot produce a B child; an A_1 woman and an A_1 man cannot produce an A_2 child; and an O, Rh-negative woman and an O, Rh-negative man cannot produce an O, Rh-positive child. Blood group testing can only exclude a putative father from fatherhood; this is now generally accepted in courts of law. By means of similar tests "mixed babies" in the newborn nursery often can be identified as belonging to a specific mother-father combination. Because of the far greater number of histocompatibility antigens compared to blood group antigens, histocompatibility typing is replacing blood group serology as the method of choice in resolving cases of disputed parentage or unidentified babies (see Chapter 15).

Another forensic application of blood grouping occurs in cases of violent deaths with loss of blood. As described in the previous chapter, serologic testing with specific antisera can identify the species and blood type of stains that are days, weeks, or even years old.

Passive hemagglutination and passive agglutination

The type of hemagglutination described in the previous paragraphs may be categorized as immune, direct hemagglutination. This implies two other forms of hemagglutination: nonimmune and indirect. Actually a few examples of the former already have been presented. The agglutination of erythrocytes by phytoagglutinins or lectins is accomplished via a nonimmune mechanism. To this could be added hemagglutination by viruses, especially the myxoviruses such as influenza virus and Newcastle's disease virus.

Indirect, or passive, hemagglutination is based on the red blood cell as an inert carrier (Schlepper) of antigens (Fig. 13-3). Erythrocytes often are preferred to other particles as the carrier because hemagglutination is a familiar serologic test and the results are easily interpreted. Hemagglutination tests are easily converted to hemolytic tests by the addition of complement, and hemolytic tests are adaptable to exact quantitation by colorimetry or spectrophotometry. Of course spontaneous lysis of erythrocytes is one complaint about passive hemagglutination testing. This

RBC with attached antigen   Antibody

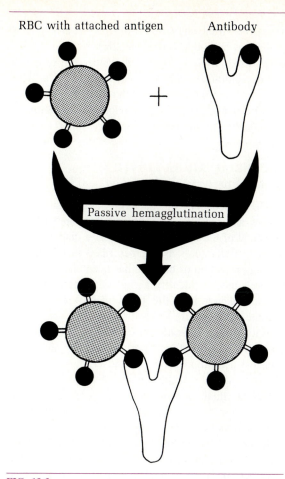

Passive hemagglutination

FIG. 13-3
Passive hemagglutination by using the erythrocyte as an inert carrier of an antigen.

of various sizes can be purchased in a concentrated stock preparation dyed a light blue to make them more visible. These can be diluted, coated with antigen, and used very simply in passive agglutination tests.

There are many variations of the passive hemagglutination test. In the simplest form the antigen is incubated with the erythrocytes, and antigen adsorption takes place spontaneously. The antigen-coated erythrocytes are washed to remove excess free antigen and then are incubated with antiserum to the adsorbed antigen to produce hemagglutination. The biochemical class of molecule most easily adsorbed on erythrocytes is polysaccharide or polysaccharides that are conjugated with lipids or proteins. LPS is a typical example. Pure protein antigens cannot be used in this type of test because they do not attach to the red blood cells.

Another handicap of simple adsorptive coating of erythrocytes by antigen is that the antigen-erythrocyte bond is strictly a physical bond, and the antigen can dissociate easily from the cell. This is of special concern because any antigen released into solution will "tie up" antibody and prevent its combination with the antigen present on the red cells. The consequence of this is that the free antigen behaves as a blocking antigen and seriously reduces the hemagglutinating titer of the antiserum.

Protein antigens can be complexed with erythrocytes that have been pretreated with tannic acid according to the technique of Boyden. These tanned erythrocytes do not lose their polysaccharide receptors, so they still will bond to these antigens as well. Tannic acid, in a final concentration of 1:20,000 to 1:40,000, is used to alter the cell and reveal new protein receptors. Spontaneous agglutination of the red cells occurs if they are overexposed to tannic acid. Buffers containing colloids prevent this. Tanned cells are especially liable to lysis, so formalinized cells are recommended. Certain metals (for example, chromium salts) will complex proteins to erythrocytes and provide a more stable antigen preparation than is afforded by the usual adsorption process.

The principal disadvantage of the aforementioned tests, from an immunologic point of view, is that the

handicap has been overcome in two ways: by the use of glutaraldehyde- or formaldehyde-treated erythrocytes as the antigen carrier and by the use of carrier particles that are less fragile or totally resistant to osmotic lysis. Aldehyde-treated cells take on a brown color and resist lysis. They even can be frozen and thawed or lyophilized so that an antigen-coated red blood cell can be preserved almost indefinitely. Other types of materials such as polystyrene spheres, polyacrylamide, and particles of latex or of charcoal, which are more osmotically resistant and in some cases easier to prepare, are replacing erythrocytes as the carrier. For example, polystyrene latex particles antigens are only loosely bound to the erythrocyte carrier. Dissociation of the antigen from the ordinary or the tanned erythrocyte can occur without notice and can invalidate the red blood cells as the "antigen." To overcome this deficit, methods designed for covalent bonding of antigens to erythrocytes have been developed. Dinitrodifluorobenzene, bisdiazotized benzidine, toluene diisocyanate, and other dually reactive compounds, such as those applied to ferritin labeling of antibodies, have been used. The antigen, erythrocyte, and coupling reagent, when mixed in the correct proportions, will yield a covalently linked red cell-antigen conjugate of almost interminable life expectancy. Such a preparation can be lyophilized in small portions and rehydrated for use, which obviates the repeated preparation and standardization of smaller, individual batches of antigen.

One useful modification of the passive hemagglutination technique is the reversed passive hemagglutination test, whereby the antibody is united covalently with the carrier and is used to detect antigen. Inhibition tests also can be devised wherein free antigen reacts with antibody to prevent its agglutination of antigen-coated erythrocytes.

The principal purpose of all passive hemagglutination tests is to convert precipitation reactions to hemagglutination reactions and to increase the sensitivity of the test. Passive hemagglutination tests are among the most sensitive serologic procedures available; under ideal conditions as little as 0.003 µg of antibody nitrogen will yield a positive test. Consequently passive hemagglutination titers of 1:1,000,000 and higher are not unusual.

The passive agglutination inhibition test for human chorionic gonadotropin has become the most rapid, least expensive, and most popular test for this hormone. Several forms of the test are available commercially; in one kit two main reagents are provided. The first is an antiserum to the hormone, which has a molecular weight of 30,000 and is an acceptable antigen. The other reagent is a formalinized erythrocyte preparation to which the hormone is attached. A mixture of the two reagents will produce a passive hemagglutination. Preincubation of fluids containing the hormone (urine or serum of pregnant women) with the antiserum will cause a serologic reaction (invisible because of the concentration of antiserum used) which will bind the antiserum so that it cannot agglutinate the hormone-bearing cells. This test is so simply performed that self-test kits now have been marketed. With obvious modifications it is adaptable to the measurement of other antigens and haptens.

BACTERIAL AGGLUTINATION
H and O bacterial agglutination

The discovery of bacterial agglutination by Grüber and Durham in 1896 and the popularization by Widal of the agglutination test as a diagnostic aid for bacterial infections are described in Chapter 1. The agglutination of bacteria has been one of the key methods used to identify and classify these microorganisms which lack the gross identifying features present in higher life forms.

Bacterial agglutination tests may be performed in tubes or on slides (Fig. 13-4). In the tube agglutination test a dilution series of antiserum is prepared, and, to each tube, a suspension of bacteria is added so that the final concentration of the organisms is approximately 900×10^6 per milliliter. The tubes are incubated and examined. Agglutination frequently is difficult to detect at this time, and so refrigeration of the test overnight often is practiced to allow further aggregation. At this time the titer can be determined by merely examining the tubes to see which still contain a cloudy suspension and which are clear; agglutinated cells do not remain in a uniform suspension and will settle to the bottom of the tube. This can be confirmed by tapping the tubes and looking for aggregates of bacteria, which rise from the sediment in the tubes exhibiting agglutination.

In the slide agglutination test small volumes of the antiserum are dispensed onto a slide and mixed with a dense suspension of organisms. The slide is tilted gently to and fro or rotated for 3 to 5 minutes. Agglutinated cells are seen as large clumps of bacteria. The slide test is more rapid and economic but is less precise than the tube test.

In either the tube or the slide test a difference in the physical size of the clumped bacteria may be noted, depending on the nature of the organism and the

≣ SITUATION

A PEACH OF A PEAR

It was Bob G. from the horticulture department. "Dave, I thought I'd give you a call about this discovery we've made. You dummies kept telling me my pear trees couldn't make antibodies, right? Even if they were resistant to the bacterial infections that killed the other pear trees, right? Well, we just did an agglutination test, and my resistant trees were positive, and the sensitive trees were negative. Now tell me again about plants not making antibodies."

Further discussion with Bob revealed that he had made an extract of pear leaves from his resistant line and from his sensitive line a few hours after infecting each with the bacterial pathogen. The extract from the resistant tree agglutinated the bacterium, a gram-negative bacillus, but the other extract did not. Extracts from the resistant tree line made prior to infection failed to clump the organisms.

I asked him a few questions about controls and gave him my advice.

Questions

1. What is nonimmune agglutination of bacteria, and how does it differ from immune?
2. What substances are capable of nonimmune bacterial agglutination?
3. What types of experiments or controls are used to distinguish nonimmune and immune agglutination?
4. What are lectins? Will they agglutinate bacteria?

Solution

Spontaneous agglutination of bacteria is a common finding in the study of certain species or genera and is separated easily from nonimmune agglutination. Spontaneous agglutination describes the clumping of bacteria, such as that seen with several corynebacteria and mycobacteria, which takes place in ordinary buffers or saline. This phenomenon makes it almost impossible to use these organisms in agglutination tests, since they already are clumped.

Nonimmune agglutination is defined as the agglutination of cells by nonantibody forces. This has been most extensively studied in the form of hemagglutination, but many of the same principles apply to nonimmune bacterial agglutination. Unsuitable pH, metal ions, and other forces that influence the ionic condition of the bacterial cell may cause agglutination. Thus clumping of red blood cells and bacteria often can be induced by mixing them with electropositive proteins—histones, lysozyme, protamines, etc. These materials bind firmly to the electronegative bacteria and neutralize their repellant electric charge. The bacteria are enabled to contact each other and remain attached, particularly if there is an adhesive structure such as a polysaccharide capsule on their surface.

Since immune agglutination is a property of immunoglobulins, it is possible to identify this type of agglutination by identifying the proteins responsible for it. If one removes all the proteins or only the globulins from a serum, it should no longer agglutinate. Sera that have agglutinated will leave a coat of γ-globulin on the bacteria. These antibodies can be recognized by various antiglobulin tests such as enhanced agglutination by the antiglobulin, fluorescent antiglobulin, and enzyme-labeled antiglobulin. This aspect of the present problem was investigated, but it was not possible to identify any adsorption of globulins by the bacteria.

The adaptive nature of the agglutinating response developed by the pear trees in this problem is characteristic of the immune response. Since no new globulins could be detected on the surface of the agglutinated bacteria, the cells were examined for their adsorption of other substances. This resulted in the finding that a protein high in polysaccharide content, a glycoprotein, seen in the extract as small structures almost viral in dimension, had attached to the bacteria. This substance in the pear leaf extracts was assumed to be lectin. When the extract was tested for its ability to agglutinate close relatives to the bacterial pear tree pathogen, they all were agglutinated. Other, more distantly placed taxonomic bacteria occasionally were agglutinated.

Further studies indicated that this agglutination was caused by a pear lectin that was normally present in the plant but which accumulated in leaves and twigs heavily parasitized by bacteria because of fluid imbalances created in these tissues during the infection. Lectins (phytoagglutinins, PHAs) are known to be normal constituents of plants that have an affinity for polysaccharides found on the surface of erythrocytes, tissue culture cells, bacteria, and other sources. Some of the lectins are multivalent and can bridge to cells (or two sites on the same cell) to hold them together. Agglutination of *Escherichia coli* by Con A and the agglutination of other bacteria by lectins have been reported. The genetics of this has been studied by using bacterial mutants.

antiserum used. If the antiserum is prepared against a whole, intact, motile organism, such as *Salmonella typhi,* and if the same organism is used in the agglutination test, the clumps will be rather large and light or snowflake in appearance. This is referred to as the H type of bacterial agglutination; H is taken from the German word *Hauch,* which means a film, breath, or haze, much as one might see on a steamed glass. Motile bacteria will produce a thin, nearly transparent type of growth on a moist agar plate. This loose flocculant type of agglutination is indicative of the operation of flagellar antigens (H antigens) and their respective antibodies in the test. The flagella, extending as they do some distance from the bacteria, are "glued" to each other by antibody molecules. This unites the bacteria into an agglutinate even though the bacterial cells proper are still some distance from each other. The result is a loosely woven lacework of clumped cells, which produces a light snowflake type of agglutination.

Quite the opposite occurs in the O type of agglutination (O from the German *ohne Hauch,* meaning without a film, hence aflagellate). In this instance agglutination is the result of antibodies to somatic (cellular) antigens, which hold the cell walls of the bacteria very closely together (Fig. 13-4). The consequence of this is the formation of a very compact, granular or hailstonelike mass of agglutinated bacteria.

Bacterial agglutination results largely from antibodies of the IgM class. In describing H and O agglutination or H and O antigens it is necessary to distinguish between human blood cell antigens and bacterial agglutination systems.

Bacterial antigens

It is obvious that the chemical nature of the agglutinogens will vary as widely as the bacteria that produce them. For this reason only the O antigens on the genus *Salmonella* are considered in detail, with a more general discussion of those of gram-positive bacteria.

Antigens of gram-positive bacteria

The chemistry of the cell walls and plasma membranes of gram-positive bacteria is dominated by the teichoic acids, which are absent from gram-negative bacteria. Teichoic acids are polymeric phosphate esters of glycerol and ribitol substituted with alanyl and glycosyl groups. The teichoic acids found in the cell membrane are always of the glycerol type and covalently joined to a glycolipid. For this reason they are designated as lipoteichoic acids. Teichoic acids of the cell wall may be based on either a glycerol or ribitol structure covalently linked to a peptidoglycan. Cell wall teichoic acids and some lipoteichoic acids are sufficiently surface oriented to combine with antibodies. For example, the group D antigen of streptococci is a lipoteichoic acid that is not found in cell walls, only the plasma membrane, yet it participates in agglutination reactions.

Lipoteichoic acids are responsible for many of the cross-reactions of gram-positive bacteria, but this does not mean that the teichoic acids are identical among all cross-reacting bacteria. These acids contain several antigenic determinants, including the glycerol phosphate backbone of the polymer, the alanyl and glycosyl side groups, and the glycolipid, although antibodies directed against the latter are rare. Those determinants need not be all identical in cross-reacting species. In some instances, as in the group D and also the group A, F, and N streptococci, lipoteichoic acids common to members of the group form the basis for the serologic grouping. Other streptococci possess other teichoic acids, and this is expressed by the failure of them to cross-react with the antilipoteichoic sera used to establish the separate antigenic groups.

Antigenic classification of *Salmonella*

The antigenic complexities of the enteric bacilli have been the most thoroughly studied of all bacteria, both on a serologic and on a chemical basis. As a result of systematic serologic experiments, largely by Kauffmann and White, approximately 1,100 serotypes within the genus *Salmonella* alone have been distinguished. These are determined on the basis of somatic, or O, antigens, flagellar, or H, antigens, and virulence, or Vi (somatic), antigens. A unique combination of these in an organism creates a unique serotype.

On the basis of common somatic O antigens the individual serotypes (species) of the genus *Salmonella* are placed in groups designated by the letters A to I. All group B species, for example, contain somatic antigen 4, and all group C_1 members contain antigens 6 and 7. There are actually some 60 different O antigens used to define the 40 groups. These serogroups are divided into serotypes on the basis of their H antigens. The virulence antigen is not used in the construction of either serogroups or serotypes. The Vi antigen is a somatic antigen situated external to the O antigens and may prevent bacterial agglutination by anti-O sera. The Vi antigen is destroyed easily by mild heating, by dilute acid, or by repeated transfer of the organism on artificial media. The H antigens are destroyed by alcohol or by extensive heating. To prepare an antiserum that contains anti-

Vi globulins, a fresh isolate of the organism must be used. Of course the antiserum also will contain antibodies to the H and O antigens. An antiserum that contains only anti-H and anti-O immunoglobulins can be prepared by using mildly heated, acid-exposed, or repeatedly transferred cells as the vaccine. Such cells are referred to as H cells. O cells can be prepared by alcohol treatment of H cells.

Agglutinin adsorption and cross agglutination

By proper adsorption experiments pure antisera against the Vi or H antigens can be prepared. It is not necessary to resort to agglutinin adsorption to prepare O antisera, since O cells contain only O an-

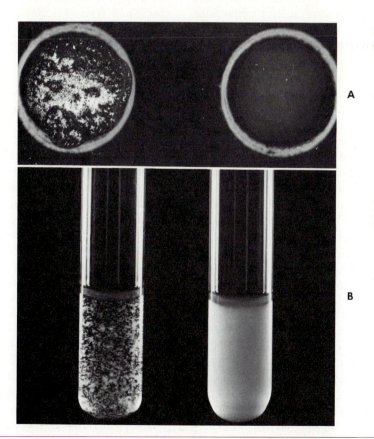

FIG. 13-4

A, Slide agglutination of bacteria is a rapid method of identifying unknown bacteria with known antisera or the reverse. **B,** Tube agglutination can be used for the same purpose and to quantitate the antibody content in an antiserum. In each case the positive test is seen at left and the negative control at right.

tigens unless one wishes to have an antiserum specific for a single O antigen.

If an antiserum against the Vi cell is incubated with the H organism, the H and O antibodies will attach to the bacteria. If the bacteria are removed by centrifugation, these H and O antibodies also are removed. This leaves only pure Vi antibody in the solution. This process is called agglutinin adsorption. Pure H antibody can be prepared by agglutinin adsorption with O cells and antiserum to the H cells. Note that one cannot prepare pure flagella by mixing H cells with anti-O sera, since all parts of the cell are removed when the cells are agglutinated and removed.

As discussed earlier, all the species of the genus *Salmonella* in one group share at least one somatic antigen. Consequently an O antiserum against the antigen will agglutinate all the bacteria in that group. Several unshared antigens also may exist between any two organisms. These shared and unshared O antigens have been identified and arbitrarily assigned numbers on the basis of cross agglutination tests and agglutinin adsorption experiments with anti-O sera. From these sources it has been possible to assign an antigenic formula to the somatic (and by the use of specific anti-H sera, to the flagella) antigens of each organism. *Salmonella typhi* is designated as 9, 12, Vi, and d; 9 and 12 represent the two ordinary somatic antigens, Vi the virulence antigen, and d a certain flagellar antigen. Antigenic formulas are exactly known for all the *Salmonella* species, since it is on the basis of an individual combination of antigens that new species were created in the past.

Salmonella O antigen chemistry

Polysaccharides from all salmonellae, regardless of their O antigenic grouping, contain five common monosaccharides. These are D-glucose, D-galactose, D-glucosamine, L-glycero-D-mannoheptose, and 2-keto-3-deoxyoctonic acid. This suggests that a unit polysaccharide core is present in all *Salmonella* species. This core may be modified by the addition of other monosaccharides to create the specific O antigens for that organism. Proteins and lipids are not involved in O antigen specificity, since all O activity is present in the pure polysaccharides. Studies of R

(rough) mutants, which lack the O antigen, support this hypothesis. Several R chemotypes have been identified that lack one or more of the five core constituents.

Attached to each core are the unique and specific monosaccharides for the individual O antigens. These may consist of additional hexoses or substituted hexoses (D-mannose, D-galactosamine), methyl pentoses (L-fucose, L-rhamnose), and ribose in unique combinations with or without a 3,6-dideoxyhexose. The 3,6-dideoxyhexoses originally were isolated from *Salmonella* species; four of these novel sugars are related to specific O antigens. The four sugars are abequose (3,6-dideoxy-D-galactose), colitose (3,6-dideoxy-L-galactose), paratose (3,6-dideoxy-D-glucose), and tyvelose (3,6-dideoxy-D-mannose); their structures are presented in Fig. 13-5. Serologic analysis reveals that these dideoxy sugars are part of the immunodominant group of O antigens. This indicates their terminal, external location in the oligosaccharide chain. Hapten inhibition studies with specific O antisera have shown that abequose contributes strongly to antigens 4 and 8, paratose to antigen 2, tyvelose to antigen 9, and colitose to antigens 35 and 40. Additional sugars contribute to these antigenic determinants. Other somatic antigens contain more common sugars in their immunodominant center: for example, glucose in antigens 1, 12, 19, and 37.

The flagellar antigens (flagellins) are usually pure proteins of 20,000 mol wt *(Proteus vulgaris)*; 20,000 to 30,000 molecules may be associated into the flagellar structure itself. Tryptophan often is missing, and unusual amino acids, for example, ϵ-N-methyl lysine, may be present.

The availability of antisera that are specific for pathogenic bacteria makes it possible to perform bacterial agglutination tests to identify microorganisms isolated from patients with infectious diseases. Moreover, when pathogenic bacteria cannot be isolated from patients, it is possible to make a serologic diagnosis of the disease. This is done by drawing two samples of blood from the patient, the first during the acute phase of the illness, usually when the patient first seeks medical assistance, and the second, or convalescent, sample 1 or 2 weeks later. Sera from the acute and convalescent samples are

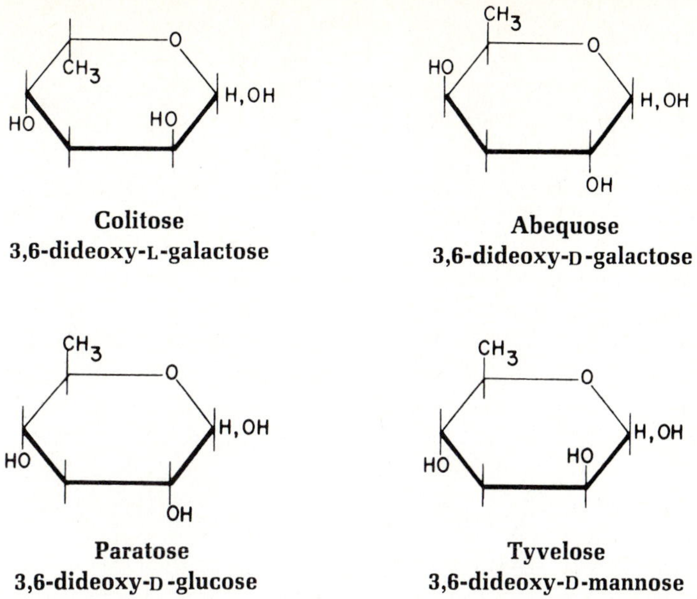

Colitose
3,6-dideoxy-L-galactose

Abequose
3,6-dideoxy-D-galactose

Paratose
3,6-dideoxy-D-glucose

Tyvelose
3,6-dideoxy-D-mannose

FIG. 13-5

Structures of colitose, paratose, abequose, and tyvelose. These unique dideoxy sugars are part of the immunodominant portion of several *Salmonella* species somatic antigens.

tested for their agglutinating capacity with known bacteria. The species of bacteria selected are those which produce an illness similar to that the patient has or had. A difference in agglutination titer of fourfold between the acute and convalescent serum samples with a specific bacterium is accepted as evidence of an antigenic exposure to that organism. This in turn is taken as proof of the cause of the disease. This evidence is only usable when both the acute and convalescent serum samples are analyzed. Patients may have a high agglutinating titer against a certain organism as the result of a cross-reaction, prior disease, or immunization with that organism; so single, high values are not easily interpreted. Among the pathogenic bacteria analyzed in this way are *Escherichia, Hemophilus, Brucella, Listeria, Corynebacterium, Leptospira, Bordetella, Shigella, Staphylococcus, Streptococcus, Proteus,* and *Salmonella* and many more outside the realm of human medical microbiology.

Special terms are used in clinical serologic laboratories to describe these agglutination tests. A test for febrile agglutinins usually means for agglutinins against *Salmonella typhi, Salmonella paratyphi* A (and possibly *Salmonella paratyphi* B), and *Brucella* and *Francisella* organisms. The Widal test refers to agglutination of *Salmonella* species. A Weil-Felix test refers to agglutinins for *Proteus* species and is used to investigate the possibility of rickettsial disease since several rickettsia cross react with *Proteus*.

REFERENCES

Bryant, N.S.: An introduction to immunohematology, 2nd edition, Philadelphia, 1982, W.B. Saunders Co.

Engelfreit, C.P., van Loghem, J.J., and von dem Borne, A.E.G.K., editors: Immunohematology, Amsterdam, 1984, Elsevier Science Publishers B.V.

Issit, P.D., and Crookston, M.C.: Blood group terminology: current convention, Transfus. **24:**2, 1984.

Lockyer, W.J.: Essentials of ABO-Rh grouping and compatibility testing, Bristol, 1982, John Wright and Sons, Ltd.

Salmon, C., editor: Blood groups and other red cell surface markers in health and disease, New York, 1982, Masson Publishing USA, Inc.

Weisz-Carrington, P.: Principals of clinical immunohematology, Chicago, 1986, Year Book Medical Publishers.

IMMUNITY

Natural resistance and acquired immunity

≡ GLOSSARY

acquired immunity　Immunity developed after birth, as opposed to inherited immunity.

cell-mediated immunity　Immunity dependent on T lymphocytes and phagocytic cells.

CMI　Cell-mediated immunity.

humoral immunity　Immunity resulting from immunoglobulins.

immunity　Condition of being resistant to an infection.

inherited immunity　Immunity conferred by one's genetic constitution, not acquired by exposure to infectious agents.

natural resistance　Inherited, not acquired, immunity.

passive immunity　Immunity contributed to one individual from another.

vaccine　A suspension of living or dead organisms used as an antigen.

The defense of an animal against infectious organisms or their toxic products can be considered from several viewpoints which include (1) whether it is a naturally existent or acquired characteristic, (2) whether it is based on humoral or cellular factors, and (3) whether it is external or internal in location. In this chapter, all of these topics will be discussed, in addition to a description of vaccines and immunizations, both present and projected.

NATURAL RESISTANCE

Natural resistance or natural immunity, known also as innate immunity, native immunity, or inherited immunity, should not be confused with naturally *acquired* immunity. Innate immunity refers to that type of resistance which each individual has by virtue of being the individual he or she is in terms of species, race, sex, or other factors associated with genetically controlled resistance. Natural immunity, unlike acquired immunity, commonly is thought of as a nonspecific barrier that is effective against many different kinds of infectious agents. Because of this, some prefer the term *natural resistance* to *natural immunity,* the word *immunity* often connoting specificity.

Examples of natural resistance
Species

Fowl malaria, dog tapeworm, avian tuberculosis, canine distemper, mouse pox (but not chickenpox), fowl typhoid, and many similar terms indicate the host range or species specificity which certain pathogens possess. This also suggests that other species of animals are resistant to the infectious agent mentioned. This fact is easily supported by simple observation; humans get mumps, but dogs and cats do not; mammals may contract anthrax, but birds do not; amphibia are resistant to tetanus and diphtheria. Exactly *why* one species contracts a certain disease when other species are resistant is not always explainable. In certain cases the body temperature of the animal will not permit growth of the pathogen;

for example, if the body temperature of chickens is lowered from 39° to 37° C, they become susceptible to anthrax.

Race or strain

It always has been difficult to evaluate differences that the human races seem to have in susceptibility or resistance to certain diseases. Unequal economic and social opportunities almost always have resulted in gross variations in exposure to most infectious agents. Only in limited segments of our population in which all persons share the same environment (for example, military installations, prisons, and mental hospitals) do we find that exposure for all individuals has been nearly the same. Under these conditions, racial differences can be detected. It appears that blacks are more susceptible than whites to tuberculosis. Conversely, blacks appear more resistant than whites to diphtheria, influenza, and gonorrhea.

Natural resistance of several mouse strains to the murine pathogen *Corynebacterium kutscheri* has been genetically analyzed. The $\log_{10}$ of the number of organisms consisting of the LD_{50} (lethal dose for 50% of the mice) varied from 3.8 to 5.8 (Fig. 14-1).

When the C57BL/6 resistant mice were bred with the susceptible Swiss Lynch strains, the LD_{50} of the F_1 hybrids and back crosses agreed with the predicted values. For example, the calculation for the C57BL/6 × Swiss Lynch mating is

$$F_1 = \frac{5.8 \times 3.8}{2} = 4.8$$

which was the observed value.

Sex

As mentioned for racial differences, apparent differences in susceptibility of the two human sexes have been clouded by the improbability of equal exposure; in laboratory animals, however, such differences have been demonstrated repeatedly. BALB/c female mice are more resistant to *Listeria monocytogenes* infection than males, but male and female C57BL/6 mice are equally susceptible.

Nutrition

Another quality that influences resistance and susceptibility is an individual's nutritional status. Protein-calorie malnutrition lowers the level of C3 and

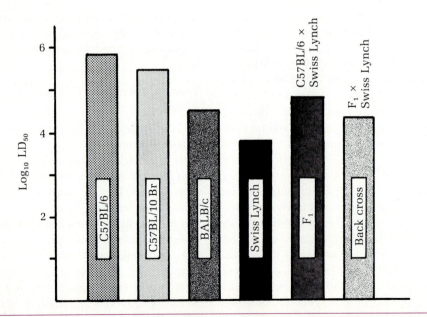

FIG. 14-1
The natural resistance of mouse strains to *Corynebacterium kutscheri* is genetically controlled. Mating of C57BL/6 and Swiss Lynch mice produced offspring with the expected susceptibility.

factor B of the complement system, decreases the IFN response, penalizes the neutrophil's activities, and seems to stress the T cell more than the B cell system. Low-protein diets alone are not invariably detrimental; the NZB mouse on a 6% protein diet may develop lower IgG1 and IgM levels but maintains its IgA level. The lymphocytes of these mice actually responded better to Con A and PHA than the cells of control mice on ad libitum diets. The lethal autoimmune disease that typically develops in NZB mice was slowed or prevented by low-intake diets.

Vitamin deficiencies often exhibit significant effects on host defense. Vitamin A deficiency affects epithelial cell integrity and allows more skin infections to develop. Folic acid deficiencies lower T cell numbers, whereas vitamin B_2 and B_1 deficiencies lower B cell activities. Vitamin C deficiencies have been related to increased or more severe bacterial infections in a number of studies. Zinc deficiency recently has been related to impairment of thymic development and thus T cell insufficiency.

Overnutrition also may be harmful. Many bacteria must scavenge iron from the body fluids in which they grow. When transferrin and lactoferrin, the body's natural iron transport compounds, are saturated by an excess of this metal, free iron is available for bacterial growth. When iron is in short supply, bacterial growth is restricted. Limited overnutrition may increase susceptibility to viral diseases. The logic used to explain this is that more virus is produced (and hence more disease) when a virus invades a healthy cell than when it infects a cell whose metabolic rate has been slowed by malnutrition.

Hormone-related resistance

Hormone imbalance (such as insulin diabetes) has a direct effect on susceptibility to a number of infectious diseases. Staphylococcal, streptococcal, and certain fungal diseases definitely occur more frequently in diabetics. The hormonal changes that occur in females at the time of puberty are responsible for a thickening of the vaginal epithelium and for the production of more intracellular glycogen and lactic acid in the adult vagina. Therefore the adult woman is more resistant than the young girl to local vaginal infections. Pregnancy is associated with marked hor-

monal alterations and an increase in urinary tract infections and poliomyelitis. The latter seems not to be related to any direct effect pregnancy might have on the female genitourinary system.

Miscellaneous

The age of an individual has a marked effect on innate immunity also. The very young and the very aged always have more infectious diseases than the middle-aged groups, possibly because of less phagocytic activity. Likewise, fatigue, climate, including simply climatic variation, and numerous other factors can significantly alter host resistance.

Mechanisms of natural resistance

The basis for natural resistance of a host to infectious or toxic agents is, like acquired immunity, based on the activities of specialized cells (cellular immunity) and the properties of certain molecules (humoral immunity). Cellular and humoral immunity do not always act independently; indeed, the attack of cells on foreign agents is often enhanced by prior molecular events, such as those involving the complement and blood clotting systems.

Natural cellular resistance

Cellular defense rests most obviously with the phagocytic cells of the mononuclear and granulocytic systems, but also with important contributions from LGL (NK) cells. In addition, the physical arrangement of cells into keratinized epithelial surfaces, or their physiologic cooperation, as in peristaltic motion of the bowel, should not be ignored as cellular events.

The marked eosinophilia associated with helminth infections prompted investigation of the contribution of eosinophils to parasite immunity. Granules within eosinophils contain a protein of 11,000 molecular weight, the major basic protein (MBP) that accounts for nearly 55% of the total granular protein. MBP released from eosinophils binds to and causes disruption of the outer membrane of *Schistosoma mansoni* schistosomules. *Trichinella spiralis* larvae become immobile when placed in a medium containing MBP. The blood stream form of *Trypanosoma cruzi* is killed by MBP. In addition to eosinophil derived MBP, a peroxidase of eosinophils kills *Staphylo-*

coccus aureus, Escherichia coli, and other bacteria, and aids killing of *Toxoplasma* and *Trypanosoma* in a cooperative event with macrophages. (Cationic proteins from macrophages are probably essential to their participation). These data reveal that eosinophils, though often ignored in cellular immunity, are important, especially in resistance against helminths.

The most significant phagocytic cell is the macrophage. The technique used by the macrophage for cell killing was described in detail in Chapter 5.

Another cell population that contributes to natural resistance is the LGL lymphocyte. Though non-phagocytic, these cells are able to secrete several cytotoxic proteins—perforins, lymphotoxins, cytolysins and others—possibly in combination with cytotoxic forms of oxygen. The LGL are noted for their attack on self cells bearing foreign (viral, tumor) antigens. These activities are described in Chapter 6.

External defense factors

The first barrier that most microbes encounter against their successful invasion (Fig 14-2) is the in-tact skin or mucous membranes. Intact skin represents a formidable mechanical barrier that can be penetrated by only a few organisms, such as the *Treponema* organisms of syphilis, *Francisella tularensis,* and certain fungi that enter at the hair roots. While being held outside the body, the microorganisms are exposed to drying, which alone may be enough to cause their death. In addition, lactic acid, caproic acid, and caprylic acid of the sebaceous glands have a proven antibacterial effect. Especially on the scalp and possibly other hairy parts of the human body, saturated C7, C9, and C11 fatty acids are present in the skin secretions. These are distinctly fungistatic and are important in the control of fungi that cause superficial skin and hair infections. Fungal infections more often begin on areas of the body devoid of sebaceous glands, for example, between the toes.

The upper respiratory tract may be considered as no more than a major invagination into the body and as such does not represent a truly internal environment. Although it is true that the very uppermost

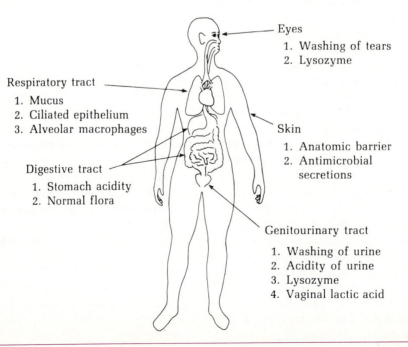

Eyes
1. Washing of tears
2. Lysozyme

Respiratory tract
1. Mucus
2. Ciliated epithelium
3. Alveolar macrophages

Skin
1. Anatomic barrier
2. Antimicrobial secretions

Digestive tract
1. Stomach acidity
2. Normal flora

Genitourinary tract
1. Washing of urine
2. Acidity of urine
3. Lysozyme
4. Vaginal lactic acid

FIG. 14-2

Natural resistance factors that function on external surfaces of the body.

portion of the respiratory tract is lined with visible hairs to exclude particles of great size, these will not remove particles with microbial dimensions. As a consequence, droplets in the range of 0.5 to 2 μm in diameter are inhaled somewhat more deeply than larger particles. Fortunately, the entire respiratory tract is bathed with a mucus secretion that acts as a glue on which these small particles impinge. This mucus is swept upward at a rate of 10 to 20 mm/minute by the action of the ciliated epithelial cells lining the respiratory tree and usually is swallowed. In a healthy person this mucous coat clears 90% of the deposited material every hour. Description of four patients who had abnormal cilia has emphasized the importance of these structures to normal health. All four patients suffered from recurrent episodes of bronchitis and sinusitis as well as frequent pneumonias and ear infections. No ciliary action could be noted in biopsy specimens, nor could mucociliary clearance of inhaled, aerosolized particles 6 μm in diameter be detected within a 2-hour test period. All evidence pointed toward a failure to form complete cilia, a fault that rendered the cilia immobile.

Unfortunately the mucous membranes do not trap all droplet nuclei; those less than 0.5 μm in diameter may be inhaled deeply into the pulmonary alveoli and there initiate an infection, provided that the pathogens can escape the alveolar macrophages. These macrophages roam over the respiratory mucosae and phagocytose inhaled particles. Alveolar macrophages of the rat can kill 99% of a dose of microorganisms that is reduced only 50% by blood phagocytes. These phagocytes killed 88% of pathogens such as *Streptococcus pneumoniae* within a 3-hour test period.

The microbes in the mucus that are swallowed or which enter the digestive system through food or water find very little in the upper alimentary canal that is detrimental to their growth. Lower in the digestive system the microorganisms encounter the tremendous acidity of the stomach, bordering on pH 1 because of the hydrochloric acid secreted from the parietal cells. Only markedly aciduric organisms or those embedded deeply in food particles can escape the protein-precipitating capacity of this acidity. As the microbes pass into the small intestine, an alteration in pH to the slightly alkaline side occurs because of the pH of the entering pancreatic and biliary fluids. In this section of the digestive system the microbial population is still rather low. A remarkable increase in this population takes place in the large intestine. The tremendous numbers of nonpathogens are undoubtedly of great importance in regulating the population of any pathogens or potential pathogens which have survived this far. When the normal flora is suppressed, as by broad-spectrum antibiotic therapy, intestinal yeast infections may ensue. This classic example of iatrogenic illness emphasizes the role of the natural flora in maintaining body health.

Little is known about any protective functions other than the slight acidity, lysozyme content, and flushing action of urine, all of which help cleanse the urinary system. Those urine samples most lethal to the gonococcus were also the most acidic. The exterior portions of the female reproductive system also are held at a low pH because of the lactic acid in the secretions.

The human eye is not protected by a third eyelid, or nictitating membrane, like that of certain lower animals. Crying has a simple mechanical benefit: it washes both small and large particles from the eye. A selective and very active antibacterial substance, lysozyme, found in tears is of much greater value. Lysozyme is a bactericidal enzyme first found in tears by Sir Alexander Fleming in 1922. Lysozyme has an isoelectric point at about pH 11. It has been suggested that it is this alkaline isoelectric point which permits its firm combination with bacteria, which have acid isoelectric points. After this combination, lysozyme begins a hydrolytic digestion of the bacterial cell wall. The cell walls of gram-positive and, to a lesser extent, gram-negative bacteria, are susceptible to this enzymatic erosion. In strict biochemical terms, lysozyme is a muramidase and cleaves the β-1,4-glycoside bond that unites *N*-acetylglucosamine and muramic acid, the backbone of the bacterial cell wall. Lipids in the cell walls of gram-negative bacteria tend to mask the substrate from lysozyme and protect these organisms.

Internal defense factors

Phagocytosis is a vital part of the internal defense system (Table 14-1). The major phagocytic cells are the neutrophils (Fig. 14-3) and the monocytes of blood and the monocytes and macrophages in tissues. The neutrophils also may enter tissues as part of the inflammatory response. These cells are drawn to areas of inflammation by various leukotactic substances and lymphokines. Opsonins such as C3b and immunoglobulin molecules augment phagocytosis. The behavior of the major phagocytic cells was described in Chapter 5.

Basic polyamines, polypeptides, and proteins display antibacterial activity. Histones, protamines, spermine, and spermidine are examples; these function by combining electrostatically with negatively charged bacterial cells and altering in some unknown way the vital cellular functions of the bacteria. Unsaturated lactoferrin in milk is one of its key protective agents. Several glycoproteins of serum, of which fetuin, transferrin, and α-1-glycoprotein are examples, inhibit attachment of viruses to susceptible cells and thus aid in termination of viral infections.

TABLE 14-1
Natural internal defense systems

Phagocytosis	Neurophils
	Monocytes
	Macrophages
Leukotaxis	C5a
	C(5,6,7)
Opsonins	C3b
	Miscellaneous proteins
Complement activation	Alternate pathway (polysaccharides)
Macromolecules	Glycoproteins
	Transferrin
	Lysozyme
	Various polyamines

ACQUIRED IMMUNITY

Acquired immunity refers to that immunity which a person develops during a lifetime. It is antigen (pathogen) specific and may be based on antibodies (humoral immunity) or may be cellular in origin and more closely associated with the activities of macrophages and T lymphocytes.

Humoral immunity

Immunity based on antibodies is probably the single most formidable type of immunity. This form of immunity is conveniently subdivided into that which is actively acquired and that which is passively acquired.

Acquired immunity
A. Actively acquired
   1. Natural
   2. Artificial
B. Passively acquired
   1. Natural
   2. Artificial

In active immunity the individual synthesizes his or her own antibodies, whereas in passive immunity the individual receives these antibodies from some other individual, either a human or a lower animal. Both active and passive immunity are subdivisible into two categories, depending on whether the immunity is acquired by natural or artificial means. Naturally acquired immunity should not be confused with natural immunity.

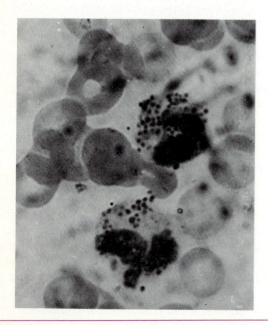

FIG. 14-3
The two phagocytic cells have engulfed numerous *Staphylococcus aureus* cells.

Actively acquired immunity

A degree of naturally acquired active immunity results from any infection from which a person recovers, whether the illness is serious or subclinical. During the illness the individual receives an antigenic stimulus which initiates antibody production against that specific pathogen. On a subsequent visitation by this same or an antigenically related pathogen, these antibodies will assist in the body's defenses. Because many microbes produce diseases with a high mortality, this is not a very satisfactory way of developing immunity.

A major goal of immunologists interested in preventing infectious diseases has been the development of vaccines or toxoids that can be used in immunization. The immunity resulting from the injection of these immunogens is said to be of the artificially acquired type, since it is a man-made procedure. Killed and attenuated strains of bacteria and viruses now are used widely for immunization against many diseases; for example, tuberculosis, mumps, poliomyelitis, yellow fever, and measles. Attenuated vaccines contain viable but weakened organisms and will produce a mild infection of little danger to the host. It has the advantage, however, of producing a much more permanent form of immunity than killed vaccines. Toxoids, that is, the detoxified but still antigenically active poisons excreted by certain bacteria, are also excellent antigens. Antibodies against toxoids are fully reactive with the native toxin and provide an excellent immunity against diseases caused by toxigenic bacteria (tetanus and diphtheria).

Passively acquired immunity

Passive immunity also may be acquired by natural means or by artificial means. Naturally acquired passive immunity, usually refers to the transplacental passage of antibodies from the mother to her unborn child during the latter part of pregnancy. This is caused almost entirely by IgG, since other immunoglobulin isotypes do not pass the placental barrier. Colostrum contains secretory IgA and secretory IgM but very little IgG. Since the digestive system of the newborn infant is poorly developed, breast-fed babies can absorb these immunoglobulins directly from the gastrointestinal system. Even if not absorbed, these antibodies may passively coat the infant's digestive tract and ward off intestinal infections. Naturally this system cannot operate in bottle-fed babies.

Artificial passive immunity refers to the original production of antibodies in some other individual (either human or lower mammal) and the acquisition of these antibodies through a needle and syringe. Injections of hyperimmune serum pooled γ globulin, or serum represent this type of immunization. Several pharmaceutical companies are involved in the production of antibodies in horses and cows by active immunization so that these antibodies may be used later to modify or prevent human diseases by passive immunization. A more limited program of hyperimmunization of humans is used for this same purpose.

A special form of antibody-related passive immunity is exemplified by adoptive immunity with B lymphocytes. If such cells or (more commonly) bone marrow is successfully grafted into a B cell–deficient person, the recipient will form antibodies that he or she previously could not. (See Chapters 16 and 20.) This usually is not done in human medicine, since the simpler injections of pooled human γ-globulin serve the same purpose.

Another form of passive immunity involves the use of monokines and lymphokines. Particularly in persons who have a T cell immunodeficiency, treatment with IL-1, IL-2, supernatant fluids from Concanavalin A treated T cell cultures, γ-IFN, and TF has been implemented with the goal of restoring T cell function. At the present time, these efforts can be considered potentially successful, but no dramatic, long-term cures have as yet been observed.

Comparison of active and passive immunity

Active and passive immunity must be compared on a broader basis than whether a person makes his or her own antibodies. There are other important and sometimes subtle differences between the two, most of which are summarized in Table 14-2.

The comparative effectiveness of active and passive immunity is heavily weighted in favor of the former. This is related to several factors, one of which is the duration of the immunity. Active immunity is known to persist for relatively long periods,

TABLE 14-2

Comparison of active and passive antibody-mediated immunity

	Active immunity	Passive immunity
Source	Self	Some other human or lower animal
Effectiveness	High	Moderate to low

Method	1. Disease itself, clinical or subclinical
	2. Immunization
	  a. Vaccines: killed or attenuated
	  b. Toxoids
		Administration of antibody by
		1. Maternal transplacental transfer
		2. Injection

Time to develop	5 to 14 days	Immediate on injection
Duration	Relatively long, perhaps years	Relatively short, a few days to several weeks
Ease of reactivation	Easy (by booster)	Dangerous, possible anaphylaxis
Use	Prophylactic	Prophylactic and therapeutic

usually years, without reactivation through booster immunization. This is true because, once the plasma cells of the animal are activated to produce antibodies, they, or their memory cell progeny, continue to do so for the lifetime of the cell. In passive immunization this does not happen. The injected antibodies are removed from the circulation without internal replacement, and the immunity then can be directly correlated with the amount of antibodies injected and their half-life. The half-life of human IgG in a human is about 25 days, but the half-life of equine or bovine antibodies in a human is nearer 7 days. It must be remembered that foreign serum proteins, including γ-globulins, are antigenic to the human being. Consequently the human recipient will make antibodies against the administered foreign antibodies, which results in their speedy elimination.

Passive immunity can be quickly restored or maintained by repeated injections of the antiserum. This is satisfactory when a human antiserum is employed but not when an antiserum from a foreign species is used. In this instance the possibility of anaphylaxis or serum sickness is great, anaphylaxis itself being a life-threatening proposition. (See Chapters 17 and 18.) On the other hand, the reactivation of active immunity by booster injections of the vaccine or toxoid is a comparatively risk-free method and one that is commonly used.

It must be pointed out that active immunity of

high efficiency requires 5 to 14 days to develop after the primary immunization. This is the time it takes for protective quantities of antibodies to appear in the serum. After booster injections of antigen only 1 to 3 days are required. On passive immunization, protection is provided immediately on completion of the injection.

Active immunization usually is restricted to prophylactic (preventive) applications, by which the person receives the immunization in advance of the exposure to the infectious agent. Under special conditions (rabies or smallpox), when the incubation time of the disease is longer than the time required for antibody formation, it is possible for the individual to be immunized after exposure. Passive immunization also can be used prophylactically, that is, prior to or immediately after exposure, in individuals who have not been actively immunized. Passive immunization (but not active immunization) also can be used therapeutically. Unfortunately this is a relatively inefficient process because the organisms or their toxins may have created considerable undetected cell damage prior to the administration of the antiserum. None of this damage is repairable by antiserum alone.

Cell-mediated immunity (CMI)

The classic example of CMI as a mechanism of acquired immunity is the Koch phenomenon. Koch observed that the responses of normal guinea pigs and tuberculous guinea pigs to an injection of tubercle bacilli were grossly different. In the former there is a gradual swelling of the lymph nodes near the site of a subcutaneous injection. These nodes may become caseous within about 2 weeks, and the animal usually will die after 6 to 8 weeks. If during the course of this infection a second injection of tubercle bacilli is given, the injection site will appear red and indurated within a few days. This area will necrose, and the dead tissue and injected bacilli will be sloughed. The elimination of the bacilli is clear evidence of a developing resistance. This acquired resistance is not caused by circulating antibodies and cannot be transferred to other animals with immune serum. It can be transferred by T lymphocytes, and the term cell-mediated immunity refers to T cell dependent immunity. Since animals with an immunity based on T cells will usually display a delayed type hypersensitivity (see Chapter 18), this type of hypersensitivity reaction is considered an index of cell-mediated immunity. Cell-mediated hypersensitivity and cell-mediated immunity are not identical. The cellular hypersensitivity seen in the Koch phenomenon is highly specific and relatable only to tubercle bacilli. The sensitized guinea pigs have a delayed skin reaction only to tuberculin and not to the products of antigenically unrelated bacteria. The T_{DTH} cells that are responsible for expressing this hypersensitivity excrete macrophage chemotactic factor and migration inhibition factor. Macrophage neighbors to the T_{DTH} cell are thus activated and able to remove other, even antigenically unrelated bacteria. Thus, the afferent phase of cell-mediated hypersensitivity, the T_{DTH} phase, is antigen specific but the efferent, macrophage phase is not.

It is always difficult to entirely separate the protective role of antibodies and cellular immunity under natural circumstances. The acid test for identifying antibodies as the cause of an immune condition is to prove that antiserum can transfer the immunity to a normal recipient. This requires that the passively immunized animal be challenged to see if it is immune. To prove that the immunity is T cell dependent, these cells must be demonstrated to transfer immunity from the resistant to the normal animal. However, the recipient animal may reject the donor's T cells through graft rejection events. Consequently, T cell transfer experiments must be conducted with this possibility in mind.

IMMUNITY TO INFECTIOUS DISEASES
New approaches to vaccine development

The application of genetic, biochemical, and immunological principles to the construction of new vaccines offers a promise for successful immunization against several diseases that have heretofore escaped conquest (Table 14-3). The methods now under investigation are the use of recombinant DNA technology, the chemical synthesis of vaccines, and the use of anti-idiotype sera. These procedures have already proven successful on an experimental basis in the development of immunity against malaria, trypanosomiasis, and hepatitis B.

Anti-idiotype vaccines

As described in an earlier chapter, an idiotypic determinant of an immunoglobulin is that portion of the variable region that contains the antigen binding site. Each idiotope, which we can call this region, corresponds with a unique epitope of the antigen. The idiotope itself is recognizable as a unique antigenic portion of the immunoglobulin, and serves as the stimulus for the formation of the anti-idiotypic antibodies in the Jerne network control system of immune regulation. Thus, an epitope is reflected by the idiotope, which is in turn reflected by another idiotope in the anti-idiotype. In this way, the anti-idiotype and epitope can be considered as mirror images of the idiotype and thus similar to each other. Does this mean that an anti-idiotype globulin can substitute for an epitope in the sense of a vaccine?

In some instances the answer is "yes"; an anti-idiotype can replace the original antigenic epitope. Anti-idiotypic antibodies used as vaccines for the surface glycoprotein antigen of the sleeping sickness trypanosome, *Trypanosoma rhodesiense,* protected mice against challenge with the parasite (the original epitope). In a separate study, mice responded to antibodies that reacted with the important *a* antigen of hepatitis B virus after receiving anti-idiotype sera. Pretreatment of animals with the anti-idiotypic serum enhanced their response to the standard hepatitis B vaccine or the peptide vaccine derived from it. In

TABLE 14-3

New vaccines under development

Disease	Pathogen	Potential vaccine
Whooping cough	*Bordetella pertussis*	Toxin free
Pneumonia	*Streptococcus pneumoniae*	Additional capsular types
Meningitis	*Hemophilus influenzae*	Type b polysaccharide
Hepatitis	1. Hepatitis B	DNA recombinant or synthetic peptides
	2. Hepatitis A	DNA recombinant or synthetic peptides
Chickenpox	Herpes virus	Attenuated virus
Influenza	Influenza viruses	DNA recombinant or synthetic peptides
Diarrhea	Rotavirus	Attenuated virus
Malaria	*Plasmodium* species	Synthetic peptides or DNA recombinant
AIDS	HIV	???

this example, the virus itself served as the booster antigen for the anti-idiotype vaccine.

Anti-idiotypic vaccines should prove most useful when the original antigen is difficult to prepare, contains some toxic component, or reverts from an attenuated state to one of full virulence. One current disadvantage is that anti-idiotypic sera of human origin have not been generally available or widely tested. Anti-idiotypic sera of lower animal species have a half-life of only one or two weeks in man, thus diminishing their effectiveness. The risk of provoking serum sickness to lower animal sera used in human treatments is real (Chapter 18). Both these handicaps would be relieved by human anti-idiotypic globulins prepared either from human sera or human hybridomas.

Synthetic vaccines

A second approach to the construction of new vaccines is based on peptide synthesis. From sequence analyses of DNA or messenger RNA for a protein, or by sequencing the protein itself, the complete structure of antigens can be determined. This is not always necessary, since the important epitopes in antigens can be determined by their techniques, but once these epitopes have been identified, peptide

synthesis is useful in providing a supply of these antigenic determinants.

Human patients recovering from hepatitis B virus infections have a good antibody response to the *a* determinant. This is also true of persons receiving the standard or anti-idiotypic hepatitis B vaccine mentioned above. Since the hepatitis B vaccine is expensive and difficult to prepare (it is comoposed of viral particles harvested from the blood of carriers) hepatitis B has been the target of several investigations with the construction of a synthetic vaccine as the goal. Chemical modification of lysines in the *a* determinant, a protein containing 226 amino acid residues, renders it inactive as an antigen. All the lysines in the *a* determinant are between residues 121 and 160. An examination of the immunogenicity of synthetic peptides in this region revealed that the sequence 139 to 147 represented all or the essential part of the determinant. This decapeptide contains only one lysine and has the sequence Cys Thr Lys Pro Thr Asp Gly Asn Cys Thr. Specificity for the *dy* variant of determinant *a* encompasses residues 110 to 137. Passive immunization with experimentally produced antisera specific for synthetic peptides containing these determinants afford partial protection of chimpanzees to viral challenge.

The diphtheria toxin (molecular weight 62,000) is another antigen that has been studied from the viewpoint of a synthetic vaccine. The complete amino acid sequence of the toxin is known and is determined to have two Cys-Cys loops. One of these loops bridges residues 188 to 201. A hexadecapeptide of amino acids 186 to 201 has been linked to a protein carrier and used to immunize guinea pigs. Antibodies in the resulting antiserum bind to the complete toxin and neutralize its dermonecrotic and lethal activity for guinea pigs. Protection of this quality is firm evidence of the vaccine's potency.

The circumsporozoite (CS) proteins of the malarial parasites are a prime example of how successful a synthetic vaccine can be. The CS proteins are present on the outer surface of the sporozoite stage, the infecting stage that man receives when the mosquito feeds. *Plasmodium vivax, Plasmodium falciparum, Plasmodium knowlesi* and probably other plasmodial species have closely related, if not identical, CS proteins. Antisera with the capability of neutralizing sporozoite infectivity cause the release of the CS protein from the parasite surface, a factor that suggests a critical role of CS proteins in immunity. Monoclonal antibodies specific for the CS from *P. knowlesi* have identified that this large protein (42,000 molecular weight) contains but a single epitope that is repeated several times. This determinant has been sequenced, and consists of the dodecapeptide—Gln, Ala, Gln, Gly, Asp, Gly, Ala, Aspn, Ala, Gly, Gln, Pro. A dimeric form of this sequence has been linked to bovine γ globulin and keyhole limpet hemocyanin as complete antigen carriers, and is used to immunize rabbits. A mixture of the anti-dimer serum with sporozoites prevented their infectivity for monkeys.

One minor disadvantage of synthetic peptic vaccines is that they often represent only a single epitope, and are thus haptenic. This requires that neoantigens be constructed, and some care is essential in selecting the carrier molecule to prevent the appearance of undesired antibodies in the vaccine recipient.

Recombinant vaccines

Undoubtedly, the most dramatic approaches to the development of new vaccines reside in the field of recombinant DNA technology. The basis for the method is that genomic DNA containing the structural gene for important antigens from virtually any source can be transferred into plasmid or viral vectors. Infection of bacteria, yeasts, or mammalian cells with the appropriate vector is followed by expression of the DNA in the form of its gene product (antigen). In this way, easily cultivated cells excrete large quantities of important antigens.

The vaccinia virus is a useful carrier for exogenous DNA because it has a large DNA genome; its naked DNA is not infectious, and can be manipulated safely in the laboratory; it has transcriptional ability built into its own genome; and it replicates in the cytoplasm of cells rather than in the nucleus, where it might more easily alter the host cell. The use of vaccinia virus for nearly 200 years to prevent smallpox caused it to gain wide public acceptance as an immunizing agent.

The order of manipulations may be varied from one investigator to another, or from one vector to another in the preparation of a recombinant DNA vaccine. Usually, one of the first steps is to purify vaccinia virus DNA and cleave it with an endonuclease. Hepatitis B DNA containing the genome for the surface antigen (HBsAg) previously cleaved with the same endonuclease is ligated to the vaccinia DNA. This is done so that each end of the HBsAg sequence has vaccinia virus DNA attached to it. This segment of vaccina-HBsAg-vaccinia DNA is then inserted into a plasmid vector by endonuclease cleavage and religation (Fig. 14-4). This construct is used to transfect a cell line that is simultaneously infected with vaccinia virus. When recombination occurs as a result of crossing over, the HBsAg sequence is implanted into the vaccinia virus. The recombinants can be selected on the basis of HBsAg secretion from a second cell culture infected by virus harvested from the primary culture. When this was done, small particles 22 nm in diameter, identical to the hepatitis B surface antigen in the blood of hepatitis carriers, were observed. Rabbits immunized with the derived vaccinia virus produced antibody levels 10 or more times the level considered protective in man. This indicates that the recombinant vaccinia virus synthesized and secreted HBsAg during

Vaccinia virus

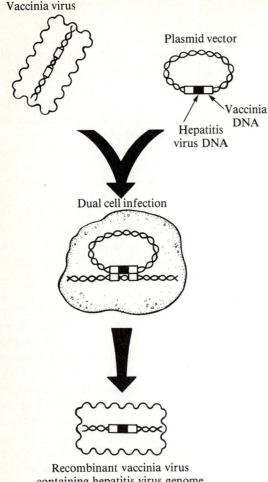

FIG. 14-4

Vaccina virus at the upper left and a vector (upper right) containing vaccinia DNA (open rectangle) on each side of hepatitis B DNA (solid rectangle) are used to infect a cell. Within the cell, the complementary vaccinia DNA sequences of the virus particle and the vector align themselves. By cross over recombination a vaccinia virus containing hepatitis B sequences is produced. This agent can then be used to immunize against hepatitis B.

what was predominantly a vaccinia virus infection.

This procedure has also been applied to herpes simplex virus (HSV) glycoprotein D. Mice immunized with the vaccinia-based vaccine were resistant to challenge with HSV. Influenza vaccines have also been prepared in this manner. Because there is space

within the vaccinia virus for 25,000 additional base pairs (bp) of DNA, and since the sequences for antigens are often less than 2,000 bp, vaccinia virus may be used as a polyvalent vaccine bearing antigens from many different pathogens.

Viral diseases

Before considering specific instances of viral disease and their immunologic prevention, a number of special features of viral disease first should be considered. The mechanism of virus infection is an important factor to be considered. Many viruses produce only local infections that tend to shield them from the full play of the host's defense system. Many of the respiratory viruses are of this type, causing infection only of the superficial tissues of the lung. Reinfection with identical virus serotypes indicates that the earlier infections promoted only a very shallow antigenic stimulus.

A second type of evasion by viruses is by their intracellular latency. Herpes simplex virus (cold sores, fever blisters) invades host cells and remains dormant and protected there from host immunity. High levels of circulating antibody may be present, but these antibodies cannot enter the virus-containing cells. Many virus particles may be neutralized by these antibodies when the virus erupts and spreads to new cells, but every person with recurrent herpes is witness to the success of intracellular hibernation by the virus.

Another distinction that must be made concerning viral diseases is the difference between producing active immunity to a specific virus and producing immunity to a type of viral disease. In general, there are few novel problems encountered in making effective vaccines against a specific virus; most of the problems have been encountered before, although not always solved to perfection. The problems of virus production, purification, preservation, and attenuation, theoretically at least, can be solved for any virus. These procedures are of no avail in disease prevention when the disease is produced by a multiplicity of distantly related viruses and are often unsuitable even when antigenically related viruses are involved. More than 100 serotypes of rhinovirus and an uncertain number of coronaviruses are involved in the common cold, and numerous strains of Coxsackie

TABLE 14-4

Immunity to various pathogens provided by B and T lymphocytes

Source of infection	B lymphocytes	T lymphocyte
Bacterial	Streptococcal, staphylococcal, neisserial, hemophilus infections	Tuberculosis, leprosy, treponematosis
Viral	Enteroviruses, poliomyelitis	Herpes viruses, measles, vaccinia, cytomegalovirus
Fungal	Few, if any	Candidiasis, cryptococcosis, histoplasmosis, etc.
Parasitic	Trypanosomiasis, malaria(?)	Leishmaniasis, pneumocystic disease, Chagas' disease

viruses cause pharyngitis in children and young adults. To halt the common cold by immunoprophylaxis would require a polyvalent vaccine containing well over 100 different viruses, a problem of considerable magnitude.

Immunity to reinfection after a viral disease or successful immunization often can be correlated with the development of specific circulating immunoglobulins. The protection afforded by these antibodies against viruses that must pass through the blood to their target tissue is the whole key to immunity. On the other hand, there are many illustrations that circulating antibodies are only indirectly related to viral immunity and simply arise as one index of an immune response to the virus. In herpes simplex and herpes zoster recurrent disease takes place in the presence of high levels of neutralizing antibody. CMI may be more critical to the resistant state than antibodies of the blood (Table 14-4). Agammaglobulinemic children develop and recover from most childhood viral diseases with the same sequence of events depicted by normal children. These two illustrations support the contention that CMI is extremely important to virus immunity.

Smallpox

Jenner's historic experiment revealed that smallpox virus was closely related to cowpox or vaccinia virus and that immunity to one was cross protective against the other. After Jenner's time person-to-person transmission of infectious vaccinia virus was the method for preventing smallpox for nearly a century. By that time the possibility of transferring syphilis, leprosy, malaria, or other diseases was sufficiently recognized, so that domestic animals were selected as the source of the virus. The method of preparing smallpox vaccine has not changed appreciably in the past 75 years. Healthy calves are vaccinated several times over a large area of freshly shaved, scrubbed flank. After 4 to 6 days the area is washed, and the animal is sacrificed. The infectious lymph is scraped from the skin and usually treated with a disinfectant. In most modern production schemes the virus is partially purified and preserved by the addition of glycerol. Such preparations must be stored in the cold, so for tropical use lyophilized virus vaccines are prepared. The vaccine is administered by multiple skin punctures; the virus grows locally and develops a systemic immunity.

Due to the heroic effort of many physicians and scientists, coordinated through the efforts of the World Health Organization (WHO), the world has been declared free of smallpox since 1979. The success of this program inaugurated in 1967 was based on several important principles, among the most important being (1) that smallpox is a natural disease only of humans, and animal reservoirs are non-existent, and (2) the remarkable history of Jennerian vaccination. The initial WHO program of mass vaccination was later replaced by a containment immunization program. The latter was chosen because smallpox spreads slowly from the initial case and vaccination is successful even after exposure. Immunization of contacts and others within a defined geographic area of the initial patient contained the infection within an immune perimetry, thus eliminating the case as a source of further disease. The last case of naturally transmitted smallpox was diagnosed in Somalia in 1977, although laboratory incidents causing transmission have occurred since that time, some with fatal results.

Rubella

The rubella virus causes a mild infection in children and adolescents known as the German measles. The agent is not as transmissible as regular (hard) measles virus; this results in a large population who escape the disease as children and remain susceptible as adults. Immunization against this seemingly benign disease assumed importance when it was recognized that rubella infections of women in the first trimester of pregnancy produced congenital defects in approximately 16% of all fetuses. The fetus of a nonimmune mother is highly susceptible to the virus, and any and all tissues may be infected. Infants who acquire the virus in utero are totally lacking in any defensive system to eliminate it. The virus continues to reproduce and invade new tissues. If the infant is not stillborn, one or more of the following conditions may be noted: cataract, deafness, heart abnormalities, microcephaly, hepatomegaly, splenomegaly, and anemia, caused by virus alteration of tissue during development. These children excrete rubella virus at birth and may continue to shed viruses for as long as 2 years.

Since between 15% and 35% of pregnant women are not immune to rubella, considerable need exists for vaccination. After it was recognized that serious fetal deformities arose from rubella and before a vaccine became available, rubella parties were held for young girls prior to puberty. It was hoped that close contact of the girls with the person who had rubella would overcome the low infectivity of the virus and cause the disease necessary to protect them and their future children.

An attenuated rubella virus vaccine was marketed in 1969 in the United States, at a time when there were nearly 28 cases per 100,000 population. Within 10 years, the incidence was reduced by 80%. The vaccine is recommended for all pre-pubertal females.

Unexpected immunization of pregnant women with the attenuated virus vaccine has not yet been proven to cause congenital abnormalities.

Influenza

Viral influenza continues to be a serious health threat and substantial epidemics appear nearly every winter. Immunity following influenza or immunization is relatively short lived and reimmunization each year, even with a vaccine of the same composition as the previous year, is recommended for persons at high risk.

The virus strains most commonly causing disease in man are type A or type B, which are distinguished serologically. Within these antigenic types, subtypes exist based on differences in the hemagglutinin (H1, H2 or H3) and neuraminidase (N1 or N2). The characteristic known as antigenic drift—a subtle, slight alteration in antigenic composition—can result in the appearance of a subtype variant for which little or no immunity exists. Antigenic drift or antigenic shift—a major alteration in antigenic composition—are responsible for epidemics and pandemics that may involve, as did the U.S. pandemic of 1968, one quarter or more of the population.

Because of epidemiologic monitoring of influenza outbreaks on a world-wide basis, new antigenic forms of the influenza virus are quickly identified. Then, the appropriate vaccine can be prepared in the succeeding weeks to protect the susceptible population. As in the case with other infectious diseases, young children, the aged, and the chronically ill are at the highest risk. Although the antigenic composition of the vaccine will differ from year to year, 1 or 2 intramuscular injections of "split" virus vaccine, depending upon the age of the recipient, is advised. The vaccine contains viral particles of both A and B type that have been disrupted.

Poliomyelitis

Successful active immunization against poliomyelitis was based first on formaldehyde-inactivated virus developed by Salk. A polyvalent vaccine containing a representative from each of the three antigenic types was administered in three intramuscular injections over a 3-month period to develop high levels of humoral antibody. Now a fourth booster dose is scheduled 6 to 12 months after the third injection. These antibodies afford complete protection against paralytic or systemic poliomyelitis, but protection against polio virus infection is not achieved by this vaccination scheme. The polio virus is basically an enteric virus; it gains entrance to the body by the oral route and infects and multiplies in the mucosa of the intestinal tract. From its intestinal phase it enters into the viremic or blood phase, from which it progresses to the central nervous system. By developing high levels of neutralizing antibody in the bloodstream the vaccine halts the virus at the blood level, which ably prevents the dreadful paralytic threat of poliomyelitis.

Immunization with active attenuated polio vaccine by the oral route (three doses over a 3-month period) is presumed to provide better protection, since both an intestinal and humoral immunity are developed. The intestinal immunity may serve very little additional benefit to the immunized person compared with the Salk vaccine, but this immunity probably removes that person as a potential carrier of virulent virus. Dissemination of the attenuated virus from the immunized person to close associates, with subsequent development of their immunity is a benefit of live virus immunization. Since continued transfer of the virus provides a better opportunity for reversion to virulence, this is also a hazard of active virus immunization. This has been observed at a rate of about 4 cases of vaccine-associated paralytic disease per year in the United States.

Statistics reveal the success of both the Salk and Sabin live vaccines. In 1955, the first year of inactive virus vaccination, 28,985 cases of polio were reported in the United States. In 1961 live virus vaccination was approved, and in 1964 there were only 121 cases of polio reported. Since polio is exclusively a human ailment, it is theoretically susceptible to total eradication; however, public apathy and failure to be immunized prevent the realization of this goal.

Hepatitis B

A hepatitis B virus vaccine was approved in the United States in 1981. This virus, described as the Australia antigen in 1965, when it was found to be common in the blood of Australian aborigines, causes a long-term carrier state in about 10% of the infected persons. In Africa, Asia, and certain populations in Australia the endemicity of the disease can reach 60% to 80% of the population. Chronic hepatitis B infections are known to increase susceptibility to hepatocellular carcinoma.

The major hurdle to vaccine production was the inability to perpetuate hepatitis B virus in tissue culture. Several forms of the virus are present in the blood of its victims, and these were separated, purified, treated with formaldehyde, and tested for efficacy. The hepatitis virus B surface antigen, HBsAg, which consists of spherical and tubular structures only 20 nm in diameter, will convert virtually 100% of all vaccinates given three doses of the vaccine with adjuvant. HBsAg from human donors is safe—it has not been proven as a source of acquired immune deficiency disease (AIDS) or other diseases. A recombinant vaccine may eventually replace the current human-source vaccine.

Rabies

All rabies viruses are of a single antigenic type, which was very critical to the success of Pasteur's experiments in 1885 and always simplifies the production of vaccines. This antigenic constancy of rabies virus is clouded by the terms *street virus* and *fixed virus,* which refer not to changes in antigenicity but to changes in infectivity. Street virus is rabies virus freshly isolated from natural infections. When first transferred to laboratory animals, street virus will have a long incubation time, will be more apt to produce furious rabies infections, and will produce numerous Negri inclusion bodies. As it is transferred, its incubation time shortens to a fixed period (hence the name fixed virus). Negri bodies are less often produced, and infectivity by the subcutaneous route is diminished.

Pasteur's vaccine was from spinal cords of rabbits infected with fixed rabies virus, considered as a live or active attenuated strain. Cords dried for 1 week are normally noninfective and presumably contain no active virus. Infected cords dried for shorter periods contain active virus, the quantity being inversely proportional to the length of the drying period. The early Pasteur immunization schedules required 11 subcutaneous injections of vaccine, one injection daily, beginning with vaccine dried for 2 weeks. The drying period was gradually shortened until the last injection was of infected cord dried for only 1 day. This method was obviously inexact, since there was no standardization of virus potency, but it was effective, if not without hazard.

The primary hazard of the Pasteur vaccine is the production of postvaccinal encephalitis. This is an allergic reaction, of the cell-mediated type, to the rabbit neural tissue of the vaccine. The lengthy immunization schedule and the high content of rabbit spinal cord antigens in the vaccine induce an allergic encephalitis that is easily reproduced experimentally. The incidence may be as low as 1 in 8,500 uses of vaccine. Unfortunately the Semple vaccine, which followed the Pasteur vaccine, did not eliminate the possibility of neural complications following immunization. Rabies virus vaccines prepared from chicken or duck eggs were less involved but did not totally eliminate neurologic symptoms. Now a vaccine from virus grown in nerve tissue–free human diploid fibroblast cell culture is the preferred vaccine.

Immunity to rabies is based on a high content of humoral antibody. The pathogenesis of rabies virus is based on its entrance and spread through neural tissue until involvement of the central nervous system occurs. After rabies virus enters the spinal cord, it is protected from antibody, but if high levels of antibody are present before this stage of disease, immunity is the result. On this basis prophylactic immunization for veterinarians, kennel employees, and others at high risk is recommended. Rabies immunization after exposure is practiced successfully, apparently because the long incubation time of street virus allows time for immunoglobulin synthesis before virus invasion of the central nervous system occurs. IFN induction by vaccine also may contribute to this protection, but this has not yet been proved.

Measles

The paramyxovirus that causes ordinary measles (rubeola) is one of the most infectious and easily transmitted pathogens known. Natural measles is often a mild disease, but the risk for death is 1 in 3,000 cases. The risk for permanent brain damage and mental retardation is 1 in 2,000 cases. A progressive chronic form of measles—subacute sclerosing panencephalitis or SSPE—may develop in persons who are unable to rid themselves of the virus acquired in early childhood or in utero when their immune system is poorly developed. SSPE is a serious disease with progressive mental and neurologic deterioration.

Attenuated strains of active measles virus protect approximately 95% of all 1-year-old children receiving the vaccine. The original attenuated Edmonston B strain of measles virus has been further reduced in virulence to eliminate the incidence and degree of febrile episodes that follow vaccination. All human measles virus isolates are of one antigenic type.

The use of the live attenuated vaccine, first licensed in 1963, reduced the incidence of measles from about 500,000 to 3,000 cases per year by 1981. A requirement for all states to mandate measles vaccination of children prior to their entry into school was designed to eliminate measles in the U.S., but this goal has not yet been achieved. Children should be given a single dose of the vaccine at about 15 months of age. Vaccination earlier than 3 months of age is not recommended due to a detrimental effect of passively acquired maternal antibodies on the success of the immunization. Protection may persist for 16 years. It is possible to vaccinate successfully within 72 hours of natural exposure, or to passively protect against natural measles with 0.25 ml/kg immune globulin if the exposed person cannot receive the vaccine due to concurrent febrile illness, allergy to egg proteins, etc. Immune globulin need not be administered with the new attenuated virus preparation.

Mumps

The mumps virus is also a paramyxovirus and exists as a single antigenic type. Mumps is not as contagious as other paramyxo- or myxoviruses. Nevertheless, mumps is an important disease since orchitis develops in 20% of postpubertal males, and benign, temporary meningitis develops in 15% of all persons contracting mumps.

An attenuated live mumps virus vaccine was licensed in the United States in December of 1967, a year when 185,691 cases were reported. By 1982, the number of cases was reduced to 5,270, and it was estimated that more than 59 million doses of vaccine had been administered. The mumps vaccine can be given at any age after 12 months. A single dose of vaccine will confer protection on 95% of all recipients.

Hazards

Immunologists and virologists are often prone to hail the advantages of immunization without citing the hazards, which *do* exist and include the reversion of active attenuated viruses to virulent forms, the spread of attenuated viruses to undesired parts of the body, immunization of immunodeficient individuals, and allergic reactions to contaminating antigens in the vaccine. An additional illustration is provided by mice infected as adults with lymphocytic choriomeningitis (LCM) virus. This infection usually is acquired by newborn mice from their mothers or other adult carriers, and the disease in this instance is mild. The mice survive the infection, which passes quickly, but they become chronic carriers of the virus. LCM virus can be isolated from any tissue of the mouse. The mice are devoid of humoral antibodies and cannot be induced to make antibodies against the virus; they are in a state of complete tolerance to the virus.

Healthy adult mice, who never have been exposed to LCM virus, develop a serious disease if virus is administered intracerebrally or intraperitoneally. Central nervous system disorder, pleural effusions that are predominantly lymphocytic in nature, and dense viral burdens in the associated tissues are typical, with death ensuing in about a week. This all can be prevented if the mice are treated with immunosuppressive drugs. The virus is present and continues to reproduce, and the animals develop into chronic carriers like infant mice, but the drug totally prevents any outward signs of the disease, and the mice survive the infection. Immunosuppression ap-

parently has halted an immune (allergic) response necessary for manifestation of the disease. This is truly a startling example of how the immune response can serve as a detriment rather than a benefit to health.

Bacterial diseases

Immunity to bacterial diseases is based on circulating antibodies to bacterial toxins or specific cellular antigens, and except for mycobacterial diseases and a few others the contribution of CMI has been debatable (Table 14-4).

Tetanus and diphtheria

Tetanus and diphtheria are two bacterial diseases clearly caused by potent exotoxins that the bacteria excrete. Tetanospasmin, the exotoxin of *Clostridium tetani* that is responsible for muscular contraction, is a neurotoxic protein with a molecular weight of 55,000. The exotoxin of *Corynebacterium diphtheriae* has a similar molecular weight, 62,000, but its action is on the protein-synthesizing machinery of host cells. Behring and Erhlich received Nobel prizes in part for their study of these toxins and their protective antitoxins. Although it was learned about this same time that formaldehyde treatment of toxins would destroy their toxicity while preserving their antigenicity, it was not until 1923 that toxoids produced in this fashion were used in human immunization. In the first World War the United States' rate of tetanus was 16 in 100,000 wounds. In World War II it was 0.44 in 100,000, or 12 cases in 2.5 million injuries. Of these 12, eight has not been properly immunized.

Currently in the United States a combined diphtheria and tetanus toxoid preparation absorbed to an adjuvant is used for routine immunization against these two diseases. The usual adjuvant is an aluminum hydroxide or aluminum phosphate gel; such preparations are unequivocally superior to fluid preparations. An alternative preparation contains the two toxoids and killed *Bordetella pertussis* cells in what is known as the DPT vaccine, the P standing for pertussis.

Normal human skin reacts slowly to injections of

diphtheria toxin with the development of a tender erythematous area, the positive Schick test. If a person has a sufficient level of antitoxin (more than 0.03 unit of antitoxin per milliliter of serum), the test is negative. The Schick test is exceptionally valuable in assaying the efficacy of immunization and in screening large populations for those who are susceptible to diphtheria. Interpretation of the test can be hindered in those persons who have developed a cell-mediated hypersensitivity to the toxin, since the delayed hypersensitive skin reaction and the positive Schick test closely mimic one another in appearance. Persons who are allergic to the toxin can be detected by the injection of toxoid, which is innocuous to normal skin (the Moloney test).

Pertussis

The vaccine against whooping cough (pertussis) contains killed phase I *Bordetella pertussis* cells. This vaccine is routinely administered as a component of the DPT vaccine to provide protection against diphtheria, pertussis and tetanus. Infants are often protected against whooping cough because of their transplacentally derived maternal antibody. When the titer of this antibody has waned—after 6 months of age until 7 years of age—the children are at their greatest risk for pertussis infections. Central nervous system damage, secondary bacterial infections, and hemorrhage during pertussis are serious side effects which prompted development of the vaccine.

Recently the pertussis vaccine has come under attack because of the high rate and seriousness of its side effects, including gran mal seizures. This prompted the cessation of vaccination in England, which then resulted in a sharp upsurge of disease. The ambition of immunologists to produce a less toxic, but still effective vaccine has not yet been fulfilled. Protection after vaccination correlates well with the circulating antibody titer, so the efficacy of trial vaccines will be easy to evaluate.

Tuberculosis

BCG vaccination against tuberculosis is the only example of an attenuated bacterial vaccine that has stood the test of time. As is widely known, BCG is the abbreviation for Bacille Calmette Guérin, a strain of *Mycobacterium tuberculosis* variety *bovis,* attenuated by 13 years of cultivation on media containing bile salts by Calmette and Guérin. Since its initial trial in 1921 it has received widespread adoption throughout the world except in the United States. The vaccine is a lyophilized culture that is given intradermally only to tuberculin (OT or PPD)-negative individuals. Immunization of persons who already display a positive tuberculin skin reaction is not only needless but may activate old, healed lesions. The injected bacteria multiply feebly at the point of inoculation, frequently causing a small ulcer that does not heal completely for 4 to 6 weeks and leaves a small scar. On successful immunization the recipient is converted to a tuberculin-positive skin reactor. This is taken as external proof of a specific CMI.

Numerous statistical analyses have proved the effectiveness of the vaccine, and new uses are being found in immunization against leprosy, dermal infections caused by *M. ulcerans,* and cancer. The first two examples may be based on cross-immunity resulting from shared antigens, but the last appears to function through a nonspecific mobilization of macrophages. Leprosy has been reduced by 87%, and *M. ulcerans* infections have been reduced by 18% to 74%, depending on the trial. BCG vaccination near melanomas has been known to totally clear the skin of tumor cells.

Meningococcal disease

Neisseria meningitidis is the second leading cause of meningitis affecting 3,000 to 4,000 persons in the U.S. each year, with a fatality rate of about 10%. This bacterium is classified on the basis of different polysaccharide capsular antigens. Serogroups A, C, Y and W-135 produce 1, 10, 20 to 25 and 15%, respectively of all infections. Cells of serogroup B strains produce 50 to 55% of the cases. A quadrivalent vaccine of 50 μg of polysaccharides A, C, Y and W-135 is now available and recommended for those at special risk, but not as a routine immunization. Those at risk include those recently exposed, those with deficiencies of the late-acting complement components, travelers to endemic regions, and others. The polysaccharide antigen of type B is poorly immunogenic and has not been included in the vaccine for that reason.

Pneumococcal disease

As late as 1982, it was estimated that 500,000 cases of pneumococcal disease occurred annually in the United States, with a fatality rate of 25% in persons older than 50 years, or those with systemic illness. Pneumococcal meningitis is still a serious disease with an attack rate of approximately 2 per 100,000 population. *Streptococcus pneumoniae,* the etiologic agent of these diseases, exists in 83 capsular serotypes. Of these, a group of 14 of these serotypes cause over 90% of the illnesses. The polysaccharide of each of these 14 has been incorporated into a single vaccine that is recommended for the elderly. Use of the vaccine has reduced the attack rate by 76% to 92% in separate trials. Currently, a vaccine containing the capsular antigens from several more serotypes is under trial and may replace the original vaccine.

Hemophilus influenzae

Antigenic types of *Hemophilus influenzae* are differentiated on the basis of the composition of their polysaccharide capsule. Of the six serotypes a through f, type b is the most common encapsulated isolate from human disease. The most serious of these diseases is meningitis, which causes a mortality of 5% in the 12,000 cases reported annually in the United States. Neurological sequelae are observed in 25-35% of the cases, the greatest majority of which are in children under 5 years of age.

An *H. influenzae* b polysaccharide vaccine holds great promise in preventing hemophilus meningitis in children beyond 18 months of age. Children younger than this respond poorly, or not at all to the vaccine. After vaccination, protection is observed at a 90% level for a 4-year period. Beyond 5 years of age, resistance against *H. influenzae* infections is quite high, so the vaccine is targeted for the most susceptible population.

IMMUNIZATIONS

Since most active immunizations are begun and completed in childhood, the American Academy of Pediatrics has established a schedule of such immunizations for normal infants and children dwelling in the United States.

Active immunization

The Academy advises protection against the following diseases through a prophylactic immunization program: diphtheria, tetanus, whooping cough (pertussis), poliomyelitis, measles, rubella, and mumps (Table 14-5). Routine smallpox vaccination is no longer recommended.

It is interesting to note that no other vaccines against bacterial diseases are recommended by the American Academy of Pediatrics. In the case of the vaccines for several enteric diseases this is understandable; the vaccine for typhoid and paratyphoid fevers is of dubious value, and modern sanitation probably has done as much to reduce the incidence of typhoid fever in the United States, as has immunization. The risk for cholera is low, and its vaccine confers only a tenuous immunity, and even that has an expected duration of only 3 to 6 months.

Passive immunization

Passive immunization continues to play a significant role in infectious disease control, but there have

---

TABLE 14-5

Recommended active immunizations*

Vaccine	Time administered
DPT	At 2, 4, and 6 months with boosters at 1½ years and at entrance to school; tetanus booster at 16 years
Oral polio	As with DPT
Measles†	At 1 year
Rubella	After 1 year, before puberty in females
Mumps	After 1 year

*Yellow fever, cholera, BCG, and other vaccinations recommended for international travel, medical personnel, and other conditions.
†May be given with rubella and mumps.

TABLE 14-6

Passive immunizations

Disease	Immunization
Measles	Hyperimmune globulin immediately after exposure or with weakly attenuated vaccines
Rubella	Pregnant women exposed to rubella
Infectious hepatitis	Immediately after exposure
Tetanus	Immediately after injury if not immunized or if immunization is outdated
Rh disease	Within 72 hours after delivery
Hypogammaglob-ulinemia	Pooled human γ-globulin

been obvious adjustments in its application in the last two decades. Prior to recent times passive immunization was limited almost exclusively to tetanus and diphtheria with occasional uses in cases of botulism or gas gangrene.

Newer developments in immunoglobulin therapy include the preparation of human hyperimmune sera and the consequent decrease in allergic reactions from their use. A second development is the use of hyperimmune sera against measles, mumps, vaccinia, and rubella viruses to modify the severity of the responses to attenuated vaccines or to modify the severity of disease in very young infants exposed to or developing these infections (Table 14-6). The recognition of hypogammaglobulinemic persons has created a continued need for antiserum therapy. Perhaps most dramatic of all, since it is outside the realm of infectious disease, is the use of human anti-Rh sera to prevent the development of Rh antibodies in women delivering Rh-positive babies. This is an expected part of perinatal medical care and should greatly reduce HDN caused by maternal-fetal Rh incompatibility.

REFERENCES

Albright, J.F., and Albright, J.W.: Natural resistance to animal parasites, Contemp. Topics Immunobiol. **12:**1, 1984.

Allen, J.C., editor: Infection and the compromised host, ed. 2, Baltimore, 1981, Williams and Wilkins Co.

Arnon, R., Shapira, M., and Jacob, C.O.: Synthetic vaccines, J. Immunol. Meth. **61:**261, 1983.

Basu, R.N., Jezek, Z., and Ward, N.A.: The eradication of smallpox from India, New Delhi, 1979, World Health Organization.

Biesel, W.R.: Single nutrients and immunity, Amer. J. Clin. Nutr. **35**(Suppl. 2):417, 1982.

Cinader, B.: Aging and the immune system, Clin. Biochem. **16:**121, 1983.

Cohen, S., and Warren, K.S., editors: Immunology of parasitic infections, ed. 2, Oxford, 1982, Blackwell Scientific Publications.

Committee on Issues and Priorities for new vaccine development: New vaccine development: establishing priorities, Washington, 1985, National Academy Press.

Cooper, E.L., editor: Stress, immunity, and aging, New York, 1984, Marcel Dekker, Inc.

Dick, G.: Practical immunization, Lancaster, 1986, MTP Press Limited.

Dreesman, G.R., Bronson, J.G., and Kennedy, R.C., editors: High technology route to virus vaccines, ASM, 1985, Washington.

Egwang, T.G., and Befus, A.D.: The role of complement in the induction and regulation of immune responses, Immunol. **51:**207, 1984.

Ennis, F.A., editor: Human immunity to viruses, New York, 1983, Academic Press, Inc.

Friedman, R.M., and Vogel, S.N.: Interferons with special emphasis on the immune system, Adv. Immunol. **34:**97, 1983.

Fulginiti, V.A., editor: Immunization in clinical practice, Philadelphia, 1982, J.B. Lippincott Co.

Gallin, J.I., and Fauci, A.S., editors: Mucosal immunity, New York, 1985, Raven Press Books, Ltd.

Germanier, R., editor: Bacterial vaccines, Orlando, 1985, Academic Press, Inc.

Gershwin, M., Beach, R., and Hurley, L., editors: Nutrition and immunity, Orlando, 1985, Academic Press, Inc.

Jacobson, I.R., and Dienstag, J.S.: Viral hepatitis vaccines, Ann. Rev. Med. **36:**241, 1985.

Lichtenstein, L.M., and Fauci, A.S., editors: Current therapy in allergy and immunology 1983-1984, St. Louis, 1983, The C.V. Mosby Co. (B.C. Decker, Inc.)

Quinnam, G.V., Jr., editor: Vaccinia viruses as vectors for vaccine antigens, New York, 1985, Elsevier Science Publishing Co., Inc.

Roitt, I.M.: Immune intervention, vol. 1, New trends in vaccines, London, 1984, Academic Press, Inc. (London) Ltd.

Stewart-Tull, D.E.S., and Davies, M., editors: Immunology of the bacterial cell envelope, Chichester, 1985, John Wiley & Sons, Ltd.

Strober, W., Hanson, L.Å., and Sell, K.W., editors: Recent advances in mucosal immunity, New York, 1982, Raven Press Books Ltd.

VanRegenmortel, M.H.V., and Neurath, A.R., editors: Immuno-chemistry of viruses. The basis for serodiagnosis and vaccines, Amsterdam, 1985, Elsevier Science Publishers B.V. (Biomedical Division).

Watson, R.R., editor: Nutrition, disease resistance, and immune function, New York, 1984, Marcel Dekker, Inc.

Yamamura, Y., Hayashi, H., Honjo, T., Kishimoto, T., Muramatsu, M., and Osawa, T., editors: Humoral factors in host defense, Tokyo, 1983, Academic Press Japan, Inc.

Yunis, E.: The cellular and humoral basis of the immune response, Seminar Arthrit. Rheum. **13** (Suppl. 1):89, 1983.

See related **Reading 7,** page 431.

CHAPTER

15

Transplantation and tumor immunology

≡GLOSSARY

ADCC Antibody-dependent cell cytotoxicity.

adjuvant therapy The nonspecific stimulation of macrophages as an avenue for immunotherapy of cancer.

allogenic Of a different genetic structure than another individual in the same species.

allograft A grafted tissue that contains antigens not present in a recipient of the same species.

autograft A graft of tissue from one location to another in the same individual.

Burkitt's lymphoma A B cell tumor associated with an infection caused by Epstein Barr virus.

carcinoembryonic antigen (CEA) An antigen secreted by fetal and cancerous adult intestinal tissue.

carcinofetal antigen A generic term for an antigen found in fetal and cancerous adult tissues.

congenic Genetically identical to another individual except at one allele.

first set rejection The rejection of an allograft after its first transplantation.

graft-versus-host reaction (GVH reaction) The attack of immunocompetent tissues in a graft against an immunocompromised host.

haplotype The genes present on one of the two chromosomes.

histocompatibility antigen An antigen on the surface of a cell that induces the response leading to graft rejection; synonymous with transplantation antigen.

Human leukocyte antigen (HLA) The major human histocompatibility system.

hyperacute rejection An accelerated rejection of a graft due to the presence of preformed antibodies.

immune enhancement Improved survival of a transplant in hosts possessing antibodies against antigens in the transplanted tissue.

immunotoxin A covalent combination of a toxin with an immunoglobulin.

microcytotoxicity test A test to determine histocompatibility by measuring antigens on donor and recipient lymphocytes.

mixed leukocyte reaction A test to determine histocompatibility by co-cultivation of donor and recipient lymphocytes.

oncofetal antigen Synonym for carcinofetal antigen.

tumor necrosis factor A protein from macrophages that is toxic to tumor cells.

tumor specific transplantation antigen A surface antigen specific for a tumor cell that behaves as a transplantation antigen.

transplantation antigen Histocompatibility antigen.

TRANSPLANTATION IMMUNOLOGY

The scientific history of transplantation immunology really did not begin until the 1950s, although organ grafting was studied extensively by Carrell and others prior to 1920. Even blood transfusions, which can be considered a form of tissue transplantation, were not practiced extensively until after 1940, although much of the immunologic basis, at least for the ABO blood group system, was well delineated prior to this time. In the 1950s the rebirth of genetics and the availability of inbred mouse lines opened tissue transplantation as a new subject for immunologic investigation, which itself was undergoing a renaissance.

Another force that has favored a more diligent study of transplantation is the subject of tumor immunity. Although tissue transplantation and tumor immunity seem to be opposites, they share many characteristics. In the development of tumors the host is exposed to new antigens in the malignant tissue that do not exist in the host's normal cells. If the host's immune system permits the continued reproduction and growth of the neoplastic tissue, then in effect the host is accepting foreign tissue. This does not differ in immunologic principle from the acceptance of tissue from a second antigenically unrelated individual. Yet in transplantations it seems the cells with the foreign antigens are often rejected. Individuals who can reject malignant cells when they arise in the body are similar to those who reject graft tissue; it is therefore appropriate that tissue transplantation and tumor immunity be considered together.

Terminology

The nomenclature of tissue transplantation has its origins in three different sciences: surgery, immunology, and genetics. The result of this has been the emergence of a multiple nomenclature system, which now is able to include terms based on the genetic relationship of tissues (Table 15-1).

When tissue is transplanted from one location to another within or on the same individual, the prefix *auto-* is used, as in the terms *autograft, autologous graft, autochthonous graft,* and *autogenous graft.* The tissue is said to be autogenic, meaning that it is genetically identical to that of the recipient, who, as defined by auto- (self), is also the donor.

When tissue is transplanted between two genetically identical, yet separate individuals, the tissue is described as syngenic or congenic. The prefix *syn-* means with or together, and congenic means of the same kind. In many genetic studies congenic means identical except for the gene or gene set under investigation. The graft is referred to as a syngraft or congraft, although the latter term is not in widespread use. In human transplantation immunology, a syngraft would refer to a graft between identical twins. In closely inbred animals, grafts made within the strain can be referred to as syngrafts or congrafts.

When tissue grafting is performed between two non-identical individuals within the same species, the tissue is described as *allogenic;* the process as *allografting.* Grafts between individuals from different species are rarely made; however, when this is the case, it is possible to use the term *xenograft* and *xenogenic* tissue.

All these terms are applicable when the graft is of tissue that must remain alive, even grow, in the recipient. This is not true of homostatic grafts, in which the tissue often serves as a structural support on which or through which host tissue grows to reestablish the original structure. Among homostatic

TABLE 15-1

Tissue transplantation nomenclature

Type of transplantation	Type of tissue	Older term	Genetic and antigenic relationships
Autograft	Autogenic	Autologous	Identical: donor and recipient are same individual
Syngraft	Syngenic, congenic	Isologous	Identical, but between different individuals
Allograft	Allogenic	Homologous	Different: genetically different individuals within one species are involved
Xenograft	Xenogenic	Heterologous	Different: individuals from different species are involved

grafts, transplantations of blood vessels, bone, and cornea are examples. The following discussion is concerned primarily with homovital transplants, in which tissue viability is demanded.

Graft rejection

Acute rejection

After allografting tissue, one of three sequences may be observed. The first of these is the hyperacute or acute rejection reaction, caused by the presence of preformed antibodies with a specificity for the transplanted tissue (Fig. 15-1). This can be the case when the donor and the recipient have not been matched for the ABO blood group antigens. These antigens are present on all cells of the body, and if cells bearing the A antigen are transferred to a group O or B individual, the anti-A hemagglutinin initiates cytotoxic destruction of the transplanted tissue. Or the recip-

ient may have developed a resistance to the new tissue from prior grafts. In either case the reaction involves the components of the complement system, polymorphonuclear phagocytes, and macrophages which function so quickly in tissue destruction that the tissue never really "takes." In the case of skin the transferred tissue remains as a "white graft"—one in which revascularization never occurs. In the case of organs in which the major vascular connections are achieved surgically, stasis of blood flow, engorgement of the organ with blood, and even coagulation of blood in the donor organ may occur so rapidly that it is obvious the graft will fail, and the organ is transplanted and removed in the same surgical procedure.

First set rejection

The usual sequence of events seen in the unsensitized recipient is less rapid and is known as the first

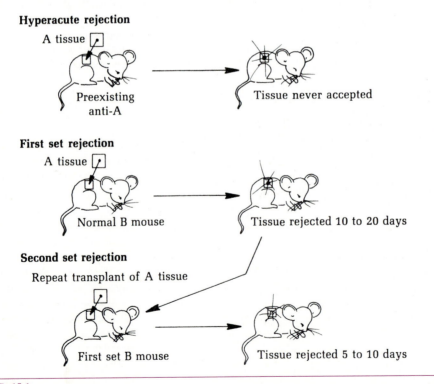

Hyperacute rejection
A tissue
Preexisting anti-A
Tissue never accepted

First set rejection
A tissue
Normal B mouse
Tissue rejected 10 to 20 days

Second set rejection
Repeat transplant of A tissue
First set B mouse
Tissue rejected 5 to 10 days

FIG. 15-1

Hyperacute rejection results from placement of tissue in an animal already possessing antibodies to antigens of grafted tissue. Second set rejection is an accelerated first set reaction and is seen in animals that have already rejected tissue at least once.

set rejection or first set reaction. Within the first few hours or days after relocation of the allograft all outward signs belie the knowledge that the graft will be rejected. Revascularization appears to proceed normally, and skin assumes its normal healthy color. Solid tissues or organs assume their typical functions of hormone production, urine excretion, pumping of blood, etc. But within a few days skin takes on a darker, purplish hue that proceeds in the ensuing days to absolute necrosis, and by the end of the eleventh to seventeenth day, depending on the animal species and other factors, the graft will be rejected. In the case of solid organs, signs of tissue rejection will include loss of vital function of the organ, fever, and malaise. Histologically the tissue becomes heavily infiltrated with mononuclear cells of several varieties: macrophages, lymphocytes, and plasma cells. By the end of the first week, fibrin accumulation and loss of blood flow and/or vascular integrity foreshadow the eventual complete loss of nutritive supply to the tissue and its death.

The actual time of graft survival varies with the species, size of the graft, tissue, and other variables. Rats reject very small skin grafts in about 21 days, but larger grafts are rejected in 8 days. Extremely large grafts may induce tolerance and survive for weeks. Kidneys often survive longer than skin.

Second set rejection

If a graft from the same donor and recipient is repeated, the first set sequence is repeated at an accelerated pace (Fig. 15-1). This second set rejection reflects the previous exposure and sensitization to the donor antigens.

The evidence is now unassailable that graft rejection or acceptance relies on immunogenetic principles, as attested by the following:

1. Antigen specificity. Tissue transplanted between antigenically identical individuals (syngraft) or autografted tissue does not undergo rejection if surgical and septic procedures meet accepted standards. In these two situations there is no exposure to new antigens and therefore no immune response.

2. Immunosuppression. In the case of allografts the onset of first set and second set rejection can be prolonged by suitable immunosuppressive treatments.

3. Immunologic memory. The accelerated second set rejection applies to a repeated transplant from the same donor but does not apply to tissues from a second donor who is antigenically unrelated to the first.

4. Immunopathology. The histologic responses occurring during rejection are typical of immune crises, involving macrophages, lymphocytes, and plasma cells.

5. Transfer. Adoptive immunization with presensitized T cells will cause the rejection of tissues matched between donor and recipient.

6. Tolerance. Grafts between monozygotic twins or antigen-tolerized persons are not rejected.

Mechanism of graft rejection

The relative role of immunoglobulins and sensitized lymphocytes in graft rejection differs considerably according to the circumstances. In the rejection of dispersed cellular grafts, humoral immunity may dominate the rejection process. In such instances the donated cells—erythrocytes, leukocytes, platelets, etc.—are fully exposed to the developing immunoglobulin response. These cells are highly susceptible to membrane damage by complement activated by the initial serologic reaction. If cytolysis does not occur immediately, the immunoglobulins may function as opsonins to encourage the phagocytic destruction of the transfused cells. Humoral immunity also is suspected of playing a major role in the rejection of xenografts and in hyperacute rejection of transplanted tissue. Xenografts possess a large number of antigens not shared between donor and recipient. Frequently one species will possess agglutinins for cells of distantly related species, which can attack the xenogenic tissue as soon as it is transplanted.

In contrast to these circumstances, the activation of cellular immunity by the T lymphocytes is the predominant cause of the first set allograft rejection. As described in several earlier chapters, such lymphocytes may directly attack cellular antigens to which they are sensitized by previous exposure, or they may attack these cells by means of cytotoxic *lymphokines*. The first few days after grafting, when the tissue may appear perfectly normal, is a sufficient time period for sensitization to occur. Thereafter the effector phase follows, causing loss of the tissue in 10 to 20 days. When sensitized lymphocytes are already present in an animal from a prior graft rejection, an accelerated rejection of tissue results from regrafting—the second set rejection. Lymphoid cells from a sensitized animal transferred to a first graft recipient will accelerate rejection of the graft. Thus graft rejection is primarily a T cell function with some assistance from immunoglobulins. The responsible T cell is the Tc.

Immunosuppression

In the early 1950s transplantation of kidneys from cadavers into patients with renal failure was initiated. Some of these patients lived as long as 6 months without treatment with cytotoxic drugs, but low dosages of steroids, probably too low to be effective immunosuppressants, were used for some patients. By 1960 it was documented that 6-mercaptopurine would prolong rabbit and dog renal allografts, and since that time virtually all human transplant patients have received some form of suppressant therapy.

Radiation

The status of radiation in prolonging allograft survival can be summarized by stating that, as a single agent, it is relatively ineffective, but when combined with chemical and ALG treatment it is beneficial. Irradiation suffers the handicap of being totally nonspecific and may lead to prolonged paralysis of nearly all aspects of the patient's immune response. The utility of irradiation has been closely related to the success of newer cytotoxic chemical agents, which have essentially replaced radiation treatments.

Cytotoxic drugs

The chemical compounds most frequently used to prolong allografts are alkylating agents (nitrogen mustards), purine and pyrimidine analogs, folic acid analogs, and the alkaloids. Specific compounds that can be mentioned, excluding the alkylating agents, are azathioprine, 6-mercaptopurine, 6-thioguanine, 5-fluorouracil, cytosine arabinoside, methotrexate and aminopterin, and vinblastine and vincristine. Activity before or after transplantation is exhibited by cyclophosphamide, a potent alkylating agent, and

to a much lesser degree by steroids and a few other agents.

Another product that has shown great promise is cyclosporin. Cyclosporin is an eleven-amino acid cyclic peptide, at first believed to have useful antibiotic properties. Although this hope proved to be unfounded, the compound was then found to have a potent immunosuppressant activity upon T cells, and was found to reduce the release of IL-2 by the T_H cells. At first, it was thought that the T cell was the only target of cyclosporin, but now it is known that the activity of other lymphocytes is influenced by cyclosporin. Cyclosporin has a very low level of toxicity and has markedly extended the survival of allografts.

A combination of azathioprine 2 to 4 mg/kg/day, steroid with dosage dependent on the steroid selected, and cyclosporin 6 to 8 mg/kg/day with ATG is now being used in some surgery units to minimize renal transplant rejection. Several steroids reduce IL-1 release by macrophages.

The immunosuppressant therapy given recipients of transplanted tissue will vary according to the surgical unit, the patient's well-being, the tissue transplanted, and other factors. Among the chemical immunosuppressants, azathioprine and methylprednisolone frequently are used in combination with ALG and/or radiation.

ATG

ALS and ALG are discussed previously, especially the problems encountered in determining the source of the lymphocyte, choice of animal to be used, choice of assay for activity, and mechanism of action. From the present literature it appears that ATG is widely used in transplantation surgery, but patient records reveal that treatment with ATG often is terminated after about 2 weeks. By this time a large percentage of patients develop severe local reactions in the form of edema, induration, erythema, and pain when the ATG is given intramuscularly. When it is given intravenously, fever and mild anaphylactic shock have been recorded as distinct hazards. Many patients produce precipitating antibodies to ATG or ATS preparations, which may contribute to allergic reactions and neutralize their effectiveness. These factors plus the more general hazards of suppressant therapy contribute to its withdrawal from the treatment regimen of most patients after a few weeks.

A prime hazard of all immunosuppressant treatments is their general depressive activity on the immune system. The incidence of infections by all classes of organisms is increased in patients receiving this type of therapy. Among the bacteria, the pyogenic cocci and *Pseudomonas* infections become more frequent. Intracellular protozoa, including *Pneumocystis* and *Toxoplasma* organisms, emerge as important pathogens. Among the viruses, whose defense relies heavily on an intact Tc system, increased herpes simplex, herpes zoster, Epstein-Barr virus (EBV), and cytomegalovirus infections are noted. Among the fungi, *Candida, Cryptococcus,* and *Aspergillus* infections are more common in the immunosuppressed patient. More startling has been the discovery that about 2% of immunosuppressed human patients develop oncogenic complications. When the immune surveillance system for neoplastic cells is thwarted by these treatments, these aberrant cells find the compromised host an ideal tissue culture incubator for proliferation.

Graft-versus-host reactions

When tissue is transplanted from one individual to another, there are actually two rejection processes to be considered. The first and traditionally most studied is the host rejection of grafted tissue, but the reverse of this is also a distinct possibility and is known as the graft-versus-host (GVH) reaction. GVH reactions may develop when immunocompetent tissues are transferred to an immunologically handicapped host. This form of adoptive immunization results in a host-directed rejection process. This may occur under natural circumstances when maternal lymphoid tissues are transferred to the fetus during pregnancy. Artificially these reactions may develop when adult tissues are injected into unborn or newborn animals or when lymphoid tissue is transferred to adults who have been irradiated or heavily immunosuppressed with chemical agents.

The situation in the newborn or fetal animal develops into the condition known as runt disease (homologous disease); the animal fails to grow, develops a distinct splenomegaly, diarrhea, and anemia, and often dies. All young animals with runt disease do not die, however; those which survive may progress through a transitory period of only a few days in which splenomegaly and hepatomegaly, an erythematous skin, and fever are the major signs that a reaction is taking place. Mild, reversible GVH reactions are more frequent when the donor and host share a good degree of histocompatibility but are not syngenic. It is this fact which gave courage to those pediatricians and surgeons who transplanted bone marrow and/or thymus tissue into young children with proved genetic immunodeficiencies. Some of these children did progress through a GVH reaction, but both tissues survived the reaction with the desired repopulation of the host with immunocompetent cells. GVH reactions are not seen when skin or other tissue lacking mature lymphoid cells is transferred, for example, transfer of fetal cells to adult animals or the transfer of tissues that have been treated with x rays to destroy immunologically capable cells.

Privileged sites and privileged tissues

Although allografts of tissues are routinely lost through the rejection process when they are placed in their normal location, they may persist almost indefinitely in certain abnormal or heterotopic sites. Heterotopic grafting is convenient in experimental transplantation studies, since the transferred tissue may be placed where its survival can be easily monitored by external observation. Through experimental studies in laboratory animals several immunologically privileged sites, that is, sites where allografted tissue is protected from the rejection process, have been detected. The best known of these sites is the hamster cheek pouch, although the brain and anterior chamber of the eye also have been described as privileged sites.

The hamster cheek pouch is exactly what its name indicates, a saclike cavity running along each cheek or jaw line of the hamster for approximately 5 cm.

The length of the pouch places its distal end over the shoulder of the hamster. These pouches are used by the animal for food storage or transport. The inner surface of the pouch is well endowed with vascular tissue and has a layer of connective tissue. Implantation of normal or neoplastic tissues from other hamsters or even from foreign species, including humans, into the pouch is followed by their long-term survival. The tissues become vascularized and grow rapidly, whereas the same tissues placed elsewhere in the hamster are quickly destroyed. The striking anatomic feature of the hamster cheek pouch, and of other immunologically privileged tissues, is its paucity of a lymphatic drainage system. This fact, coupled with the known abundance of T lymphocytes in lymph, was useful in developing our present concept that CMI is responsible for first set allograft rejection. The absence of lymphoid tissue in the hamster cheek pouch is the key to long-term graft survival.

The cornea is one of the best-described privileged sites. When transferred from one host to another, under ideal surgical conditions when the vascular bed is not damaged, the cornea is accepted and can successfully restore vision lost from corneal defects. This standard ophthalmologic surgical procedure is almost invariably successful. If the cornea is placed elsewhere in vascularized tissue, it is rejected in the usual fashion. This seems sufficient evidence to negate the presumption that the cornea is nonantigenic or resistant to the allograft rejection process, ideas that were forwarded to explain the easy success of corneal transplants.

Tissues from a variety of anatomic locations that appear to escape the usual allograft rejection process have been described as immunologically privileged tissues. These, in contrast to privileged sites, are tissues which are not rejected, regardless of where they are relocated. Among these are bone, cartilage, heart valves, sections of the aorta or other major blood vessels, and tendon; the developing fetus also can be added to this list. The first mentioned group of tissues—bone, cartilage, etc.—can be preserved indefinitely in the lyophilized state or frozen, and when needed, they can be rehydrated or thawed and are immediately ready for use. Chemical sterilization of these tissues is also practical, even with solutions that contain as much as 4% formalin. It is obvious that these procedures are lethal to the living constituents of these tissues, and this makes it essential to consider them for what they really are: physical structures with little if any cellular vitality that, when allografted, provide a matrix of the size and shape desired about which new host tissue can form during its regeneration. This type of repair has little if any real advantage over the use of steel pins, plastic tubes or valves, or other synthetic parts for the replacement or repair of vital tissue. In fact the use of artificial devices will avoid the possibility of sensitizing the recipient to antigens of the natural tissue, which might interfere with a later medical procedure.

The developing fetus is considered the example par excellence of an immunologically privileged tissue. With the exception of completely syngenic laboratory animals, natural fertilization demands that each cell of the developing embryo contain antigens unique to the male. In outbred animals potent antigenic differences between the male and female should hazard the success of the pregnancy on the grounds of histoincompatibility, but it is known that even females preimmunized with tissues of the male will still bear that male's offspring without incident. Transplantation of other tissues to the uterus of nonpregnant animals results in graft rejection, however, and this clearly indicates that the nonpregnant uterus behaves the same as other tissues. Thus there must be some specific property of the pregnant uterus that accounts for survival of the fetus. This special property is believed to reside in the trophoblast. The trophoblast is a layer of tissue that physically separates the uterine wall from the tissues of the fetus. Each cell in this membrane appears to surround itself with a mucoprotein, and the amount of this substance formed is proportional to the antigenic distance of the mother and fetus. In syngenic relationships very little of the mucoprotein is formed. Consequently a general impermeability of the trophoblastic layer is credited with the protective role that is provided the fetus. This is operationally the same condition which exists in the hamster cheek pouch.

Immunologic tolerance and immunologic enhancement

The prolongation of transplant viability may occur as the result of a host failure to respond to antigens of the tissue (immunologic tolerance) or from the production of enhancing antibodies (immunologic enhancement or immunologic blockade). Although immunologic tolerance customarily has been examined through the use of purified antigens, its principles also apply to transplantation and tumor immunology. Immunologic enhancement has been studied primarily in the domain of tumor immunology but can be applied equally as well to the study of tissue rejection or survival.

Immunologic tolerance is described in Chapters 8 and 9, so only brief attention will be given to this subject in this section. A state of tolerance to foreign histocompatibility antigens is developed easily in fetal or newborn animals by an exposure to tissue (nonlymphoid tissue will avoid GVH reactions) containing foreign antigens. The unresponsive condition can best be detected by reexposure to the antigens in the form of a skin graft. Such grafts persist almost indefinitely in the recipient. This state is related primarily to an induction of Ts cells and down regulation of the immune response. This procedure has been applied to human transplantation successfully by giving the recipient a large-volume blood transfusion (of the donor's blood type) prior to the transplantation of tissue.

Immunologic enhancement refers to the active prolongation of tissue life by antibodies to antigens of the tissue. This has been so intimately connected with tumor immunology that it is discussed later in this chapter.

Transplantation antigens

The chemistry and genetic origin of the major histocompatibility antigens was described in Chapter 4, and only a brief restatement will be presented here. The class I genes A, B, and C on human chromosome 6 have many alleles; consequently, many proteins similar in structure, yet antigenically different, are possible. Each person has the possibility of producing two proteins of each series unless homozygous at one allele. These proteins have a molecular weight of 45,000. The 345 amino acids comprising an HLA-A, -B, or -C protein can be divided into five discrete domains. The three sections of the protein exterior to the cytoplasmic surface are referred to as the $\alpha1$, $\alpha2$ and $\alpha3$ domains. Of these, the $\alpha1$ domain is most exterior, displays substantial variation in amino acid sequence from one specimen to the other, and is thus the sector most apt to display antigenic specificity. Domain $\alpha2$ probably also contributes to the antigenic novelty of an HLA protein, but the $\alpha3$ domains are quite similar to one another and are believed to have a minor role in antigenic specificity. A transmembranic sequence and cytoplasmic anchor complete the five domains. A $\beta2$ microglobulin of 12,500 molecular weight is ionically associated with the HLA protein, but does not contribute to the antigenic specificity of the complex, since these proteins are virtually identical in amino acid sequence.

Numerous other proteins contribute to graft rejection, including the class II proteins of the MHC and others. The antigenic potency of these, and hence their position in transplant rejection, is less than that of the HLA-A, -B, and -C antigens.

Genetic relationships and their application

In humans the HLA-A, -B, and -C genes exist as multiply varied alleles of a paired chromosome system. Because one antigen of each set is transmitted through the germ cells, the genetic composition of progeny can be described in terms of their paternal and maternal haplotypes. The gene products of each A, B, and C gene set are numbered (Table 15-2). These numbers are not sequential within the A, B, or C series because they were numbered prior to knowledge of their gene association.

Because so many different antigens are involved, most haplotypes are rare except within a specific line of inheritance. Mathematically the chance for two persons to have a common phenotype is less than 1 in 20 million. As a consequence of this, any haplotype that is common between a child and a putative father is nearly absolute evidence of parentage (Table 15-3). Because of its mathematic superiority,

TABLE 15-2

Human HLA antigen specificities and frequencies*

HLA-A	Frequency (percent)	HLA-B	Frequency (percent)	HLA-C	Frequency (percent)
A1	15.8	B5	5.9	Cw1	4.8
A2	27.0	B7	10.4	Cw2	5.4
A3	12.6	B8	9.2	Cw3	9.2
A9	11.2	B12	16.6	Cw4	12.6
A10		B13	3.2	Cw5	8.4
A11	5.1	B14	2.4	Cw6	12.6
A23		B15	4.8	Cw7	Unknown
A24		B17	5.7	Cw8	Unknown
A25	2.0	B18	6.2		
A26	3.9	B21			
A28	4.4	B27	4.6		
A29	5.8	B35			
A30		B37	1.1		
A31		B40	8.1		
A32		Plus 28 Bw antigens			
Plus 8 Aw antigens					

*Includes antigens not precisely identified, as designated by the gene letter plus *w* (for workshop).

HLA typing is destined to replace blood grouping to identify individuals in cases of disputed parentage, unidentified infants, violent death, etc. The major application of the HLA system at the current time is in histocompatibility testing preparatory to tissue transplantation.

HLA and disease

Since the genes that regulate the synthesis of the HLA antigens and those which govern the immune response are positioned so close to one another on the chromosome, it has been interesting to examine the relationship of HLA antigens to various forms of disease. The diseases investigated have been for the most part those with some presumed immunologic origin: neoplastic disease, autoimmune disease, and allergies. These are described in Chapter 19 and summarized in Table 19-2.

Histocompatibility testing

There are two basic procedures employed to determine the suitability of tissue for grafting purposes. In one system the histocompatibility antigens of both the donor and recipient are determined by microcyto-

toxicity testing, and tissues that share common histocompatibility antigens are considered suitable for use in transplantation. In the other method lymphocytes of the donor and recipient are placed together in culture and observed for antagonistic reactions. When these are not noticed, the tissues are considered histocompatible. Some investigators prefer the second system, since it is a "natural" system and may measure antigenic disparities for which no antisera are yet known, but microcytotoxicity testing is a far more common procedure.

Microcytotoxicity tests

Although agglutination tests and complement fixation tests have been used to detect histocompatibility antigens on leukocytes or to quantitate HLA antisera, the lymphocyte toxicity test is now the most widely applied method for this purpose. To identify the HLA antigens, a reasonably pure preparation of lymphocytes is prepared from heparinized blood. Whole blood may be added to commercially available solutions, which on standing or light centrifugation will stratify the lymphocytes in an isolated band. The lymphocytes are then adjusted to 10^6 cells

TABLE 15-3

Genetic transmission of HLA antigens and haplotypes

	A antigens						B antigens					
	1	2	3	9	11	25	5	7	8	12	13	14
Father	+	−	+	−	−	−	−	+	+	−	−	−
Mother	−	+	−	+	−	−	+	−	−	+	−	−
Children												
First	+	+	−	−	−	−	+	−	+	−	−	−
Second	+	−	−	+	−	−	−	−	+	+	−	−
Third	−	+	+	−	−	−	+	+	−	−	−	−
Fourth	−	+	+	−	−	−	+	+	−	−	−	−

	Interpretation	
	Phenotypes	Haplotypes
Father	A1, 3/B7, 8	A1, B8/A3, B7
Mother	A2, 9/B5, 12	A2, B5/A9, B12
Children		
First	A1, 2/B5, 8	A1, B8/A2, B5
Second	A1, 9/B8, 12	A1, B8/A9, B12
Third	A2, 3/B5, 7	A3, B7/A2, B5
Fourth	A2, 3/B5, 7	A3, B7/A2, B5

per milliliter. A few microliters of the cell suspension are added to each of many histocompatibility antisera that have been dispensed in microliter droplets in a multiconcavity test tray. Serum complement is added, and incubation, usually for 1 hour at room temperature or 37° C, is allowed before staining the dead cells with eosin or trypan blue. Living cells do not take up these dyes; so by microscopic evaluation one can determine if a certain antiserum-complement combination was cytotoxic for the lymphocytes (Fig. 15-2). When this is the case, then the antigen corresponding to that antiserum was present on the lymphocyte surface. By performing this test on lymphocytes of both donor and recipient with a battery of antisera, one can determine their histocompatibility antigen composition.

Naturally there are many subtle variations to the microcytotoxicity test. The lymphocytes may be labeled with ^{51}Cr by incubating them briefly with Na_2 $^{51}CrO_4$, followed by a centrifuge washing to remove the excess isotope. This ^{51}Cr is released by cells undergoing membrane damage and is a rapid and sensitive test for cytotoxicity. Viable lymphocytes also can be labeled with a fluorescein dye; when the integrity of their cell membrane is lost, the dye leaks out. In this test the presence of unstained cells is an index of cytotoxicity. Regardless of the system employed, the cytotoxic assays are the most generally used of the histocompatibility tests.

Data collected over the past decade clearly demonstrate the relationship of HLA antigen matching with transplantation success. In the case of HLA matched siblings, the survival of kidney grafts reached 90% in one study over a one year span, and 80% over five years. In semi matches, kidney survival is 75% and 55% over the same two time periods. Because of the gene frequency of some antigens, a perfect HLA-A and B match is virtually impossible, except between parents and children, or between siblings. The size of families in many countries limits the possibility of tissue grafts between brothers and sisters, but kidney graft survival in 4 way matches (two A and two B antigens) approaches 100%.

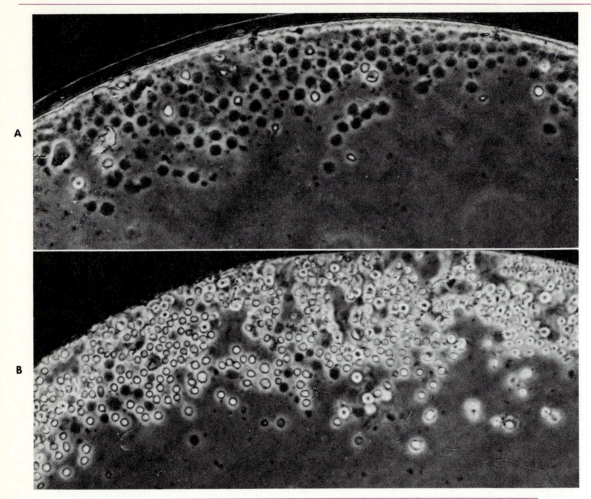

FIG. 15-2

A, The dark stained lymphocytes represent a positive microcytotoxicity test. **B,** A negative test in which the refractile living lymphocytes remained unstained. (Courtesy Dr. A. Luger.)

It is interesting to note that the success of heart transplants correlates less with HLA matching than it does with matching of other tissues but, fortunately, this permits the successful transfer of tissue against the histocompatibility barrier.

Mixed lymphocyte cultures

From studies conducted in the early 1960s it was realized that the in vitro culturing of peripheral blood leukocytes from two separate donors was an assay for histocompatibility differences between the two individuals. The test does not attempt to measure the antigenic composition of donor and recipient, only their compatibility. Cells from unrelated donors undergo lymphocyte transformation, as evidenced by intensive nucleic acid metabolism, enlargement of the cell nucleus with an accompanying increase in mitotic figures, and an increase in cell size before division. Such is the result of an MLC or MLR. These changes can be detected cytologically (Fig. 15-3),

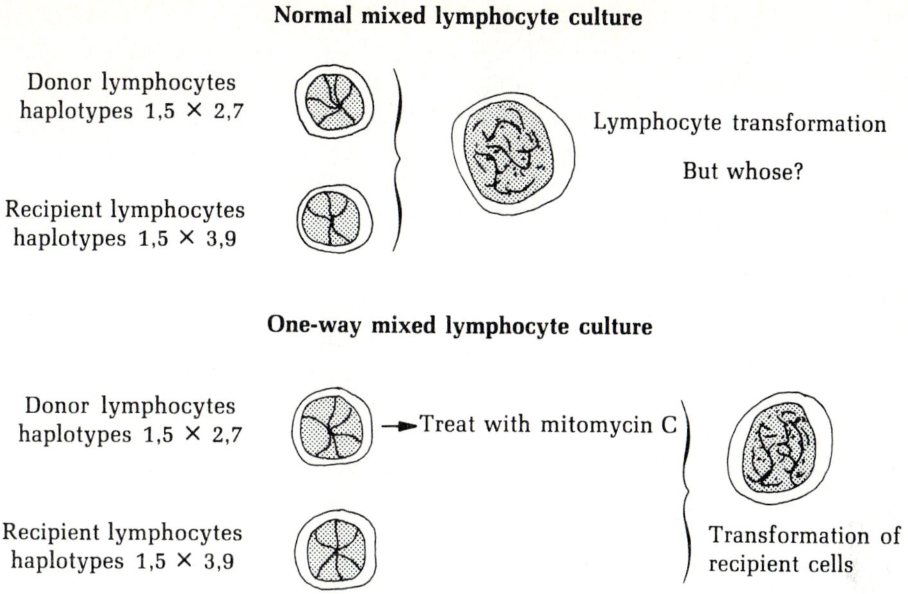

Normal mixed lymphocyte culture

Donor lymphocytes
haplotypes 1,5 × 2,7

Recipient lymphocytes
haplotypes 1,5 × 3,9

 Lymphocyte transformation

But whose?

One-way mixed lymphocyte culture

Donor lymphocytes
haplotypes 1,5 × 2,7

 → Treat with mitomycin C

Recipient lymphocytes
haplotypes 1,5 × 3,9

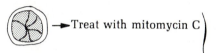

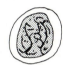 Transformation of
recipient cells

FIG. 15-3

Poisoning donor lymphocytes ensures that a positive MLC is the result of recipient lymphocyte transformation.

but because this requires tedious microscopic observation, resort to radioassay has been necessary to expedite data collecting. The basis of the radioassay is that tritiated thymidine added to the cultures is incorporated into the nuclear DNA of rapidly proliferating cells but not into unstimulated control cultures. Fixation of the radiolabel by the cultures can be determined by scintillation counting and used as an index of histocompatibility difference between the two persons.

The MLC reaction is a response of T cells to antigens on B cells. When the HLA-A, B, and C antigens are identical, the MLC is a measure of D-region disparity between the donor and recipient cells. Antisera which inhibit the MLC in these instances are sources of antibodies to the D-region antigens.

The MLC reflects primarily incompatibilities of the major transplantation antigens; the "weak" antigens often go undetected. The maximal MLC response may require 5 days cultivation of the cells, an obvious handicap when donor tissues are already available. Although donor tissues may be preserved

a few days at 4°C in maintenance buffers, it is generally agreed that no advantage in transplant success is derived from tissue storage.

To expedite MLC testing, some laboratories maintain a panel of primed lymphocytes, a panel of cells that have already had an exposure to cells with a specific D region heritage. Upon re-exposure to the antigen to which they were previously exposed, the cells rapidly enter into transformation. This approach to an abbreviation of the time necessary to complete MLC testing is very expensive, and most laboratories have continued with microcytotoxicity testing. Results of MLC tests agree closely with those of cytotoxicity studies for nonidentity of the major HLA antigens but may detect some antigens missed by the cytotoxicity test because of the lack of antisera for all antigens.

Since circumstances could exist in which only the lymphocytes of a donor could react to antigens of the recipient and thus give a false view of potential grafting success, the one-way MLC was developed. In this modification the lymphocytes of the donor are poisoned with mitomycin C (20 μg/ml) or irradiation (4,000 rad for 6½ minutes) before mixing them with the recipient's cells. Such donor cells are incapable of incorporating tritiated thymidine after these treatments and thus cannot contribute to positive tests. Under these circumstances the test becomes solely a measure of the recipient's response to the donor's transplantation antigens and a predictor of transplant success.

TUMOR IMMUNOLOGY

The similarities of transplantation immunology and tumor immunology are truly astounding. In each instance a host is confronted with a set of tissue cells similar in antigenic composition to the autologous cells. Through the normal events of transplant rejection the histoincompatible cells activate the immune response. This embodies all aspects of the defense system—macrophages, B cells, and T cells. In transplantation immunology every effort is made to suppress this immune response so that the grafted tissue can survive.

In neoplastic disease, tumor cells appear spontaneously in the host, probably from only a single or a few transformed cells. These tumor cells, like allografts, have some antigenic similarity to host cells but are not antigenically identical to them. For reasons that still escape a precise delineation, the host's immune response is either not fully activated and fails to reject the tumor tissue or develops in such an imbalanced pattern (enhancing or blocking antibody) that growth of the tumor not only is permitted, it is even encouraged (Fig. 15-4).

It is apparent that common immunologic events are shared by tumor immunology and transplantation immunology. Why the outcomes of these events are so distantly polarized from each other—the survival of oncogenic tissues on one hand versus the death and rejection of transplanted cells on the other—is the mystery that immunologists must try to solve.

Tumor antigens
Chemical versus viral induction

As the neoplastic cell arises from the normal cell, antigens not previously recognized or not produced become detectable on the cell surface. Tumors of lower animals can be placed into one of two categories in regard to these antigens. In the case of chem-

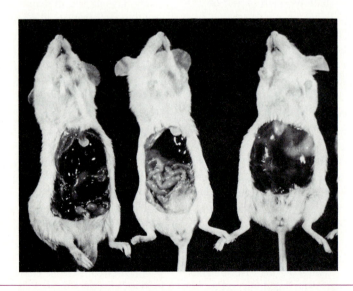

FIG. 15-4
Normal mouse in the center is flanked on the left by a mouse with a large subcutaneous plasmacytoma (IgA type) seen as a large, dark mass. The mouse on the right has an ascites, a dispersed cell tumor distributed throughout the peritoneal cavity. (Courtesy H. Gebel and M. Daley.)

ically induced tumors the new antigens are different for each tumor. For example, a tumor induced on a mouse by painting its skin with methylcholanthrene will have a different antigenic composition than the tumor of a partner mouse treated with the same carcinogen. In fact two anatomically distinct tumors induced on a single mouse by the same chemical carcinogen will be antigenically distinct. Exceptions do occur, but the antigenic cross-reactions between chemically provoked cancers arise by chance and are mathematically unpredictable.

Tumor-specific transplantation antigens

Viral induced tumors express unique antigens, but these tumors, unlike those induced by chemicals, are antigenically constant from specimen to specimen. This is true even though the tissue origin or even the species origin of the tumor may differ. These constant antigens are known as tumor-specific transplantation antigens (TSTA). The constant expression of an identifiable antigen is a useful diagnostic aid and has been used to suggest that a tumor of unknown cause is of viral origin. Either DNA or RNA viruses may induce these antigen-specific tumors.

Among the DNA viruses that can code for new antigens in host cells are herpesviruses, adenoviruses, and the papovaviruses, formerly known as the polyoma and papilloma viruses (Table 15-4). Specific examples of the herpesvirus group are Marek's disease of chickens, Lucké's carcinoma of frogs, and Burkitt's lymphoma of humans, the most convincing candidate to be the first proved virus-induced tumor of humans. Adenoviruses from humans, notably types 12 and 18, will cause cancers in laboratory mice. Simian virus SV40 and Shope papilloma virus are examples from the papovavirus group. These DNA viruses are tiny and can carry only sufficient genetic information to code for approximately a half dozen proteins. Most of these proteins are involved with virus replication, but at least one of them is the TSTA.

RNA viruses are usually larger and can code for a variety of proteins. Here again at least one is a TSTA of the cell surface, unique to each virus. It seems that the leukemia viruses of practically every species have this property, as do the Rous sarcoma virus and mouse mammary tumor virus.

The antigens associated with viral transformed cells are of three types: (1) those which are associated with the infective virion, (2) the tumor (T), or nuclear, antigens, and (3) the TSTA, or cytoplasmic membrane antigens. A discussion of the viral antigens is beyond the scope of this chapter; however, it is clear that the presence of antibodies or T cell responses to known oncogenic viruses could bear importantly on the diagnosis of the cancerous condition they cause.

The T antigens first detected in transformed cells following viral infection are located in the nucleus. These antigens are specific for the inducing virus and

---

TABLE 15-4

Oncogenic viruses

Type of virus	Animal involved
RNA	
Leukemia: sarcoma viruses	Bird, mouse, cat, rat, guinea pig, hamster, cattle, monkey, and possibly human
Mammary tumor viruses	Mouse, monkey, and possibly human
DNA	
Herpesviruses	Frog: Lucké's kidney carcinoma; bird: Marek's lymphomatosis; monkey: malignant lymphoma; human*: nasopharyngeal carcinoma and Burkitt's lymphoma
Adenoviruses	Monkey, avian, and human viruses in cell cultures; hamsters
Papovaviruses	Rabbit: Shope papilloma; mouse: polyoma, monkey: SV40, bovine: papilloma, human: wart

*Evidence very good but circumstantial.

not for the malignant cell. These antigens are detectable in all cells infected by the virus even though the cell may not become transformed, but the T antigens persist in malignant cells. These antigens are not identical with antigens of the virus particle, and some of them may be virus-induced enzymes. These T antigens are immunogenic for the tumor-bearing animal, and high levels of circulating anti-T globulins follow oncogenic conversion by adenoviruses, polyoma, and SV40 viruses. Because of the intracellular location of the T antigen, these antibodies are not able to react with the antigens in vivo and thus cannot contribute to tumor immunity, only to tumor diagnosis.

The most important antigens from the standpoint of availability as targets for the immune response are the TSTAs of the cytoplasmic membrane. The TSTAs, also known as TSA-tumor specific antigens, have been recognized in the adenovirus, papovavirus, herpesvirus, and leukemia-sarcoma virus systems. Antibodies to these antigens are found in the circulation of tumor-bearing animals; however, the titer of these antibodies does not correlate well with resistance to the tumor or regression of the tumor. How tumor cells with specific TSTA escape the rejection process, which to all purposes should be identical to an HVG rejection, is not yet clear. T cells that are responsive to these TSTAs also are generated by infections with these viruses.

Burkitt's lymphoma

Natural regression of Burkitt's lymphoma and chemotherapeutic cures of this malignancy have been of great interest to immunologists and tumor biologists. Burkitt's lymphoma is presumed to have a viral origin, a suggestion made in 1958 when Burkitt noted a high incidence of this cancer across the mosquito belt of central Africa. This disease is predominantly a malignancy of the jaw and associated facial bones and the abdominal tissues of children. Histologic examination of the tissue allows it to be classified as a lymphoma. The disease may run a fatal course, although spontaneous cures have been noted. Treatment with the alkylating agent cyclophosphamide will produce long-term remission.

Interest in Burkitt's lymphoma stems from several features of the disease: its cause, its cytology, and its immunology. The epidemiologic pattern of Burkitt's lymphoma indicated a potential arthropod vector in its cause. The disease has its highest incidence in the malarial regions of Africa where the mosquito population is highest. Examination of Burkitt's cells in culture with the electron microscope has revealed that some of the cells contain viruslike particles which are indistinguishable from those of the herpes group (DNA viruses). Nearly 90% of African Burkitt's patients have these viral particles in their tumor cells. Some cells produce and release these viral particles, which are known as Epstein-Barr virus (EBV). Several EBV antigens have been identified in these cells, including the nuclear antigen (EBNA) and viral capsid antigens. Many investigators are now willing to accept EBV as the first proved viral agent to cause human cancer, but much of the data to support this is circumstantial and based on immunologic analyses.

Before considering the serologic status of Burkitt's lymphoma it is important to emphasize that the tumor cells represent an immunoproliferative activity of the immune system. Lymphomas are malignancies of lymphocytes or their precursor cells. If the cell line producing the lymphoma is sufficiently differentiated toward the T or B cell line, it can be classified as such. Waldenström's macroglobulinemia, for example, is often classified as a B cell immunoproliferative disease because the cells involved are morphologically distinct from plasma cells, and their IgM product is easily demonstrated. Burkitt's lymphoma is classified as a proliferative disease of B cells that are at an early stage in the maturation sequence, that is, lymphoblastoid cells; thus no immunoglobulin product in blood is associated with the disorder. These cells often will produce antibodies in culture. As aberrant B cells, Burkitt's lymphoma cells would be expected to contain unique or unusual antigens.

One of the novel antigens in Burkitt's cells is the EBV agent. Patients with the lymphoma have higher than normal levels of antibody to EBV capsid antigens and to cell membrane antigens of the lymphoma cells. They also possess high titers of EBV-neutralizing antibodies. In the examination of sera for EBV antibodies it was discovered that persons recently recovered from infectious mononucleosis were those with the highest titers. In fact 80% of Africans have EBV antibodies, although only a few have Burkitt's lymphoma. These antibodies do not differ from those found in patients with Burkitt's lymphoma. The links between infectious mononucleosis, Burkitt's lymphoma, and EBV are not yet completely understood, but their association is unique in viral oncogenesis. It may be that persons who develop infectious mononucleosis do so as the normal course of EBV virus infection. An unfortunate few are unable to respond in this normal way to the infection, and they develop Burkitt's lymphoma. Fortunately Burkitt's lymphoma is treatable with cytotoxic drugs, and spontaneous cures, evidence of a self-generated immunity, are known.

Genetic studies in Burkitt's lymphoma have revealed some exciting facts about the neoplastic origin of the disease and its relationship to immunoglobulin genetics. Approximately 75% of all Burkitt's patients demonstrate a translocation of a portion of chromosome 8 to chromosome 14 and vice versa (Fig. 15-5). Chromosome 8 normally contains a silent myc gene and chromosome 14 is the residence of the genes for the H chains of the immunoglobulins. The effect of this dual translocation is to place the myc gene under the influence of the H gene promoter, resulting in its activation. The remaining 25% of Burkitt's patients have a similar event occur between chromosome 8, and either chromosome 2 or 22. Chromosome 2 is the site of κ chain genes and chromosome 22 of λ chain genes.

Nasopharyngeal carcinoma

Another neoplastic disease associated with the EBV particle is nasopharyngeal carcinoma. This cancer is common in southern China but rare in other parts of the world, including central and northern China. Serologic studies of these patients have revealed that they more frequently have elevated titers to the EBV particle than do Burkitt's lymphoma patients. Unlike Burkitt's lymphoma, viral particles have not been observed in cells of patients with nasopharyngeal carcinoma, but viral DNA has been identified in these cells. The expression of EBV antigens, including EBNA and capsid and membrane antigens, occurs in the tumor cells.

Nasopharyngeal carcinoma and Burkitt's lymphoma are thus ideal candidates for the first human cancers to be induced by a virus, but the associations thus far established are not critical proof despite the knowledge that EBV is oncogenic for some laboratory animals. EBV could be an innocent passenger virus needed for the oncogenic expression of some as yet unidentified virus. In addition, environmental and genetic factors may be involved. This is suggested by the geographic distribution of the EBV-associated tumors and by the damage to chromosome 14 in Burkitt's lymphoma.

Human T cell leukemia viruses

In 1980 and 1981, the first isolations of a retrovirus from a small population of black subjects with a T cell lymphoma occurred. Shortly thereafter, the virus was isolated from cultured cells of several patients with adult T cell leukemia. Since then, a close association of the virus with leukemic patients in the endemic regions of Japan and the Carribean have been reported. In 1982, a second retrovirus virus, antigenically related to that discovered in adult T cell leukemia, was isolated from patients with hairy cell leukemia. In 1984, a third retrovirus antigenically related to the two just mentioned was isolated from patients with AIDS (see Chapter 20). Most investigators accept that these three, identified as HTLVI, II, and III, are capable of transforming T cells, the first two to a neoplastic state, and the third to a fatal state. HTLV III has recently been renamed as HIV—human immunodeficiency virus.

Carcinofetal antigens

A second type of TSA exists in the form of antigens known as carcinofetal, carcinoembryonic, or regression proteins. The synthesis of these proteins is unrelated to viral oncogenesis and is an expression of the metabolic shift of cancerous cells from an adult to an "immature" pathway of protein synthesis.

7 to 8. It has a molecular weight near 200,000 and exists as a β-glycoprotein with its major saccharide being *N*-acetylglucosamine. It is an unusual protein, since it contains 40% to 80% carbohydrate by weight. Its normal function in the fetus and the signal to halt or to renew synthesis in the malignant state are unknown.

Alpha fetoprotein

An α-globulin found in fetal serum but not in the adult serum of several species is known as the α-fetoprotein (AFP). The organ source of AFP is the liver. In fetal plasma AFP may reach a concentration of 3,000 ng/ml. Pregnancy sera levels may reach 500 ng/ml. The normal adult level is 5 to 10 ng/ml.

It now is recognized that nearly all primary hepatomas result in a metabolic shift of liver tissue to the fetal state and the synthesis of AFP. The detection of AFP, like that of CEA, is of potential diagnostic and prognostic significance in human oncology.

The history of AFP parallels closely that of CEA. At first relatively insensitive serologic procedures such as gel diffusion were used for its identification. This meant that rather significant quantities of the antigen had to be present in sera to produce a positive test. Such persons usually had hepatomas of substantial size so that positive tests for AFP correlated nicely with the incidence of hepatocarcinoma. With the development of RIA and the capacity to detect AFP in nanogram quantities per milliliter of serum it was found that AFP persisted in small quantities into adult life. Normal adult serum levels are only 5 to 10 ng/ml. AFP levels significantly above 10 ng/ml are considered a diagnostic level, are reached in 94% of patients with hepatoma and in 68% with teratoma. The diagnostic range is exceeded 12% of the time in patients with acute hepatitis, 67% with chronic hepatitis, and 49% with alcoholic cirrhosis. AFP also was detected above the normal level in some patients with extrahepatic tumors such as those of the stomach, lung, and pancreas and in patients with ataxia telangiectasia. AFP determinations as an aid to the diagnosis of liver cancer must be used in company with diagnostic aids for other forms of liver disease and for cancers of other organs.

AFP is a glycoprotein that behaves electrophoretically like an α_1-globulin. It has a molecular weight near 70,000, of which about 4% is carbohydrate. It is so similar in its biophysical properties to albumin that is has been difficult to secure the highly purified preparations needed to develop antisera for RIA.

The normal biologic function of AFP is unknown. The globulin fraction of serum is immunosuppressive, and this may have some importance to the maternal-fetal relationship and to the cancerous state. T lymphocytes bind AFP, and this may block proper recognition of antigen by T cells, thus allowing the cancer to grow.

A very successful use of AFP is in the monitoring of neural tube malformations (spina bifida) in fetuses by measuring the AFP level in amniotic fluid, which is normally 1.5 to 26 μg/ml at the fifteenth week of gestation. Excesses of this concentration correlate well with serious defects, including anenecephaly.

Other carcinofetal proteins

The α_2-hepatic protein (AHP), a globulin with a high iron content and synonymous with α_2-hepatic globulin or α_2-ferroglycoprotein, first was associated with cancer of the liver in 1965, when it was extracted from the hepatomas. AHP also is extractable from liver tissue of persons with tumors in other anatomic locations. Although 50% of adult cancer patients have positive RIA tests for α_2-hepatic ferroprotein in their serum, 20% of patients with nonmalignant disease are also positive. The figures are more impressive in juveniles with cancer: 80% of children with cancer have positive RIA tests for AHP versus an incidence of only 8% in healthy children. AHP and ferritin are closely related proteins. Both are found in liver, and both are rich in iron, with AHP containing 15% to 25% iron in the ferrous state. Ferritin also contains about 23% iron, but this is in the ferric state. The molecular weight of AHP is estimated at 600,000, and ferritin has a molecular weight of 465,000. The normal physiologic function, if any, of AHP is unknown, but it is believed to be identical to β-ferritin, a carcinofetal form of ferritin. A γ-ferroprotein also has been identified in fetal serum and in the serum of adults with malignancies.

A sulfated glycoprotein antigen that can be iso-

phoma cells. They also possess high titers of EBV-neutralizing antibodies. In the examination of sera for EBV antibodies it was discovered that persons recently recovered from infectious mononucleosis were those with the highest titers. In fact 80% of Africans have EBV antibodies, although only a few have Burkitt's lymphoma. These antibodies do not differ from those found in patients with Burkitt's lymphoma. The links between infectious mononucleosis, Burkitt's lymphoma, and EBV are not yet completely understood, but their association is unique in viral oncogenesis. It may be that persons who develop infectious mononucleosis do so as the normal course of EBV virus infection. An unfortunate few are unable to respond in this normal way to the infection, and they develop Burkitt's lymphoma. Fortunately Burkitt's lymphoma is treatable with cytotoxic drugs, and spontaneous cures, evidence of a self-generated immunity, are known.

Genetic studies in Burkitt's lymphoma have revealed some exciting facts about the neoplastic origin of the disease and its relationship to immunoglobulin genetics. Approximately 75% of all Burkitt's patients demonstrate a translocation of a portion of chromosome 8 to chromosome 14 and vice versa (Fig. 15-5). Chromosome 8 normally contains a silent myc gene and chromosome 14 is the residence of the genes for the H chains of the immunoglobulins. The effect of this dual translocation is to place the myc gene under the influence of the H gene promoter, resulting in its activation. The remaining 25% of Burkitt's patients have a similar event occur between chromosome 8, and either chromosome 2 or 22. Chromosome 2 is the site of κ chain genes and chromosome 22 of λ chain genes.

Nasopharyngeal carcinoma

Another neoplastic disease associated with the EBV particle is nasopharyngeal carcinoma. This cancer is common in southern China but rare in other parts of the world, including central and northern China. Serologic studies of these patients have revealed that they more frequently have elevated titers to the EBV particle than do Burkitt's lymphoma patients. Unlike Burkitt's lymphoma, viral particles have not been observed in cells of patients with nasopharyngeal carcinoma, but viral DNA has been identified in these cells. The expression of EBV antigens, including EBNA and capsid and membrane antigens, occurs in the tumor cells.

Nasopharyngeal carcinoma and Burkitt's lymphoma are thus ideal candidates for the first human cancers to be induced by a virus, but the associations thus far established are not critical proof despite the knowledge that EBV is oncogenic for some laboratory animals. EBV could be an innocent passenger virus needed for the oncogenic expression of some as yet unidentified virus. In addition, environmental and genetic factors may be involved. This is suggested by the geographic distribution of the EBV-associated tumors and by the damage to chromosome 14 in Burkitt's lymphoma.

Human T cell leukemia viruses

In 1980 and 1981, the first isolations of a retrovirus from a small population of black subjects with a T cell lymphoma occurred. Shortly thereafter, the virus was isolated from cultured cells of several patients with adult T cell leukemia. Since then, a close association of the virus with leukemic patients in the endemic regions of Japan and the Carribean have been reported. In 1982, a second retrovirus virus, antigenically related to that discovered in adult T cell leukemia, was isolated from patients with hairy cell leukemia. In 1984, a third retrovirus antigenically related to the two just mentioned was isolated from patients with AIDS (see Chapter 20). Most investigators accept that these three, identified as HTLVI, II, and III, are capable of transforming T cells, the first two to a neoplastic state, and the third to a fatal state. HTLV III has recently been renamed as HIV—human immunodeficiency virus.

Carcinofetal antigens

A second type of TSA exists in the form of antigens known as carcinofetal, carcinoembryonic, or regression proteins. The synthesis of these proteins is unrelated to viral oncogenesis and is an expression of the metabolic shift of cancerous cells from an adult to an "immature" pathway of protein synthesis.

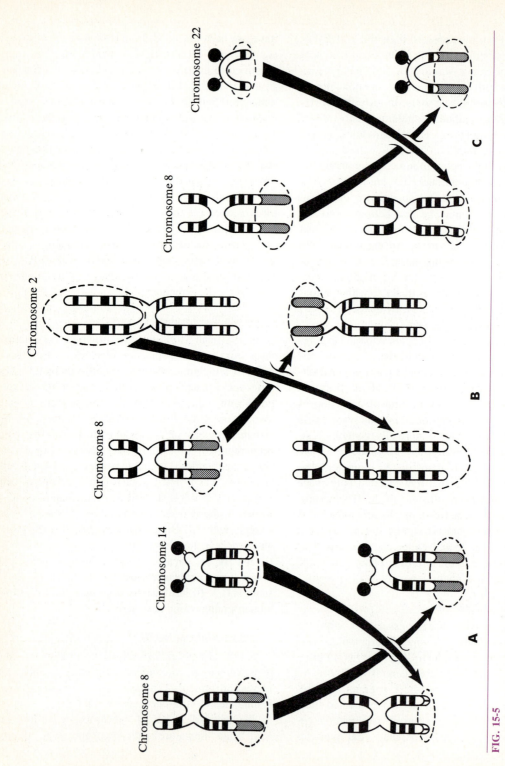

FIG. 15-5

The three panels in this illustration portray the chromosomal translocations that occur in Burkitt's lymphoma. **A** shows the rearrangement between chromosomes 14 and 8 that occurs in most patients. **B** and **C** represent changes seen in about 25% of the patients. In all three instances, the movement of a silent myc gene from chromosome 8 places it under an immunoglobulin chain promoter, leading to the malignancy.

The carcinofetal proteins are synthesized by normal fetal tissues and by tumors of these same tissues in adults. Whereas the TSAs are specific for a particular oncogenic virus, the carcinofetal proteins are not. Although once thought specific for anatomic locations of cancers, the carcinofetal antigens now are believed to be general expressions of cell reversion to a more primitive metabolic pathway (Table 15-5).

Carcinoembryonic antigen

In 1965 Gold and his co-workers began a series of investigations of an antigen they isolated from a human cancer of the colon. This antigen was not present in the normal tissue surrounding the tumor, but it was found in tumors of the digestive tract, including the small intestine, liver, pancreas, stomach, and rectum, in addition to the colon. This antigen also was found in human embryonic gut and gut-associated organs during the first two trimesters in utero, after which the antigen became more difficult to demonstrate. These facts led to the description of the antigen as the carcinoembryonic antigen (CEA).

Since the first descriptions of CEA based on immunodiffusion studies more and more sensitive serologic tests have been used to identify it. The current method of choice is radioimmunoassay (RIA). This test can identify nanogram quantities per milliliter of this antigen. One of the results is that a greater percentage of patients with gastrointestinal tumors can be identified as CEA positive, as follows: rectal and colonic, 56%; stomach, 67%; and liver and pancreas, 73%. At the same time it became evident that persons with other carcinomas were positive for CEA in significant percentages; breast cancer, 47%; prostate, 40%; lung, 77%; and gynecologic tumors as a group, 65%. These figures vary from study to study but reveal the nonspecificity of CEA for colonic tumors and gastrointestinal tumors and that CEA titrations might indicate cancer of a more expansive group of tissues. Unfortunately the use of CEA was further clouded by the finding that many nonmalignant conditions produced RIA-positive tests for CEA. These conditions include cigarette smoking (19% compared with 3% nonsmokers), chronic lung disease (57%), cirrhosis of the liver (45%), and ulcerative colitis (32%). Even 21% of healthy donors were positive in one report.

These data have not denied an important use of CEA in human medicine. It is now accepted that CEA titrations must be evaluated carefully in cancer diagnosis, and such tests may be a very useful prognostic index of the success of surgery or chemotherapy of cancer. The normal adult blood level of CEA is about 2.5 mg/L. Levels significantly higher than this are a good index of cancer and CEA levels usually become elevated 2 or 3 months before other signs of cancer become positive. Likewise, continued high levels of CEA, above 5 mg/L after therapy, are indicative of a poor prognosis. If preoperative CEA titers persist after surgery, it can be presumed that the surgery was incomplete. Perhaps significant metastases precluded a surgical cure of the patient. If the CEA titers fall and then rise, this would indicate a failure to completely remove the tumor, followed by its regrowth, CEA production, and an increase in titer. Similar evaluations would apply to the treatment of cancer with cytotoxic drugs.

The CEA antigen is a β-globulin with an $S_{20,w}$ of

TABLE 15-5

Characteristics of carcinofetal antigens

Synthesis	By embryonic and fetal tissues and cancers in adult tissues; fetal synthesis diminishes near birth
Source	Embryonic organs, cancerous organs, blood
Specificity	Slight specificity for organ system producing them
Chemistry	Proteins or glycoproteins; some are enzymes
Identification	Immunoassay with antisera rendered specific by adsorption with normal tissues
Value	Possibly in cancer diagnosis; definitely in prognosis

7 to 8. It has a molecular weight near 200,000 and exists as a β-glycoprotein with its major saccharide being *N*-acetylglucosamine. It is an unusual protein, since it contains 40% to 80% carbohydrate by weight. Its normal function in the fetus and the signal to halt or to renew synthesis in the malignant state are unknown.

Alpha fetoprotein

An α-globulin found in fetal serum but not in the adult serum of several species is known as the α-fetoprotein (AFP). The organ source of AFP is the liver. In fetal plasma AFP may reach a concentration of 3,000 ng/ml. Pregnancy sera levels may reach 500 ng/ml. The normal adult level is 5 to 10 ng/ml.

It now is recognized that nearly all primary hepatomas result in a metabolic shift of liver tissue to the fetal state and the synthesis of AFP. The detection of AFP, like that of CEA, is of potential diagnostic and prognostic significance in human oncology.

The history of AFP parallels closely that of CEA. At first relatively insensitive serologic procedures such as gel diffusion were used for its identification. This meant that rather significant quantities of the antigen had to be present in sera to produce a positive test. Such persons usually had hepatomas of substantial size so that positive tests for AFP correlated nicely with the incidence of hepatocarcinoma. With the development of RIA and the capacity to detect AFP in nanogram quantities per milliliter of serum it was found that AFP persisted in small quantities into adult life. Normal adult serum levels are only 5 to 10 ng/ml. AFP levels significantly above 10 ng/ml are considered a diagnostic level, are reached in 94% of patients with hepatoma and in 68% with teratoma. The diagnostic range is exceeded 12% of the time in patients with acute hepatitis, 67% with chronic hepatitis, and 49% with alcoholic cirrhosis. AFP also was detected above the normal level in some patients with extrahepatic tumors such as those of the stomach, lung, and pancreas and in patients with ataxia telangiectasia. AFP determinations as an aid to the diagnosis of liver cancer must be used in company with diagnostic aids for other forms of liver disease and for cancers of other organs.

AFP is a glycoprotein that behaves electrophoretically like an α₁-globulin. It has a molecular weight near 70,000, of which about 4% is carbohydrate. It is so similar in its biophysical properties to albumin that is has been difficult to secure the highly purified preparations needed to develop antisera for RIA.

The normal biologic function of AFP is unknown. The globulin fraction of serum is immunosuppressive, and this may have some importance to the maternal-fetal relationship and to the cancerous state. T lymphocytes bind AFP, and this may block proper recognition of antigen by T cells, thus allowing the cancer to grow.

A very successful use of AFP is in the monitoring of neural tube malformations (spina bifida) in fetuses by measuring the AFP level in amniotic fluid, which is normally 1.5 to 26 μg/ml at the fifteenth week of gestation. Excesses of this concentration correlate well with serious defects, including anenecephaly.

Other carcinofetal proteins

The α₂-hepatic protein (AHP), a globulin with a high iron content and synonymous with α₂-hepatic globulin or α₂-ferroglycoprotein, first was associated with cancer of the liver in 1965, when it was extracted from the hepatomas. AHP also is extractable from liver tissue of persons with tumors in other anatomic locations. Although 50% of adult cancer patients have positive RIA tests for α₂-hepatic ferroprotein in their serum, 20% of patients with nonmalignant disease are also positive. The figures are more impressive in juveniles with cancer: 80% of children with cancer have positive RIA tests for AHP versus an incidence of only 8% in healthy children. AHP and ferritin are closely related proteins. Both are found in liver, and both are rich in iron, with AHP containing 15% to 25% iron in the ferrous state. Ferritin also contains about 23% iron, but this is in the ferric state. The molecular weight of AHP is estimated at 600,000, and ferritin has a molecular weight of 465,000. The normal physiologic function, if any, of AHP is unknown, but it is believed to be identical to β-ferritin, a carcinofetal form of ferritin. A γ-ferroprotein also has been identified in fetal serum and in the serum of adults with malignancies.

A sulfated glycoprotein antigen that can be iso-

lated with a high frequency from stomach cancers is a TSA also found in fetal tissues. This fetal sulfoglycoprotein is antigenically related to CEA.

Several enzymes described as carcinoplacental or carcinoembryonic enzymes and originating from trophoblastic tissues have been associated with a broad range of cancers. The best known of these are the isozymes of alkaline phosphatase, particularly the Regan isozyme. This enzyme is present in the sera of persons with various forms of cancer and is not restricted to those with placental or trophoblastic tissue tumors, although the enzyme from all these sources is indistinguishable from the enzyme produced by normal placenta. The enzyme is present in about 20% of persons with cancer. Other isozymes associated with cancerous states include aldolase, glycogen phosphorylase, glucosamine 6-phosphate synthetase, and amino acid transaminase. Virtually all these have been studied in relation to hepatomas. As the hepatoma develops, there is an expression of altered gene behavior in the excretion of the fetal isozyme form of each of the isozymes just mentioned. The adult or mature isozyme is produced by the remaining normal liver tissue, but when electrophoretic and immunologic studies are performed, the shift toward the immature carcinofetal type of enzyme is detectable.

TUMOR IMMUNITY
Immune surveillance and immune enhancement

There is no single satisfactory explanation for the success of tumors in escaping the rejection process. Many theories have been forwarded, practically all of which have been based on immunologic observations surrounding the development of a limited number of neoplastic conditions. Many of the earlier hypotheses were naive and have been discarded. For example, it was suggested that cancerous tissue was nonantigenic and that tumors lost their antigens, thereby escaping the host's immunologic defense system. Certain tumors do definitely lose some of their antigenic components, for example, tumors of endocrine tissue often lose their ability to produce hormones. It is also known that the normal histocompatibility antigens may be more diluted on the surface of tumor cells as they are replaced or crowded out by TSTA, but these are examples of antigenic drift and not of total nonantigenicity. Antigenic drift also has been suggested as an escape mechanism for tumors, but it is doubtful that this antigenic change is sufficiently rapid to protect the cancer cells from the host's immune response.

In transfer experiments it is known that the quantity of tumor tissue injected is very instrumental in predicting cancer development. Low doses of tumor cells are easily eliminated; larger doses are not. When an animal acquires the ability to reject a small dose of tumor cells, it usually is equipped to reject continually larger and larger doses. This information has been used to support the concept of specific immunologic tolerance as the means for graft survival. The hypothesis is that a sufficiently large dose of tumor cells inoculated into an animal deletes the normally expected rejection response. These is good evidence that tumor patients do not respond to their tumor antigens. Only a low percentage of these patients produce circulating antibodies in any quantity to the tumor antigens, and their lymphocytes tend not to be cytotoxic to tumor tissue in vitro.

The emergence of tumors is regularly cited as evidence of a failure of the immune surveillance system. Immunologists are reluctant to accept this and cite the possibility that the body may be producing oncogenic cells every day. For weeks, months, or years the immune surveillance system successfully contains these aggressive cells. Then on a later single occasion when this does not occur, the immune surveillance system is described as faulty.

Recent evidence with hybridoma antibodies originally believed to be specific for tumor antigens has revealed an unexpected incidence of cross-reactions with normal tissues. This has raised the question as to whether true TSTAs actually exist. Perhaps tumors have only an uneven distrubution of normal antigens, with greater concentrations of some and lower concentrations of others, which has given the appearance of a unique antigenic composition. This cannot be answered until more definitive studies of the specificity of these antitumor hybridomas are completed, but if these indicators prove true, then the immune surveillance system cannot be expected to control cancer.

Hellström KE & Hellström I.

Lymphocyte-mediated cytotoxicity and blocking serum activity to tumor antigens.

Advan. Immunol. **18**:209-77, 1974.   [Depts. Pathology, Microbiology, and Immunology, Univ. Washington Medical School, Seattle, WA]

This paper reviews evidence that lymphocytes from animals and human patients with tumor are specifically reactive to cells from the same tumor in vitro *and that their reactivity can be prevented by circulating 'blocking factors' such as tumor antigens and antigen-antibody complexes. [The SCI® indicates that this paper has been cited a total of 653 times of which 8 occurred in 1974, 74 in 1975, 119 in 1976, 113 in 1977, 126 in 1978, 87 in 1979, 66 in 1980, and 60 in 1981.]*

Karl Erik Hellström and Ingegerd Hellström
Fred Hutchinson Cancer Research Center
University of Washington
1124 Columbia Street
Seattle, WA 98104

January 25, 1982

"In 1966, we both started working at the University of Washington Medical School in Seattle, having left George Klein's group at the Karolinska Institute in Stockholm, where we got our training. The project on which we embarked concerned lymphocyte reactivity to tumor-associated antigens as assayed *in vitro*.

"We found, rather to our surprise, that lymphocytes from mice with growing, chemically induced sarcomas were often as reactive to cells from the same sarcomas *in vitro* as were lymphocytes from mice whose tumors had been removed. Similar findings were made with other experimentally induced tumors and with human neoplasms.

In an attempt to learn why tumors can grow progressively *in vivo*, in spite of the fact that the tumor-bearing individuals' lymphocytes can kill plated tumor cells *in vitro*, we tested serum from the respective tumor-bearers for any adverse effect on the ability of the lymphocytes to react. We observed that tumor-bearer serum could suppress ('block') lymphocyte reactivity, and we attributed this to circulating 'specific blocking factors.'[1] These factors were able to bind to tumor cells from the donors of the respective sera and they disappeared shortly after tumor removal. In 1971, we obtained evidence that the circulating blocking factors were circulating antigen-antibody complexes and that free antigen could also serve as a blocking factor.[2]

"The findings that we had obtained were confirmed and extended in other laboratories.[3] They contradicted the prevailing view that lymphocyte clones that are reactive to a given tumor antigen are absent ('forbidden') from the tumor-bearing host. They indicated, instead, that lymphocyte reactivity must be regulated, and we proposed that the 'blocking factors' play an intricate part in this regulation. Further evidence supporting the view of regulation of lymphocyte activity rather than clonal loss came from studies which we performed on rats that had been made tolerant to skin allografts. These rats had lymphocytes that were reactive *in vitro* to the tolerated tissue, and they also had circulating blocking factors, inhibiting this reactivity.[4]

"Our 1974 paper in *Advances in Immunology* reviewed these findings. We believe that the reason our paper has been much cited reflects both the great amount of interest and the considerable controversy which our rather unexpected observations caused. Today, it is generally accepted that reactive lymphocytes occur in tumor-bearing animals, that their activity is subject to close regulation, that blocking factors in the form of tumor antigens and complexes turn on suppressor T cells, and that other blocking factors are the products of such cells.[5] The greatest advancement since 1973 is that it has become possible, using proper cell surface markers, to dissect subsets of lymphocytes with distinct functions, while in 1974 we did not know of NK cells and of various types of T killer, helper, and suppressor cells. Thus, the phenomenological framework in which we and others were then working is gradually being replaced by knowledge at the cellular and even at the molecular level."

1. Hellström I, Hellström KE, Evans CA, Heppner G, Pierce GE & Yang JPS. Serum mediated protection of neoplastic cells from inhibition by lymphocytes immune to their tumor specific antigens. *Proc. Nat. Acad. Sci. US* **62**:362-9, 1969.
2. Sjögren HO, Hellström I, Bansal SC & Hellström KE. Suggesting evidence that the 'blocking antibodies' of tumor bearing individuals may be antigen-antibody complexes *Proc. Nat. Acad. Sci. US* **68**:1372-5, 1971.
3. Baldwin RW, Price MR & Robins RA. Inhibition of hepatoma-immune lymph node cell cytotoxicity by tumor-bearer serum, and solubilized hepatoma antigen. *Int. J. Cancer* **11**:527-35, 1973.
4. Bansal SC, Hellström KE, Hellström I & Sjögren HO. Cell-mediated immunity and blocking serum activity to tolerated allografts in rats. *J Exp. Med.* **137**:590-602, 1973.
5. Hellström KE & Brown JP. Tumor antigens. (Sela M. ed.) *The antigens*. New York. Academic Press, 1979. Vol. 5. p. 1-82

The recognized anergic state of many T cell-dependent responses in cancer patients, some of which can be overcome with adoptive immunization and transfer factor treatment, indicates that tumors themselves may be immunosuppressive. The chemically induced fibrosarcoma in the A/J mouse strain elicits a potent Ts response that, when negated by anti-J protein serum, decreases the rate of tumor growth. Even alterations of macrophage metabolism may abet rather than hinder tumor growth. Activated macrophages release argininase, an enzyme with a long history as an immunosuppressant because of its degradation of arginine, which is required by lymphocytes. Oxidation of free amino groups of protein or of amino acids by macrophage polyamine oxidase creates aldehyde groups that possess a cytostatic effect by reacting with nucleic acids.

To these suggestions, we also can add immunologic enhancement as a means of encouraging tumor survival. Immune enhancement can be defined as the enhancement of tumor growth by specific antibodies. This phenomenon stands in contrast to immunologic tolerance, in which specific antibodies and sensitized T lymphocytes simply are not formed in response to an antigen. Although immune enhancement could be applied to many situations such as the fetus as an allograft and to normal graft rejection or survival, it is considered here only as it may be applied to tumor immunology.

Immune enhancement was discovered through the transplantation of tumors to recipients that had been preimmunized to produce circulating antibodies to the tumor tissue. Rather than observing a hastened rejection and elimination of the tumor, it was noted that the tumor had an increased growth rate. Further experiments of this type in laboratory animals have been supported by human studies which have demonstrated conclusively that certain immunoglobulins were not cytotoxic but were growth promoting instead. These antibodies have been purified and have the following characteristics: (1) sedimentation values and molecular size consistent with their inclusion among the IgG antibodies, (2) an enhancing activity when in low titer or when transferred in small quantities to a recipient, but a cytotoxic activity when present in high titer, (3) a failure to appear in the cir-culation until several days or a few weeks after exposure to tumor antigens (this is typical of IgG), (4) an antigenic specificity typical of all antibodies that can be measured by fluorescent antibody studies which detect the enhancing antibody bound to tumor cells, and (5) a high avidity for antigens on the tumor cell surface.

Several of these features have been incorporated into a theory that does much to explain the immune enhancement phenomenon. First, the enhancing antibody may be considered as an immunosuppressor via the mechanism of feedback inhibition, which prevents the formation of more actively cytolytic antibodies. Second, it may attach to the tumor cells, and because of its high avidity, it may create a firm antigen-antibody complex, which serves as a physical blockade to prevent the attachment of cytolytic antibodies. In this sense enhancing antibodies can be listed among the blocking antibodies. If the host response to tumor antigens is dictated by genetic control mechanisms to produce large amounts of cytolytic antibody and low amounts of enhancing antibody, the tumor regresses. In the opposite circumstance the tumor growth is enhanced.

Cells active in tumor immunity

As might be expected from the previous paragraphs, combined with the knowledge that cells dominate the rejection process that leads to the elimination of foreign tissue, cells rather than immunoglobulins are believed to dominate tumor immunity. The LGL cells, ADCC effector cells, and cytotoxic T cells all participate.

LGL cells are present in nude mice, which are T cell deficient, and unlike T cells, LGL cells need no previous exposure to antigens of the target cell before they become active. LGL cells are not target cell or antigen specific, although their indiscriminate activity could result from the combined activity of several LGL subsets, each of which has a restricted target cell specificity. Another distinguishing feature is that target cells are more quickly destroyed by LGL cells than by T cells.

Among the criteria supporting a tumoricidal role for LGL cells is (1) their presence in nude mice and the surprising resistance of nude mice to transplantable tumors in view of their lack of T cells, (2) the decreased numbers of LGL cells in the beige mouse line coupled with its heightened sensitivity to tumors, (3) the loss of LGL cells as mice age concomitant with an increased incidence of tumors, and (4) the protection against transplantable tumors afforded by adoptive immunization with an enriched population of LGL cells.

The cytotoxic activity of specific antibody acting with any of several cell types has been labeled anti-

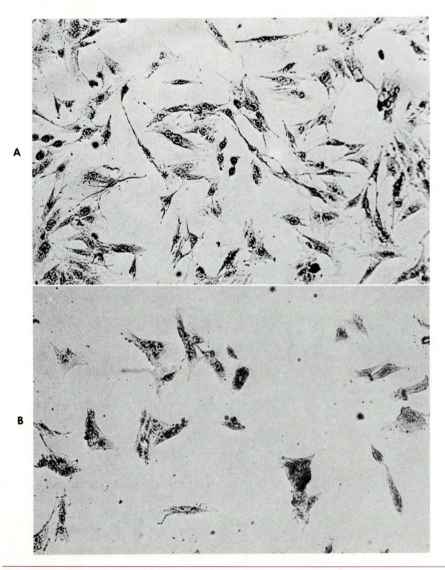

FIG. 15-6

The effects of cytotoxic lymphocytes on tumor cells can be seen here. **A,** The tumor cells prior to contact with the immune lymphocytes. **B,** The tumor cells after this contact. Notice that many cells have detached from the surface, some cells are swollen, and few cells show the morphology of the normal cells. (Courtesy Dr. J. Berkelhammer.)

body-dependent cell cytotoxicity (ADCC). The antibody is usually, if not always, an IgG and may be of any subclass. Complement is often present in the assay but is not required. The major source of confusion about the ADCC test is in deciding which cells contribute to target cell lysis. It is generally agreed that the effector cell must have receptors for Fc regions of IgG. Macrophages and granulocytes, especially neutrophils, have these receptors and are accepted as participants in ADCC; platelets and B cells do not participate even though they have Fc receptors. Macrophages and neutrophils do not phagocytose the target cell during ADCC and must be cytocidal by other means. Since these cells undergo the oxidative burst typical of activated phagocytes when they contact the target cell, ADCC may result from the secretion of toxic forms of oxygen.

Certain lymphocytes that cannot be identified as T or B cells are active in ADCC. These cells lack the Thy 1 antigens typical of T cells and are devoid of surface immunoglobulin characteristic of B cells. These cells have been described as null cells to reflect their independence from both B and T cells. They also have been designated as K cells to reflect their killer activity on foreign cells.

The cytotoxic T cells, prior to exposure to antigen, have no inherent cytocidal activity. Just as is the case with the ADCC active cells, T_C participates in the acquired phase of tumor immunity, not in natural resistance to tumors. The sensitized T_C cell is able to recognize the foreign nature of the TSTA in association with self class I MHC determinants and attack the tumor cell (Figs. 15-6, 15-7, and 15-8). Histologic examination of tumors will often demonstrate an infiltration of T_C lymphocytes. It is believed that these cells release lymphotoxins, or other cytotoxic lymphokines, in an effort to remove the tumor cells. Certainly, these tumor infiltrating lymphocytes are more effective versus tumors in culture than are peripheral blood lymphocytes.

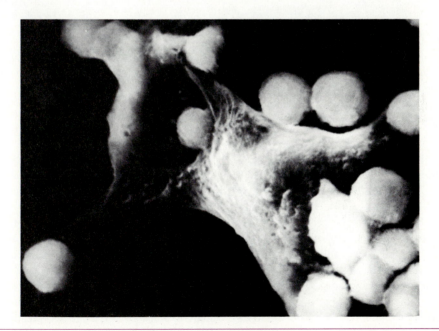

FIG. 15-7
The white spheres seen in this scanning electron microscope view are T lymphocytes attacking a much larger Walker carinoma cell. T lymphocytes are a significant part of our defense against foreign, including cancer, cells. (Courtesy Dr. E. Adelstein.)

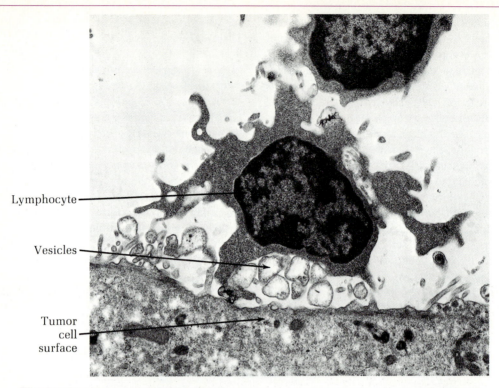

Lymphocyte

Vesicles

Tumor
cell
surface

FIG. 15-8

Transmission electron microscopy reveals the initial stages of the attack of a cytotoxic lymphocyte on a tumor cell, only a portion of which is seen. Notice the vesicles and blebs of cytoplasm that are being shed by the lymphocyte. (Courtesy Dr. E. Adelstein.)

Immunotherapy
Adjuvant therapy

One avenue of tumor immunotherapy is the catalysis of natural resistance through nonspecific immunization with BCG vaccine (an attenuated strain of *Mycobacterium tuberculosis* variety *bovis*). Cell fractions of the BCG organism and other potentiators of nonspecific resistance such as *Propionibacterium acnes* also can be used successfully. The greatest success with these vaccines applied as nonspecific adjuvants has been observed when the vaccine is deposited in the immediate vicinity of the tumor. Within a few weeks the tumor can be observed to diminish in size, and this regression continues in some instances until the tumor is no longer detectable. Intradermal BCG vaccination near melanomas on the skin has proved successful in both experimental animals and humans. This therapeutic mode is unsuccessful for disseminated or internally located tumors.

Five separate mechanisms have been advanced to explain the immunopotentiation of tumor immunity by BCG vaccine. These include (1) the enhancement of macrophage cytotoxicity, (2) a stimulation of lymphocyte trapping, (3) an activation of T lymphocytes, (4) a direct influence on B lymphocytes, and (5) the existence of shared antigens between the mycobacteria and certain tumors. There is evidence to support each of these. When the ability of macrophages from BCG-vaccinated, tumor-bearing animals to release ^{51}Cr from isotopically labeled cells was compared with the same activity of normal macrophages, it was found that the immune macrophages were twice as active. It was necessary to harvest the macrophages at 14 days after BCG immunization to show this effect, which was very time dependent.

When ^{51}Cr lymphocytes were infused into BCG-treated and normal animals, the amount of radioactivity in lymph nodes in the region of the subcutaneous injection of BCG increased sharply for up to 35 days after immunization until it reached three times the values observed in the normal animals. No such effect was noted in the contralateral lymph nodes or when the BCG vaccine was given intravenously. Local trapping of lymphocytes is presumed to ensure their exposure to tumor antigens that drain into the lymphatic system near the tumor.

Although the experimental efficacy of BCG vaccination as an antitumor agent is well established, how well it works in human cancers other than melanoma is still to be determined. Two approaches have indicated limited success. One of these was a retrospective comparison of a large population of blacks in Chicago for their incidence of death from cancer and leukemia and their status as BCG vaccinates. Of 83,356 subjects who had received BCG, 13 deaths were attributed to leukemia and other forms of cancer, for a rate of 1.2 per 100,000. The "non-BCG group" consisted of 534,820 persons. Their cancer mortality was 4.4 per 100,000, or a total of 306 deaths. Although environmental factors were beyond control, both groups were of the same race, encompassed the same socioeconomic groups, and were from the same area of the city.

BCG vaccination of patients with active malignant lymphoma or acute myelogenous leukemia was not helpful. However, in one study of 100 patients with acute lymphoid leukemia no relapses were observed in a 48-month follow-up period after BCG and chemotherapy. With the chemotherapy alone the relapse rate was 35% in the same period.

Immunotoxins

A novel approach to immunotherapy that has proven exceptionally effective against dispersed tumors is the use of immunotoxins. Immunotoxins are conjugates of an antibody and a toxin. Several different toxins have been used, including ricin, abrin, and diphtheria toxin. These toxins are of the A-B type in which A is the active, toxic part of the molecule, and B is a cell binding portion (Fig. 15-9). Diphtheria toxin kills cells that it enters by causing a ribosylation of peptide elongation factor 2 (EF2)

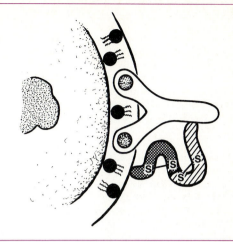

FIG. 15-9

This immunotoxin is a conjugate of an immunoglobulin versus a TSTA of a tumor cell and diphtheria toxin. The cell-binding portion of the bacterial toxin enhances entrance of the complex into the cell, which is then killed by the toxin.

which renders it inactive and halts protein synthesis.

In a limited number of human patients with leukemia or lymphoma, it has been possible to remove bone marrow, then lethally irradiate the patient, often simultaneously adding cytotoxic drug therapy. The bone marrow is purged of tumor cells by incubation with an immunotoxin and then re-implanted. Six patients with adult T cell leukemia have been treated in this way and two escaped the early relapse that affected the other four. Eleven patients with a B cell type non-Hodgkin's lymphoma have been so treated, and six had no relapse within 14 months, the normal time for relapse to occur after other treatments.

Immunotoxins may be useful in bone marrow transplants, since it should be possible to remove the T_C cells responsible for graft versus host reactions.

LAK

Peripheral blood lymphocytes exposed in culture to IL-1 and/or IL-2 and IFN have been reinfused into animals with cancers. These lymphokine-activated killer or LAK cells have effected a few cures and have been especially valuable in preventing metastases. Human trials are now in progress.

REFERENCES

Althouse, R., and others, editors: Some antineoplastic and immunosuppressive agents, Switzerland, 1981, International Agency for Research on Cancer, WHO.

Blasecki, J.W., editor: Mechanisms of immunity to virus-induced tumors, New York, 1981, Marcel Dekker, Inc.

Boss, B.D., Langman, R., Trowbridge, R., and Dulbecco, R., editors: Monoclonal antibodies and cancer, Orlando, 1983, Academic Press, Inc.

Bril, H., and Benner, R.: Graft vs. host reactions: mechanisms and contemporary theories, CRC Crit. Revs. Clin. Lab. Sci. 22:43, 1985.

Calne, R.Y., editor: Transplantation immunology. Clinical and experimental, Oxford, 1984, Oxford University Press.

Ceriani, R.L., editor: Monoclonal antibodies and breast cancer, Boston, 1985, Martinus Nijhoff Publishers.

Cohen, D.J., and others: Cyclosporine: a new immunosuppressive agent for organ transplantation, Ann. Intern. Med. 101:667, 1984.

Evered, D., and Whelan, J., editors: Fetal antigens and cancer, London, 1983, Pitman Books, Ltd.

Fefer, A., and Goldstein, A.L., editors: The potential role of T cells in cancer therapy, New York, 1982, Raven Press.

Foon, K.A., and Morgan, A.C., Jr., editors: Monoclonal antibody therapy of human cancer, Boston, 1985, Martinus Nijhoff Publishers.

Gill, T.G., III: Immunity and pregnancy, CRC Crit. Rev. Immunol. 5:201, 1985.

Hall, B.M., and Dorsch, S.E.: Cells mediating allograft rejection, Immunol. Rev. 77:31, 1984.

Hancock, B.W., and Ward, A.M., editors: Immunological aspects of cancer, Boston, 1984, Martinus Nijhoff Publishing.

Herberman, R.B., editor: Cancer immunology: innovative approaches to therapy, Boston, 1986, Martinus Nijhoff Publishers.

Herberman, R.B., Reynolds, C.W., and Ortaldo, J.: Mechanisms of cytotoxicity by natural killer (NK) cells, Immunol. Rev. 4:651, 1986.

Jacoby, D.R., Olding, L.B., and Oldstone, M.B.A.: Immunologic regulation of fetal-maternal balance, Adv. Immunol. 35:157, 1984.

Jones, S.E., and Salmon, S.E., editors: Adjuvant therapy of cancer IV, Orlando, 1984, Grune and Stratton, Inc.

Mason, D.W., and Morris, P.J.: Effector mechanisms in allograft rejection, Ann. Rev. Immunol. 4:119, 1986.

Mitchell, M.S., and Oettgen, H.F., editors: Hybridomas in cancer diagnosis and treatment, New York, 1982, Raven Press Books, Ltd.

Nieburgs, H.E., Birkmayer, G.D., and Klavins, J.V., editors: Human tumor markers, New York, 1983, Alan R. Liss, Inc.

North, R.J.: The murine antitumor immune response and its therapeutic manipulation, Adv. Immunol. 35:89, 1984.

Purtilo, D.T., editor: Immune deficiency and cancer, New York, 1984, Plenum Publishing Corporation.

Ray, P.K., editor: Immunobiology of transplantation, cancer and pregnancy, New York, 1983, Pergamon Press, Inc.

Reisfeld, R.A., Harper, J.R., and Bumol. T.F.: Human tumor-associated antigens defined by monoclonal antibodies, CRC Crit. Rev. Immunol. 5:27, 1984.

Reisfeld, R.A., and Ferrone, S., editors: Melanoma antigens and antibodies, New York, 1982, Plenum Press.

Reisfeld, R.A., and Sell, S., editors: Monoclonal antibodies and cancer therapy, New York, 1985, Alan R. Liss, Inc.

Riviere, G.R., and Hildemann, W.H., editors: Oral immunogenetics and tissue transplantation, New York, 1982, Elsevier North Holland, Inc.

Rogers, G.T.: Carcinoembryonic antigens and related glycoproteins. Molecular aspects and specificity, Biochim. Biophys. Acta. 695:227, 1983.

Schatten, S., Granstein, R.D., Drebin, J.A., and Greene, M.I.: Suppressor T cells and the immune response to tumors, CRC Crit. Rev. Immunol. 4:335, 1984.

Sell, S., and Wahren, B., editors: Human cancer markers, Clifton, NJ, 1982, The Humana Press, Inc.

Serrou, B., and Rosenfeld, C., editors: Human lymphocyte differentiation: its application to cancer, Amsterdam, 1978, Elsevier/North-Holland Publishing Co.

Serrou, B., and Rosenfeld, C., editors: Suppressor cells in human cancer, Amsterdam, 1981, Elsevier/North-Holland Press.

Serrou, B., Rosenfeld, C., Daniels, J.C., and Saunders, J.P., editors: Current concepts in human immunology and cancer immunomodulation, Amsterdam, 1982, Elsevier Biomedical Press.

Shevach, E.: The effects of cyclosporin A on the immune response, Ann. Rev. Immunol. 3:297, 1985.

Shively, J.E., and Beatty, J.D.: CEA-related antigens: molecular biology and clinical significance, CRC Crit. Rev. Oncol. Hematol. 2:355, 1985.

Sikora, K., editor: Interferon and cancer, New York, 1983, Plenum Press.

Sulitzeanu, D.: Human cancer-associated antigens: present status and implications for immunodiagnosis, Adv. Cancer Res.44:1, 1985.

Tiwari, J.L., and Terasaki, P.I.: HLA and disease associations, New York, 1985, Springer-Verlag New York, Inc.

Tosato, G., and Blaese, R.M.: Epstein-Barr virus infection and immunoregulation in man, Adv. Immunol. 37:99, 1985.

Vitetta, E.S., and Uhr, J.W.: Immunotoxins, Ann. Rev. Immunol. 3:197, 1985.

Waters, H., editor: Tumor antigens: structure and function, New York, 1981, Garland STPM Press.

Welsh, R.M.: Natural killer cells and interferon, CRC Crit. Rev. Immunol. 5:55, 1984.

Zmijewski, C.M.: HLA and disease, CRC Crit. Rev. Clin. Lab. Sci. 20:285, 1984.

See related **Reading 8,** page 434.

IMMUNOPATHOLOGY

Introduction to allergy

≡ GLOSSARY

allergen A substance (antigen or hapten) that causes an allergy, that is, stimulates IgE synthesis or causes a delayed hypersensivity.

allergy An altered state of reactivity to an antigen or hapten; used synonymously with *hypersensitivity*.

anaphylactic allergy An allergy caused by IgE.

anergy The inability to respond to an antigen, especially in the allergic sense.

cytotoxic allergy An allergy dependent on an antibody- and complement-mediated cell toxicity.

delayed hypersensitivity Synonym of *cell-mediated hy-*

persensitivity; a form of allergy expressed by T lymphocytes, not involving immunoglobulins, and developing slowly when provoked dermally.

hypersensitivity An unexpected, exaggerated reaction to an antigen or hapten.

immediate hypersensitivities Allergies relatable to IgE, or similar immunoglobulins in lower species, such as hay fever, food allergies, and certain drug allergies.

immune complex disease A disease caused by or associated with the formation of antigen-antibody complexes, for example, glomerulonephritis and serum sickness.

T cell–mediated allergy An allergy expressed by antigen-sensitized T cells.

IMMUNOLOGIC BASIS OF THE HYPERSENSITIVITIES

Immunization and the formation of antibodies does not uniformly lead to a state of resistance or immunity. This is most obvious when the antigen employed in the immunization has nothing to do with infectious organisms or their toxins: for example, immunizations with bovine γ-globulin, sheep red blood cells, or ragweed pollen. Many times the synthesis of specific immunoglobulins and the later reaction of these antibodies with the antigen can be detrimental to the host's well-being. In such cases the immunization may be referred to as a sensitization, which more accurately describes the result of the antigenic exposure than does immunization. Whether the term *immunization* or *sensitization* is used is largely dependent on the response of the treated animal to a subsequent exposure to antigen and not to any substantial difference in the cellular and chemical events that follow the injection of the antigen. Certain manipulative procedures such as the administration of rather small quantities of an antigen may favor sensitization by restricting the quantity of antibody formed, but this only emphasizes that the difference between immunization and sensitization is more quantitative than qualitative.

The untoward or unusual reaction that is seen following the second exposure of the animal to the antigen reveals the existence of the sensitization. This is the allergic or hypersensitive response. *Allergy* is defined as an altered ability to react; in immunology this means an altered reactivity to an antigen or a hapten. Strictly interpreted, *hypersensitivity* means a heightened reactivity and is not synonymous with *allergy,* but on the basis of common usage the terms are interchangeable. Hyposensitivity is defined as a condition of diminished reactivity, and anergy refers to an absolute failure to react when a reaction otherwise would be expected.

Allergic or hypersensitive responses are unquestionably immunologic in origin. The initial stage in their development is an exposure to an antigen or an autocomplexing hapten. This is the sensitizing exposure. The animal is not immediately capable of displaying its sensitivity; an immunologic waiting period of 5 to 10 days must elapse before the sensitization is expressible. This is the interlude customarily associated with the production of antibodies. After the animal is sensitive, the sensitivity can be demonstrated by the injection of a second, or shocking, dose of antigen. The manifestation of shock will vary according to the condition used to elicit it, including the kind of sensitivity the animal has developed, the route, form, and dosage of antigen, plus other variables. Provided the shock has been of sufficient yet sublethal intensity, the animal will progress into a temporary state of hyposensitivity. This condition can be induced deliberately, without serious harm to the animal; it is described as desensitization.

In all these events (sensitization, shocking, and desensitization) the ground rules of immunologic specificity apply. Antigenic and haptenic materials are required for sensitization. The shocking dose is ineffectual until an immunologic waiting period has expired. The shocking antigen must be the one initially used in the sensitization or one that is serologically cross-reactive with that antigen. Specific desensitization is possible only with the sensitizing antigen or known cross-reacting antigens. These factors all point to an immunologic origin of the hypersensitivities.

CLASSIFICATION OF THE HYPERSENSITIVITIES
Immunoglobulin relationships

The immunoglobulins that are associated with allergic diseases fall into two classes: the heat-stable and the heat-labile immunoglobulins (Table 16-1). The heat-stable antibodies are the ordinary immunoglobulins considered in detail earlier (Chapter 3) and represented by IgG, IgA, and IgM. It is uncertain what role IgD may take in the hypersensitivities. The "classic" immunoglobulins resist destruction when held at 56° to 60° C for periods of 30 minutes to 4 hours.

TABLE 16-1

Comparison of the properties of classic immunoglobulins and IgE

	Classic immunoglobulins	IgE
Immunoglobulins included	IgG, IgA, IgM, IgD (?)	IgE (reagin)
Stability at 56° to 60° for 30 minutes to 4 hours	Stable	Labile
In vitro reactions with antigens	Yes: precipitation, agglutination, complement fixation, etc.	Combination but no directly observable reaction
Associated class of allergy	Cytotoxic and immune complex	Immediate or atopic
Types of antigens involved	Ordinary, including hapten-antigen conjugates, cellular for cytotoxic reactions, soluble for immune complex reactions	Chemistry poorly understood but probably not unusual, often in a cellular form (spores, pollens, etc.)
Placental passage	IgG	No; does not pass to fetus from mother
Fixation to skin on passive transfer	Relatively short time	Relatively long time (several days)
Desensitization	Difficult, seldom attempted	Yes, by hyperimmunization to form blocking antibody; temporary

Allergies caused by IgG can be passively transferred through the placenta. When passive transfer is made with serum from the allergic individual to the skin of a normal individual, it is found that these antibodies remain fixed to the skin for only a few hours. During this time a local skin reaction can be produced in the recipient by the injection of the offending antigen into the skin site, but thereafter the dermis returns to its usual nonreactive state typical of the nonallergic individual.

The term *reagin* was used prior to 1970 to describe a heat-labile (56° to 60° C for up to 3 hours) serum reagent, immunoglobulin-like in nature, that was correlated with a second type of hypersensitivity. Now reagin has been positively identified as IgE. IgE is responsible for the immediate type hypersensitivity reactions including hay fever, food allergies, insect sting allergies, and the atopic allergies. The word *atopy* means foreign, unusual, or out of place and indicates that the allergy has arisen from a rare or even unknown antigenic stimulus. Now it is generally agreed that the IgE-dependent allergies result from natural oral or respiratory immunizations from food- or air-borne antigens.

Since IgE does not pass the placental barrier, an allergic mother will not give birth to a passively sensitized child. The child may have a hereditary disposition to form IgE against naturally occurring antigens in the environment because of his or her inheritance of specific Ir genes. Passive transfer of serum IgE from sensitized individuals to the skin or normal persons will sensitize the recipient for several days after the transfer, that is, IgE fixes for relatively long periods to the skin on transfer. Desensitization of the atopic allergies is dependent on the production of high levels of circulating immunoglobulins of the usual type. In this instance these antibodies which minimize or prevent the allergy are referred to as blocking antibodies.

Temporal relationships

The hypersensitivities traditionally have been separated on the basis of the time they appear after exposure to the shocking dose of antigen. On this basis there are two types of hypersensitivities: immediate and delayed. The immediate hypersensitivities are IgE mediated, whereas the delayed, or cell-mediated, allergies depend on the activities of sensitized T cells. Decades of study have revealed that immediate and delayed hypersensitivities differ in more fundamental respects than the times of their appearance (Table 16-2). Hypersensitivities also are classified on an immunopathologic basis (Table 16-3).

Immediate hypersensitivity

The immediate response appears within a few seconds or a few minutes after the administration of the shocking dose of antigen. This reaction fades or disappears rapidly so that in a few hours there may be no obvious external indication that the reaction even occurred. If a systemic response is evoked by the shocking dose of antigen, the symptoms of the immediate hypersensitivity will be noted to affect special target tissues. The exact tissue involved will vary but usually will include smooth muscle. These reactions may terminate fatally, so care must be taken to prevent their development.

The immediate allergic reaction results from the presence of specific IgE in the sensitized individual. For this reason cells are involved in creating the sensitivity only in the requirement of plasma cells to produce the antibody. This means that the sensitivity can be passively transferred by serum. It also means that, to demonstrate an immediate hypersensitivity on a local or an isolated tissue basis, a vascularized tissue must be chosen. If this tissue is skin, and if the change in histology of the reaction site is observed over a period of time, it will be noted that neutrophils migrate quickly into the affected tissue. Eosinophils also aggregate in large numbers. Mononuclear cells are relatively rare early but increase in number later in the reaction sequence. This skin reaction in its outward physical appearance is very similar to that which follows the intradermal injection of small amounts of histamine. The triple response of erythema accompanied by edema and wheal formation is typical in both cases. Other vasoactive substances also may produce the triple response; in some animal species these substances (serotonin, kinins, leukotrienes) may be more responsible for the hypersensitive response than is histamine itself. These compounds usually arise from mast

TABLE 16-2

Comparison of IgE- and T cell–mediated hypersensitivities

	IgE mediated	T cell mediated
Timing of response after shocking exposure	Appears within a few minutes, fades within a few hours; immediate	Develops and fades gradually; maximum at 24 to 72 hours; delayed
Special target tissue	Usually smooth muscle, but organ varies with species	Generalized tissue involvement
Tissue death	May occur; variable	Occurs but not typical of ordinary reaction
Humoral factor involvement	Yes; IgE	None yet identified
Cellular factor involvement	Only in that immunoglobulins are produced by B lymphocytes and plasma cells; mast cells	T lymphocytes, directly, not via immunoglobulin
Passive transfer	With immunoglobulins	With T lymphocytes
Type of tissue involved	Vascular	Vascular, but relatively avascular suitable also
Histology of skin reactions	Predominantly neutrophils and eosinophils; edema obvious, with wheal and erythema	Tendency toward mononuclears, with some neutrophils; species variation; less edema and wheal; erythema and induration
Mediators	Histamine, serotonin, kinins; species variation	Lymphokines
Moderators	Antihistamines and smooth muscle relaxants (adrenergic compounds)	Steroids (antiinflammatory compounds)
Immunotherapy (desensitization)	Yes; relatively easy, temporary; via neutralizing antibodies or formation of blocking antibodies	Yes; with difficulty, temporary; usually not attempted

cells, basophils, or platelets; therefore a cellular participation at this level is required.

Chemotherapy and chemoprophylaxis of the immediate hypersensitivities are logically based on three classes of drugs: those which oppose the action of histamine as competitive metabolites (antihistamines), those which physiologically oppose the physiopharmacologic action of histamine (smooth muscle relaxants such as adrenaline and other adrenergic compounds), and those which stabilize mast cells. Desensitization is relatively easy as far as the immediate hypersensitivities are concerned; it depends on the cautious neutralization of antibody and the formation of blocking antibody. The desensitized state is only temporary.

Delayed type hypersensitivity

The behavior of the delayed hypersensitivities is almost always the opposite of the immediate hypersensitivities for each of the criteria listed in Table 16-2. To begin with, the shock response in delayed hypersensitivities is slow in developing and does not reach its maximum until sometime between 24 and 72 hours after the exposure to antigen. On a whole animal basis no special target organs seem to be involved; rather vague, generalized symptoms are observed, such as headache, fever, backache, and malaise. In this reaction cell death is uncommon.

The delayed hypersensitive reaction does not depend on circulating immunoglobulins but is dependent on specifically sensitized T lymphocytes; there-

TABLE 16-3

Classification of hypersensitive reactions

	Anaphylactic (type I)	Cytotoxic (type II)	Immune complex (type III)	T cell dependent (type IV)
Immunoglobulin	IgE	IgG, possibly other	IgG, IgM, etc.	None
Complement involved	No	Yes	Yes	No
Cellular involvement	Mast cells and basophils	Red and white blood cells, platelets	Host tissue cells	T cells and macrophages
Chemical mechanism	Mast cell products and others	Complement-dependent cytolysis	Complement-dependent reactions	Lymphokines
Examples	Anaphylaxis, hay fever, food allergy	Transfusion reactions, Rh disease, thrombocytopenia	Arthus reaction, serum sickness, pneumonitis	Allergy of infection, contact dermatitis

fore the passive transfer of this kind of allergy to a normal recipient requires the transfer of lymphocytes. It is possible to effect this transfer in some species with soluble products from the T cells. Since delayed hypersensitivity does not depend on free proteins of the circulatory system, the reaction can be evoked in relatively avascular tissue, such as the external layers of the dermis. The major requirement is simply that the tissue be situated close enough to the vascular system that lymphocytes can emigrate from it to the point of antigen deposition.

The ordinary locus for detecting delayed hypersensitivity is the skin. Compared with the immediate skin reaction there is less edema and virtually no wheal, only erythema and induration. In delayed hypersensitivity the cellular infiltrate is dominated by mononuclear cells and less by granulocytes. Variation in the cellular response from species to species has been noted. The lymphokines are chemical associates of the reaction, but the biochemical basis for the activity of these compounds has only recently come under investigation. Since their exact chemical mechanism is unknown, it has been impossible to devise a logical chemoprophylactic or chemotherapeutic suppression of the delayed hypersensitive state. Steroids and other antiinflammatory drugs will minimize the shock reaction but cannot totally prevent it. Desensitized individuals will display no shock reaction; this condition is relatively difficult

to create, and since the delayed hypersensitivities are seldom life threatening, desensitization is seldom attempted.

When sensitization to an antigen develops, it does not develop solely in the form of an immediate hypersensitivity with the exclusion of any delayed or cell-mediated component. One or the other form may very well dominate the allergic state, but the two forms are usually mutually present. It is often the method of testing that causes one form of hypersensitivity to be detected in the absence of the other.

Immunopathologic relationships

An alternative system of classification for hypersensitive responses was forwarded by Gell and Coombs in England over two decades ago (Table 16-3). Although four types of hypersensitive reactions are included in this system, the first three are subdivisions of the immunoglobulin-dependent hypersensitivities, and the fourth is the cell-mediated, or delayed hypersensitivity.

The anaphylactic type of reaction is that in which homocytotropic or heterocytotropic immunoglobulins of the IgE type, synthesized by plasma cells, become attached to mast cells and basophils via their Fc portion. The two Fab regions protrude from the cell surface and, when combined with antigen, alter the permeability of these cells. Pharmacologically active substances, such as histamine and the leukotrienes, released by the cells affect the shock tissues, primarily smooth muscles. Serum complement is not required in this reaction. The immunoglobulins are described as cytotropic or homocytotropic antibodies because of their affinity for tissue cells.

In the cytotoxic allergies, antibodies of the IgG and possibly other classes react directly with antigens or hapten-antigen complexes on the surface of the tissue cell. Complement participates in this reaction and promotes cytolysis or cytotoxic reactions such as those seen in hemolytic reactions and thrombocytopenic purpura. Elements of this type of reaction may be present in several autoimmune diseases, drug allergies, and allograft rejection.

In the immune complex reaction antigen-antibody complexes form in the soluble or fluid phase of tissues or in blood and then deposit on vessel walls, glomerular membranes, and elsewhere to interrupt normal physiologic processes. These immunoglobulins may be of the IgG, IgM, or possibly other classes. Complement becomes activated in many of these reactions and releases chemotactic factors. The attracted leukocytes release enzymes and possibly other agents that injure local tissues. Immune complex reactions are typified by the Arthus reaction, portions of serum sickness, and aspects of autoimmune disease such as SLE and glomerulonephritis.

The delayed type reaction is the cell-mediated hypersensitive reaction involving antigen-sensitized T cells, which respond directly or by the release of lymphokines to exhibit contact determatitis and allergies of infection.

REFERENCES

Altman, L.C., editor: Clinical allergy and immunology, Boston, 1984, G.K. Hall Medical Publishers.

Beal, G.N., editor: Allergy and clinical immunology, New York, 1984, John Wiley & Sons.

Kaplan, A.P., editor: Allergy, New York, 1985, Churchill Livingstone, Inc.

Korenblat, P.E., and Wedner, H.J., editors: Allergy, theory and practice, Orlando, 1984, Grune and Stratton, Inc.

Lessof, M.H., editor: Allergy, immunological and chemical aspects, Chichester, Eng, 1984, John Wiley & Sons, Ltd.

Lockey, R.F., and Bukantz, S.C., editors: Principles of immunology and allergy, Philadelphia, 1987, W.B. Saunders Co.

Middleton, E., Jr., Reed, C.E., and Ellis, E.F., editors: Allergy, principles and practice, 2nd ed., St. Louis, 1983, The C.V. Mosby Co.

Ring, J., and Burg, G., editors: New trends in allergy II, Berlin, 1986, Springer Verlag.

Sly, M.R.: Textbook of pediatric allergy, New Hyde Park, NY, 1985, Medical Examination Publishing Company, Inc.

Anaphylaxis and IgE-mediated hypersensitivities

≡ GLOSSARY

adrenergic drugs Drugs such as adrenalin that constrict blood vessels, relax smooth muscles, and in general function in the opposite way as histamine; synonym of β-adrenergic drug.

anaphylactoid reaction A pseudoanaphylactic reaction and similar to it in all respects except that it is not created by antigen-antibody reactions.

anaphylaxis An unexpected, detrimental reaction to a second exposure to antigen in which histamine, serotonin, etc. are released by reaction of the antigen with IgE on the surface of mast cells (*ana,* without; *phylaxis,* protection).

antihistamine A drug that is an inhibitor, usually a competitive inhibitor, of histamine.

atopy An IgE-dependent allergy often arising from unknown exposure to an antigen or autocoupling hapten.

blocking antibody An antibody that prevents the action of another antibody, as exemplified by antibodies formed during desensitization against atopic allergies.

bradykinin A specific peptide of nine amino acids formed during anaphylaxis.

catecholamine An adrenergic drug such as adrenalin.

cromolyn A mast cell stabilizing drug.

cytotropic antibody An antibody that attaches nonspecifically to mast cells and basophils.

desensitization Elimination or reduction of allergic sensitivity, usually through a programmed course of antigen treatment.

ECF-A Eosinophilic chemotactic factor of anaphylaxis.

heterocytotropic antibody An antibody from one species that will attach to mast cells of another species.

histamine A specific chemical compound released from

mast cells and producing vasodilation, smooth muscle contraction, and edema during anaphylaxis.

homocytotropic antibody An antibody that will attach to the mast cells of the species producing it.

kallidin Lysylbradykinin or kinin 10.

kallikrein Protease(s) that releases kinins from kininogen; synonymous with *kininogenase.*

kininogenase *see* Kallikrein.

kininogens α-Globulin proteins of serum that are precursors to kinins.

kinins Peptides or polyamines released during anaphylaxis that possess vasodilating and muscle-contracting activity.

leukotriene *see* Slow-reacting substance of anaphylaxis.

mast cell A cell found in connective tissue in which heparin and histamine are stored in numerous intracytoplasmic granules.

PAF Platelet-activating factor from basophils.

Prausnitz-Küstner (P-K) test A test for immediate hypersensitivity performed in a normal subject who has been passively sensitized by immunoglobulin from the allergic individual.

prekallikrein Prokininogenase.

prokininogenase The proenzyme precursor to kininogenase.

prostaglandin A derivative of arachidonic acid.

reagin Antiquated name for IgE.

Schultz-Dale reaction An in vitro anaphylactic response of sensitized uterus or gut when exposed to antigen.

serotonin A chemical mediator of anaphylaxis (5-hydroxytryptamine).

slow-reacting substance of anaphylaxis (SRS-A) A material that causes a slow or prolonged contraction of

smooth muscle released during anaphylaxis; leukotrienes C, D, and E.

vasoactive amine   An amine or peptide that produces
vasodilation.

■   ■   ■

Hypersensitivities caused by IgE may assume any
of several forms from the life-threatening anaphylactic reactions to the milder discomforts associated
with food allergies. Regardless of their severity,
these depend on the presence of an IgE with a serologic specificity for the offending allergen. The combination of the allergen with IgE on the surface of
mast cells and basophils releases pharmacologic
agents that trigger an immediate physiologic response. These immediate hypersensitivities or
anaphylactic hypersensitivities are compared with
other forms of allergy in Chapter 16, which should
be consulted for review.

ANAPHYLAXIS
Systemic anaphylaxis

Systemic anaphylaxis is the most devastating
form of the IgE-mediated hypersensitivities. The first
complete description of this phenomenon was given
by Portier and Richet in 1902. These investigators
attempted to immunize dogs against the toxins of the
sea anemone by administering spaced injections of
small, nonlethal quantities of the toxin. When the
animals received secondary injections of sublethal
quantities of the toxin, at a time when it might be
expected that they would be immune, the dogs entered the shock syndrome that Richet designated as
anaphylaxis. This word indicates that the prior injections of the antigen had produced the converse of the
expected situation, prophylaxis.

The initial injection of the toxin must be considered as the sensitizing exposure, which was followed
by an immunologic waiting period necessary for immunoglobulin synthesis. For the easiest provocation
of systemic anaphylaxis the shocking dose of antigen
should be given in fluid form directly into the circulation so that it can be rapidly distributed throughout
the body. For this reason the intramuscular injection
of bacterial vaccines or precipitated toxoids rarely
causes anaphylaxis.

The symptoms of anaphylaxis vary from species
to species because of the central involvement of different shock organs. In virtually every instance
smooth muscle contraction, dilation of the vascular
system, and edema are among the major changes.

The symptoms of anaphylaxis in the guinea pig
first appear as ruffling of the hair on the back of the
neck, restlessness, sneezing, and pawing at the nose.
These quickly progress to coughing and retching,
combined with gasping for air. Tremors may course
through the animal's body. Cyanosis is evident by
the pallor or bluish cast assumed by the mucous
membranes. Defecation, urination, and collapse of
the animal followed by convulsive kicks and continued respiratory failure lead to death, frequently
within 5 to 10 minutes after the injection of the antigen. The most obvious finding at autopsy is the
marked inflation of the lungs from constriction of the
bronchial musculature. Hemorrhages may be noted
in the viscera and on the diaphragm, but the animal
dies of asphyxiation.

The symptoms of anaphylactic shock in humans
are more similar to those in guinea pigs than in any
other animal. Shortness of breath, increased heart
rate, and a tingling in the throat precede collapse.
Death may follow within a few minutes. Edema of
the throat, brain, and lungs and inflation of the lungs
are observed at autopsy.

Some species, such as the rat, mouse, and hamster, are quite refractory to lethal anaphylaxis, but
anaphylactic sensitivity can be induced by repeated
exposures to antigen. Anaphylaxis has been demonstrated in virtually all species tested, provided the
species is capable of immunoglobulin synthesis.

Active sensitization to anaphylactic shock can be
induced by any antigen; proteins, polysaccharides,
conjugated antigens, and autocoupling haptens have
been used. The amount of antigen needed for sensitization depends on the species of animal, the antigen, and the manner of sensitization. Large amounts

of antigen or intensive immunization (sensitization) schedules usually should be avoided, except in markedly resistant animals. A single injection of 0.001 to 1 mg of soluble proteins given intraperitoneally will provide uniform sensitivity in guinea pigs, which usually are not susceptible to shock until the eighth day after antigen exposure and display maximal sensitivity at 21 days.

Rapid and immediate saturation of the animal with antigen by the shocking dose of antigen favors lethal anaphylaxis. For this reason it is important that the antigen be fluid and that it be given by the intravenous or intracardial route. A total amount of 0.1 to 1 mg of antigen is adequate, but since a prozone phenomenon with excess antigen is not observed, larger quantities of antigen can be used.

Animals that escape death after the administration of the shocking dose of antigen are specifically desensitized for a period of several days to several weeks, after which their sensitivity returns.

Variants of anaphylaxis

Cutaneous anaphylaxis is merely the provocation of the immediate type of skin reaction in a sensitized individual by injecting the allergen responsible for the sensitivity into the skin. This can be accomplished by intracutaneous injection, prick, or scratch testing. A skin test of this sort should be conducted if it is necessary to administer an antigen systemically to a person, because it will reveal if the person is susceptible to anaphylactic shock.

To perform the passive cutaneous anaphylactic (PCA) reaction, serum from an anaphylactically sensitized animal is injected into the skin of a normal animal. When antigen is injected systemically several hours later, an edematous and erythematous reaction develops at the skin site. In fact one may delay the antigen injection for several days and still elicit the immediate skin reaction. When the PCA reaction is conducted in man, it is known as the Prausnitz-Küstner (P-K) reaction, named for the German physicians who first performed this test. Küstner was allergic to cooked fish. If Küstner's serum was injected into the skin of the nonallergic Prausnitz, and this was followed the next day by the injection of an extract of cooked fish into the same site rather than

systemically, an immediate skin reaction developed. It is interesting that extracts of raw fish did not elicit the reaction, which indicates that Küstner was allergic to a heat-denatured antigen.

The original experiment that illustrated the necessity of cell-bound (cytotropic) antibody for anaphylaxis was the Schultz-Dale reaction. Schultz and Dale found that the uterus or a segment of ileum removed from a sensitized guinea pig, if heavily perfused, can be washed free of circulating immunoglobulins. When suspended between a fixed and a movable pole in an isotonic bath solution, muscles in these tissues will contract when the sensitizing antigen is added to the bath. This contraction is recordable by contact of a pen on the movable pole against a turning drum (kymograph). The Schultz-Dale reaction is thus an in vitro anaphylactic reaction that proves the need of cell-bound antibody to produce anaphylaxis.

Pathway to anaphylactic shock
Immunoglobulin formation and fixation

The immunologic basis for anaphylaxis is antibody of the reaginic type, that is, IgE. Three conditions offer strong evidence against a dependence of anaphylaxis on circulating antibody. One of these is that an actively sensitized animal can be placed in shock even though it has no detectable antibody in its blood. A second line of evidence is that animals with a high titer of circulating antibodies are quite refractory to shock. That circulating immunoglobulins are involved at all is demonstrable by passive sensitization experiments. When antiserum with a good reaginic titer is taken from an actively sensitized animal and injected into a normal animal, the recipient becomes sensitized to anaphylaxis. The recipient is not immediately susceptible to anaphylactic shock, however. It is necessary to allow the fixation of serum antibody to tissue cells.

The IgE that is free in the circulation of allergic persons thus is not the cause of their allergic condition; it is the IgE that has become bound to cells. IgE is a cytophilic, or cytotropic, antibody. In the guinea pig and mouse their IgG1 is the primary cytotropic analog to human IgE. A homocytotropic antibody is one that binds to cells of its own species.

Wide L, Bennich H & Johansson S G O.

Diagnosis of allergy by an in-vitro test for allergen antibodies.
Lancet **2:**1105-7, 1967.   [Dept. Clinical Chemistry and Blood Centre, Univ. Hosp., and Inst. Biochemistry, Univ. Uppsala, Sweden]

An in vitro method, the radioallergosorbent test (RAST), was developed for the detection and assay of allergen-specific antibodies of a new immunoglobulin class, later termed IgE. The method was a noncompetitive radioimmunoassay using labeled antibodies. [The SCI® indicates that this paper has been cited in over 740 publications since 1967.]

Leif Wide
Department of Clinical Chemistry
University Hospital
S-751 85 Uppsala
Sweden

November 12, 1984

The conception of this paper was the result of some remarkable coincidences. My interest in the development of a test for the diagnosis of an allergy arose from a seminar presented at our hospital. Lennart Juhlin, a dermatologist, held the seminar when he returned from the US in August 1966. He described the basophil degranulation tests[1] and discussed the need for very high sensitivity in measuring reagins in serum. At that time, I had developed the prototype of an extremely sensitive new principle for radioimmunoassay (RIA), which was noncompetitive and used a labeled binding reagent. I suggested that this method might be used for the assay of reagins, and we decided to collaborate using penicillin allergy as a model.

At about the same time, Hans Bennich and Gunnar Johansson informed me that they had tested a large number of sera with a single radial immunodiffusion test (SRD) and failed to find a normal counterpart to a myeloma protein called ND. We decided to try a solid-phase competitive RIA, the radioimmunosorbent technique,[2] which was about 1,000 times more sensitive than the SRD. With their collaboration, I labeled the ND protein with ^{125}I and coupled the antibodies to Sephadex. About six months later, we concluded that a protein corresponding to ND was present in all human sera tested and that it represented a new class of immunoglobulins.[3]

One serum specimen had a remarkably high level of the protein. The individual it represented turned out to be hypersensitive to dog epithelium. As it was a possibility that this elevated protein level in the serum specimen arose as reaginic antibodies to dog epithelium, I constructed a noncompetitive sandwich RIA to detect allergen-specific antibodies of the new immunoglobulin class in the serum. The presumptive reagins were first bound to a solid phase-coupled aller-gen and then detected by binding ^{125}I-labeled antibodies to the ND protein. An increased amount of radioactivity was bound to the solid phase when the serum was tested with dog epithelium, and all controls were negative. Sera from patients with hay fever and allergic asthma were tested with different allergens, and the results correlated well with those of provocation tests. These results, together with a number of other observations, indicated that the reagins belonged to the new immunoglobulin class and that this class was related to the gamma-E (later IgE) described by Ishizaka et al.[4]

The noncompetitive sandwich technique combined two important properties: a very high sensitivity and a two-sided specificity. Used as an allergy test, only antibodies against a particular allergen were detected, and only those belonging to IgE. The method was called the radioallergosorbent technique (RAST). For the next few years, I examined the clinical significance of RAST and summarized the results in 1973.[5]

I believe that this paper is frequently cited for two reasons. First, RAST has become extensively used as a test for diagnosis of allergy and for quantitation of allergen-specific IgE. RAST is also used as a method for control of allergen extracts. Second, it was the first noncompetitive RIA and the first quantitative assay using labeled antibodies. Similar sandwich techniques have come to be used more and more in many different fields of research as well as routinely in the clinical laboratory.

Honors received for the studies include the Anniversary Medal of the Swedish Society of Medicine, in 1969, for the allergy test and, in 1983, the Clinical Ligand Assay Society Senior Investigator Award for the noncompetitive "sandwich" ligand-binding assay.

1. Shelley WB & Juhlin L. A new test of detecting anaphylactic sensitivity: the basophil reaction. *Nature* **191:**1056-8, 1961. (Cited 85 times.)
2. Wide L & Porath J. Radioimmunoassay of proteins with the use of Sephadex-coupled antibodies. *Biochim. Biophys. Acta* **130:**257-60, 1966. (Cited 480 times.)
3. Johansson SGO, Bennich H & Wide L. A new class of immunoglobulin in human serum. *Immunology* **14:**265-72, 1968. (Cited 295 times.)
4. Ishizaka K, Ishizaka T & Hornbrook MH. Physico-chemical properties of reaginic antibody. IV. Presence of a unique immunoglobulin as a carrier of reaginic activity. *J. Immunology* **97:**75-85, 1966. (Cited 305 times.)
5. Wide L. Clinical significance of measurement of reaginic (IgE) antibody by RAST. *Clin. Allergy* **3:**583-95, 1973. (Cited 50 times.)

This distinguishes it from a heterocytotropic antibody, which will bind to cells of other species. The third line of proof is the Schultz-Dale reaction cited immediately above.

Quantitation of IgE

Because of the paucity of IgE in normal human serum, sensitive serologic procedures must be used for its quantitation. These include the radioimmunosorbent test (RIST), the radioallergosorbent test (RAST), and enzyme immunoassays. The Mancini radial diffusion and nephelometric precipitation tests also may be used, since potent antisera now have been prepared against IgE myeloma proteins.

The RIST procedure is dependent on the availability of an ^{125}I-labeled IgE myeloma protein and its specific antibody, the latter used in the solid phase of this RIA procedure. Competition of IgE in an unknown serum sample with the radiolabeled myeloma protein is measured as a decrease in bound label and is a direct measure of the IgE in the sample. This test measures total serum IgE and is a typical competitive inhibition RIA test.

The RAST test uses a specific allergen bound to a solid phase carrier, which then is incubated with a serum sample containing an unknown amount of IgE specific for the allergen. When radiolabeled anti-IgE specific for the ϵ chain is added, the amount of label bound is a measure only of the allergen-specific IgE in the serum. IgG or other antibodies to the allergen could be detected by specifically labeled antibodies for IgG, etc. Both the RIST and RAST tests have been adapted to enzyme immunoassays.

By these procedures it has been determined that the healthy adult usually will have 61 to 100 ng of IgE per milliliter of serum. IgE in cord sera of newborn infants averages 37 ng/ml, or about 35% of the adult average. There is no correlation between the maternal and newborn serum IgE levels, which indicates that fetal IgE synthesis can occur. From infancy to puberty the IgE levels progress gradually toward the adult norm. In various atopic allergic diseases, especially hay fever and asthma, IgE levels may rise to nearly 6,000 ng/ml of serum, with a mean value of 1,191. Consequently values over 1,000 are considered pathologic. Very high levels have been noted in children with roundworm infection. Hyposensitization therapy for hay fever also increases the serum levels, which seem to remain high for several months. The effectiveness of hyposensitization obviously is not through its effect on IgE levels.

Since IgE occurs in only minute quantities in normal sera (16 to 97 ng/ml of serum), critical biochemical studies were hampered for several years after its discovery. Even though serum levels of IgE in allergic individuals may be elevated to 50 times the normal serum levels, sera from these allergic persons simply are not available in quantity. This dilemma was circumvented by the discovery in Sweden of a patient with a unique myeloma protein, originally designated as the ND myeloma protein. This paraprotein was not antigenically related to any previously known myeloma protein or immunoglobulin H chain, although it was related to immunoglobulins by virtue of its λ L chain determinants. This ND protein soon was proved to be serologically identical to IgE. This discovery and the attendant availability of large quantities of IgE opened the way to a precise biophysical characterization of this new immunoglobulin.

Examination of the blood of animals undergoing anaphylactic shock reveals that the blood has an extended clotting time and is toxic to the skin of normal animals given intradermal injections of the blood. It also has been noted that anaphylactic shock in the guinea pig has many points in common with histamine shock. In the late 1920s the triple response of skin to histamine injections was observed to parallel very closely the immediate hypersensitive skin response of sensitized guinea pigs to intradermal injections of the offending antigen. This response consists of immediate erythema and edema at the injection site followed by wheal and flare, or pseudopodial spread, of the reaction. Subsequent inquiries now have defined histamine as a primary pharmacologic mediator of anaphylaxis in guinea pigs. Other compounds with profound physiopharmacologic activity also are released during anaphylaxis. Tissue mast cells and basophils are two important cell sources of these molecules.

Mast Cells

Mast cells were discovered and named by Ehrlich. These cells are widely distributed throughout the body but are especially populous in connective tissues, in lung and uterus, and around blood vessels. They are abundant in liver, kidney, spleen, heart, and other organs. The individual mast cell is ovoid and about 10 to 15 μm in diameter (Fig. 17-1). It has a poorly developed endoplasmic reticulum, contains only a few mitochondria, and has a heavily granulated cytoplasm (Fig. 17-2). The granules are about 0.5 to 2 μm in diameter, stain unevenly, and are surrounded by a limiting membrane. These granules may be so numerous as to totally obscure the cell nucleus in stained preparations, and it is not unusual for a single cell to contain 200 to 500 of these granules. The tissue mast cell is similar in appearance to the basophilic leukocyte. The granules in both cells consist of a complex of heparin, histamine, and zinc ions, with the heparin existing in an approximate ratio of 6:1 with histamine. The actual heparin content is about 70 to 90 μg/10^6 cells, and the histamine content is about 10 to 15 μg/10^6 cells.

Basophils

The basophil is the least common of the blood granulocytes. There are only about 40 such cells per cubic millimeter of human blood, in which the basophils constitute about 2% of the cells. Basophils are the smallest of the granulocytes with a range in diameter from 8 to 18 μm. The nucleus is not as well segmented as in the neutrophils and eosinophils. The cytoplasm of basophils contains a few mitochondria and other structures but is most noted for its numerous round or ovoid granules, which are basophilic in their staining properties. These granules average 0.5 μm in diameter and under electron microscopy are observed to have an internal subgranular structure composed of particles of only 100 to 150 Å in diameter. The morphologic resemblance of basophils and mast cells is very striking and accounts for the description of the mast cell as the tissue basophil and

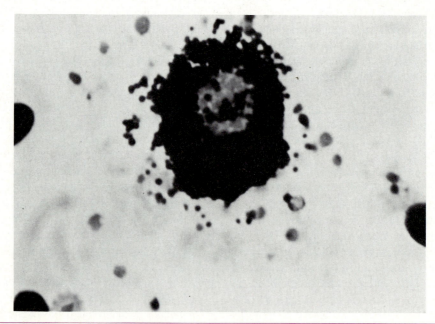

FIG. 17-1

A mast cell that has begun to discharge its granules. The light area in the center of the cell, partially shielded by granules, is the nucleus.

of the basophil as the circulating mast cell (Fig. 17-3). This is an oversimplification, since these cells arise from separate stem cells.

The morphologic unity of mast cells and basophils is repeated in their chemical composition. Basophils contain several enzymes, but as with mast cells, the most important is histidine decarboxylase. This enzyme is the catalyst for the formation of the biogenic amine found in the basophil, just as it is in the mast cell. The histamine content of basophils is some 20 to 50 times less than in mast cells, seldom exceeding 2.5×10^6 μg/cell.

Cell receptors for IgE

The attachment of IgE to cells is made possible by the presence of IgE receptors on the outer surface of these cells. Two separate molecular forms of these receptors are known. These are designated FcεR1 and FcεR2, since binding involves the Fc fragment of the IgE molecule. It is uncertain whether the CH3 or the CH4 domain is the primary attachment site of the receptor.

FcεR1 is present on mast cells, basophils, platelets, and macrophages. It is estimated that 10^4 to 10^6 receptor molecules are present on a single mast cell. This would place the molecules only 50 nm apart, and since molecules on the cell surface are subject to lateral movement, this too would ensure the reaction of two IgE molecules with antigen. The R1 receptor is a four-protein complex of three different polypeptides (Fig. 17-4). The most externally positioned is the α peptide of 45,000 molecular weight. The next

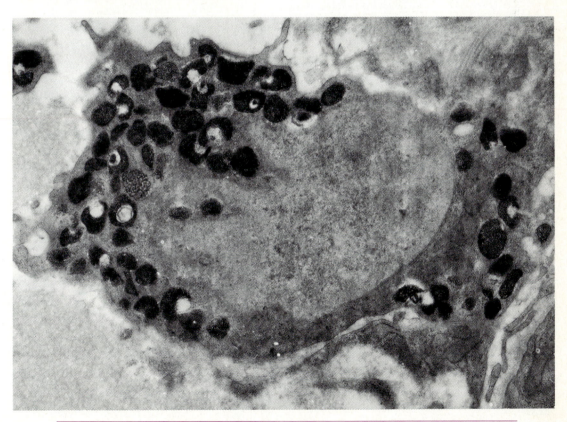

FIG. 17-2
Electron micrograph of a human mast cell. Note the fine granular structure of the numerous cytoplasmic granules, which store histamine and heparin. (Courtesy Dr. E. Adelstein.)

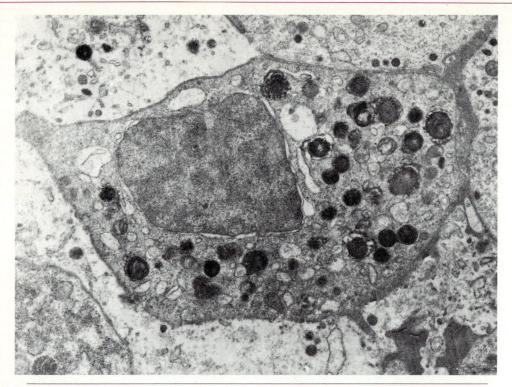

FIG. 17-3

This electron photomicrograph of a basophil in bone marrow should be compared with that of a mast cell in Fig. 17-2. The granules in basophils contain histamine. (Courtesy Dr. E. Adelstein.)

most internal is the β molecule with a molecular weight of 33,000 and extending through the lipid bilayer into the cytoplasm. Two γ molecules with molecular weights of 9,000 are linked by a disulfide bond and serve as anchors for the complex. The evidence indicates that only the α peptide functions in IgE binding.

Crosslinking of two IgE molecules by the R1 receptor is necessary to initiate mediator release from mast cells. Proof of this is found in experiments in which haptens or single epitopes, or Fab fragments of IgG specific for IgE, fail to stimulate mediator release, whereas divalent epitopes or F(ab')₂ fragments of antibodies specific for IgE are successful releasers.

The R2 receptor for IgE has a wide distribution, being identified on macrophages, eosinophils, plate-

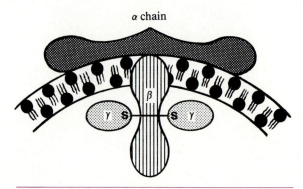

FIG. 17-4

The Fc receptor for the ε chain of IgE consists of an externally located α chain that binds to the immunoglobulin. The α chain is noncovalently associated with the β chain and two γ chains.

lets, and both T and B lymphocytes. These cells have approximately 10^3 to 10^5 receptor molecules each. The R2 protein consists of one α peptide of 45,000 to 50,000 molecular weight, and one β peptide of 25,000 to 33,000 molecular weight. The physical arrangement of these in the cell membrane is under study.

Mass cell degranulation
General immunology

The histamine and heparin held within the granules of mast cells and basophils are released when these cells are exposed to specific immunologic or chemical agents.

Mast cell degranulation can be accomplished in any of three immunologic ways. The first of these is to use mast cells as the antigen for immunizaton of a heterologous species of animal. Passive administration of the anti–mast cell serum to the species that was the source of the mast cells will initiate a complement-dependent immunolytic reaction that will destroy the mast cell and release histamine and heparin.

The second method is by the passive administration of antibody to the animal's IgG, IgA, or IgE. The reaction of antiglobulins with κ, λ, or ϵ chains of antibodies on the mast cell surface activates the complement cascade and results in a typical complement-dependent immunocytolytic anaphylactic reaction.

The third method depends on the fixation of IgE to the cell surface and the reaction of these cell-bound antibodies with antigen. The subsequent release and dissolution of granules does not depend on the fixation of complement or on mast cell lysis.

Cellular events during mast cell degranulation

The molecular events that follow mast cell activation and that terminate in the release of mediators of the immediate hypersensitivity reaction are complex, and occur within a few seconds. For these reasons, the exact sequence of biochemical events is uncertain. Moreover, the known behavioral differences of rat peritoneal mast cells, human mast cells, and basophils has complicated the synthesis of a unit mechanism. Nevertheless, the flux of calcium into the cell, the formation of cyclic AMP (cAMP), the activation of phospholipases, protein kinases, and methyl transferases have all been associated with mast cell degranulation.

In harmony with the first and second messenger hypothesis for the release of storage materials from other secretory cells, the first message to the mast cell is the bridging of two IgE molecules by antigen (Fig. 17-5). Both mathematical and immunologic evidence reveal the need for two IgE molecules, but these need not react with the same epitope, though this may be the case when the same epitope is repeated in an allergen. This is probably the case in anaphylactic drug allergies. Allergen binding to IgE may release Ca^{2+} from its internal storage pool, thereby influencing the stability of the mast cell granule by direct ionic forces. Since calcium uptake in IgE sensitized-antigen exposed cells is so pronounced, calcium admitted through transmembrane channels, rather than released from intracellular storage depots, may be sufficient to increase the calcium pool to the critical concentration. Several lines of evidence support an early participation of calcium. The Ca^{2+} ionophore A23187 will transport Ca^{2+} into cells and this initiates degranulation in mast cells. Calcium-bearing liposomes also cause degranulation when they fuse with mast cells.

The influx of calcium into mast cells may be preceded or accompanied by other important steps—the kinetics are not yet entirely clear. The activation of a decarboxylase that converts phosphatidylserine to phosphatidylethanolamine is one of the first reactions. This may be preceded by a conversion of a nucleotide regulatory unit to an activated "on" position. The phosphatidylethanolamine is doubly methylated by a methyltransferase to produce phosphatidyl choline. It is probably here that the calcium becomes important by activating phospholipase A2. Phospholipase A2 then releases arachidonic acid from the cell membrane lipid, simultaneously producing lysophosphatidylcholine (LPC) as an end product. Phospholipase C is also activated and produces 1,2 diacylglycerol (DAG). LPC and DAG are both described as fusogens because they are lipid solvents

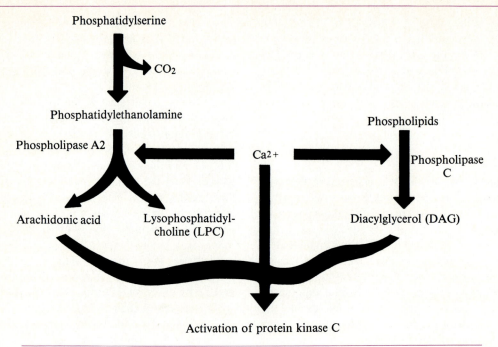

Phosphatidylserine

CO_2

Phosphatidylethanolamine

Phospholipids

Phospholipase A2

Ca^{2+}

Phospholipase C

Arachidonic acid

Lysophosphatidyl-choline (LPC)

Diacylglycerol (DAG)

Activation of protein kinase C

FIG. 17-5

The central role of calcium in stimulating phospholipase A2, phospholipase C, and protein kinase C in mast cells leads to an alteration of granule and cell membranes as the fusogens DAG and LPC are produced.

and can derange membranes. Both may be important in the fusing of the membrane of mast cell granules with the cell membrane, thus permitting degranulation. Arachidonic acid and DAG cooperate with calcium ions to activate protein kinase C. Protein kinase C phosphorylates, and thereby activates several enzymes, including proteases and lipases that may be involved in the degranulation reaction. The evidence for this pathway has support in the finding that exogenous phosphatidylserine stimulates histamine secretion and calcium uptake. Opposed to this hypothesis, one can cite the feeble inhibition of degranulation by inhibitors of methylation.

Another starting point in the biochemistry of degranulation is related to the cAMP system (Fig. 17-6). Within seconds after the crosslinking of membrane bound IgE by antigen, the intracellular cAMP level increases as the result of an activation of adenyl (adenylate) cyclase. This burst may activate cAMP-dependent protein kinases. As stated above, protein kinases phosphorylate proteins, and this may affect the permeability of the granule or cell membrane and allow more Ca^{2+} to enter the cell. Another role of calcium not mentioned above is its requirement for the conversion of actinomyosin to actin. Intracellular actin fibers may provide the avenues for the displacement of the mast cell granules to the cell perimeter, where they discharge their contents. It is known that the Fc_ϵ receptor is phosphorylated during mast cell degranulation; however, this is associated with a decrease in calcium permeability, rather than an increase. A support for the cAMP cycle is that theophylline, an inhibitor of the phosphodiesterase that cleaves one of the phosphoesterase bonds to form "normal" adenosine monophosphate, also inhibits the immediate hypersensitivity reaction. Thus, high mast cell levels of cAMP may be stabilizing, whereas high intracellular cAMP in other cells usually stimulates secretion.

Anaphylactic shock, then, is the summation of

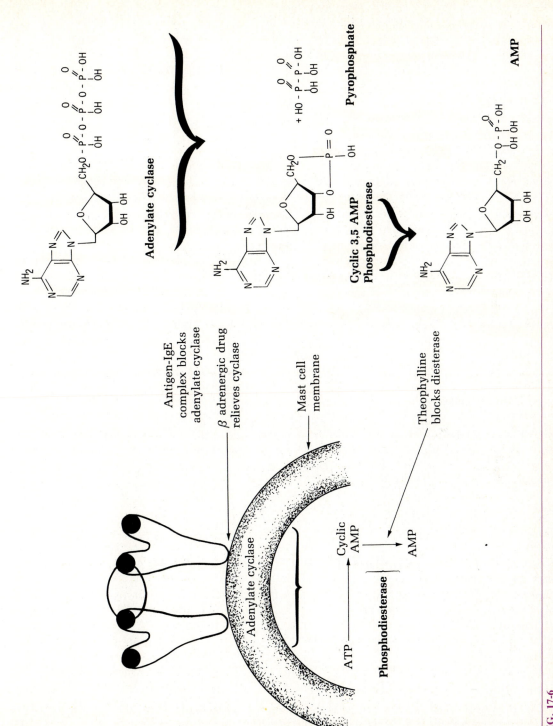

FIG. 17-6

Inhibition of the enzyme adenylate cyclase in the membrane of the mast cell by IgE-antigen combination on its surface reduces the intracellular level of cyclic 3,5-AMP. This is associated with mast cell degranulation.

IgE formation, the fixation of these IgE molecules to mast cells and basophils, an in vivo antigen-antibody reaction, and the degranulation of mast cells and basophils.

Mediators of anaphylaxis

Several important pharmacologically active compounds are discharged from mast cells and basophils during anaphylaxis (Table 17-1). These include histamine, heparin, serotonin, ECF-A, and the leukotrienes formerly known as SRS-A. Additional substances also are known to participate. Histamine, serotonin (in some species), heparin, and the eosinophil chemotactic factor of anaphylaxis (ECF-A) are preformed substances that are stored in mast cell granules. Other mediators, such as platelet activating factor (PAF), the prostaglandins, and the leukotrienes or slow reactive substances of anaphylaxis (SRS-A), are generated by the mast cell as part of the degranulating reaction. The importance of each

of these is directly correlated to its relative proportion (in a physiopharmacologic sense) in the mixture of substances liberated during anaphylaxis, to the sensitivity of smooth muscle and vascular tissue of the animal species involved to the specific action of the compound, and to the rate and mechanism of its detoxification or degradation.

Histamine

Histamine is a simple chemical with a molecular weight of 111. It is formed by the action of the enzyme histidine decarboxylase and its cofactor, pyridoxal phosphate, on histidine (Fig. 17-7). The required enzyme is abundant in tissue mast cells and basophils.

Human lung and skin are well endowed with mast cells, and contain 1 to 10×10^6 mast cells per gram of tissue. The histamine content of the human mast cell is 1 to 5.5 pg, generally less than that of other species. Rat mast cells contain 7 to 10 pg of hista-

TABLE 17-1
Mediators of immediate hypersensitivities

Mediator	Description	Primary activity	Antagonist
Histamine	From histidine in mast cell, 111 mol wt, a heterocyclic amine	Contracts smooth muscle	Antihistamines
Serotonin	From tryptophan in mast cells, 171 mol wt, an aromatic amine	Contracts smooth muscle	Methysergide
ECF-A	From mast cells, about 380 mol wt, a peptide	Attracts eosinophils	None known
SRS-A	Leukotrienes	Prolonged contraction of smooth muscle	Arylsulfatases
Bradykinin and related kinins	From plasma kininogens, near 1,000 mol wt	Contracts smooth muscle slowly	None known
Anaphylatoxins	C3a, 8,900 mol wt C4a, 9,000 mol wt C5a, 16,000 mol wt (not involved in IgE-regulated activities)	Release histamines	Ana INH
PG	Twenty-carbon unsaturated fatty acids, connection to allergy uncertain	Increase cAMP, dose-dependent effect on histamine release, contract smooth muscle	Indomethacin, aspirin
Platelet-activating factor	Substituted phosphorylcholine	Causes platelet degranulation	Phospholipases

mine, and dog and guinea pig mast cells have 7 to 34 pg of histamine per mast cell; both clearly exceed the human level.

In the mast cell, histamine is held in an ionic complex with heparin in the mast cell granules. Heparin is a substituted polysaccharide consisting primarily of alternating units of α-D-glucuronic acid-2-sulfate and α-D-glucosamine-3,6-disulfate united by a 1,4-glycosidic bond. Heparin has a molecular weight of approximately 17,000. The ionized sulfate and carboxylate groups in heparin hold histamine in an ionic complex through its protonated nitrogen atoms. Degranulation of mast cells dissociates this complex and releases heparin and histamine. As a consequence, the anticoagulant activity of heparin and the vasodilating and smooth muscle contracting properties of histamine are identified easily in the individual suffering from anaphylactic shock.

Histamine constricts smooth muscle (Fig. 17-8), and in humans the musculature of the respiratory system and the smooth muscle of the venules are highly sensitive to histamine. Serious allergic reactions are accompanied by respiratory distress in which the individual takes rapid, short inhalations

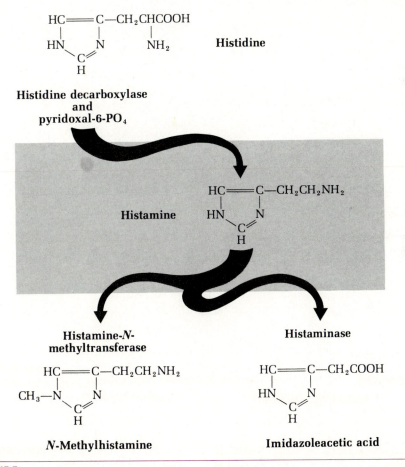

FIG. 17-7
Histamine is formed in the mast cell, as indicated in upper portion of diagram. Two methods of detoxifying histamine are indicated in lower portion.

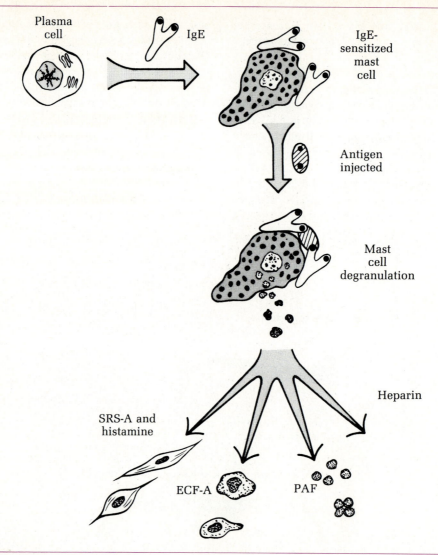

FIG. 17-8

Pathway to anaphylactic sensitivity. Plasma cells are responsible for synthesis of the immunoglobulins that are released and circulate through the blood. The homocytotropic immunoglobulins attach to mast cells. On injection of antigen a cell-fixed antibody-antigen reaction releases histamine and SRS-A to contract smooth muscle, ECF-A to attract eosinophils (eosinophil chemotaxis), PAF to aggregate platelets, and heparin to affect blood clotting.

without an equal exhalation phase. The blood pressure may drop as the capillaries expand, a compensatory action for venule constriction. This forces fluids into the tissue bed (edema), and the accompanying capillary engorgement is observed as erythema.

These activities eventually subside as histamine is detoxified by methylation and oxidation to methylhistamine and imidazoleacetic acid, which do not have the pharmacologic activity of their precursor amine (Fig. 17-7).

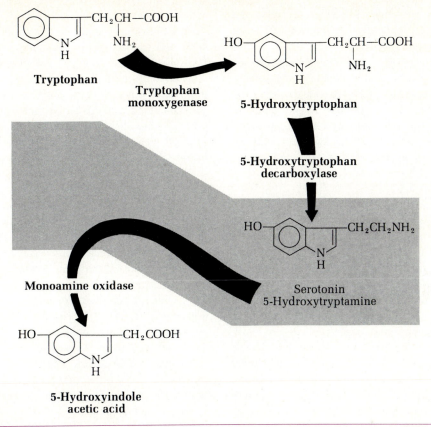

FIG. 17-9

Biochemical pathway for formation of serotonin in the mast cell is indicated in upper half of diagram. Lower half illustrates how detoxification of serotonin occurs.

A role for histamine as a mediator of the inflammatory reaction received its first significant support from the studies of Lewis, who described the triple response of the skin to the intradermal injection of histamine. This response included an immediate edema, erythema, and wheal or spread of these effects into the surrounding tissues. It was recognized that these were the exact characteristics of the immediate hypersensitivity reaction which could be provoked in allergic individuals by the intradermal administration of the offending antigen. It also was known that during anaphylaxis a substance appeared in blood which could be injected into the skin of a normal animal and elicit the triple response. Not until 1953 was it

possible to associate this activity with histamine. Even at that time it was recognized that histamine probably was not the sole mediator of the immediate allergic response.

Serotonin

Serotonin (5-hydroxytryptamine) is derived from the amino acid tryptophan after two enzymatic reactions, the first being a hydroxylation at the 5 position in the ring and the second being the decarboxylation of 5-hydroxytryptophan (Fig. 17-9). Species variation in the distribution and content of serotonin is marked. Most mammals have appreciable serotonin in the gastrointestinal tract and brain. Serotonin is present in the mast cells of many species but not those of the human, mouse, dog, or cat. Platelets are a human source of serotonin.

Serotonin has basically the same pharmacologic action as histamine; it causes a rapid contraction of smooth muscles and increases vascular permeability. Rodents seem especially sensitive to its action; in both rats and mice there are data that definitely implicate serotonin as a primary mediator of anaphylactic shock. This is not true for humans, guinea pigs, or dogs.

Eosinophil chemotactic factor of anaphylaxis

A third product of mast cells that contributes to the immediate hypersensitive response is a chemotaxin for eosinophils (Fig. 17-10).

Its activity has been attributed to two tetra-peptides from mast cells: Val-Gly-Ser-Glu and Ala-Gly-Ser-Glu. Both molecules are very active on eosinophils, less chemoattractant to neutrophils, and have no influence on monocyte motility.

Several other chemotaxins have been described as mast cell products in addition to the low molecular weight ECF-A. An intermediate sized ECF-A with a molecular weight between 1,500 and 3,000 is attractive to eosinophils. Neutrophils respond to a molecule of greater than 75,000 mol wt, described as a high molecular weight neutrophil chemotactic factor (HMW-NCF, or NCF). The chemistry of these molecules is under further study.

Leukotrienes

The treatment of guinea pig lung with cobra venom will release a substance that produces a slow contraction of guinea pig ileum. This material was designated as SRS (for slow-reacting substance) by Feldberg and Kellaway, its discoverers, in 1938. Since that time similar substances elaborated during anaphylaxis also have been noted, and it was suggested that these be designated SRS-A to denote their anaphylactic origin. SRS-A has now been identified as a family of three leukotrienes designated LTC_4, LTD_4, and LTE_4, all of which originate from arachidonic acid. Each leukotriene possesses the ability to cause the prolonged contraction of certain smooth muscles, to produce increases in vascular permeability as measured in skin, and to be synthesized and released on immunologic order. LTC_4 is 200-fold more active than histamine in the smooth muscle contraction of the guinea pig ileum. These molecules do not exist preformed in mast cells.

Arachidonic acid is found in the cytoplasmic membrane of cells where it is esterified into the structure of sphingomyelin. When liberated from sphingomyelin, by the phospholipases involved in mast cell degranulation, arachidonic acid becomes subject to alteration by two principal pathways: the cyclooxygenase or lipoxygenase pathway. The prostaglandins and several chemotactic molecules (thromboxanes) are produced in the former pathway. In the lipoxygenase pathway additional chemotaxins (HETE) and the leukotrienes are synthesized. Arachidonic acid (Fig. 17-11) is oxidized to 5-hydroperoxyeicosatetraenoic acid, which decomposes spontaneously to form leukotriene A (LTA). LTA itself is unstable but becomes stabilized by the addition of glutathione to form LTC_4. This is accomplished by the enzyme glutathione S transferase. The loss of glutamic acid forms LTD_4, and the further loss of glycine from the remainder forms LTE_4, which has only cysteine as its amino acid substituent.

The leukotrienes are liberated from mast cells, basophils, neutrophils, and even macrophages when these cells are stimulated by either IgE- or IgG-mediated serologic reactions on their cell surface. The muscle-contracting property of LTC_4, LTD_4, and LTE_4 is inactivated by arylsulfatase A and B, found in eosinophils to regenerate the inactive LTA, which is degraded further by other enzymes.

Prostaglandins and prostacyclins

The confirmation that SRS-A activity was resident in the leukotriene derivatives of arachidonic acid stemmed from earlier suggestions that prostaglandins were involved in IgE-mediated reactions. The prostaglandins (PG), so named because they were first identified in the prostate gland, are 20-carbon unsaturated fatty acid derivatives of arachidonic acid. Prostaglandins A, B, E, and F are identified according to the position of keto or hydroxyl substitutions

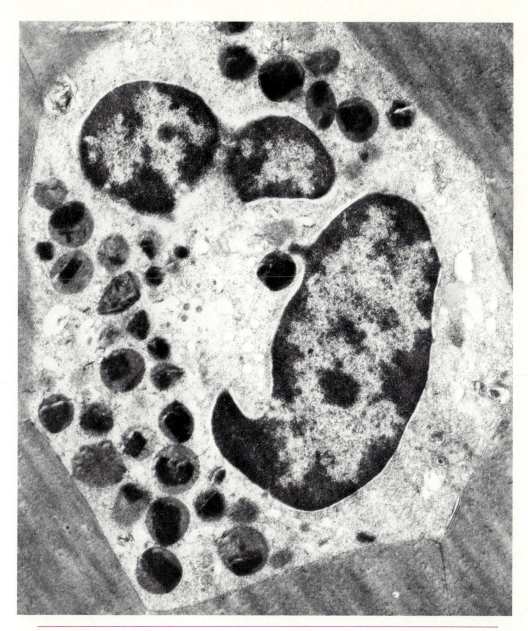

FIG. 17-10

Angular structure of the eosinophil in this electronmicrograph is an artifact created by the dense red cell population surrounding it. Notice that the eosinophil is polymorphonuclear, and its cytoplasm contains many granules. These granules contain a crystalloid bar, which allows them to be distinguished from basophilic or neutrophilic granules. Other than their response to ECF-A, the role of eosinophils in IgE-mediated reactions is uncertain. (Courtesy of Dr. E. Adelstein.)

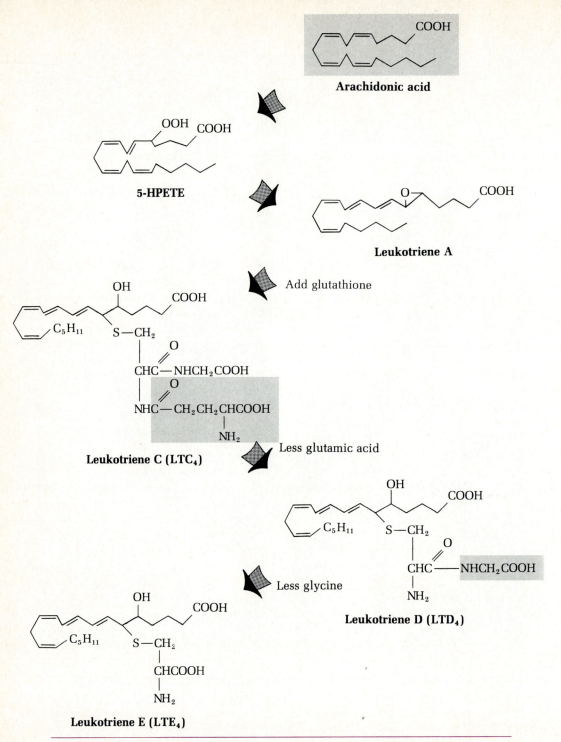

Arachidonic acid

5-HPETE

Leukotriene A

Add glutathione

Leukotriene C (LTC₄)

Less glutamic acid

Leukotriene D (LTD₄)

Less glycine

Leukotriene E (LTE₄)

FIG. 17-11

The leukotrienes with SRS-A activity are created from the metabolism of arachidonic acid via the lipoxygenase pathway. LTC, LTD, and LTE all participate in anaphylactic reactions.

and unsaturated bonds. PGE and PGF compounds are the two best known series in terms of their biologic activity.

During degranulation, the human mast cell releases PGD predominantly, in company with the leukotrienes and histamine. Histamine then acts on lung tissue to cause the release of PGE and PGF_{2a}. PGE causes vasodilation, increases vascular permeability, and lowers the intracellular concentration of cAMP. This, in turn, stimulates more histamine release and continues the cycle. PGF_{2a} causes bronchospasm, bronchodilation and increases vascular permeability, all of which are characteristic of anaphylaxis. The first prostaglandin in this system, PGD, is chemotactic for neutrophils, and causes wheal and flare reactions when injected into skin.

Additional products of arachidonic acid metabolism that may relate to the immediate allergic reaction are the prostacyclins. In the cyclooxygenase pathway of arachidonic acid metabolism, two unstable intermediates, prostaglandin G_2 and prostaglandin H_2, are formed. In lung tissue, PGH_2 is preferentially degraded to PGI_2 which is also unstable. Of importance, however, is that mast cells and macrophages synthesize PGI_2 and this compound is a potent vasodilator, increases vascular permeability, produces pain when injected into the skin, and potentiates the vascular permeability produced by other agents. Although these are familiar activities noted in many inflammatory mediators, the contribution of the prostacyclins to the immediate hypersensitivity reaction is yet to be determined.

Platelet-activating factor

Human mast cells, basophils, monocytes, macrophages, neutrophils and other cells have been identified as sources of 1-0-alkyl-2-acetyl-glyceryl-3-phosphorylcholine, better known as platelet activating factor, or PAF (Fig. 17-12). The biochemical pathway used by these cells to synthesize PAF during the anaphylactic reaction is not yet known, but PAF does not exist in these cells preformed.

The influence of PAF on platelets, particularly rabbit platelets which are more sensitive than their human counterpart, is characterized by a rapid change in shape, a release of serotonin from the

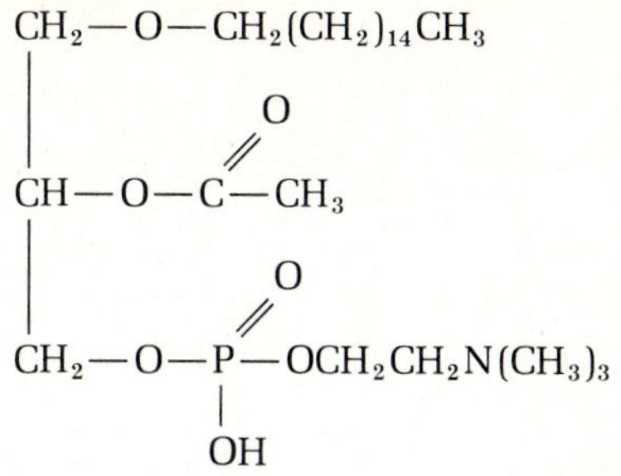

$$CH_2-O-CH_2(CH_2)_{14}CH_3$$
$$|$$
$$\qquad\qquad O$$
$$\qquad\qquad \diagup\!\diagup$$
$$CH-O-C-CH_3$$
$$|$$
$$\qquad\qquad O$$
$$\qquad\qquad \diagup\!\diagup$$
$$CH_2-O-P-OCH_2CH_2N(CH_3)_3$$
$$|$$
$$OH$$

FIG. 17-12
PAF is substituted phosphorylcholine whose alkyl group has a carbon length of 16 to 18 carbons.

platelet granules, and platelet aggregation (Fig. 17-13). *In vivo,* a thrombocytopenia is demonstrable. PAF has other inflammatory activities, including the activation of polymorphonuclear neutrophils, causing their degranulation and shift to oxidative metabolism, the contraction of smooth muscle, and an alteration of vascular permeability. In the last of these PAF has been found to be 100 to 1000 times more potent than histamine. These activities of PAF are destroyed by phospholipases A_2, C, and D.

Bradykinin and other kinins

The term *kinin* was applied to a number of vasoactive substances on the basis of their similar activity long before their chemical structures were known. This activity includes the slow contraction of smooth muscle (*brady,* slow; *kinin,* to move), an extremely potent vasodilating effect, and an enhancement of capillary permeability. The first of these compounds to be characterized chemically was bradykinin itself (Fig. 17-14). It is a peptide composed of only nine amino acids. Closely related to bradykinin in structure are two other compounds, lysylbradykinin (kallidin) and methionyl-lysylbradykinin, also known as kinin 10 and kinin 11, respectively. They all are formed from the same parent compound(s) by what is proving to be a complex biochemical pathway. Not only is the pathway intrinsically complex, involving several compounds in an interrelated sequence of enzyme activation steps (Fig. 17-15), but it also involves a confusing set of nomenclature.

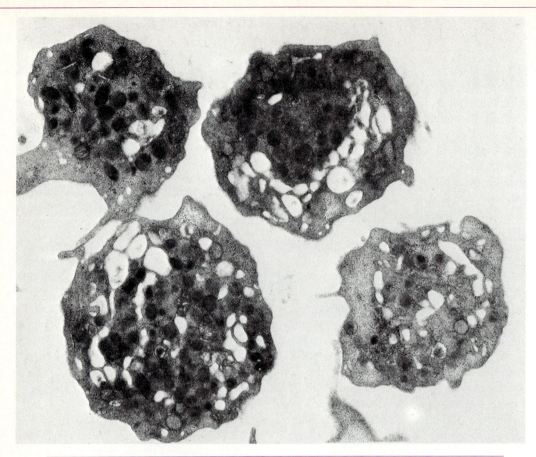

FIG. 17-13
Platelets have numerous granules and vacuoles, as is apparent in this electron micrograph. (Courtesy Dr. E. Adelstein.)

The generation of these kinins begins with the Hageman factor. Hageman's factor, known as factor XII in the blood clotting cascade, is a globulin with a molecular weight of approximately 80,000. Hageman's factor is enzymatically inert until it is activated by contact with a negatively charged surface or antigen-antibody aggregates to become a proteolytic enzyme. In this activation, a serine protease activity is generated. This enzyme is capable of activating plasminogen proactivator and prekallikrein (prokininogenase). Activation of plasminogen proactivator forms plasminogen activator. This enzyme and its proenzyme are both γ-globulins with molecular weights near 100,000. Plasminogen activator converts plasminogen, a β-globulin with a molecular weight of 80,000, into plasmin, an active proteolytic enzyme. Plasmin converts a proenzyme, prokininogenase, also known as prekallikrein, into its enzymically active form kininogenase, or kallikrein. This involves a peptide bond cleavage in the 108,000 mol wt proenzyme (also cited to exist in two forms with molecular weights nearer 90,000) to produce its enzyme. Hageman's factor is also able to effect this hydrolysis to form kininogenase.

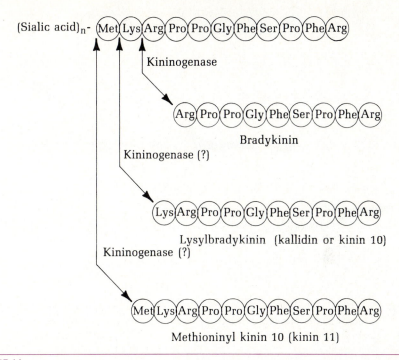

Human kininogen I

FIG. 17-14

Several kininogens and kininogenases in human tissues are known. This diagram suggests how bradykinin and its related kinins may be formed from kininogen I.

The substrates for kininogenase are the kininogens. These are naturally occurring serum proteins separated into high molecular weight and low molecular weight subclasses. These differ in size from species to species and from report to report, but the high molecular weight molecules range between 80,000 and 125,000 mol wt, and the low molecular weight forms are near 50,000 mol wt. Both types of kininogen contain the sequence of bradykinin within their structure; bradykinin is situated centrally in high molecular weight and terminally in low molecular weight kininogens (Fig. 17-16). Thus the activation of four proenzymes, all found in plasma, culminates in the generation of the kinins.

Various peptidases, which can use kinins as substrates, destroy their biologic activity. Kininases in certain tissues may be highly specific; for example, a specific oligoendopeptidase in brain hydrolyzes only bradykinin and not other substrates.

Anaphylatoxins

Anaphylatoxins are, by definition, molecules of biologic origin that can induce the release of histamine from mast cells. Three anaphylatoxins are known to originate from complement: C3a, C4a, and C5a. These molecules produce edema and erythema in human skin. Their vasoactive property is dependent on a terminal arginine and is lost when this arginine is removed. The knowledge that the activation of complement by nonantibody mechanisms through the properdin or alternate pathway would release C3a, C4a, and C5a suggests these anaphyl-

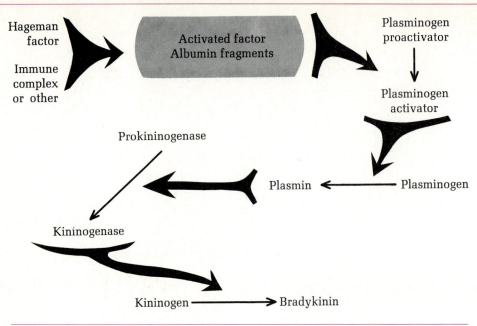

FIG. 17-15

Multistage proenzyme-enzyme reactions through which bradykinin and other kinins are released begin with the activation of Hageman's factor by immune complexes or enzymes, starch, agar, drugs, and other substances that produce anaphylactoid reactions. (From Barrett, J.T.: Basic immunology and its medical application, ed. 2, St. Louis, 1980. The C.V. Mosby Co.)

atoxins may be very important in nonantibody-mediated immediate allergic reactions (anaphylactoid reactions).

Anaphylactoid reactions

Anaphylactoid reactions can be produced by the injection of agar, starch, india ink, colloidal iron, barium sulfate, and several other nonantigenic materials. These immunologically inert materials activate serum and tissue proteases and the alternate pathway of the complement system. This is the basis of anaphylactoid reactions.

Direct chemical degranulation of mast cells may be the cause of anaphylactoid reactions resulting from the injection of complex macromolecules, or these may function by first causing anaphylatoxin formation. Several low molecular weight agents, including the calcium ionophore A 23187, guanidine, aromatic and aliphatic monoamines, diamines, and quaternary amines, opiates, and radiocontrast me-

dias, will liberate histamine from mast cells. The most thoroughly studied of these is probably 48/80, a condensation product of p-methoxyphenethylmethylamine and formaldehye, which is an extremely potent histamine releaser. The administration of large quantities of 48/80 will throw an animal into a synthetic duplicate of anaphylactic shock. The injection of 48/80 into the skin produces the triple response typical of immediate hypersensitive skin reactions. Examination of biopsy tissue specimens after either experience reveals that mast cells indeed are degranulated. If the chemically initiated release of histamine in a sensitized animal is continued until the histamine storage depots are exhausted in a nonlethal reaction, then the animal is desensitized to anaphylactic shock by specific antigen.

Moderators of anaphylaxis

Since such a variety of chemical substances are involved in the immediate allergic reaction, and

High molecular weight kininogen

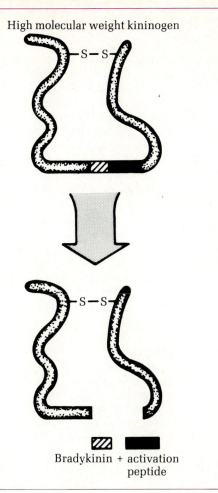

Bradykinin + activation
peptide

FIG. 17-16
High molecular weight kininogen contains a centrally located bradykinin *(striped bar)*, which is liberated with an activation peptide by kininogenase.

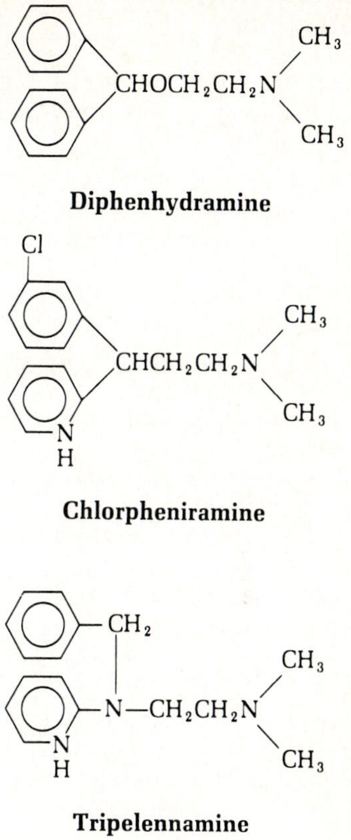

Diphenhydramine

Chlorpheniramine

Tripelennamine

FIG. 17-17
Structures of three antihistamines. These compounds all are substituted diamines. Literally dozens of compounds with antihistaminic activity are known.

since smooth muscle is an important target organ, it is clear that antagonists of those chemicals and smooth muscle relaxants would be superior combatants of these reactions. The body's natural moderators of anaphylaxis are the enzymes that decompose the mediators of anaphylaxis.

Antihistamines

Histamine acts on mammalian cells by combining with histamine receptors on their cell surface, of which there are two distinct types, H1 and H2. The H1 receptor is more important in immunology than the H2 receptor, since it is associated with smooth muscle contraction, venule dilation, and pruritus. The classic antihistamines competitively inhibit this receptor. The H2 receptor is associated with nonimmunologic events such as histamine-induced gastric secretion and mucous secretion, but it also may be important in suppressing T cell activities.

Antihistamines frequently are substituted amines or ethanolamines that have only a vague resemblance to the structure of histamine (Fig. 17-17). Nevertheless these compounds plus certain substituted piperazines, phenothiazines, and hydroxyzines are compet-

☰ SITUATION

ANAPHYLACTIC OR ANAPHYLACTOID?

The elevator for employees stopped on the fifth floor, and I expected to see one of my friends from the physiology department get on. Sure enough, John S., pushing a cart ahead of him, stepped on and pushed the ground floor button. As we started down, I asked him how his research was going.

"You've got the answer right in front of you. On that cart is the sixth animal in a row that died before we could complete the experiment. Every one of them lately has died of anaphylaxis."

"How do you know it's anaphylaxis? What's your experimental set up?"

"Well, we've been wanting to check the effect of a new drug used for parasite infections on kidney function. We've set up a series of intravenous injections of the compound, increasing the dose stepwise. At various times we give them tests for kidney function and take kidney biopsies. Now that we have increased the dose to 5 mg the animals all roll over dead in about 10 minutes."

"I don't know, John. It might be anaphylaxis, and it might not. Let me check you out on a few things. You know what an anaphylactoid reaction is, don't you?"

Questions

1. What is an anaphylactoid reaction?
2. What types of agents cause anaphylactoid reactions?
3. What are the major characteristics that distinguish anaphylactoid and anaphylactic reactions?
4. How can anaphylactoid reactions be prevented or treated?

Solution

An anaphylactoid reaction may be defined as any reaction having the characteristics of anaphylaxis but not based on immunologic phenomena. Anaphylactoid reactions are acute, life-threatening reactions that follow the intravascular administration of nonantigenic materials. Substances that provoke anaphylactoid reactions also lack the qualities of autocoupling haptens. Nevertheless in sufficient doses these agents through direct actions on the kinin system of the blood, or on basophils and mast cells, cause the release of histamine, serotonin, kinins, and other mediators that are responsible for the anaphylaxis-like reaction. Small quantities may produce symptoms so mild as to go unnoticed by inexperienced observers, and larger doses may produce pronounced symptoms or death. A direct-dose response relationship is not a constant observation in anaphylactoid reactions, however. A dose of a given magnitude may produce an anaphylactoid reaction on one occasion and fail to do so at another time.

Anaphylactic reactions are dose dependent, but this is difficult to demonstrate, since such tiny amounts of antigen can elicit the full response. An important feature which distinguishes these two reactions is the failure to observe antibodies in individuals who demonstrate anaphylactoid reactions.

Among the substances causing anaphylactoid reactions, starch, organic iodine, agar, bromphenol blue, and contrast media used in urographic analysis can be mentioned. The latter are important human causes of anaphylactoid reactions. These reactions are so unpredictable and rare (only 0.05% of all patients subjected to intravenous pyelography had acute reactions) that little is done to prevent them. Treatment is also uncertain, but corticosteroids, fluid replacement, and adrenergic drugs have been used.

In this situation the death of the animals almost certainly was caused by anaphylactoid reaction to the large doses of the drug used in the later injections.

itive inhibitors of histamine. Antihistamines have no effect on histamine release from mast cells or basophils. In humans antihistamines are effective antagonists of edema and pruritus, and this is probably related to their blockage of histamine-induced increases in capillary permeability. Antihistamines are relatively less effective in humans in preventing bronchoconstriction.

The competitive function of histamine analogs is best displayed when they are administered prior to the release of histamine. Since this is rarely the case in human allergies, these drugs have been thought less effective than experimental situations indicate. Drug effectiveness always must be evaluated in terms of side effects, and sedation is a major undesired effect of many antihistamines.

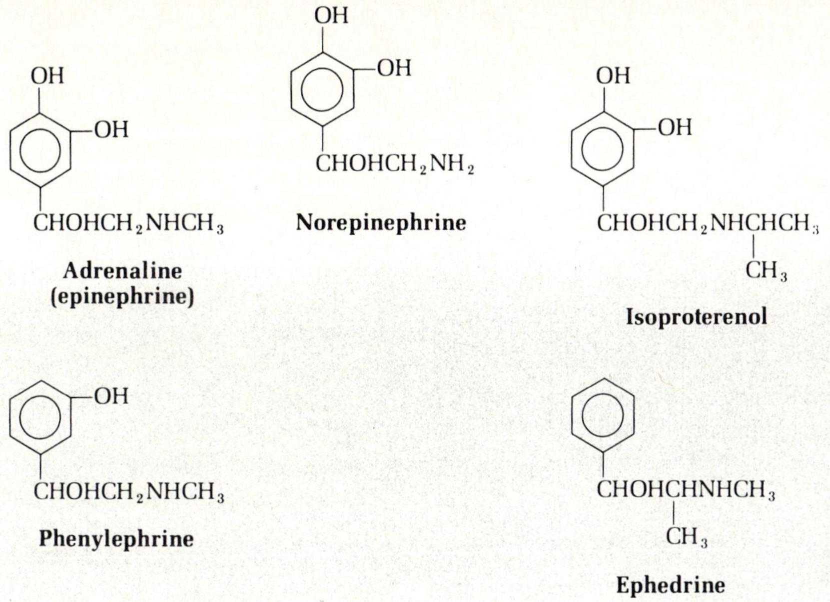

OH

OH

$CHOHCH_2NHCH_3$

**Adrenaline
(epinephrine)**

OH

OH

$CHOHCH_2NH_2$

Norepinephrine

OH

OH

$CHOHCH_2NHCHCH_3$

CH_3

Isoproterenol

OH

$CHOHCH_2NHCH_3$

Phenylephrine

$CHOHCHNHCH_3$

CH_3

Ephedrine

FIG. 17-18
Adrenaline and several related adrenergic drugs.

Catecholamines

The terms *adrenergic* drug, *sympathomimetic drug,* and *catecholamines* are used interchangeably to describe a series of substituted amines that have a potent bronchodilating and smooth muscle relaxant activity. The physiologic response to these compounds is best explained on the basis of the concept of the α, β, and $β_2$ receptors on the effector cells. The α receptors govern muscle constriction; the $β_1$ receptor regulates lipolysis and cardiac muscle responses, and the $β_2$ receptor is concerned with bronchodilation and vasodilation. Various adrenergic drugs differ in their affinity for these three receptors, and thus may differ significantly in their effect on the immediate hypersensitive response. The preferred drugs are those that influence the $β_2$ receptors. The best known of these are adrenaline (epinephrine), ephedrine, and isoproterenol, but many structurally related compounds are available (Fig. 17-18). Preferential attachment to the $β_2$ receptor relaxes smooth muscle, thus reversing the effect of histamine and other mediators of anaphylaxis. These drugs also act directly on mast cells to increase cAMP levels and thus stabilize mast cells against further degranulation. Consequently, the $β_2$ adrenergic drugs have both prophylactic and therapeutic applications.

Cromolyn

Extracts of the seeds of the plant *Ammi visnaga* contain a complex heterocyclic compound—cromolyn sodium—that has been tested and proven effective in modifying allergic reactions. The compound is absorbed poorly from the intestinal tract (Fig. 17-19), therefore it is administered by inhalation. The field trial successes can be attributed to its prevention of histamine and leukotriene release from mast cells, which cannot degranulate in the presence of cromolyn. Cromolyn also retards calcium accumulations by mast cells and elevates their cAMP by inhibiting phosphodiesterase. Cromolyn is a prophylactic drug and is not antagonistic to leukotrienes or histamine.

A specific cromolyn binding protein (CBP) of 50,000 to 55,000 molecular weight is the key Ca^{2+} channel forming protein on the mast cell. Reaction

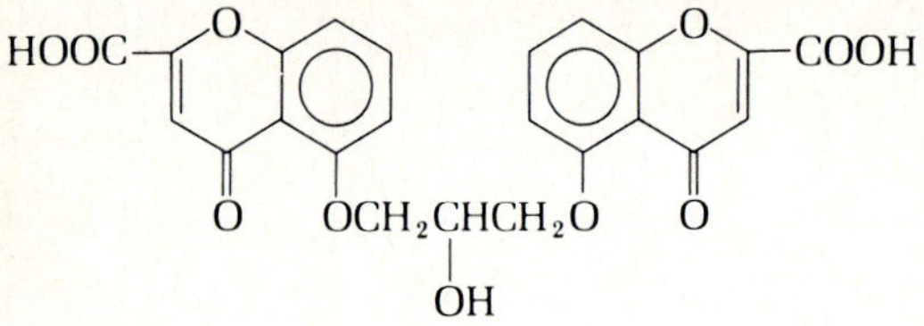

Cromolyn

FIG. 17-19
Structure of cromolyn.

of surface IgE with antigen aggregates the CBP to permit the calcium flux into the cell that precedes degranulation. This is blocked by combination of CBP with cromolyn.

Methyl xanthines

Relaxation of smooth muscle by the methyl xanthines caffeine, theophylline, and theobromine has encouraged their use as bronchodilators. These compounds also function at the level of the mast cell by increasing the concentration of cAMP and reducing mast cell degranulation. An undesirable effect of the methyl xanthines is their diuretic function.

Antiserotonins

Inhibition of 5-hydroxytryptophan-induced constriction of smooth muscle is possible with lysergic acid derivatives, but because of the hallucinogenic activity of these compounds, they are not used.

Desensitization

When skin tests reveal that an intended recipient is allergic to an antigenic injectable or inhalant allergen, the existing cellbound IgE can be neutralized. This can be accomplished and yet avoid the life-threatening hazard of a massive release of histamine if minute and increasing dosages of the antigen are injected over a few hours. The first small amounts of antigen provoke only a minimal amount of histamine release, and this is rapidly converted to the inert imidazoleacetic acid. When the symptoms of mild histamine shock have disappeared, another dose of antigen is given, and this is continued until the individual can tolerate the therapeutic dose of the injectable.

Before IgE neutralization is attempted, it is prudent to administer antihistamines and to have adrenaline ready to reverse any accidental severe shock. This desensitization is temporary and in fact consists of booster exposures to the antigen. A week or so after neutralization has been completed, the production of IgE may restore the original hypersensitivity.

It does not necessarily follow that repeated exposure to an allergen will accentuate the hypersensitivity. Specific desensitization procedures are based on booster injections of antigen spaced over periods of weeks rather than hours to prompt the formation of blocking antibodies. These blocking antibodies are circulating IgG antibodies which combine with the antigen in the vascular system and prevent antigen diffusion into the tissues where IgE-coated mast cells reside. This mechanism of action for blocking antibodies was first proved in desensitization to insect stings, where the level of IgG blocking antibodies is well correlated with the degree of protection against the allergic reaction. Blocking antibodies now have been proved to be the protective antibodies formed by desensitization to several allergens. It does not matter that the desensitization increases IgE levels; there was previously sufficient IgE present to render the individual seriously allergic. What is important is that cellbound IgE has less chance to react with allergen in the face of high levels of circulating IgG.

ATOPY

Approximately 10% to 20% of the population in the United States has some type of allergy. Of these, it has been estimated that 8,000,000 persons have hay fever, 3,000,000 have asthma, and 9,000,000 have atopic allergies to other agents—certain foods, animal dandruff or feathers, dust, antibiotics, wool, insect stings, and a countless variety of other substances. These atopic allergies (*atopy,* a strange disease) are for the most part naturally occurring conditions for which the antigenic exposure is not always known.

Atopic illnesses were among the first antibody-associated diseases noted to have a strong familial or hereditary tendency. More than 60 years ago hay fever, bronchial asthma, and food allergies were observed to be family-associated in almost half the reported instances. About 58% of all allergic children had parents who were both allergic, and only 12.5% of such children had allergy-free parents. Knowledge of the genetic basis for allergies thus has a long history.

Genetic studies in humans first suggested specific haplotypes were associated with atopic allergy to ragweed, but this was not supported by subsequent analyses. Nevertheless genetic studies in mice have determined that poor IgE responders are under Ir gene control via Ts cells.

Inhalant allergy

Probably the most common offending inhalant antigens are pollens or spores of higher plants and molds. Animal danders, vegetable and cereal dusts, and house dust should not be excluded from this list of excellent natural sensitizers. The pollens of higher plants such as the several species of ragweed (genus *Ambrosia*), many different trees, and grasses are responsible for the condition known as hay fever. It has been estimated that a single ragweed plant produces as many as 1,000,000 pollen grains annually. A square mile of ragweed would liberate about 16 tons of pollen into the air in one season (Fig. 17-20). The pollen grains are very light and can be carried for miles by a gentle summer breeze. Contact of the pollen with the mucous membranes of the eye, nose, and throat is the normal manner of sensitization. Reexposure of these surfaces, perhaps in a subsequent pollen season, causes the local allergic reaction known as hay fever. Sneezing, watery reddened eyes, an itching and running nose, and respiratory distress are all part of the usual episode. Although this might be described as a mild form of anaphylaxis, local in nature because of the mode of contact and insoluble state of the pollen, hay fever sufferers certainly would not refer to their condition as a mild illness.

It would be impossible to consider the chemistry of the many pollen antigens, even if they were known. The principal antigens of the low ragweed plant, *Ambrosia elatior,* are two proteins designated as antigens E and K. Studies with antigen E and its reaginic antibody led to the designation IgE for that antibody. These have been purified by a combination

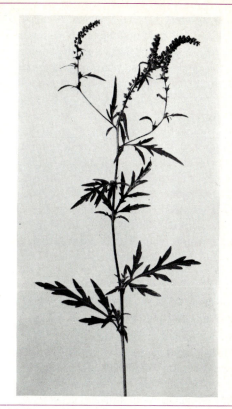

FIG. 17-20

Ragweed plant with pollen-bearing stems at the top.

of ammonium sulfate precipitation, Sephadex filtration, and ion exchange chromatography. Both antigens have molecular weights of about 38,000, and both are pure proteins containing less than 1% carbohydrate. Antigen E represents 6% of the total protein in the pollen and antigen K about 3%. These two antigens, which are not cross-reactive, represent the two most important allergenic proteins in low ragweed. Although other antigens are present in the pollen, they have a much weaker sensitizing ability.

Other offending pollens include those of *Ambrosia trifida* (giant ragweed), those of most trees, including elm, oak, and pines, and those of grasses such as rye, timothy, and bluegrass. Many flower pollens are allergy inducers.

Allergy to house dust is surprisingly constant over widely dispersed geographic areas where the dust has clear differences in composition because of the nature of the soil itself and the plants which grow in these areas. A common feature of house dust is its population of dust mites, which live in carpets and soil. Many persons allergic to house dust react to extracts of the mites *Dermatophagoides farinae* and *D. pteronyssinus*.

The respiratory allergies are often divided into those with a seasonal and those with a nonseasonal frequency. This is useful to physicians in identifying the source of the allergy. Obviously, those allergies with a nonseasonal pattern are due to substances to which we are constantly exposed—house pets, house dust, down-filled pillows, occupational dusts, etc. Allergens whose production is controlled by climate are the usual offenders in the case of nonseasonal allergies.

Ingestant allergy

Food allergies represent another major class of atopic allergies. An allergy to food may arise at any age; it may be expressed locally by oral inflammation, canker sores, cramping, by nausea, gaseous distention, and diarrhea. The symptoms may erupt in the skin as splotches of urticaria known as hives. Respiratory symptoms also may develop, especially with dry foods to which respiratory exposure is almost guaranteed. Based on skin sensitivity testing of 200 allergic children below the age of 8 years, the following percentages of allergy were determined for these foods: chocolate 19%, cow's milk 15%, wheat or wheat products 26%, orange 25%, strawberries 33%, and codfish 45%. Other "good" allergens include tomatoes, peanuts, egg, and rye and other cereals. Food avoidance rather than desensitization is recommended to prevent recurrence of food allergies.

Injectant allergy

Anaphylactic allergy arising from the injection of antigens also can exist as an atopic allergy. In the United States about 40 deaths are reported each year as the result of insect stings. The principal insects involved are represented by the common honey bee, yellow jacket, yellow hornet, paper wasp, and others in the order *Hymenoptera*. Only the females of these insects sting, and when they do so, several different proteins, including the enzymes phospholipase, hyaluronidase, and phosphatase, may sensitize the individual by stimulating an IgE response. A repeated sting may incite a serious, even lethal anaphylactic response to these enzymes contained within the venom. Bee keepers who are insensitive to bee stings have high levels of IgG, in the company or absence of high circulating levels of IgE.

Although penicillin is undoubtedly one of the least toxic of all drugs used in the therapeusis of human and animal diseases, it has been responsible for an increasing number of allergic reactions and anaphylactic deaths since its introduction on the pharmaceutical market approximately 45 years ago. It now is estimated that over 300 anaphylactic deaths occur each year from treatment with penicillin.

Penicillin is a complex, although relatively low molecular weight, compound that is subject to decomposition by several different routes to a diverse array of products. Most intermediates and end products have been isolated or synthesized and used as haptenic sensitizers of humans and experimental animals. Immunization with hapten-antigen conjugates also has been practiced. Studies of the dermal sensitivity or antiserum reactivity with specific degradation products have indicated that penicilloic acid derivatives, and to a lesser extent derivatives of penicillamine and penicillenic acid, are the key sensitizing agents (Figs. 2-5 and 17-21). All these are capable of covalent bonding with proteins, the latter two through sulfhydryl exchange reactions. Penicilloyl conjugates are formed by amidination reactions which open the oxazole ring of penicillenic acid.

Detection of anaphylactic sensitivity to one or another of the haptenic metabolites of penicillin is complicated by several problems associated with skin tests with haptens. One of these is that the hapten alone is incapable of releasing the pharmacologic mediators of immediate hypersensitivities because haptens cannot bridge two IgE molecules. Second, on combination with the antibody the free hapten may block the binding of any in vivo–formed hapten-protein conjugate and thus mask the hypersensitivity that is present. A third problem is that in vivo formation of the hapten-protein conjugate may be so

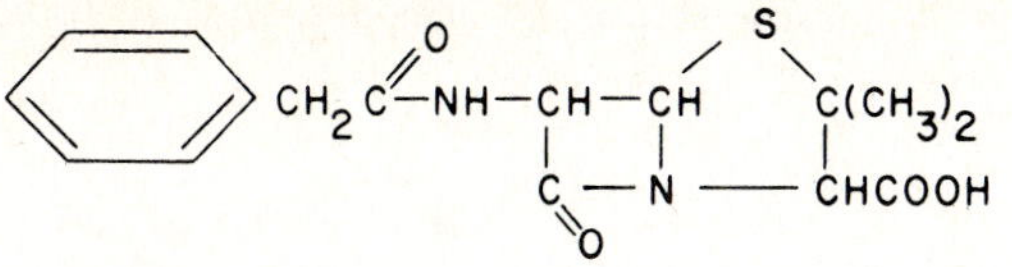

Penicillin G

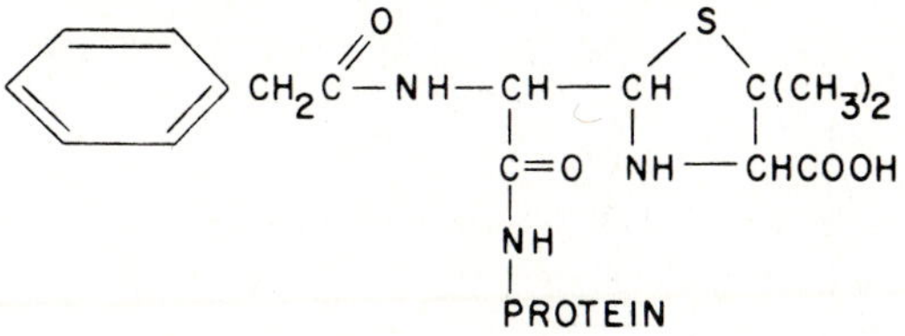

Penicilloic acid–protein complex

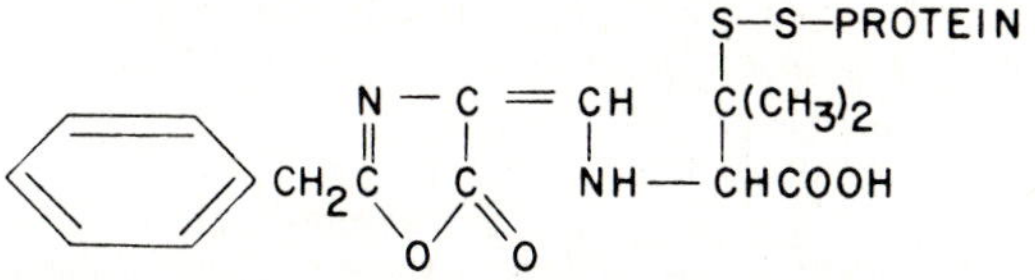

Penicillenic acid–protein complex

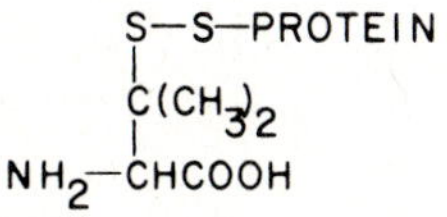

Penicillamine–protein complex

FIG. 17-21

Three hypersensitizing derivatives of benzyl penicillin (penicillin G). The penicilloic acid compound is formed by opening of the oxazolone ring of penicillenic acid during conjugation.

rapid and extensive that systemic anaphylactic shock rather than a mild skin reaction may be elicited. A fourth factor is that the skin test with the hapten may serve as a hypersensitizing experience and produce sensitivity in a previous nonsensitive individual.

It is clear that the use of hapten-protein conjugates would eliminate some of the faults of testing with pure haptens alone, since it could be made multivalent with respect to penicillin determinants and used in a standardized fashion. Testing with hapten alone always leads to some confusion, since the amount of autocoupling from person to person varies considerably. One major fault inherent in the use of conjugates is that one can become sensitized to the protein carrier. Egg albumin, milk casein, and certain other proteins that humans regularly contact in their diet should not be used as carriers. A clever solution to this dilemma was realized when penicilloyl poly-D-lysine became available. After testing it was found that this reagent is a very sensitive detector of penicillin hypersensitivity in the human when other tests are negative. Furthermore it does not induce penicillin allergy or allergy to poly-D-lysine, since this carrier is nonimmunogenic. The use of this reagent has greatly reduced the incidence of allergic reactions to penicillin, since individuals whose skin test results are positive now can be selectively excluded from the anaphylactic risk group by being given an alternative therapeutic.

Miscellaneous allergies

Physical allergies to heat, cold, sunlight, and pressure are not as life threatening as those related to injectables. Heat, cold, and ultraviolet light are believed to cause a physicochemical derangement of proteins or polysaccharides of the skin and transform them into autoantigens that are responsible for the allergic reaction. Prevention of these allergies is based on avoidance of the incitant. Dermographism (dermatographism, or skin writing) is seen as edematous and mildly erythematous eruptions in the track of mild pressure applied to the skin. Most if not all of these are due to the action of a self-directed IgE.

DETECTION OF THE IgE-DEPENDENT HYPERSENSITIVITIES

Diagnosis of atopic allergies is dependent on the specificity of the immediate skin reaction observed after the intradermal exposure to the allergen. This may be done by scratch, prick, or intracutaneous testing. A droplet of the allergen extract is placed in a superficial scratch on the skin and observed for local edema. Literally, a score of such tests can be applied to the back and forearms of a patient at one sitting. In prick testing, a series of small skin punctures is made with a needle, and a droplet of allergen is placed on the skin. Scratch and prick testing are about a hundred times less sensitive than intracutaneous testing. Ophthalmic testing, with observation for conjunctival irritation, is little better than intracutaneous testing, although it may involve slightly less risk. Diagnosis is also possible on the basis of the P-K test. The P-K test now is used only when it is necessary to avoid multiple skin testing of a child or of a seriously ill individual.

With the knowledge that IgE is the allergic antibody, in vitro testing procedures for total IgE content of sera (RIST) or IgE specific for specially selected antigens (RAST) are available to replace the skin testing currently used in diagnosing atopic allergies. However these tests are relatively expensive. The radial quantitative immunodiffusion test is a less expensive substitute. After diagnosis of the allergy, desensitization can be initiated if needed.

REFERENCES

Ahlstedt, S., and Kristofferson, A.: Immune mechanisms for induction of penicillin allergy, Prog. Allergy 30:67, 1982.

Becker, E.L., Simon, A.S., and Austen, K.F., editors: Biochemistry of the acute allergic reactions, New York, 1981, Alan R. Liss, Inc.

Breneman, J.C.: Basics of food allergy, ed. 2, Springfield, 1984, Charles C. Thomas Publisher.

Buckle, D.R., and Smith, H., editors: Development of antiasthma drugs, London, 1984, Butterworth and Co. Publishers, Ltd.

Froese, A.: Receptors for IgE on mast cells and basophils, Prog. Allergy 34:142, 1984.

Galli, S.J., Dvorak, A.M., and Dvorak, H.F.: Basophils and mast cells: morphologic insights into their biology, secretory patterns, and function, Prog. Allergy 34:1, 1984.

Gershwin, M.E., and Keslin, M.H., editors: Allergic emergencies, Clin. Rev. Allergy 3:1, 1985.

Gibson, G.G., Hubbard, R., and Parke, D.V.: Immunotoxicology, London, 1983, Academic Press, Inc.

Gorevic, P.D., and Levine, B.B.: Penicillin allergy: prediction, prevention, diagnosis, treatment and desensitization, Clin. Immunol. Update 1985, New York, 1985, Elsevier Science Publishing Company, Inc.

Heiner, D.C., editor: Food allergy, Clin. Rev. Immunol. 2:1-95, 1984.

Homburger, H.A.: Diagnosis of allergy: in vitro testing, CRC Crit. Rev. Clin. Lab. Sci. 23:279, 1986.

Ishizaka, K.: Isotype-specific T cell factors for the IgE response, CRC Crit. Rev. Immunol. 5:229, 1985.

Ishizaka, K.: Regulation of IgE synthesis, Ann. Rev. Immunol. 2:159, 1984.

Lichtenstein, L.M., and Fauci, A.S., editors: Current therapy in allergy, immunology and rheumatology, Toronto, 1985, B.C. Decker, Inc.

Lieberman, P.L., and Crawford, L.V.: Management of the allergic patient, New York, 1982, Appleton-Century-Crofts.

Malmsten, C.L.: Leukotrienes: mediators of inflammation and immediate hypersensitivity, CRC Crit. Rev. Immunol. 4:307, 1984.

Metzger, H., Alcaraz, G., Hohman, R., Kinet, J.-P., Pribluda, V., and Quarto, R.: The receptor with high affinity for immunoglobulin E, Ann. Rev. Immunol. 4:419, 1986.

Newball, H.H., editor: Immunopharmacology of the lung, New York, 1983, Marcel Dekker, Inc.

O'Flaherty, J.T., and Wykle, R.L.: Biology and biochemistry of platelet-activating factor, Clin. Rev. Allergy 3:353, 1983.

Parker, C.W.: The chemical nature of slow-reacting substances, Adv. Inflamm. Res. 4:1, 1982.

Samuelsson, B.: Leukotrienes: a new class of mediators of immediate hypersensitivity reactions and inflammation, Adv. Prostagland. Thrombox. and Leukotriene Res. 11:1, 1983.

Samuelsson, B., and Paoletti, R., editors: Leukotrienes and other lipoxygenase products, New York, 1982, Raven Press.

Schwartz, L.B., and Austen, K.F.: Structure and function of the chemical mediators of mast cells, Prog. Allergy 34:271, 1984.

Sirois, P.: Pharmacology of the leukotrienes, Adv. Lipid Res. 21:79, 1985.

Solomon. W.R., editor: Allergens, Clin. Rev. Immunol. 3:269, 1985.

Speer, F.: Food allergy, ed. 2, Bristol, 1983, John Wright PSG, Inc.

Spiegelberg, H.L.: Structure and function of Fc receptors for IgE on lymphocytes, monocytes, and macrophages, Adv. Immunol. 35:61, 1984.

Yoshida, H., Hagihara, Y., and Ebashi, S., editors: Biochemical-immunological pharmacology, Oxford, 1982, Pergamon Press, Ltd.

Cytotoxic, immune complex and delayed type hypersensitivities

≡ GLOSSARY

allergy of infection An allergy, often of the delayed type, resulting from an infection.

Arthus reaction A necrotic, dermal reaction caused by antigen-antibody precipitation, complement fixation, and neutrophilic inflammation in tissues of an animal inoculated intracutaneously with antigen.

CBH Cutaneous basophilic hypersensitivity.

cell-mediated hypersensitivity A T cell hypersensitivity of the delayed type.

contact dermatitis A delayed or cell-mediated hypersensitivity response to cutaneously applied allergens.

Coombs test An antiglobulin test to detect the presence of a nonhemagglutinating antibody on the surface of erythrocytes.

cutaneous basophilic hypersensitivity A T cell hypersensitivity characterized by a basophilic infiltration.

delayed hypersensitivity (DH) Synonym for *cell-mediated hypersensitivity;* a form of allergy expressed by T lymphocytes, not involving immunoglobulins, and developing slowly when provoked dermally.

erythroblastosis fetalis A hemolytic disease of the newborn due to the acquisition of maternal antibodies specific for fetal erythrocyte antigens.

HDN Hemolytic disease of the newborn: see *erythroblastosis fetalis.*

immune complex pneumonitis An alveolar Arthus reaction with many synonyms.

Jones-Mote reaction An older synonym of cutaneous basophilic hypersensitivity.

Koch's phenomenon Rejection of subcutaneously placed tubercle bacilli by tuberculous animals as an expression of CMI.

OT Old tuberculin.

passive cutaneous anaphylaxis A form of anaphylaxis caused by dermal injection of cytotropic antibodies followed by systemic injection of antigen.

PCA Passive cutaneous anaphylaxis.

PPD Purified protein derivative of tuberculin.

reversed passive Arthus An Arthus reaction provoked by an intradermal injection of antiserum and intravenous injection of antigen.

RPA Reversed passive Arthus.

serum sickness An allergic reaction caused by the presence of antigen at the time that antibody is being formed.

Shwartzman reaction A necrotic reaction in tissue produced by endotoxins.

T_{DTH} cell The T cell responsible for delayed hypersensitivities.

transfer factor (TF) A ribonucleotide (700 to 4,000 mol wt) that can transfer (in some species) the cell-mediated hypersensitivities of the lymphocytes from which it is extracted.

tuberculin A concentrate of the growth medium of *Mycobacterium tuberculosis* used to test skin for delayed hypersensitivity to this organism.

urushiols Catechols found on poisonous plants, responsible for contact dermatitis.

According to the Gell and Coombs classification of hypersensitivity the cytotoxic and immune complex reactions depend on heat-stable antibodies, in contrast to the anaphylactic allergies associated with the heat-labile IgE described in the preceding chapter. The cytotoxic allergies of alloimmune origin include conditions such as transfusion reactions, hemolytic disease of the newborn (HDN), and components of graft rejection. Autoimmune cytotoxicity, described in Chapter 19, is seen in several blood-vascular conditions, including autoimmune hemolytic disease, autoimmune thrombocytopenia, and autoimmune granulocytopenia. The immune complex reactions also develop from either alloimmune or autoimmune phenomena, but this chapter includes a discussion of only immune complex phenomena related to foreign antigens.

Historically, the cytotoxic and immune complex allergies have been categorized as precipitin allergies because the antigens involved normally precipitate with the fluid antigen. The term *precipitin allergy* seldom is used today.

CYTOTOXIC HYPERSENSITIVITY

Only two examples of alloimmune cytotoxic allergic reactions will be described here and both have erythrocytes as the target cell. Graft rejection as a cytotoxic response to alloantigens is described in Chapter 15.

Blood transfusion reactions

Mismatched blood transfusions involving the ABO or other blood group systems where preformed antibodies are present in the recipient will produce an immediate and severe reaction. This usually includes a mixture of fever and chills, lowered blood pressure, back pain near the location of the spleen and kidneys, and other symptoms. In the later stages, jaundice will develop.

The immunoglobulin responsible for this reaction is IgG, although IgM antibodies undoubtedly contribute to some extent. Since the immunodominant portion of many blood group antigens is polysaccharide in nature, an IgM response accompanies the IgG response. Binding of these antibodies with infused red cells activates the complement system. Lysis of the complement sensitive erythrocytes ensues and the transfusion reaction begins. This is clearly an example of a cell-directed cytotoxic allergy. Due to the deposition of erythrocyte antigen-immunoglobulin complexes in the kidney, aspects of immune complex hypersensitivity are also seen in transfusion reactions.

Blood transfusion reactions historically have been thought of as resulting only from mismatched red blood cells interacting with immunoglobulins. This is still the major cause of hemolytic transfusion reactions, but reactions caused by foreign white blood cells or platelets are a common cause of transient fever after transfusion. An awareness of previous immunization to plasma proteins such as IgA is also necessary to ensure safe transfusions.

Hemolytic disease of the newborn

Erythroblastosis fetalis, one of the more severe forms of HDN, is frequently the result of a so-called Rh incompatibility. The conditions for development of HDN exist when an Rh-negative mother carries an Rh-positive child and through alloimmunization produces antibodies to the Rh antigen. This antibody, if of the IgG class, can pass the placental barrier and react with the fetal erythrocytes (Fig. 18-1). These erythrocytes are removed from the circulation and lysed, causing a hemolytic condition in the fetus. An attempt by the erythropoietic tissue of the fetus to compensate for this loss of mature red blood cells results in an outpouring of immature erythrocytes (erythroblasts) into the blood. From this the name of the condition is derived. Depending on the severity of the disease, the fetus may be aborted, may be stillborn, or may be born alive with evidence of a hemolytic disease.

Until recently there has been little agreement on the origin of maternal Rh alloimmunization. Earlier it had been noted that the first Rh-incompatible pregnancy rarely resulted in HDN but that the risk for erythroblastosis fetalis steadily increased with each succeeding pregnancy. From this it was deduced that the greatest opportunity for maternal immunization was associated with the trauma of childbirth, and there are methods by which fetal contamination of maternal blood can be detected. For example, the

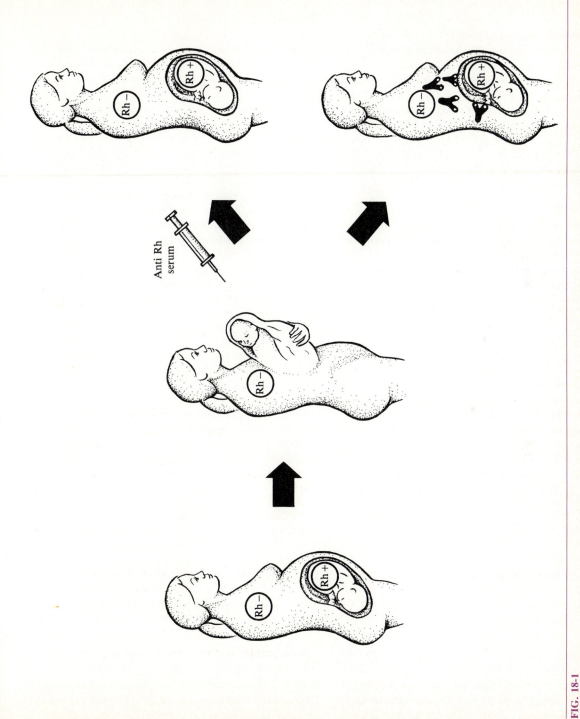

FIG. 18-1

The Rh⁻ mother is exposed to Rh⁺ antigens during the birth of her Rh⁺ child. If passively immunized with anti-Rh sera immediately after delivery, the maternal anti-Rh immune response is suppressed. A subsequent Rh⁺ fetus is uncomplicated by HDN (*upper right*). When passive immunization is not practiced, erythrocytes of an Rh⁺ fetus are subject to destruction by maternal antibodies and complement (*lower right*).

Anti Rh serum

☰ SITUATION 1

THE WORRIED BRIDEGROOM

Your roommate has just returned to the dormitory and announced that he and Louise, his steady since they were sophomores, are pinned. It looks like a summer marriage. After congratulations and a quick trip to The Pub for a brief celebration a sudden cloud passes over your mind, and you ask, "What's Louise's blood type?" Your roommate doesn't know, but then it hits him: "That's right—when we took Immunology 420 I checked out group A,M,Rh+(D). What if she's Rh negative?"

Questions

1. What is an "Rh-incompatible" marriage?
2. Is an Rh-negative mother doomed to produce children with hemolytic disease?
3. Can hemolytic disease result from conditions other than Rh incompatibilities?
4. How is HDN caused by Rh antigens prevented?

Solution

When an Rh(D)-negative woman takes an Rh(D)-positive man as her husband, the possibility exists that their children will inherit the Rh(D) antigen. If the father is genetically Rh+/Rh−, then mathematically only half the children would be Rh positive. Naturally 100% of the children would be Rh positive if the father were homozygous. A marriage between an Rh-positive man and an Rh-negative woman may be described as Rh incompatible, but when the father is heterozygously Rh positive, then only half the children are "incompatible" with the mother. The incompatibility exists because the Rh(D) antigen inherited by the child is considered a foreign antigen by the immune system of the mother. Any fetal cells reaching the maternal lymphoid system will stimulate an anti-Rh(D) response.

The time of almost unavoidable immunization of the mother occurs during childbirth with an Rh-positive child. The rupture of placental membranes releases fetal Rh-positive cells into the womb and activates the immune response. Rh immunization also may result from transfusion of Rh-positive blood into an Rh-negative woman. The first Rh-positive child is unaffected by the incompatibility if his or her birth is the immunizing experience. In a second Rh-positive pregnancy the antibody titer may rise because of exposure to Rh antigens during the gestation period. There is also the possibility of a shift to IgG from IgM antibodies as a result of the booster immunization. The former class of antibodies is more dangerous, since they can migrate freely across the placental barrier. The maternal anti-D globulins move into the fetal circulation and attach to and accelerate the destruction of fetal erythrocytes. The fetus becomes jaundiced and anemic and is delivered with HDN.

Anti-D is the most common cause of HDN. In 99% of all cases of HDN anti-D immunization was known to occur. Even so only about 4% of mothers who have delivered two Rh-positive babies become immunized. Women with Rh-positive children who are compatible with their mother in the ABO or MN groups are more likely to develop anti-D than when their children are ABO incompatible. The maternal anti-A or anti-B tends to minimize immunization with the fetal erythrocytes.

These facts applied to this situation indicate a risk for HDN because of the Rh(D) antigen. If Louise is group O or B, her natural anti-A may reduce somewhat her risk for an affected child, presumably by speeding their elimination and reducing the risk for immunization.

The administration of anti-D to every Rh-negative mother within 72 hours of childbirth has proved fantastically successful in preventing HDN. In one study of 1,662 women so treated only two formed anti-D, whereas in 1,168 untreated control subjects 111 developed anti-D. The mother must be tested to ensure that she is D negative, or a serious reaction could develop when she is passively immunized with anti-D.

hemoglobin of fetal erythrocytes is quickly leached from red blood cells by dilute acid, whereas adult hemoglobin is not. Periodic examination of a mother's blood during pregnancy and especially after delivery has proved that the child's red blood cells can be present in the maternal circulation. Radiolabeled erythrocytes placed in the uterine cavity immediately after delivery were detected in the maternal circulation in 10 of 30 instances. Fluorescent antibody to human γ-globulin that is attached to Rh-positive cells can detect one antibody-coated cell in a population of 1 million Rh-negative cells. This means that as little as 0.01 ml of fetal blood can be detected as foreign in the maternal circulation. By such methods, used in different patient study groups, it has been revealed that 20% to 50% of the mothers are exposed to the blood of their children at delivery.

Rh immunoprophylaxis

To the knowledge that immunization occurred most often at delivery, additional pieces of information have been added to produce an immunologic method for the control of erythroblastosis. One of the added bits of information is that blood group O, Rh-negative mothers have fewer infants with hemolytic disease than statistics would predict. It was suggested that the maternal anti-A and anti-B combined with any A, Rh-positive or B, Rh-positive fetal cells at the moment they entered the maternal circulation and contributed to their speedy removal without antibody formation. It also was shown that Rh-negative men given Rh_0-positive cells precoated in vitro with anti-Rh_0 were protected from making anti-Rh_0. This led to experiments in which pregnant women were given anti-Rh_0 γ-globulin if immunization from an Rh-positive child was anticipated. In one of the studies conducted in the United States 0.2% of mothers passively immunized with anti-Rh_0 globulins developed anti-Rh_0, whereas nearly 7% of untreated mothers produced the antibody. In a study in England 21% of non–passively immunized controls produced anti-Rh_0, compared with only 0.6% of immunized mothers. The studies have been so convincing that passively administered anti-Rh_0 now is given at every delivery or induced abortion for an Rh-negative woman and is considered routine perinatal care for the mother. A typical recommendation is that 100 to 200 μg of anti-Rh_0 be given within 72 hours of delivery unless there is a heavy load of fetal erythrocytes entering the maternal circulation, in which case 1,000 μg of antiserum is given. Interestingly it is believed that incomplete Rh_0 antibodies are largely responsible for the protection and that complete, hemagglutinating antibodies are ineffective. The only serious risk to the procedure that has been noted so far is that recipients who are unable to

synthesize IgA may become sensitized to this immunoglobulin and be subject to anaphylactic shock on reexposure as a result of a later pregnancy. It is believed that Rh immunoprophylaxis may reduce Rh-mediated HDN to 1 in every 20,000 opportunities.

Coombs' tests

However, feedback control of Rh immunization by the passive administration of anti-Rh_0 globulins at the time of delivery only controls future Rh disease and can do little to regulate erythroblastosis when the mother already has been immunized by a previous Rh-positive pregnancy or improper blood transfusion. In these instances the attending physician must in some way measure the potential for HDN. He could assume that maternal anti-Rh could be detected by merely incubating the mother's serum with Rh-positive erythrocytes and determining if they are agglutinated. Such would be the case if the mother had produced the usual complete antibody. Experience has shown, however, that incomplete antibody is as likely as complete antibody to cause erythroblastosis, even though incomplete antibodies do not function in the ordinary hemagglutination test. Fortunately Coombs and his associates have devised a test to demonstrate incomplete antibodies in maternal sera or on fetal or newborn erythrocytes. The Coombs tests, for actually there are two, are known as antiglobulin tests or double antibody tests. In immunologic jargon such tests sometimes are described as immunologic sandwich procedures.

The direct Coombs test is used to detect monovalent maternal antibody already present on the infant's erythrocytes (Fig. 18-2). These antibodies are often anti-Rh in character but could be directed as well toward other erythrocyte antigens. For positive tests it is necessary for the maternal antibody to pass the placenta, enter into the circulation of the unborn child, and attach to his or her red blood cells. If the mother has a low titer of these antibodies, caused either by the decay of hemagglutinin titers developed from an early exposure to antigen or by recent immunization in this pregnancy, insufficient antibody may be present in the fetus to cause death or even serious hemolytic disease prior to birth. However, it is not unusual in such instances for gradual jaundice

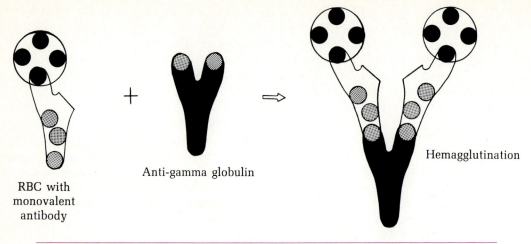

FIG. 18-2

Direct Coombs' test. Erythrocytes coated with a monovalent antibody that is incapable of hemagglutination become agglutinated by an antibody versus the antierythrocyte globulin. Although the monovalent antibody, as illustrated, lacks one Fab fragment, the evidence is that the monovalent and divalent antibodies differ only in function and not in structure.

of the baby to develop within the first few days after birth as a result of red blood cell destruction. This may require total blood exchange transfusion. Therefore it is important to test the baby's red blood cells for antibodies that might cause hemolysis. This is accomplished by the direct Coombs test, which requires only one incubation, that is, newborn red blood cells (coated with incomplete antibody) with an antibody to human γ-globulin. The latter product is available commercially and is prepared by immunizing rabbits, goats, or other animals with human γ-globulin. The Coombs antiglobulin reagent must be a divalent antiglobulin that will combine with the human γ-globulin on the red blood cells and produce hemagglutination. The incomplete anti-Rh serves as both an antibody and an antigen and is the filling in the immunologic sandwich. A negative direct Coombs test is interpreted as an absence of maternal antibody on the child's erythrocytes.

The indirect test is designed to detect the presence of incomplete anti-Rh globulins in maternal sera (Fig. 18-3). Two incubations are needed, as compared with the single incubation in the direct test. Maternal serum is incubated with known Rh-positive cells, after which the cells are washed to remove ex-

traneous serum proteins. This is followed by incubation of the coated cells (in the case of tests that will be positive) with Coombs' reagent, which then agglutinates the cells. Naturally there is no need to perform the indirect Coombs test on maternal sera that contain complete hemagglutinins.

As mentioned briefly, the Coombs test is applicable to the detection of any incomplete immunoglobulin. HDN may arise from incompatibilities between antigens other than the Rh antigen; when monovalent antibodies are incriminated, they can be measured by the Coombs antiglobulin test.

IMMUNE COMPLEX HYPERSENSITIVITY

The formation of soluble immune complexes is favored when the antigen-antibody ratio is greater than 1. When the reverse is true, the complexes continue the aggregation phase of the serologic reaction and become insoluble. In the two examples of immune complex hypersensitivity described in this chapter, serum sickness represents the soluble complex type of hypersensitivity and the Arthus reaction, the precipitated complex type of reaction. Each of these conditions in human subjects was more common in the past than at present. They are described

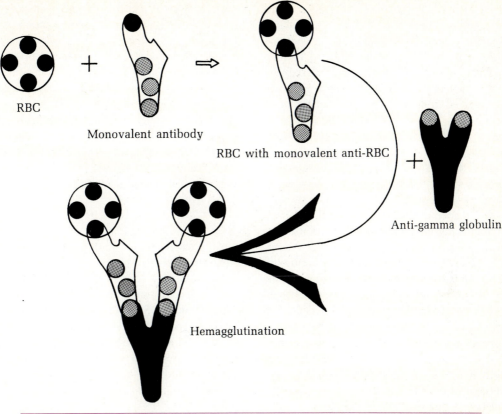

RBC

Monovalent antibody

RBC with monovalent anti-RBC

Anti-gamma globulin

Hemagglutination

FIG. 18-3

Indirect Coombs' test. This test is the same as the direct test except that the monovalent antierythrocyte globulin must be combined with the red blood cell prior to addition of the antiglobulin in the second stage of the reaction.

here because they relate to allergic pneumonitis, a type of naturally developing Arthus reaction, and aspects of certain autoimmune diseases (Chapter 19).

Serum sickness

Serum sickness develops in approximately 50% of normal human beings who receive a single injection of bovine or horse antitoxin against tetanus, gas gangrene, or other toxins for prophylactic or therapeutic purposes. Since antitoxin therapy is less frequently practiced today because of the superiority of immunity developed through active immunization with toxoids, the allergic response to serum per se as the cause of serum sickness is diminishing. An excep-

tion to this can be noted in persons receiving ALS for immunosuppression of graft rejection reactions. The majority of these patients develop serum sickness within a few weeks of therapy even though given chemical immunosuppressives simultaneously. Penicillin is now a most common causative agent of serum sickness, especially penicillin injected in long-acting repository form.

Primary serum sickness

Ordinary serum sickness, an allergic reaction to a foreign serum or an autocoupling hapten, is marked by hives, extensive edema (especially about the face, neck, and joints), joint pain, malaise, and fever.

These symptoms usually are first seen about 7 to 10 days after the injection and persist for several days, after which they gradually subside. von Pirquet and Schick presented the first full description of the disease, although it had been described previously by several investigators. von Pirquet's interest in serum sickness stemmed from his conviction that the onset of many diseases with an inflammatory quality resulted from the formation and reaction of antibodies with an antigen.

Primary serum sickness is caused by the mutual presence of antigen and antibody in the blood following the primary immunization. By about the fifth to eighth day after an initial immunization with a substantial quantity of fluid antigen a portion of the antigen still will be circulating. By this time the initial traces of antibody are detectable in the blood. IgG and possibly other immunoglobulins combine with the antigen in the circulation and are deposited at various locations throughout the body. These immune complexes can be seen in the blood vessel walls and in the kidney, where they can be stained with fluorescent anti-C3 or anti-IgG. Immune complex nephritis is a regular finding in serum sickness. These immune complexes of antigen, antibody, and complement activate the complement cascade. C5a draws neutrophils to the complex, which then is phagocytosed. The neutrophils may release lysosomal enzymes and contribute to local tissue damage. The C3a, C4a, and C5a anaphylatoxins cause degranulation of mast cells, which results in the appearance of histamine, ECF-A, and the leukotrienes in the blood. This pathway accounts for the hypocomplementemia, edema, joint pain, and eosinophilia seen in patients with serum sickness.

In addition to these symptoms relatable to IgG complex formation with antigen, IgE also contributes to serum sickness. Since each molecule of mast cell bound IgE is able to combine with antigen and release histamine at the moment the antibody molecule fixes to cells, there is never a sudden release of lethal quantities of pharmacologic amines and peptides. Moreover histamine detoxification mechanisms may be able to keep pace with its formation under these circumstances. This would also apply to the detoxification of the other molecules that contribute to IgE-based allergic reactions. Thus the symptoms of serum sickness are more chronic and less life threatening than those of anaphylaxis, even though IgE may add to the mast cell effects of the anaphylatoxins.

Since the symptoms of serum sickness do not appear until several days after the injection of the antigen, the disease has been called protracted anaphylaxis. This is a poorly chosen term. Anaphylaxis is clearly an IgE-mediated condition. Serum sickness is largely an IgG-mediated disease, although other immunoglobulin classes, including IgE, may contribute to the symptomatology.

Accelerated serum sickness

An accelerated form of serum sickness can be provoked in persons who were sensitized several years previously to an antigen that they now are given a second time. The appearance of the symptoms within 2 to 5 days is typical in these cases. The hastened onset of accelerated serum sickness compared with primary serum sickness is due to the anamnestic response which follows this second exposure to antigen.

The Arthus reaction

Local anaphylaxis was the term used by Arthus in 1903 to describe the development of dermal necrosis at antigen injection sites in rabbits that have a high level of circulating antibody. In the Arthus reaction the first indication of an allergic reaction is the development of an extensive zone of erythema and edema surrounding the bleb created by the intradermal injection of antigen. Within a few hours a cyanotic center develops within an erythematous ring. Later this assumes a deep purplish black cast indicative of cellular necrosis. Over the succeeding day or two this necrotic zone may enlarge to a few centimeters in diameter. The dead tissue dries, and over a period of a week or more healing becomes complete (Fig. 18-4).

This local reaction is caused by the deposition of an intravascular precipitate and thrombosis. Diffusion of the antigen into the vascular bed surrounding the injection site creates a zone of sufficiently high concentrations of antigen and antibody that a precip-

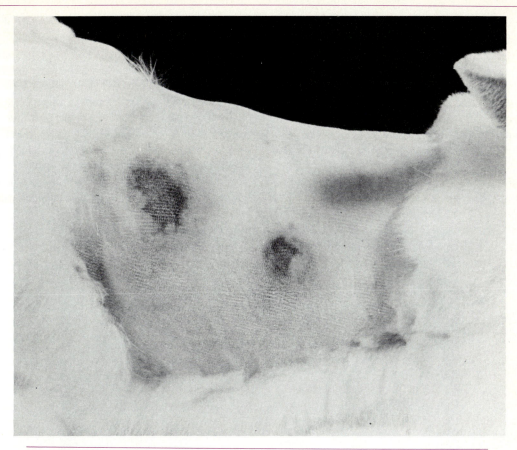

FIG. 18-4

Two Arthus reactions in rabbit skin. The larger reaction has an extensive zone of erythema and edema surrounding its necrotic center.

itate forms. This precipitate becomes so extensive as to physically blockade the small venules. Deprivation of gas exchange, coupled with the inability to adequately eliminate tissue waste products or supply nutrients, results in local tissue destruction. Tissue destruction is further favored by the participation of serum complement in the reaction and the release of chemotactic factors. Massive infiltration of PMNs follows. Within a few hours, after the dermal dose of antigen, the leukocytes begin to disintegrate and release their lysosomal enzymes, which contribute to the damage. Within 1 or 2 days most of the damage has been done, and healing begins.

The pivotal role of neutrophils in the Arthus reac-

tion is demonstrated by the effect of certain alkylating agents on the reaction. In particular the nitrogen mustards have a powerful depressing effect on the level of circulating neutrophilic leukocytes and almost totally eliminate the Arthus reaction. Since these leukocytes are attracted to the site by the action of complement-derived leukotaxins, the complement-fixing antibodies, that is, IgG and IgM, not IgE, dominate the Arthus reaction. A good appraisal of the circulating IgG titer of an animal can be determined by measuring its Arthus response to antigen.

Variants of the Arthus reaction include the passive Arthus and the reversed passive Arthus (RPA) reactions. The first of these is simply the provocation of the Arthus reaction in an animal that has been passively immunized. In the RPA reaction the antiserum is injected into the skin (rather than systematically), and the antigen then is given systemically (rather than intradermally). Both injections are made at about the same time so that a sufficient amount of antibody will remain near the injection site to precipitate with the antigen and cause local necrosis.

PCA and RPA reactions

Sensitization to systemic passive anaphylaxis results from the transfer of serum containing IgE into the vascular system of a normal recipient. When a latent period of 4 to 18 hours is allowed for fixation of the antibody to mast cells and basophils, the animal is sensitized. At that time a shocking dose of antigen given intravascularly will evoke total body anaphylaxis. If the antiserum is injected intradermally, however, only the PCA reaction follows (Fig. 18-5). This is expressed as the triple response of edema, wheal, and erythema, which is difficult to observe on the skin of some animal species. The reaction area is stained a light blue if Evans blue dye is included in the antigen solution. Since the anaphy-

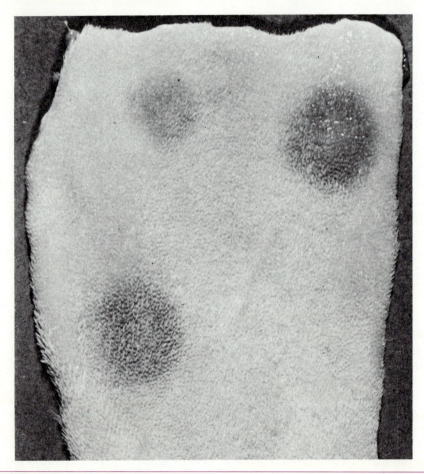

FIG. 18-5

PCA reactions in guinea pig skin. Antiserum dilutions were placed intradermally 18 hours before an intravenous injection of Evans blue dye and antigen. The skin was excised 45 minutes later. The saline control site is on lower right, where no reaction is shown. The positive sites are dark and correlate directly with the dilution of the antiserum injected.

lactic reaction increases the permeability of the vascular bed around the reaction site, blood proteins and the dye leak into and stain the surrounding tissue.

Technically, the RPA and PCA reactions are performed in the same way, that is, antibody is placed in the skin, and antigen is administered intravascularly, but the RPA and PCA reactions are distinct immunologic phenomena (Table 18-1). For the PCA reaction a period of 4 to 18 hours is necessary to allow antibody to fix to cells before a positive test can be elicited by the shocking dose of antigen. Since the Arthus reaction does not depend on mast cell degranulation and histamine release, antihistamines are ineffective in preventing the RPA reaction, but they will moderate the PCA reaction. Any species of antibody will function in the RPA test, but certain species of heterocytotropic antibodies do not fix to guinea pig tissue, and these cannot be used in the PCA test.

Immune complex pneumonitis

The human ailments referred to by the terms *hypersensitivity pneumonitis, allergic pneumonitis,* and *immune complex pneumonitis* are natural expressions of the Arthus reaction. This condition has a plethora of synonyms, most of which are derived from some occupation or avocation associated with the disease, although humidifier lung and air conditioner allergy do not have this type of origin. Thus we have farmer's lung, laundry worker's lung, pigeon breeder's disease, etc. as names for a kind of pneumonitis that is immunologically the same in all affected persons (Table 18-2).

TABLE 18-1
Distinctions between PCA and RPA reactions

	PCA	RPA
Quantity of antibody required	Very little	Large amount
Cytotropic antibody required	Yes; homocytotropic or heterocytotropic	No
Latent period after transfer	Yes	No
Histamine release	Yes	No
Antihistamines effective	Yes	No
Complement required	No	Yes

TABLE 18-2
Various forms of immune complex pneumonitis and their cause

Disease	Source of antigen	Antigen
Humidifier lung	Humidifier evaporation screens	*Thermoactinomyces candidus*
Air conditioner allergy	Dust filtering screens	*Thermoactinomyces candidus* and others
Farmer's lung	Moldy hay	*Micropolyspora faeni* spores
Mushroom worker's lung	Moldy compost	*Thermoactinomyces saccharii* spores
Bird fancier's lung	Dry bird droppings	Bird proteins
Pigeon breeder's disease	Pigeon droppings and dander	Pigeon proteins
Bagassosis	Moldy sugar cane (bagasse)	*Thermoactinomyces vulgaris* spores
Maple bark pneumonitis	Moldy maple bark	*Cryptostroma corticale* spores
Malt worker's lung	Moldy barley	*Aspergillus clavatus* spores
Miller's lung	Contaminated flour	*Sitophilus granarius* (wheat weevil)
Cheese washer's disease	Cheese casings	*Penicillium caseii* spores
Sequoiosis	Moldy redwood or other sawdust	Spores of *Graphium* and *Pullularia* species

≡ SITUATION 2

THE CHRISTMAS BREAK

It was good to be home. The semester had been rough, but three As and a B weren't bad. Dad would need the help during the holiday season, always the busiest of the year. And Mom said the old man hadn't been feeling all that well lately. A few good hard days at the bakery would be tiring, but to the body, not to the mind. I was looking forward to it this Christmas break.

It was only 2 PM, but for the early shift bakers it was quitting time. Dad and I headed for the shower. This time I was sure of it. He was having trouble breathing, not wheezing exactly, but trouble anyway. Seemed like he'd been OK after that little episode at the early coffee break. As we walked along, things began to fit into place. I didn't get that A in immunology for nothing, so I said to him, "Dad, you better check with Doc. I think you've got allergic pneumonitis."

Questions

1. What is allergic pneumonitis?
2. How does allergic pneumonitis differ from asthma and other allergic respiratory complaints?
3. What antigens are involved in allergic pneumonitis in bakers and those with other occupations?
4. Can allergic pneumonitis be treated? If so, how?

Solution

Allergic pneumonitis is only one of several synonyms for an IgG-mediated respiratory disease characterized by an Arthus-like necrosis in the alveoli. Allergic alveolitis, extrinsic allergic pneumonitis, and hypersensitivity pneumonitis are generic equivalents for specific names such as farmer's lung, pigeon breeder's disease, bird fancier's lung, and mushroom worker's disease. These conditions all were named to reflect a specific hobby or vocation associated with the disease. The common thread to all these conditions is a sporadic exposure to an atmosphere heavily contaminated with some form of dust. For the farmer it is dusty hay, straw, or silage; for the pigeon breeder and bird fancier it is the dusty atmosphere of the bird loft or coop, heavy with bird dander and pigeon droppings; and for the baker it is the flour-filled air of the bake shop. Proteins in the flour are absorbed from the inhaled particles and stimulate the production of IgG. Subsequent inhalation of the flour and absorption of the antigens into the capillary bed of the alveoli results in intravascular precipitation and the development of numerous, small Arthus lesions.

The respiratory distress associated with the necrotic Arthus lesions develops several hours after inhalation of the antigens. It is very common for an early episode of respiratory distress to precede this. The early reaction is dominated by a local IgE reaction with the antigen. This biphasic condition is characteristic of allergic pneumonitis and eases differentiation from asthma, which is more chronic and constant once symptoms are evident. Asthma is not related to IgG, as is the case here. Baker's asthma has been described as an IgE-dependent condition characterized by immediate skin tests to flour, histamine release of leukocytes incubated with flour, and positive P-K tests. Bakers are often allergic to insects found in grain or flour and may express a contact dermatitis of the delayed type to proteins from wheat, rye, or other grains.

Allergic pneumonitis cannot be treated with chemotherapeutics such as the antihistamines or adrenergic drugs. Mast cell products have little to do with the severest portions, the second necrotizing phase of the illness, so treatment with these drugs is doomed to failure. These drugs will moderate the earlier, less serious phase of the disease. The only successful treatment is avoidance of antigen exposure.

A cardinal feature shared by all persons afflicted by immune complex pneumonitis is a regular exposure to an atmosphere heavily laden with antigen. This exposure need not be constant and in fact is more often intermittent. Such an atmosphere is created, for example, by farmers working with hay or silage, by mushroom workers preparing mushroom beds, by pigeon breeders and bird fanciers as they clean the bird roosts, or by the birds as they fly in and around their coops. Such air is heavily charged with antigens that vary to some extent according to the source of the dust but usually include spores of a fungus or an excretory product from an involved animal. Media such as moist hay, silage, wood bark, cotton, and fertilized soil favor mold growth, which terminates in sporulation. Fungal spores, most of which are less than 10 μm in diameter, are inhaled deeply into the lung. Fungal spores may be present in bird manure, but it is more likely that antigens of these materials or animal dander are the offending substances.

The respiratory route is a very satisfactory avenue of immunization. Patients with hypersensitivity pneumonitis develop high levels of IgG and may have elevated levels of IgE as well. If both antibodies are present, a reexposure to the antigen will produce a biphasic response. The earliest is the IgE-dependent response characterized by sneezing, edema of the respiratory tract, increased nasal discharge, and the symptoms of an atopic respiratory condition. These symptoms typically disappear within a few hours.

The distinguishing feature of allergic pneumonitis, however, is delayed for several hours after the exposure to antigen. This reaction embodies a dry cough, shortness of breath, fever, and general malaise, all appearing within 6 to 8 hours. Within a few days the person feels perfectly healthy again. Another exposure to the antigen source will trigger another episode of disease.

The immunohistology of lung tissue from patients with allergic pneumonitis is very revealing. A neutrophilic infiltration of the alveolar capillaries, a deposition of fibrin and platelets, and the accumulation of IgG precipitates are completely harmonious with those seen in the Arthus reactions. The present opinion is that all these conditions are examples of the Arthus reaction produced in the lung because of a respiratory exposure of sufficient magnitude and frequency to stimulate high levels of IgG, which precipitate with the antigen in capillaries of the lung. In every instance removing the source of the antigen terminates the disease.

The Shwartzman reaction

The Shwartzman reaction is a dermal reaction characterized by intense hemorrhage and necrosis.

To provoke this reaction, the skin first is sensitized by the intradermal injection of a culture filtrate of a gram-negative bacterium. Almost any such organism can be chosen, including the typhoid, cholera, or common colon bacillus. This initial injection produces only a local erythema, which can be directly correlated with the LPS or endotoxin content of the injected material. Twenty-four hours later, when an intravenous injection of the same filtrate or one from a dissimilar organisms is given, the hemorrhagic necrosis at the initial skin site develops. The Shwartzman lesion can be detected within 2 hours and is usually maximal by the sixth hour.

Currently the most favored theory of the mechanism for the Shwartzman reaction is that the endotoxin contained in the first material injected causes local intravascular coagulation and gradual deposition of fibrin on the blood vessel walls. At first the cells of the RES are stimulated by the LPS and attempt to remove this debris by phagocytosis. Later the LPS depresses the RES, and this permits the accumulation of fibrin in the blood vessels. The second injection again stimulates fibrin deposition on the original fibrin matrix, creating a blockade of the small blood vessels and causing tissue necrosis. When agents other than endotoxin are used in the second injection, fibrin accumulation is also the result but by uncertain pathways, possibly by the activation of Hageman's factor and the blood-clotting sequence.

DELAYED TYPE HYPERSENSITIVITY

In the introductory pages of Chapter 16 the characteristics of the cell-mediated, or T cell-dependent, hypersensitivities are described and compared with the characteristics of the immediate, immunoglobulin-related hypersensitivities. The hallmarks of the delayed hypersensitivities, as listed in Table 16-2, include their slow development following the shocking exposure to the antigen, lack of tissue specificity, requirement for T lymphocytes and their products, collectively described as lymphokines, lack of any known dependence on humoral antibodies, tendency toward mononuclear cell infiltrates in affected tissues that can be combated by steroids, and the difficulty in achieving relief from these allergies by specific antigen desensitization. These same features characterize and identify hypersensitivities (Table 16-3) expressed by antigen-sensitized T lymphocytes. Of course lymphocytes are involved in the immediate and other immunoglobulin-mediated allergies, but these lymphocytes are of the B type. Lymphocytes involved in the cell-mediated hypersensitivities consist of the Lyt-1 or T_{DTH} subset of T cells of the mouse. The T cell subset essential to delayed hypersensitivity in humans has been identified as the $T4^+$ (Leu 3^+) lymphocyte.

A brief reminder about terminology is appropriate. The term *T cell–mediated allergy* or *hypersensitivity* has been equated with two closely related terms: *cell-mediated immunity* (CMI) and *cell-mediated hypersensitivity*. Although these three phrases customarily are interchangeable, their meanings are not exactly the same. CMI in sensu stricto should refer to protection acquired from cellular activities. This includes the bactericidal and other protective actions of blood and tissue phagocytes as well as certain activities of T lymphocytes. Activities of the phagocytes are not antigen specific. Cell-mediated hypersensitivity refers to antigen-specific properties expressed by T lymphocytes that contribute to the delayed inflammatory allergic reaction, as seen in contact dermatitis to certain chemicals and allergies of infection.

One can argue that these older terms prefixed by cell mediated should be dropped. In these hypersensitivities the lymphocytes are operating mainly through extracellular products: the lymphokines. These lymphokines differ immensely from immunoglobulins, but their existence indicates that cell-mediated hypersensitivities are really no more cell mediated than the IgE- or other immunoglobulin-mediated hypersensitivities. They merely are dependent on a different class of lymphocyte.

Allergy of infection

The discovery of the delayed hypersensitivities is credited to Koch; he described the Koch phenomenon and the unique skin reactions to tuberculin exhibited by persons who have or who previously had tuberculosis. The tuberculin reaction is considered the prototype of the delayed hypersensitive skin reaction.

Two separate materials may be used in the tuberculin skin test: OT or PPD prepared from OT. OT is prepared by first growing *Mycobacterium tuberculosis* in a special broth for several weeks (Fig. 18-6). Thereafter the broth is concentrated on a steam bath

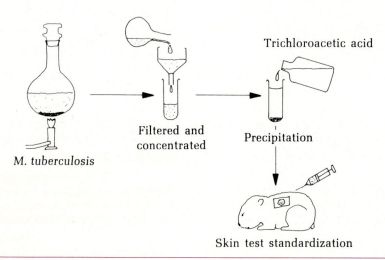

Trichloroacetic acid

M. tuberculosis

Filtered and concentrated

Precipitation

Skin test standardization

FIG. 18-6

Important stages in the preparation of PPD.

to one tenth its previous volume. The mycobacteria are removed by filtration, and the product is OT. Other tuberculin preparations, similar in nature and including extracts of the organism, have not been proved superior to the original tuberculin.

The active principal in OT can be precipitated from it by trichloroacetic acid or ammonium sulfate. One of the small proteins of about 2,000 mol wt in this precipitate contains virtually all the tuberculin activity. This fraction, PPD, is remarkably stable when dried and has a constant activity; therefore it is gradually replacing OT as the skin-testing reagent of choice.

Several different techniques are used in cutaneous tuberculin testing. In the von Pirquet test, one of the first forms of the test to be critically evaluated, tuberculin is rubbed into scarified skin. Variations of this test include the tine test, or multiple puncture method. In this procedure a drop of OT or PPD is placed on a bed of needles, which is used to puncture the skin. Two other procedures are in greater use. In the Mantoux test the allergen is injected intradermally. The Vollmer patch test is used widely for tuberculin testing of children, since no injection is necessary. The patch is simply a square of paper impregnated with OT and held to the skin with a piece of tape. The commercially available tape strip incorporates a normal broth control. A positive test develops slowly and reaches its maximum at about 48 to 72 hours after application or injection of the reagent. The skin is erythematous and indurated (hardened), and in the Mantoux test the reaction site must be at least 10 mm in diameter to be considered positive (Fig. 18-7). In highly sensitized individuals a small vesicle develops in the center of the inflamed zone. Central necrosis may develop but usually does not do so.

The skin of many animals is not adaptable to intradermal skin testing for hypersensitivities. The mouse is a prime example, having a very thin skin that is almost laminated in structure. Intradermal injections are unsatisfactory because the skin appears to split, and the fluid injected does not remain localized. Solutions injected into the footpad or into the ear remain localized and in this vascular tissue can be approached by lymphoid cells and immunoglobulins. Footpad and ear swelling, if determined after any immediate hypersensitive response has subsided,

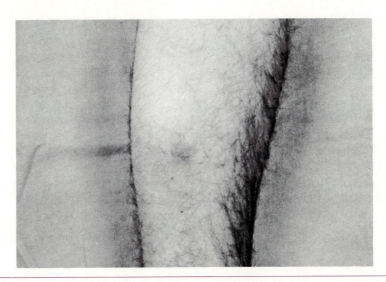

FIG. 18-7

A delayed skin reaction exhibiting an erythematous but nonedematous zone 15 mm in diameter at 48 hours. A control site, inoculated higher on the forearm, shows no reaction at this time.

can be measured exactly with calipers for a precise quantitation of the reaction. This method serves as a useful substitute for typical delayed skin reaction in other small animals, including hamsters, rats, guinea pigs, and gerbils.

Systemic reactions to tuberculin follow intravenous injections in experimental animals, and constitutional reactions have been noted in humans. A sharp rise in body temperature, malaise, and pain in the extremities are the major symptoms; these usually subside within 24 hours. Fatal tuberculin shock can be produced in laboratory animals.

The tuberculin reaction has been described as an allergy of infection. Not all allergies to infectious organisms are of the delayed type, but the tendency toward delayed reactions has been so prominent that the term *allergy of infection* is used synonymously with *delayed hypersensitivity*. Other examples are the delayed skin reactions associated with leprosy, histoplasmosis, coccidioidomycosis, blastomycosis, brucellosis, mumps, lymphogranuloma venereum, and smallpox virus (Table 18-3).

It must be remembered that positive skin reactions with PPD, lepromin, histoplasmin, etc., are not diagnostic tests for a current illness. Allergies of infection generally are persistent throughout life and remain positive long after the infection itself has disappeared. This is because of the longevity of the T_{DTH} cells responsible for the delayed hypersensitive reactions.

Another interesting aspect of these skin tests is that some of the eliciting products—histoplasmin, for example—are themselves antigenic. The consequence of this is that repeated skin testing of a nonreactor may convert him or her to a positive state and also induce the formation of antibodies. These events could confuse the diagnosis of disease on the basis of both a false positive skin test and a false positive serologic test. Since the active ingredient in OT and PPD has a molecular weight of only 2,000, these events are unlikely with the use of these reagents.

Contact dermatitis

Dermal sensitivity of the delayed type may follow contact with chemicals from many sources, includ-

TABLE 18-3
Delayed hypersensitive skin tests for allergies of infection

Disease	Skin test	Reagent
Bacterial diseases		
Tuberculosis	Mantoux, Vollmer, etc., according to method	OT or PPD
Leprosy	Lepromin (Mitsuda)	Extract of lepromatous tissue (lepromin)
Diphtheria	Moloney	Diphtheria toxoid
Brucellosis	Brucellergin	Heat-killed organism
Tularemia	Foshay	Bacterial protein antigen
Streptococcal infection	—	Streptokinase-streptodornase
Viral diseases		
Lymphogranuloma venereum	Frei	Inactive virus
Smallpox	—	Vaccinia virus
Mumps	—	Mumps virus vaccine
Fungal diseases		
Histoplasmosis	Histoplasmin	Concentrate of culture filtrate (histoplasmin)
Coccidioidomycosis	Coccidioidin	Concentrate of culture filtrate (coccidioidin)
Blastomycosis	Blastomycin	Concentrate of culture filtrate (blastomycin)
Candidiasis	Candidin	Concentrate of yeast culture

ing cosmetics, insecticides, topically applied disinfectants and ointments, metals, hair and clothing dyes, photographic chemicals, rubber goods, leather goods, and many others (Table 18-4). In many of these instances specific chemicals in the product are known to be the incitant: for example, formaldehyde, mercury, and other heavy metals in insecticides; nickel and copper in coins, metal buckles, watchbands, and jewelry; potassium dichromate in leather goods and yellow dyes; paraphenylenediamine in black, brown, and blue dyes for human and animal hair or cloth; and phenyl-β-naphthylamine in rubber goods. Allergies to "poisonous" plants such as poison ivy, poison oak, and poison sumac or primrose are caused by specific compounds, often substituted urushiols on the surface of their leaves.

Poison ivy and poison oak represent interesting examples of contact dermatitis common in the rural United States. *Rhus radicans* (poison ivy), *Rhus toxicodendron* (poison sumac), and *Rhus diversiloba* (poison oak) cause contact dermatitis because of the common catechols present in the plant sap and on the surface of bruised leaves. Urushiol is the name given to the mixture of four catechols found in the poison ivy plant. These catechols differ from each other only in the degree of saturation of their pentadecyl side chain. The fully saturated compound is 3n-pentadecylcatechol; the compound that is singly unsaturated has a double bond at position 8 to 9; the

doubly unsaturated compound has a double bond at positions 8 to 9 and 11 to 12; and the trienyl compound has a double bond at positions 8 to 9, 11 to 12, and 14 to 15 (Fig. 18-8). These compounds exist in urushiol in the ratio of 3, 15, 60, and 22, respectively; thus it is not surprising that patients show more strongly positive reactions to the latter two than to the former two compounds.

Catechols are haptenic and can couple to tissue proteins by virtue of their ready oxidation to quinones, the sensitizing form of these compounds. Blocking quinone formation by substituting the hydroxyl groups renders the catechols inert. When it is applied to skin, only 44% of pentadecyl-catechol remains at the site of application; the remainder is recoverable from feces, urine, lymph nodes, and internal organs. The exact form of the catechol-protein conjugate and the identity of specifically involved proteins are not known. (Dinitrochlorobenzene, a potent skin sensitizer, binds to 15 different proteins in skin.) Many of these low molecular weight chemicals such as the substituted nitrophenols and oxazolones are classifiable as autocoupling haptens. When these compounds contact the skin, they combine with skin or tissue antigens to form neoantigens against which the hypersensitivity develops. Langerhans cells in the skin are essential to this process, since the elimination of these cells through irradiation with ultraviolet light prevents sensitization.

TABLE 18-4

Sources of contact dermatitis and the allergens involved

Object	Sources	Compounds involved
Metal	Jewelry, belt buckles, watches, watchbands, scissors, thimbles, cosmetics	Nickel, chromium, iron, cobalt, copper, mercury
Clothing		Animal and plant fibers, anthraquinone and other dyes, vinyl, acrylate, glycol, and other permanent press agents, formaldehyde
Rubber	Swim wear, garters, shoes, condoms	Hydroquinone and other antioxidants, benzothiazole and other accelerators
Cosmetics	Rouge, lipstick, eye shadow, hair dye, depilatories, perfumes, lotions, sprays	Iron and cobalt dyes, sulfide depilatories, phenylenediamine and other dyes, balsam
Leather	Belts, shoes, leather watchbands	Potassium dichromate, dyes
Plants	Poison ivy, oak, sumac, etc.	Catechols

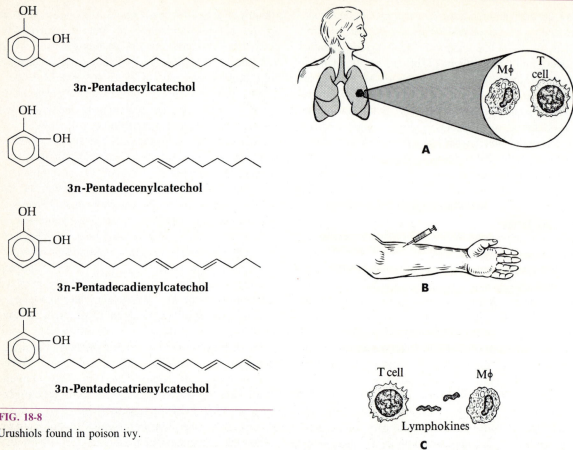

3n-Pentadecylcatechol

3n-Pentadecenylcatechol

3n-Pentadecadienylcatechol

3n-Pentadecatrienylcatechol

FIG. 18-8
Urushiols found in poison ivy.

Cellular interactions and lymphokines

Induction of delayed type hypersensitivity is possible only with T cell dependent antigens. It is generally accepted that T cell dependent antigens must be processed by I-A or I-E bearing macrophages. These cells and others such as the non-phagocytic dendritic cells present the antigenic epitopes and IL-1 to the $T4^+$ human ($Lyt1^+$ murine) T cell. It is possible to refer to this cell as either a T_H or T_{DTH} cell since they can not be distinguished. Cloned T_H cells display all the characteristics of T_{DTH} cells, i.e., principally, the production of the macrophage chemotaxin and macrophage migration inhibitor (Chapter 7) (Fig. 18-9).

Other, less well described lymphokines also participate in delayed type hypersensitivity reactions.

FIG. 18-9
The cellular interactions involved in delayed type hypersensitivity are illustrated here using tuberculosis as an example. Tubercle bacilli are engulfed and processed by macrophages in the lung (**A**). T cells become sensitized. The antigen specific component of the T cell response is seen in the delayed type skin reaction (**B**). The T cell–derived macrophage chemotaxin and macrophage inhibitory factor attract and hold macrophages at the reaction site (**C**).

Many of these are only partially described, and it is often difficult to be certain that they do not merely represent a second biological activity of a previously known lymphokine. For example, a skin reactive factor that induces a histologic picture in skin, like that seen in DTH reactions, has a molecular weight similar to the macrophage chemotaxin; e.g., 12,000.

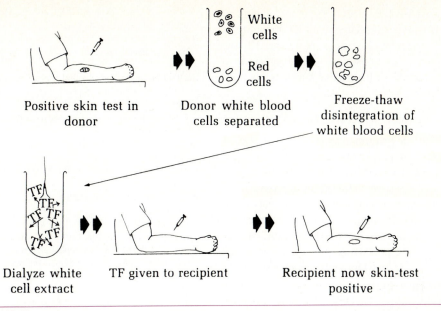

Positive skin test in donor

Donor white blood cells separated

White cells

Red cells

Freeze-thaw disintegration of white blood cells

Dialyze white cell extract

TF given to recipient

Recipient now skin-test positive

FIG. 18-10

Lymphocytes separated from peripheral blood of a person with a T cell–dependent (delayed) skin reaction to a specific antigen can be used as the source of transfer factor *(TF)*. This molecule will diffuse through the pores of a dialysis bag and can be used to convert a normal individual to the same reactive status as that of the transfer factor donor.

A leukocyte chemotactic behavior has been recovered from T cell cultures in fractions ranging from 5,000 to 300,000 molecular weight. None of these, however, seem to be identical to the earlier described neutrophil chemotactic factor.

Transfer factor

Delayed type hypersensitivity in human subjects, higher primates, cattle, dogs and a few other animals can be transferred by T cell lysates of a sensitized donor to nonsensitive individuals of the same species. This transfer is entirely antigen specific, unlike the activities of the lymphokines. Efforts to define the exact chemistry of transfer factor, though frustrating, have indicated that TF is not a protein as are the lymphokines. On the basis of this difference in chemistry and antigen specificity, TF is clearly separable from the lymphokines.

Following the successful transfer of contact dermatitis in guinea pigs with peritoneal exudate cells in

the hallmark experiment of Landsteiner and Chase, tuberculic hypersensitivity to tuberculin was transferred by the same method. The earlier effort to transfer these hypersensitivities with cell extracts failed. From the early 1940s until the early 1950s, little progress was made in the understanding of DTH until Lawrence's group found that allergy of infection to several agents—tuberculin, histoplasmin, and diphtheria toxoid—could be transferred with cell extracts prepared from the T cells of sensitive donors. Nearly two decades of work have failed to unveil the complete chemistry of TF. It is nonantigenic and found in the molecular weight range of 700 to 4000. It contains phosphate, pentoses and an unidentified purine. At one time, it was believed hypoxanthine or uracil was a part of its structure. TF has an absorption spectrum that indicates the presence of a nucleic acid-like substance combined with amino acids. The molecule is heat labile at 56° C. It is insensitive to DNAases or RNAases. Though its chemical nature is obscure, it appears to function as a semi-genetic vehicle. Recipients of TF regain their DTH, but do not retain it permanently (Fig. 18-10). Thus TF converts the existing T cell population to the effector capacity of the donor, but does not convert stem cells.

Cutaneous basophilic hypersensitivity

A form of skin reaction described as the Jones-Mote reaction and previously described as an evanescent delayed hypersensitive response now is generally known as cutaneous basophilic hypersensitivity (CBH). In experimental laboratory animals intradermal reexposure to antigen 5 to 7 days after the initial exposure initiates the CBH reaction. Within the first 24 hours a nonedematous area of erythema develops, which persists for only another 24 to 48 hours. Eosinophils are identified as the first cells to infiltrate the reaction site, and these are supplanted by basophils by the forty-eighth hour.

CBH is a transitory reaction that precedes by several days the expression of the classic delayed dermal reaction and is no longer demonstrable when the classic delayed reaction can be elicited. Nevertheless, T cells can mediate the CBH reaction; however, B cells and IgE also seem to participate. This is clearly a composite of several immunologic effector systems.

REFERENCES

Abel, E.A., and Wood, G.S.: Mechanisms in contact dermatitis, Clin. Rev. Allergy 4:339, 1986.

Adams, R.M.: Diagnosis of allergic contact dermatitis of occupational origin, Clin. Rev. Allergy 4:323, 1986.

Al-doory, Y., and Domson, J.F., editors: Mould allergy, Philadelphia, 1984, Lea and Febiger.

Basten, A.: The role of T cell subsets and Ia antigens in delayed-type hypersensitivity, Int. Arch. Allergy 66 Suppl. 1, 197, 1981.

Beall, G.N., editor: Allergy and clinical immunology, New York, 1983, John Wiley and Sons.

Claman, H.N., Miller, S.D., Conlon, P.J., and Moorhead, J.W.: Control of experimental contact sensitivity, Adv. Immunol. 30:121, 1980.

Emanuel, D.A., and Kryda, M.J.: Farmer's lung disease, Clin. Rev. Allergy 1:509, 1983.

Etain, C.: Contact dermatitis, Edinburgh, 1980, Churchill Livingstone.

Fisher, A.A.: Contact dermatitis, ed. 3, Philadelphia, 1986, Lea and Febiger.

Frigoletto, F.D., Jr., Jewett, J.F., and Konugres, A.A.: Rh hemolytic disease, Boston, 1982, G.K. Hall and Co.

Geczy, C.L.: The role of lymphokines in delayed-type hypersensitivity reactions, Springer Semin. Immunopathol. 7:321, 1984.

Holborow, E.J., and Reeves, W.G., editors: Immunology in medicine: a comprehensive guide to clinical immunology, ed. 2, New York, 1983, Grune and Stratton, Inc.

Hollan, S.R., Bernat, I., Fust, G., and Sarkodi, B., editors: Recent advances in haematology, immunology, and blood transfusion, Chichester, England, 1983, John Wiley & Sons.

Lachmann, P.J., and Peters, D.K., editors: Clinical aspects of immunology, ed. 4, Oxford, 1982, Blackwell Scientific Publishers.

Larsen, G.L.: Hypersensitivity lung disease, Ann. Rev. Immunol. 3:59, 1985.

Naguwa, S.M., and Nelson, B.L.: Human serum sickness, Clin. Rev. Allergy, 3:117, 1985.

Nishioka, K.: Allergic contact dermatitis, Int. J. Dermatol. 24:1, 1985.

Turk, J.L.: Delayed hypersensitivity, ed. 3, New York, 1980, Elsevier/North-Holland Biomedical Press.

Yoshida, T., editor: Investigation of cell-mediated immunity, Edinburgh, 1985, Churchill Livingstone.

Autoimmunity

GLOSSARY

cold agglutinin   An agglutinin or hemagglutinin that is active at 4° C but not at 37° C.

EAE   Experimental allergic encephalomyelitis.

horror autotoxicus   Fear of self-poisoning, as related to the usual inability of an antigen to serve as an autoantigen.

LATS   Long-acting thyroid stimulator.

LE   Lupus erythematosus.

LE cell   A polymorphonuclear cell that has engulfed the enlarged nucleus of another white blood cell which was distorted by antinuclear antibody.

Masugi's nephritis   A form of glomerulonephritis produced by passive immunization with antikidney serum.

MBP   Myelin basic protein.

MG   Myasthenia gravis.

MS   Multiple sclerosis.

relative risk   A calculation that relates HLA antigens with susceptibility to an autoimmune disease.

rheumatoid factor (RF)   An IgM with specificity toward IgG associated with arthritis.

sequestered antigen   An antigen not found in the circulatory system.

SLE   Systemic lupus erythematosus.

Witebsky's postulates   A set of conditions that must be met before a disease can be accepted as an autoimmune illness.

warm agglutinin   An agglutinin or hemagglutinin that is active at 37° C but not at 4° C.

The autoimmune diseases represent a group of conditions in which immunoglobulins or T cells display a specificity for self-antigens, or autoantigens. In certain situations this "forbidden" immune response can be defended as the etiologic basis of the disease, but more often this is not the case. Then one can only list these autoimmune phenomena as correlates of the disease. This is unlike the alloimmune diseases (blood transfusion reactions, HDN, graft rejection) or the diseases (serum sickness, anaphylaxis, hay fever) where the immune response is clearly the cause of the disease.

AUTOIMMUNIZATION AND HORROR AUTOTOXICUS

Autoimmunization is the use of self-antigens or autoantigens to produce circulating immunoglobulins or sensitized lymphocytes, which react with the autoantigen. According to the concept of horror autotoxicus forwarded by Ehrlich, one does not develop an immune response to the normal circulating antigens. A combination of these two definitions reveals that autoantigens must be noncirculating or abnormal. Only under those conditions can the two definitions remain intact.

A more modern view toward autoimmunity has developed recently—a view that self reactivity of the immune system is a normal event. This is seen most dramatically in the intricate interaction of the regulatory T cell subsets, where helper cells regulate several populations of T and B cells, and the suppressor and contrasuppressor cells oppose each other in their influence on the helper cell. In the idiotypic network for the regulation of immunoglobulin synthesis, self reactivity is evident at a molecular level. In other areas of immunology, particularly the complement system, a counterbalance of effectors and regulators governs the expression of the system.

Thus self reactivity for the purpose of a regulated control of immunological events is normal. When regulation fails, an autoimmune disease results. Quantitative abnormalities in the production or activity of lymphocytes, excesses in the production of immunoglobulins or effector cells, and excessive formation of immune complexes coupled with extremes in activation of the complement system are all examples of deregulated, self-directed activities seen in autoimmune disease. Either extrinsic agents (viruses, other infectious agents, chemicals) or intrinsic forces (mutation, hormones) may promote deregulation.

Etiology of autoimmune disease

Actually there are five major avenues through which an individual may develop an autoimmune response:

1. A response to antigens that do not normally circulate in the blood (the hidden or sequestered antigen theory)
2. A response to an altered antigen (The alteration could arise through chemical, physical, or biologic means, such as hapten complexing, physical denaturation, and mutation, respectively.)
3. A response to a foreign antigen that is shared or cross-reactive with self-antigens
4. A mutation in immunocompetent cells to acquire a responsiveness to self-antigens
5. A loss of immunoregulatory power by T_H, T_S, and T_{CS} cells

Sequestered antigen

An unfortunate attraction of the sequestered, hidden, or noncirculating antigen notion is that it is based on a negative concept, the inability to identify these "normally hidden" antigens in the circulation under conditions of normal health. Even our most sensitive detectors require that picogram or nanogram quantities of an antigen be present before a positive test can be observed. Consequently any antigen not found in the blood at these levels is described as a noncirculating or sequestered antigen. This can easily be a fallacious assumption.

Antigens often grouped as noncirculating antigens are lens proteins of the eye, milk casein, antigens of the reproductive system, thyroglobulin, etc. Although some antigens (lens proteins may be an example) are unusually stable and have very little metabolic turnover, others such as those of the thyroid gland or male reproductive tract might be expected to undergo degradation and elimination just like antigens of the kidney, liver, and other tissues. Under this circumstance, they could be present in the circulatory system but at levels too low to detect and be erroneously classified as hidden antigens.

Altered antigen or neoantigen

Altered antigens of neoantigens may be created by chemical, physical, or biologic means. Convincing proof that new antigens are formed by autocoupling haptens already has been advanced as a mechanism for contact dermatitis and anaphylactic sensitivity to low molecular weight compounds. When a portion of the immune response is directed against the carrier antigen, then an autoimmune disease may result. Physical autoallergies to visible light, ultraviolet light, physical pressure, and cold arise through a similar mechanism. In these instances the physical forces reform the molecule to expose or create a new antigenic determinant or determinants against which the response might be developed. By mutation in an antigen-producing cell a new and structurally different antigen might be produced that would no longer be recognized as self by one's immune machinery and thus would stimulate an immune response.

Shared or cross-reactive antigen

A third potential for autoimmunization is that exogenous antigens exist which are cross-reactive with self-antigens. Because of the size of antigenic determinants, the possibility exists that complex structures which are recognized as foreign could include simpler parts that are identical or similar to self-structures. This would result in immunologic cross-reactivity. If this is viewed in the sense of Ehrlich's lock and key hypothesis of antigen-antibody combination, it is not inconsistent with immunologic specificity. A fit of the key (autoantigen) into only a small part of the lock (autoantibody or

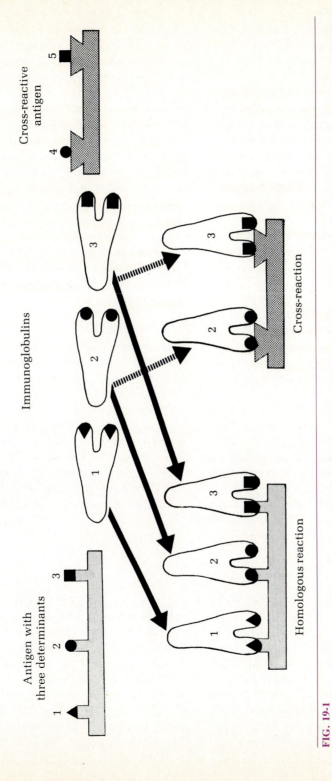

FIG. 19-1

Schematic representation showing how the cross-reactive antigen theory may function in autoimmune diseases when the first antigen is foreign and the second one is a self-antigen.

T cell receptor) might be perfectly adequate to initiate an autoimmune disease (Fig. 19-1).

Mutation

The mutation of an immunocompetent cell to acquire an unnatural responsiveness to self-antigens would be a de facto abrogation of the concept of horror autotoxicus. The inclusion of hypermutable lymphoid cells in one form of the clonal selection theory would ensure an expanded antigenic responsiveness to self-antigens in later life. The mutations responsible could occur at the level of the macrophage, T or B lymphocytes, or their progenitor cells.

The synthesis of new antigens as a result of mutation is mentioned previously under the section on altered antigen.

Loss of immunoregulation

The recognition that T_H, T_S, and T_{CS} cells have pronounced effects on B cells and certain T cell subsets suggests that diminished immunoregulatory activities would be reflected in heightened immunoglobulin levels or T cell responses. Evidence for this already exists in systemic lupus erythematosus, where a lowered T_S cell function is associated with disease. Likewise, overactive T_{CS} cells could correlate with an immunoglobulin dependent autoimmune disease, though no example of this is known at this time.

This loss of immunoregulation is synonymous with a loss of self-tolerance. Tolerance to self-antigens exists as the natural result of embryonic development. Most potential antigens are present in the fetus prior to the time of immunologic maturation and induce a tolerogenic state in the immunocompetent cells or their progenitors as they develop. The continued presence of the antigen ensures a continuation of the tolerance until such time that mutation or loss of immunoregulatory powers permits an escape from that condition and self-antigens behave as foreign antigens. This forbidden response results in autoimmune disease.

Witebsky's postulates

There are many diseases associated with autoimmune phenomena (Table 19-1). Whether these autoantibodies merely are associated with the disease or

---

TABLE 19-1

Human diseases expressing autoimmune phenomena

Disease	Antigen	Immunoglobulin and/or T cell response
Postvaccinal and postinfectious encephalomyelitis	Myelin, cross-reactive	T cell
Aspermatogenesis	Sperm	T cell
Sympathetic ophthalmia	Uvea	T cell
Hashimoto's disease	Thyroglobulin	IgG and T cell
Graves' disease	—	Long-acting thyroid stimulator (LATS)
Autoimmune hemolytic disease	I, Rh, and others on surface of red blood cells	IgM and IgG
Thrombocytopenic purpura	Hapten-platelet or hapten-adsorbed antigen complex	IgG
MG	Acetylcholine receptor	IgG
Rheumatic fever	Streptococcal cross-reactive with heart	IgG and IgM
Glomerulonephritis	Streptococcal cross-reactive with kidney	IgG and IgM
Rheumatoid arthritis	IgG	IgM to Fc(γ)
SLE	DNA, nucleoprotein, RNA, etc.	IgG

play a central role in the cause of the illness is not always easy to determine. Much the same problem confronted microbiologists in their initial efforts to identify which organisms isolated from patients actually were responsible for infectious diseases. Koch created four criteria to be used by microbiologists interested in the accurate assignation of microbes as the agents of these diseases. These standards have become known as Koch's postulates. Witebsky has erected the following very similar criteria for immunologists who wish to determine the relationship of immunologic phenomena to disease etiology.

1. The autoimmune response must be regularly associated with the disease.
2. A replica of the disease must be inducible in laboratory animals.
3. Immunopathologic changes in the natural and experimental diseases should parallel each other.
4. Transfer of the autoimmune illness should be possible by the transfer of serum or lymphoid cells from the diseased individual to a normal recipient.

Among the most obvious immunologic findings associated with autoimmune diseases are one or more of the following: general hypergammaglobulinemia, specific self-directed immunoglobulins, decrease in total serum complement levels (hypocomplementemia) or in specific complement components, increase in activities associated with the activation of complement, especially chemotactic attraction to sites where γ-globulin and complement are bound to tissues involved in the disease, and the appearance of T lymphocytes with self-directed activities. Serologic tests directed toward identification of these unusual immunologic manifestations are useful screening procedures for the diagnosis of autoimmune disease.

Replicas of most of the human autoimmune conditions described in this chapter have been developed in experimental animals. In most instances these mimics have been created by removing a portion of some tissue, treating it as an antigen, emulsifying it with adjuvant, and injecting this into the same animal which donated the tissue. This procedure is very convenient when the tissue source exists as a paired organ (such as thyroid or gonad). Half the organ then serves as the antigen and its remainder as an in-

dicator tissue for any evidence of autoimmune phenomena resulting from the autoimmunization. Injections of haptenic materials also have been used to generate autoimmune replicas.

Alloimmunization and even immunization with exogenous antigens also can produce replicas of autoimmune diseases. This is not unexpected when the antigens involved share determinants with the autoantigen. Since this has been proved in only a few instances, acceptance of these as embodying the precise phenomena of the autoimmune condition should be guarded.

Other models of human autoimmune diseases may be found in a natural autoimmune counterpart in experimental animals. Mice, rats, dogs, chickens, and other species sometimes are affected by diseases which closely parallel those observed in humans. Particularly in mice, where our depth of knowledge about the immune response often exceeds what we know about the human system, these spontaneous autoimmune diseases have been very informative. In chickens the separation of the central lymphoid tissues into the bursal and thymic compartments has been especially important in evaluating the role of immunoglobulins versus that of T cells in the cause of autoimmune disease.

The reaction of self-antigens with autoantibodies or autosensitized T lymphocytes is the natural result of their simultaneous existence in an individual. In certain instances it is believed that this reaction is the final immunologic event in the development of the disease. The autoimmune hemolytic diseases and thrombocytopenic purpura can be cited as examples. In a greater number of cases in which immunologic reactions are occurring, it is uncertain or even doubtful whether they cause the disease with which they are associated. In many instances these immunologic events appear to be only secondary aspects of the disease which, although they may contribute to the perpetuation of it, may have little or nothing to do with the origin or continuation of the illness.

One indirect line of evidence that an immunologic event is critical to the continuation of an autoimmune disease stems from the types of treatment that are most effective for the disease. In the past decade the availability of a large number of cytotoxic agents with immunosuppressive action has resulted in their therapeutic application to several autoimmune diseases. Corticosteroids, purine and pyrimidine analogs, and alkylating agents have been used successfully in diseases such as autoimmune thyroiditis, SLE, rheumatoid arthritis, and autoimmune hemolytic disease. The prolonged use of these drugs is not without hazard, since the total immune capabilities of the subject are depressed, and constant supervision of patients for the development of infectious diseases is a necessity. Temporary or intermittent treatment with the more potent drugs is necessary to avoid undesirable side effects, but, as logic would indicate, autoimmune diseases do respond favorably to these compounds.

THE MHC AND AUTOIMMUNE DISEASE

Although the major source of our knowledge about the MHC and its relationship with the immune response evolved from the study of the murine H-2 system, our knowledge about the relationship of the MHC to autoimmune disease is largely, if not entirely, the result of studying the human animal. These investigations quickly followed those in mice which correlated the susceptibility of the mouse to leukemia with its H-2 antigens and have been a steadily expanding field of study.

To determine if an autoimmune disease is a genetic trait, two approaches are possible: family studies and population studies. When family members with a presumed autoimmune disease can be identified as sharing common HLA haplotypes, then a link between the disease and HLA clearly is suggested. Because large families displaying autoimmune disease are not always available due to death or failure to recognize the disease as a family characteristic population studies must be used. In this approach antigen frequencies among large groups of patients with a specific illness are compared with those of a group of healthy control subjects. Since the frequency of most HLA antigens is 0.20 or less, statistically significant associations are frequently impossible, even when large groups are studied. Instead a calculation of relative risk is used to indicate the HLA-disease relationship. Relative risk is calculated as follows:

$$\text{Relative risk} = \frac{\substack{\text{Frequency of} \\ \text{patients with} \\ \text{the HLA} \\ \text{antigen}} \times \substack{\text{Frequency of} \\ \text{control subjects} \\ \text{lacking the} \\ \text{HLA antigen}}}{\substack{\text{Frequency of} \\ \text{patients lack-} \\ \text{ing the HLA} \\ \text{antigen}} \times \substack{\text{Frequency of} \\ \text{control subjects} \\ \text{with the HLA} \\ \text{antigen}}}$$

The autoimmune disease with the highest relative risk is ankylosing spondylitis, where the HLA-B27 antigen yields a relative risk of approximately 90% (Table 19-2).

Currently the autoimmune diseases expressing HLA associations have identified antigens in the B series as those most related to the disease. In one sense this is an artifact of the available technology. The DP, DQ, and DR region of the human MHC is the immune response region of the MHC and these genes and their protein products should be used in the analysis of relative risk. Unfortunately antisera to identify these human Ir products are available for only a few of the proteins. Until such antisera are available, relative risks must be calculated for antigens of the MHC for which antisera exist. The higher relative risk values associated with the B antigens are a result of the closer proximity of the B locus to the DP, DQ, and DR loci compared with the position of the A and C genes.

Table 19-2 presents a list of relative risk calculations for several human diseases. Although some of these conditions appear to be infectious diseases, this actually is not the case. For example, arthritides associated with bacterial infections are not the direct result of the bacterial infection but are sequelae that stem from the infection, even after the infection has been eliminated.

T CELL–ASSOCIATED AUTOIMMUNE DISEASES

In this section the human autoimmune diseases and some of their experimental counterparts that have well-documented associations with T cell phenomena are considered. It bears repeating that unexpected immunoglobulin activities often are associated with these diseases, and it may be difficult to determine

TABLE 19-2

Relationship of HLA and autoimmune human diseases

| Disease | HLA | Antigen frequency (percent) | | Relative risk |
		Patients	Control subjects	
Ankylosing spondylitis	B27	79 to 100	4 to 13	90
Addison's disease	B8	20 to 69	18 to 24	1 to 7
Reiter's syndrome	B27	65 to 100	4 to 14	36
Graves' disease	B8	25 to 47	16 to 27	1.8 to 2.4
Yersinia arthritis	B27	58 to 78	9 to 14	18
Salmonella arthritis	B27	60 to 69	8 to 10	18
Sjögren's syndrome	Dw3	68 to 69	10 to 24	8 to 16
Adult rheumatoid arthritis	Dw4	38 to 65	18 to 31	4.4
Autoimmune thyroiditis	Bw35	63 to 73	9 to 14	16.8
Anterior uveitis	B27	37 to 58	7 to 10	9.4
MG	B8	38 to 65	18 to 13	4.4
Multiple sclerosis (MS)	B7	12 to 46	14 to 30	1.7

whether the undesired T cell activities actually dominate these conditions. This is best determined by successful transfer of the disease with T cells.

Allergic encephalomyelitis

Postvaccinal and postinfectious encephalomyelitis

Postvaccinal encephalomyelitis following immunization against rabies was an undesired sequela to the use of the Pasteur rabies vaccine. This vaccine was prepared by phenolizing extracts of spinal cord of rabbits that had experimental rabies. In addition to the inactivated rabies virus, many different antigens from the central nerve tissue of the rabbit were present in the preparation. For rabies immunization, daily inoculations of this vaccine over a 2-week period were prescribed. In rare instances (1 in 4,000) symptoms of encephalomyelitis appear about 2 weeks after the immunization. Persons who survived the acute stages invariably recovered without permanent neurologic disorders. Rabies vaccines free of neural tissue have replaced the Pasteur vaccine and largely eliminated this problem.

A second form of postvaccinal encephalomyelitis is known to accompany vaccination with attenuated viruses. These vaccines for measles, rubella, mumps, and chickenpox do not contain nerve tissue antigens; however, the viruses in these attenuated vaccines are able to initiate an abbreviated, normally mild disease. These viruses may invade cells of the central nervous system during the course of their modified disease. This usually occurs early in the disease, and later, when active viral particles are no longer detectable, the symptoms of encephalomyelitis appear. These include an elevated temperature, drowsiness perhaps proceeding to a comatose state, convulsions, and paralysis of the legs. The survivors may demonstrate mental retardation, epileptic seizures, or other neurologic symptoms, although many survivors remain free of secondary effects. Incidents of postvaccinal encephalomyelitis have been the dominating force in efforts to improve these vaccines.

These examples of postvaccinal encephalomyelitis are artificially induced instances of postinfectious encephalomyelitis, which may develop after natural infections with viruses. In 1968 it was reported that 22% of all cases of encephalitis were associated with childhood diseases, practically all of which had a viral origin. Among the diseases involved are measles, mumps, rubella, influenza, chickenpox (varicella), herpes zoster and herpes simplex. The association of these childhood viral diseases with encephalomyelitis is what prompted the development of the attenuated vaccines for their prevention. This reduced the incidence of viral associated encephalomyelitis but did not eliminate it. The immunologic origin of this form of postvaccinal and postinfectious encephalomyelitis is the attack of Tc and possibly LGL cells upon host cells with viral antigens on their exterior surface.

The best model for both postvaccinal encephalomyelitis and postinfectious encephalomyelitis is experimental allergic encephalomyelitis.

Experimental allergic encephalomyelitis

The postvaccinal and postinfectious encephalomyelitides have counterparts that serve as excellent models. The best model, experimental allergic encephalomyelitis, or EAE (Fig. 19-2), is produced by the inoculation of brain or spinal cord extracts in Freund's adjuvant into the animal to be studied. There is virtually no species barrier to this disease; extracts of the brain of most common domesticated mammals are equally effective in inducing EAE in rats. The symptoms of EAE in the rat begin at about the tenth to fourteenth postsensitization day. Grossly these include an ascending, flaccid paralysis that may disappear after 2 weeks accompanied by complete recovery. Histologic lesions in the brain are variable, but focal perivascular areas of inflammation containing lymphocytes, Ia$^+$ dendritic cells, mononuclear cells, and plasma cells are common in most species. Complement-fixing anti–brain tissue globulins usually are produced in response to the immunization, but these are unable to transfer the disease. However, it is possible to passively transfer EAE with sensitized lymphocytes. These have been identified as T cells. Adult mice depleted of T cells develop EAE after reconstitution with Lyt1$^+$ cells and injection with spinal cord homogenate.

Chemical fractionation of brain extracts that successfully produce EAE in rats, guinea pigs, mice, rabbits, and other animals has incriminated the myelin basic protein (MBP) as the key encephalitogen (Fig. 19-3). This protein alone represents about 30% of the protein in the central nervous system myelin. It has a molecular weight of 18,500 and is composed of 169 amino acid residues. Its isoelectric point is 10.2 because of the presence of 31 residues of lysine and arginine. The amino acid sequence of the MBP

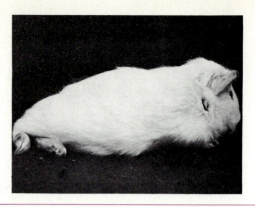

FIG. 19-2

Hind quarter paralysis in a guinea pig with EAE. (Courtesy Dr. C.W. Purdy.)

from several species has been completely determined. MBPs from the species studied are virtually identical with very few amino acid substitutions, and this permits the use of non-autologous antigens to induce the disease.

Although MBPs from diverse species are nearly identical, the encephalitogenic sequences differ for the different species. For the rabbit the encephalitogenic determinant generally encompasses amino acids 44 to 89 and specifically the region 66 to 74; for the rat the determinant includes amino acids 68 to 88, for the guinea pig amino acids 114 to 122, and for the monkey amino acids 154 to 167. In each instance, strain variations occur—Lewis strain rats recognize epitopes in the 68-88 region and BN rats, the region between 43 and 67. The Lewis strain has been the most used to examine EAE in rats. Thus, when describing EAE, one need not refer to the species source of the MBP but only to the species and strain tested, since the encephalitogenic peptide varies as follows:

1. For rabbit, 66 to 74: Thr-His-Tyr-Gly-Ser-Leu-Pro-Gln-Lys
2. For rat 68 to 88 of which 75 to 84 is: Ala-Gln-Gly-His-Arg-Pro-Gln-Asp-Glu-Asn
3. For guinea pig, 114 to 122: Phe-Ser-Trp-Gly-Ala-Glu-Gly-Gln-Lys
4. For monkey, 154 to 167: Phe-Lys-Leu-Gly-Gly-Arg-Asp-Ser-Arg-Ser-Gly-Ser-Pro

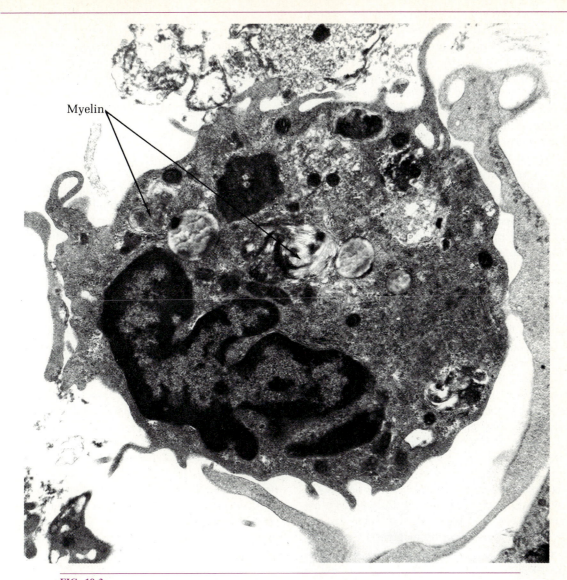

FIG. 19-3

The inclusions within this granulocyte are not all identifiable, but the ones identified by the arrows are myelin. (Courtesy Dr. E. Adelstein.)

Aspermatogenisis

Autoimmunization of guinea pigs with sperm was one of the first experimental autoimmunizations ever conducted and dates back to the work of Metalnikoff in 1900. Since spermatic and testicular antigens develop after the immunologic apparatus has matured, and since they appear to be sequestered antigens, the ability of these tissues to serve as autoantigens is not considered unusual.

Immunization of guinea pigs or rats with autologous testis extracts in Freund's complete adjuvant has been very successful in producing an experimental aspermatogenesis. As in hypothyroiditis, half the tissue system is used for immunization and the remainder for assaying the disease. Aspermatogenesis is almost the only result of testis immunization; there is very little generalized tissue damage to the gland. About 3 weeks after the immunization the seminiferous tubules are almost devoid of cells. Interstitial cell infiltration is evident, but it is localized rather than generalized. This condition persists, with some testicular atrophy, for 3 to 6 months, after which regeneration of the spermatogenic capacity occurs; after 1 year normal sperm production is regained. Since these changes can be produced by the injection of sperm just as easily as by the use of homologous or autologous testis extracts, the potential for birth control vaccines in humans exists. One advantage of such vaccines is that the interruption of sperm production is temporary.

The aspermatic condition is accompanied by circulating antibody formation and anaphylactic sensitivity, but the experimental disease is not transferable with serum. However, aspermatogenesis can be passively transferred with viable cells. Experimental aspermatogenesis thus is dependent on the cell-mediated hypersensitive response.

The potentiality of birth control of the female by immunization with sperm antigens is a second possibility. It was noted over a generation ago, before efficient chemical and mechanical control of fertilization was possible, that the incidence of pregnancy in prostitutes, was not totally compatible with their exposure. Among the suggested explanations for this was that such women produced sperm agglutinating and immobilizing antibodies as a result of immunization through the vaginal mucosa. Sperm immobilizing antibodies have been identified in human vaginal washings; these very well could protect against impregnation. Experiments with lower animals generally, but not always, have demonstrated protection of the female by immunization with homologous sperm.

Sympathetic ophthalmia

Sympathetic opthalmia is a chronic inflammatory reaction in a healthy eye that appears within a few days to a few weeks following surgical or traumatic injury to the other eye. At the cellular level this is characterized by an infiltration of mononuclear cells that engulf the uveal pigment. Clusters of lymphocytes and occasional eosinophils are seen. Attempts to demonstrate circulating antibodies in persons with sympathetic ophthalmia usually have met with failure.

Sympathetic ophthalmia appears to be representative of an autoimmune disease that is dependent on the response of antigen-exposed T cells rather than on immunoglobulin synthesis. Skin reactions of the delayed type are present in patients with the disease. The skin test intensity often parallels that of the disease, whereas antibody titers, when detected, show little correlation with the symptomatology. The ability of steroids to control the disease also is suggestive of a delayed hypersensitive mechanism. The critical passive transfer experiments in experimentally produced ophthalmia have not been performed. Reproducible animal models for sympathetic ophthalmia that might clarify its immunopathology have not been developed.

Cataract removal sometimes is followed by a postoperative intraocular complication known as phacoanaphylaxis. Histologic examination reveals that the lens is invaded by leukocytes and macrophages. It is believed that lens antigens, which escape during the surgical procedure, hypersensitize the individual. These patients exhibit immediate skin reactions when tested with lens proteins. The exact immunologic cause of this disease is uncertain, but it appears that circulating antibodies are involved.

Hashimoto's thyroiditis

A form of thyroiditis unique and readily distinguished from other types of thyroiditis on a histologic basis was the first disease that satisfied Witebsky's criteria for an autoimmune disease. Hashimoto's disease (hypothyroiditis) is characterized physiologically by a deficiency in thyroid hormone and anatomically by an enlarged thyroid gland infiltrated with plasma cells and lymphocytes (Fig. 19-4). In the sera of a certain proportion of patients with Hashimoto's disease a single gel precipitin line

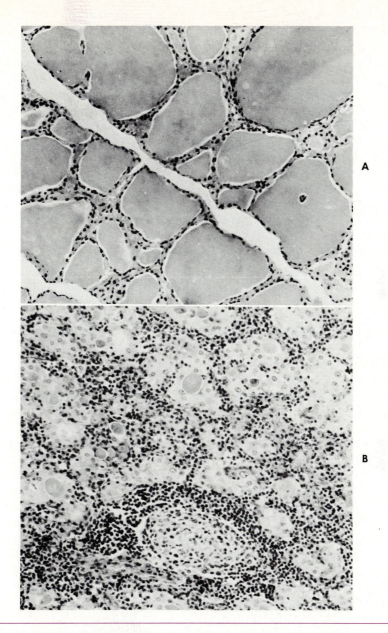

FIG. 19-4

A, Normal thyroid. **B,** Thyroid of Hashimoto's disease. In the normal thyroid the colloid fills the vesicles, whereas in the diseased gland only isolated deposits of colloid are seen. The cell infiltrate is lymphoid in nature. In the lower center is a germinal center. (From Anderson, J.R., Buchanan, W.W., and Goudie, R.B.: Autoimmunity, Springfield, Ill., 1967, Charles C Thomas, Publisher.)

between the serum and an extract of human thyroid gland is produced. This same precipitin band is produced when purified thyroglobulin is the antigen.

Thyroglobulin is stored as a distinct colloid that fills the vesicles in a normal thyroid gland and is the reservoir of thyroxin, the thyroid hormone. In Hashimoto's disease little colloid can be detected in the gland. Many plasma cells and lymphocytes are present. Formation of antithyroglobulin and the mononuclear cell population of the thyroid gland are compatible with an autoimmune origin of this disease.

Experimental thyroiditis can be produced in rabbits by autoimmunization with thyroid gland extracts emulsified in Freund's complete adjuvant. One lobe of the gland is used as the immunizing antigen, and the disease is assayed in the intact, remaining lobe. The formation of circulating antibody and the histologic changes in the rabbit thyroid parallel very closely the condition in the human. The disease now has been created in other common laboratory mammals.

It has not been possible, either in the human patient or in the experimental animal, to establish an exact correlation between serum antithyroglobulin titers and the severity of the thyroiditis. Transmission of the disease by passive immunization with serum is very difficult, and infants of mothers with Hashimoto's disease are unaffected by the maternal antithyroglobulin antibodies. Delayed hypersensitive skin reactions to thyroglobulin correlate in intensity with the severity of the disease; the transfer of the disease by lymphocytes strongly indicates a cell-mediated origin of the disease. However, the initial insult which permits that development of this autoallergic illness has not been identified yet, nor can one state unequivocally that this is a T cell–related disease.

Spontaneous autoimmune thyroiditis develops in the Obese (OS) strain chicken and the Buffalo rat. The avian model is especially interesting because of the anatomical division of the B and T cell system in birds. Neonatal thymectomy of OS chickens accelerates the onset of thyroiditis, whereas neonatal bursectomy prevents the development of autoimmune thyroiditis. The transfer of T cells from OS chickens to X-rayed normal chickens induces thyroiditis; however, the presence of B cells is required for a full expression of the disease. These data suggest that B cells are required for manifestation of the disease, i.e., it is basically an immunoglobulin mediated disease in these chickens, but the primary cause lies within the T cell compartment. Experimental studies of the Buffalo rat have led to the same conclusion, namely a loss in T_S cells resulting in the production of antibodies that are responsible for expression of disease.

These examples of spontaneous thyroiditis appear not to mimic spontaneous human thyroiditis. As stated above, newborn children of mothers with high antithyroglobulin titers do not suffer from thyroiditis. Transfers of high titered human sera to monkeys do not cause disease. Nevertheless, human antibody may be responsible for the increase in ADCC directed against cells in the thyroid, and a decrease in thyroglobulin specific T_S has been noted in Hashimoto's disease.

IMMUNOGLOBULIN-ASSOCIATED AUTOIMMUNE DISEASES
Autoimmune hemolytic disease

Autoimmune hemolytic diseases represent a complex assortment of disorders that share the major feature of anemia and accelerated blood cell loss associated with the simultaneous presence of immunoglobulins specific for the person's own erythrocytes. In a surprisingly large percentage of instances the anemia may be almost nonexistent, but in others, such as paroxysmal cold hemoglobinuria, red blood cell lysis is a striking feature of the illness. In 50% to 75% of the cases the cause is unknown; these are the so-called idiopathic acquired hemolytic anemias. In the remainder the condition develops secondary to disease of the RES, other lymphoid illnesses, or drug therapy.

The immunoglobulins associated with hemolytic diseases may be of the cold agglutinin type or the warm type (Table 19-3). The former function well at 4° C or other low temperatures but are feebly active at room temperature and almost, if not totally, inactive at 37° C. These may or may not be hemolytically active with complement. The warm agglutinins are usually poor complement fixers, which is com-

TABLE 19-3

Autoantibodies found in autoimmune hemolytic disease

	Warm antibody	Cold antibody
Immunoglobulin class	IgG	IgM
Temperature optimum	37° C	4° C
Antigen involved	Rh and other	I and other
Hemolysis	Less hemolytic	More hemolytic
Complement fixation	Less fixation	More fixation
Age attack range	Any age	Tendency toward older persons
Anemia	Variable	Variable
Associated diseases	SLE	*Mycoplasma* infection

patible with the rarity of severe hemolytic episodes in patients with this type of antibody. These warm agglutinins are also feeble agglutinators, and their presence usually is detected by antiglobulin tests for human IgG on the affected red cells. The cold agglutinins are most commonly of the IgM class, and they, too, are easily detected by antiglobulin tests of erythrocytes. Complement components also may be detected on the erythrocytes. It is not definitely known if these antibodies develop from a break in tolerance to normal antigens or if neoantigens are formed by infectious agents. Hemolytic anemias following primary atypical pneumonia or infectious mononucleosis are so common as to support a neo- or cross-reactive antigen etiology.

Autoimmune hemolytic disease caused by warm antibodies rarely occurs in childhood. The antibody is invariably an IgG and most often directed against an Rh antigen. About one third of the cases involve other than Rh antigens. The antibodies are not highly active; in vivo little anemia develops, although there are exceptions. Autoagglutination of erythrocytes from these patients is uncommon except in high-protein media (plasma).

Autoimmune hemolytic diseases caused by cold antibodies of the IgM class are often anti-I. The I antigen is formed after birth during "maturation" of red cell development. Agglutination of erythrocytes by cold agglutinins is reversed by warming the cells to 37° C. Necrosis of the fingertips, earlobes, tip of the nose, or other chilled parts of the patient's body may result from vascular plugging by the agglutinated cells. The simplest protection against these episodes is to keep warm.

Cold autoantibodies of the IgG class also are known to participate in hemolytic disease. These antibodies bind to erythrocytes at low temperature and at body temperature fix complement and function as hemolysins. This temperature dependence clearly is related to the disease with which these antibodies are most regularly associated: paroxysmal cold hemoglobinuria. After cold shock these patients experience a severe hemolytic episode. This can be duplicated by immersing the hand and forearm in ice water. The low temperature promotes antibody–red cell combination, and the warmer temperature promotes lysis. This form of hemolytic anemia is a complication of tertiary syphilis, although it may have other origins as well. The autoantibody is to the P antigen of the human red blood cell.

Drug-induced autoimmune hemolytic anemia has been associated with many different chemotherapeutics, such as quinine, quinidine, the sulfonamides, penicillin, cephalosporin, tetracycline, aspirin, antihistamines, and cytotoxic drugs used in cancer therapy. These drugs stimulate antibody formation by complexing with the erythrocyte surface to create new antigenic determinants, by forming new determinants with serum proteins, which then adsorb to the red cell surface, or by modifying the erythrocyte surface so that its new determinants are expressed. Only the latter does not contain the drug-hapten complex as an integral part. Antibodies formed against any of these would react with the antigen on the erythrocyte surface, combine with complement and cause hemolytic anemia.

Thrombocytopenic purpura

Thrombocytopenic purpura is an illness characterized by lowered platelet count (thrombocytopenia) in the circulation and the appearance of purpuric or petechial hemorrhages in the skin and tissues. The known contribution of thrombocytes to blood clotting is fully compatible with a close association of these two expressions of the disease.

Thrombocytopenic purpura in infants can arise through alloimmunization in much the same way that erythroblastosis fetalis develops, that is, the transplacental migration of maternal antifetal thrombocyte globulins. An autoimmune form of thrombocytopenic purpura is seen in adults. Invariably the afflicted persons are on a continued drug regimen of some sort. The offending drug may be aspirin, a sulfonamide, an antihistamine, quinine, digitoxin, or a tranquilizer. During the time the drug therapy is maintained, the purpura and thrombocytopenia are evident, but when the drug is withdrawn, the disease abates. Reinitiation of the therapy causes an exacerbation of the illness. The disease is truly iatrogenic in origin. An in vitro mixture of the patient's serum with human platelets plus the offending drug results in complement fixation and lysis of the platelets. If complement is absent, platelet agglutination may occur, but lysis cannot. If the offending drug is absent, the patient's serum has no effect on the platelets. These features indicate that a hapten-antigen complex in which the hapten dominates the determinant site is the incitant of the disease.

Two immunologic hypotheses have been formulated for this disease. One assumes that the hapten (inciting drug) complexes naturally with platelets to create a neoantigen and that the antibody is formed against this complex. Therefore normal platelets are not agglutinated or lysed by the antibody in the absence or presence of complement; these reactions require the drug (Fig. 19-5). The other proposal suggests that the drug binds to a serum protein to form the hapten-antigen complex. This complex adsorbs to the platelet surface and causes lysis in the presence of the specific antibody and complement. Whatever the exact mechanism, there can be no question that this is a hapten-mediated condition which is directly associated with circulating antibody. Passive transfer of the patient's serum will convey the disease to a normal person, provided the latter receives the drug also.

Myasthenia gravis (MG)

Myasthenia gravis is a disease in which a gradual progressive weakness of striated muscle is a prominent external sign and which becomes so severe that even eating is laborious. MG affects 1 in every 10,000 to 40,000 persons. About 10% to 20% of its victims have a thymoma of mixed epithelial and thymocytic nature. A number of immunologic aberrations are seen in MG patients. Germinal centers are detectable in the thymus gland, which normally is devoid of these structures. Antinuclear antibodies (ANA) are found in about 20% of the patients. RF is present in 5% to 10% of the patients, and antibodies that react with striated muscle are quite common (30% to 40% frequency). The presence of an antibody to the acetylcholine receptor in 80% of the patients is the most important of these immunopathologic features. This autoantibody is frequently of the IgG3 isotype, but other IgG subclasses and IgM occur in some patients. The failure of MG disease severity to correlate with antibody titer may relate to the avidity of the antibody.

At the normal muscle-nerve (myoneural) junction acetylcholine is released from the nerve when it stimulates the muscle to contract. The acetylcholine binds to a receptor on the muscle surface and initiates contraction of the muscle. When antibody is adsorbed to or adjacent to this receptor, this event is inhibited. Consequently muscular contraction and strength are impaired (Fig. 19-6).

Experimental models of MG can be produced in species such as chickens, rats, rabbits, mice, and monkeys by immunization with acetylcholine receptors from the electric eel. It is interesting that this receptor is antigenically similar in the eel and several mammals. The receptor molecule is composed of five peptides, two α units plus one each of the β, γ,

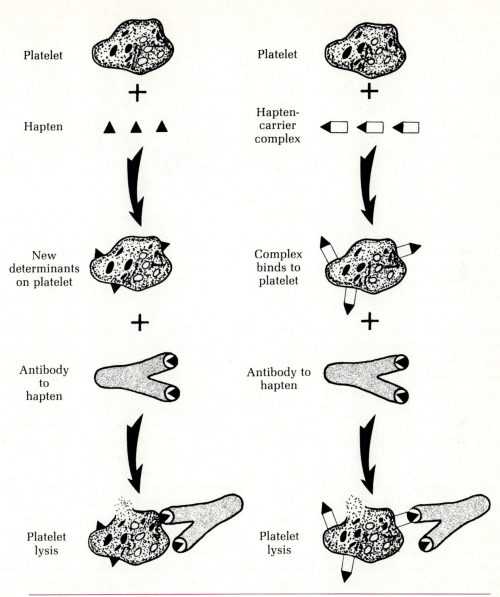

FIG. 19-5

Two hypotheses for the autoimmune origin for thrombocytopenia purpura. On the left, a hapten combines with the surface of a platelet to create new antigenic determinants. The resulting antibody reacts with the platelet and complement to cause cell lysis. On the right, the hapten combines spontaneously with a carrier molecule, which adsorbs to the surface of the platelet. The new antigenic determinant involves the hapten and carrier but not the platelet.

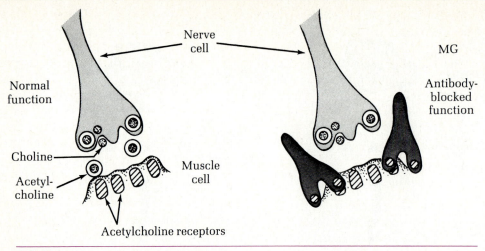

FIG. 19-6

At the normal neuromuscular junction *(left)* acetylcholine is released from the nerve cell and degraded by a cholinesterase in the acetylcholine receptor on the muscle cell. This causes the muscle to contract. This is prevented by antibody against the receptor in the person with MG *(right)*.

and δ subunits. The antibody in MG is directed toward the α units, which do not actually contain the acetylcholine binding site. MG is thus due to a loss of receptor function as a result of the blockade of antibody and not to receptor binding directly.

Multiple sclerosis (MS)

Partial loss of vision, nystagmus, facial palsy, and muscular incoordination are a few of the varied symptoms of MS. Remissions and exacerbations are characteristic of this disease, which may affect more than 250,000 persons in the United States. Dietary, infectious, and immunologic causes all have been proposed for the disease.

The major pathologic feature of MS is an inflammatory lesion of the myelin in the central nervous system. Myelin of the central nervous system and that of peripheral nervous tissues differ chemically, and this accounts for the specificity of MS for myelin of the central nervous system. Denuded foci along the nerve sheath create lesions that are characteristic of the disease and which are known as sclerotic plaques. These lesions are associated with the neuromuscular symptoms of MS.

The basis for theories of a dietary cause of MS is

based on modern diets that have a low content of polyunsaturated fatty acids, presumably leading to a defective lipid content of the myelin sheath. Evidence for a viral origin is more convincing and is based on epidemiologic studies and the reports of viruslike particles in early MS lesions.

Immunologic associations with MS include the identification of lymphocytes, plasma cells, monocytes, and macrophages in the plaques. Antibodies are present in serum and spinal fluid that react with the MBP. An increased content of IgG in the spinal fluid of MS patients is one of its most reliable clinical tests, being reported in up to 94% of the patients in some studies. Antibodies directed against the myelin-forming oligodendrocytes also may be present. Sera from MS patients are also toxic for myelinated cells in vitro, and the titer of these antibodies often correlates well with the severity of the disease. Although these facts indicate a potential immunoglobulin basis for MS, a loss of T_S cells is known to precede MS in children and would account for the changes in immunoglobulin levels. The immunologic basis of MS is still poorly defined.

The autoimmune basis of MS is indicated by its close association with HLA-B7 and HLA-Dw2. The incidence of the Dw2 antigen in MS patients is 70% versus 16% in healthy control subjects.

Numerous models of MS can be developed in laboratory animals. These demyelinating diseases include acute EAE, neurotropic virus infections, including visna in sheep, canine distemper, and encephalomyelitis virus infections in mice, and combinations of EAE with these viral infections. EAE is discussed previously with a full discussion of the MBP.

Poststreptococcal diseases
Rheumatic fever

Acute rheumatic fever has been recognized for a long time as one of two important diseases that typically follow a group A streptococcal illness. Unlike poststreptococcal glomerulonephritis, poststreptococcal rheumatic heart disease may follow infection with any one of more than 50 types of group A streptococci. The latent period for the symptoms of the rheumatic heart disease coincides roughly with the time required for the development of high anti-streptococcal titers. This has suggested an autoimmune origin of the illness, specifically, an involvement of circulating antibodies.

Among the immunopathologic changes that occur in rheumatic fever are elevated titers against streptolysin O, streptococcal DNAse B, and several other enzymes and toxins of group A streptococci. Inflammatory tissue changes in the heart include the aggregation of lymphocytes and macrophages around fibrinoid deposits to form Aschoff's bodies. These structures are almost pathognomonic of rheumatic fever. IgG and, to a lesser extent, IgM, IgA, and complement can be found deposited in the Aschoff body, in the perivascular connective tissue, and in the sarcolemma (Fig. 19-7). Many patients have antibody free in their blood plasma that is reactive with heart tissue.

Several potential mechanisms for poststreptococcal autoimmune heart disease have been suggested. The two most commonly discussed are the alteration of heart tissue by streptococci to create new hapten-antigen complexes, which initiate the formation of antiheart immunoglobulins, and the sharing of similar antigens by human heart and group A streptococci.

Most of the available information supports the second or cross-reacting antigen theory. The streptococcal groups, which are designated by the letters A, B, C, etc., are segregated according to the chemical and immunologic nature of the C carbohydrate in their cytoplasm. Within the group A organisms, serotyping is arranged on the basis of variations in the M protein. This protein is located on the cell surface, possibly in the fimbriae. More than 60 different forms, or antigenic types (designated by numbers), of this M protein are known. This protein is associated with the virulence of the group A streptococci. Many of these infections precede rheumatic fever. These infections stimulate high antibody titers to the M protein and other streptococcal antigens, but the anti-M titer is higher in those who become rheumatic than in those with uncomplicated streptococcal infections. Antibody deposits on human cardiac myofibers can be identified in these rheumatic patients with fluorescent antihuman IgG. Elevated levels of circulating immune complexes, presumably containing a soluble component of heart tissue, also occur. Complement component C3 also has been recognized in these deposits. The evidence now indicates that this antibody is specific for the M protein or another protein which is closely associated with the M protein. This streptococcal antigen is cross-reactive with human heart tissue. Rabbit antibody to group A streptococci will precipitate on human cardiac myofibers but not on fibers of the voluntary muscles. This can be prevented by adsorption of the antiserum either with bacterial cell wall preparations or extracts of human heart tissue. Monoclonal antibody versus the streptococcal M protein reacts with a 20,000 molecular weight protein of the sarcolemma. This is considered as very strong supportive evidence for the cross-reacting antigen theory of poststreptococcal rheumatic fever.

Glomerulonephritis

Basically there are three forms of immune disease that involve the glomerulus. One is associated with antecedent group A streptococcal infection; a second is involved with heterologous antibodies versus glomerular basement membrane antigens (Masugi's nephritis); the third is based on immune complex

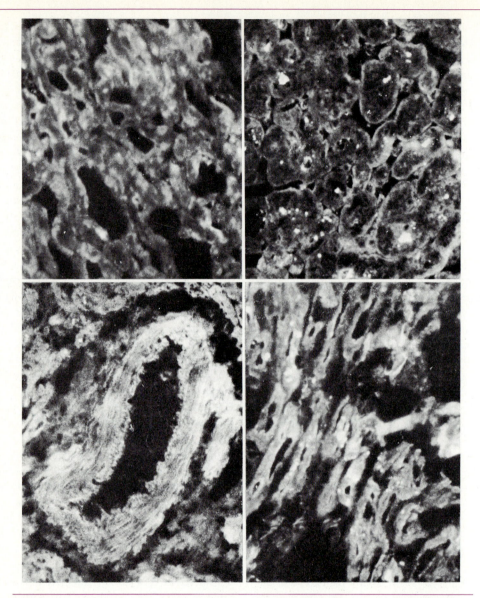

FIG. 19-7
Immunofluorescent staining of human heart tissue with antibody to group A streptococcus cell membrane; indirect fluorescent antibody procedure. (From Zabriskie, J.B.: Mimetic relationships between group A streptococci and mammalian tissues, Adv. Immunol. **7:**147, 1967.)

formation with foreign antigens, as in serum sickness, or alloantigens, as in SLE.

Autoimmune glomerulonephritis, in which edema, hematuria, and other symptoms of kidney failure become manifest, is an immune complex disease in which globulins precipitate within the kidney. This may follow staphylococcal or pneumococcal infections or malaria, but in the United States it more commonly is considered the result of a prior group A streptococcal infection. Unlike rheumatic fever, which may follow virtually any group A streptococcal infection, poststreptococcal glomerulonephritis is limited to a few serologic types. These include types 12, 4, 5, 25, 49, 52, 55, and a few others. These nephritogenic cocci synthesize a lipoprotein molecule of about 120,000 mol wt that is a part of their cytoplasmic membrane. This antigenic lipoprotein is serologically cross-reactive with kidney tissue. Just as with rheumatic fever, when symptoms of the streptococcal infection begin to subside, some 10 to 14 days after the initial infection, the symptoms of the autoimmune kidney disease begin to appear.

Fluorescent antibody and histologic studies of the kidney indicate that IgG (or sometimes IgA or IgM) and C3 are deposited in a granular distribution along the glomerular basement membrane. Activation of the complement system generates chemotaxins, which cause the entrance of PMNs into the region. Infiltration of the PMNs into the tissues contributes to the disease.

Autoimmune and alloimmune duplicates of glomerulonephritis can be produced by preparing kidney homogenates with adjuvants and using these for immunization. The passive immunization of animals with heteroantisera developed against kidney antigens causes a form of nephritis known as Masugi's glomerulonephritis. Masugi's nephritis has been provoked in most experimental animal species. The pathologic manifestations of Masugi's autoimmune, and alloimmune nephritis will vary from one species to another and are close but not exact mimics of the poststreptococcal disease. They are useful models, since streptococcal infections are not reliable incitants of glomerulonephritis in animals.

Masugi's nephritis is a closer mimic of antiglomerular basement membrane nephritis seen after unsuccessful kidney grafts than it is of poststreptococcal disease. Goodpasture's syndrome (Fig. 19-8) and rapidly progressive nephritis are like the Masugi disease in that the γ-globulin and complement deposits are linear not granular as in poststreptococcal nephritis.

Autologous antibodies made against exogenous nonglomerular antigens will complex in the circulation and become trapped in the capillary vessel walls of the kidney. Since complement is fixed in the reaction, anaphylatoxins and chemotaxins are released.

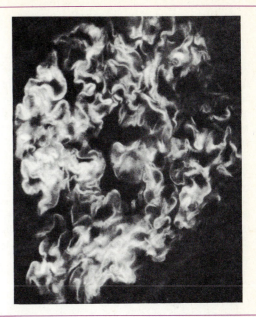

FIG. 19-8

Deposition of γ-globulin along the glomerula capillary walls in a human kidney of a patient with Goodpasture's disease; fluorescent antibody procedure. (From Lerner, R.A., Glascock, R.J., and Dixon, F.J.: The role of antiglomerular basement membrane antibody in the pathogenesis of human glomerulonephritis, J. Exp. Med. **126:**989, 1967.)

This leads to local tissue damage. This type of glomerulonephritis is produced in serum sickness and SLE.

Autoimmune glomerulonephritis is observed in both the canine and mouse models of SLE and in Aleutian mink disease. These mink, valued and bred for their unique pelt color, are infected by a virus (or cell-free agent) that promotes a sharp increase in the number of plasma cells and a hypergammaglobulinemia. The infective agent is transmitted easily to young mink, which die of glomerulonephritis within the first 6 months of life. The cause of renal failure is the accumulation of virus-antigen complexes with complement in the kidney.

A virus disease of horses is responsible for an equine form of autoimmune glomerulonephritis. This disease, like Aleutian mink disease, is characterized by an intense hypergammaglobulinemia and an accumulation of antibody-virus-complement complexes

☰ SITUATION 1

RHEUMATOID ARTHRITIS

Frank, a 53-year-old pastry worker in a small home-style bakery, contacted his physician because of pain in his wrists and thumbs. Morning stiffness in these joints was also a chief complaint, and some swelling and warmth in the wrist area was noticed. This condition had developed slowly over the past year or more, eventually causing enough distress to necessitate medical attention. The patient was informed that there was a good possibility that he was developing rheumatoid arthritis, although other diagnoses were possible. Blood was collected for serologic and hematologic studies, and x-ray films were taken of the affected joints. The findings confirmed rheumatoid arthritis, and aspirin was prescribed.

Questions

1. What serologic tests are used to aid in the diagnosis of rheumatoid arthritis?
2. What is the immunopathology of this disease?

Solution

The laboratory findings in rheumatoid arthritis often include an elevated γ-globulin level, and positive RF tests. The RF test is positive in about 80% of all patients with classic rheumatoid arthritis when the latex agglutination test is used. In this test, pooled human γ-globulin is adsorbed onto latex particles and used as the antigen in passive agglutination tests. The patient's serum contains RF, an antiglobulin, most frequently an IgM, but it may also be either an IgG or IgA, that fixes to the globulin on the latex particle, thus causing agglutination. Antigenic sites on the IgG molecule to which RF attaches are labeled as the Gm determinants. Pooled γ-globulin is used to coat the latex particles, since an individual γ-globulin may lack the Gm determinant with which the patient's RF reacts.

Positive RF tests are not diagnostic of rheumatoid arthritis, since such tests are positive in many connective tissue diseases, including lupus erythematosus, scleroderma, Sjögren's syndrome, viral hepatitis-arthritis, polyarteritis, cirrhosis, and polymyositis. Many infectious diseases also lead to false-positive RF tests, of which, leprosy, syphilis, tuberculosis, viral hepatitis, and even influenza can be mentioned. The titer of RF even in frank rheumatoid arthritis does not correlate with the intensity of the disease. As a consequence, positive RF tests must be interpreted cautiously; clinical and radiologic findings are probably more important in the diagnosis of rheumatoid arthritis.

Other positive tests in rheumatoid arthritis include ANA (incidence of 20% to 60%) and positive LE preparations (incidence of 10% to 20%).

The immunopathology of the disease is unproven, but is possibly based on an infectious joint disease, followed by an outpouring of IgG and inflammatory cells into the synovial fluid. IgG molecules become altered by lysosomal enzymes secreted by the inflammatory cells and this exposes new antigenic determinants in the Gm markers and stimulates IgM formation. This is described more fully in the chapter text.

---

in the capillary bed of the glomeruli, causing a glomerulonephritis. A cardinal symptom of the disease is a hemolytic anemia, but the exact immunologic basis of this is uncertain.

Rheumatoid arthritis

Rheumatoid arthritis is an inflammatory disease of the joints and connective tissue; amyloid deposition in tissues and permanent deformity of the joints may result. Despite intensive study of the microbial flora of joint fluids, of the sex differences in susceptibilities, and of nutritional and genetic factors, the cause of the rheumatoid disease remains unknown. The induction of arthritis in rats by the injection of adjuvant and the known association of arthritis in certain lower animals with bacterial infection have done little to clarify the cause of human rheumatoid disease. Interest in this disease as a potential allergic disease was strengthened by the discovery that sera of rheumatoid patients would agglutinate erythrocytes coated with subagglutinating quantities of antibody. The agglutinating agent is known as rheumatoid factor (RF), an antibody versus an antibody.

RF is a 19S immunoglobulin compatible in all respects with IgM. In the patient's sera RF may circulate as a 22S complex that, on dissociation, yields a molecule of IgM and one or perhaps as many as six molecules of IgG. RF is an unusual IgM antibody in only one respect—its relative lack of specificity for human IgG: it will react with rabbit IgG and that of other species. The original tests for RF depended on its ability to enhance erythrocyte agglutination with rabbit antibody; later erythrocytes or latex particles bearing pooled human IgG were used as the antigen. The sensitivities of these tests differ; in various studies between 50% and 95% of rheumatoid arthritic patients had positive RF tests. Such findings suggest that RF is an antibody to an altered form of IgG which usually is not found in the circulation.

In tests for RF pooled human IgG is the usual antigen coated on erythrocytes or latex particles. If IgG from a specific individual is used as the antigen, many RF sera, positive according to the pooled antigen test, become negative. This is due to the fact that RF reacts with specific Gm determinants and these determinants are not equally distributed among all IgG subclasses, and are in fact the basis for different allotypes of IgG. In a variation of the test based on inhibition of the agglutination reaction between RF and the pooled IgG antigen, the IgG from certain (but not all) individuals will inhibit the agglutination. This is the original method used to determine that all human IgG molecules are not antigenically identical and became the basis for the classification of the IgG-Gm allotypes.

Even though inflammatory cells, lymphocytes, and plasma cells are detectable in synovial tissue, and even though RF is present in sera, an autoimmune origin of rheumatic fever has been difficult to prove unequivocally. One conjectured mechanism is essentially as follows (Fig. 19-9). An initial joint inflammation possibly arises from some infectious agent. This stimulates an immunoglobulin response against the pathogen, and antibody of the IgG type is formed. The reaction of this immunoglobulin with the organisms releases (from the complement involved) chemotactic and anaphylatoxic reagents. These add to the inflammatory reaction with the release of lysosomal enzymes, which damage the IgG antibody and convert it to a neoantigen. This sparks an immune response of the IgM type, the product of which is RF. When RF reacts with the IgG, addi-

tional chemotactic and anaphylatoxic events occur that perpetuate the inflammation, the continued damage of IgG, and a continued recycling of these events. The theory seems quite logical, but unfortunately there is little evidence for or against it. If the facts do correspond with this theory, it will be confirmed that RF is not the direct cause of rheumatoid arthritis. Transfusion of blood with high levels of RF does not provoke rheumatoid arthritis, nor does the direct infusion of RF into joint fluid. RF is produced in the tissues of the joint, and RF-IgG-complement complexes can be detected in rheumatoid synovia. Whether these are the result or the cause of the joint disease is conjectural, but they most certainly are not the cause of other tissue aspects of rheumatoid arthritis, for example, subcutaneous nodules. There is no evidence as yet that cellular hypersensitivity contributes to this disease.

Systemic lupus erythematosus (SLE)

SLE or LE is a disease with a more certain immunologic cause. SLE is four times more common in women than in men, and many patients are HLA-B8 positive. The cardinal external sign of the disease is a red rash across the nose and upper cheeks, from which the disease gets it name (*lupus erythematosus,* the red wolf). More serious internal lesions involve the kidney, the blood vessels, the blood cells, and the heart. Several immunologic phenomena are associated with the disease, including hypergammaglobulinemia and hypocomplementemia.

One of the first immunologic changes noted was LE cell formation, first described in 1948. The LE cell is a neutrophil containing a large, pale staining structure that often fills the cytoplasm of the phagocyte. Occasionally the LE body is not engulfed but can be seen free in stained blood films, often surrounded by neutrophils, whose dark staining nuclei produce a rosettelike arrangement. Microcinematography has revealed how these structures develop. If serum from an SLE patient is mixed with whole blood, it will be noted that the nucleus of certain white blood cells undergoes a sudden explosive swelling and loses its dark staining quality, becoming paler and spherical. Unaffected phagocytes approach the LE body, strip away its cytoplasm, and

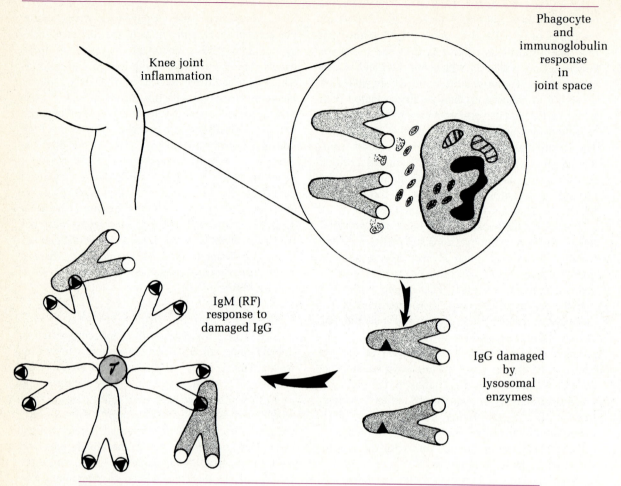

FIG. 19-9

One hypothesis for the origin of RF is related to formation of damaged IgG in infectious joint disease. RF attaches to the Fc section of the IgG molecule.

engulf its nucleus to become LE cells. Rosette formation results when the LE body is not engulfed but is surrounded by viable neutrophils, each of which apparently is competing with the others for phagocytosis of the deranged LE nucleus (Fig. 19-10).

The LE factor in serum responsible for these changes has been definitely identified as an antideoxyribonucleoprotein (anti-DNA) of the IgG isotype. This antibody will attach to nuclei from almost any source in agreement with the known nonspecificity of anti-DNA antibodies. LE cell forma-

tion is a useful diagnostic aid when positive, but many patients produce negative tests because of the difficulty in performing and interpreting LE cell tests. Consequently fluorescent antinuclear antibody (FANA) or other ANA tests have supplemented LE cell procedures. The human ANA, although usually an IgG, may be an IgM or IgA.

FANA in sera of SLE patients is identified by the indirect fluorescent antibody procedure. Yeast cells, calf thymus cells, other mammalian cells, or *Crithidia,* a protozoan with a high intracellular content of

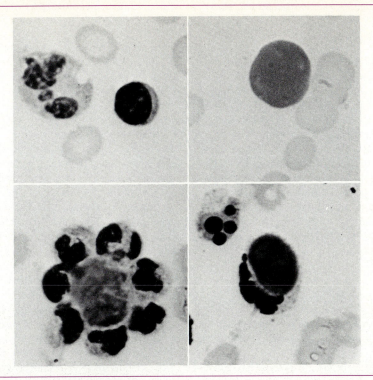

FIG. 19-10
LE cell test. Upper left quadrant, a normal neutrophil and lymphocyte; upper right, a free LE body; lower left, a rosette; and lower right, a single LE cell. (From Anderson, J.R., Buchanan, W.W., and Goudie, R.B.: Autoimmunity, Springfield Ill., 1967, Charles C Thomas, Publisher.)

DNA, are used as a source of DNA and prepared on a slide. This is developed with the patient's serum and then with a fluorescent antihuman γ-globulin. When whole cells are used, the pattern of staining will be distinctive from one patient to another. Staining of the perimeter of the nucleus indicates the serum is dominated by an anti-DNA antibody. A homogeneous staining of the nucleus indicates nucleoprotein (DNA-histone) staining. Fluorescence in the nucleolus is characteristic of an antibody specificity for RNA, and a speckled pattern reflects the presence of an antibody to an extractable nuclear antigen (ENA).

ENA is not a single antigen; rather it is a mixture of perhaps as many as 20 antigens, which are acidic. Few of these have been characterized chemically other than for the presence of dsDNA, dsRNA, ssDNA, or ssRNA and of protein. Two ENAs that appear to have a high degree of specificity for SLE are the Sm and MA antigens. Sm is an acidic glycoprotein with a molecular weight of less than 150,000. Anti-Sm is found in 24% of all SLE patients. Patients with severe SLE often have antibodies that react with the MA antigen.

Other antibodies found in SLE sera react with nRNP (nuclear ribonucleoprotein), PCNA (proliferating cell nuclear antigen), SS-S and SS-B (Sjögren's syndrome antigens A and B), H1, H3, and H4 (histone antigens), and others. Investigators are actively searching for an antigen or panel of antigens that will be of diagnostic significance for SLE.

In addition to the presence of antibodies to

≣ SITUATION 2

SYSTEMIC LUPUS ERYTHEMATOSUS

Judy, a 28-year-old employee of a local boutique, first contacted a dermatologist because of a rash that developed over the bridge of her nose and across her upper cheeks while she was on vacation in Florida. At first she masked the rash with cosmetics. However, the rash persisted, and when she began to develop other vague symptoms of illness—fever, malaise, and a slight weight loss—she contacted her dermatologist. A laboratory workup revealed a slight hypergammaglobulinemia, a low C3 component of complement, and a positive RF test. A second serum sample was analyzed for antinuclear antibodies (ANA) and found to be positive. Precipitation tests for Sm, RNP and other antigens was requested.

Questions

1. What method(s) can be used to measure total complement activity in patient sera?
2. What would be the advantages in measuring certain specific components rather than total complement activity?
3. What method(s) can be used to measure the individual complement components?
4. What results would be anticipated from serum complement studies of this patient if SLE actually were the diagnosis?
5. What other immunoassays are useful in cases of SLE?

Solution

To determine the complement level, serum in final dilutions ranging from 1:10 to 1:50 is normally added to antibody coated erythrocytes and evaluated against 100% lysis and normal cell (0% lysis) controls. The dilution of complement that will lyse 50% of the cells (the CH_{50} unit) is used to express the complement level in the serum. Normal values range between 20 and 50 CH_{50}/ml.

Assays for total hemolytic activity do not reveal whether the alternate or classic pathway is responsible for a lowered CH_{50} titer. Neither would this assist in the identification of a genetic or other loss of a specific component. Individual complement components can be measured by hemolytic assays using commercially available reagents. In general, these tests require sensitized erythrocytes and an excess of all the complement components except the one to be quantitated in the patient's serum. Radioimmunoassays are now available for some components of the complement system.

Comparative assays for C4 and C3 are always of interest. If C4 remains high in the presence of depressed C3, then an alternate pathway activation is indicated.

In the patient described, the total complement and the C3 levels were depressed. The C4 level was also low. These results are compatible with a diagnosis of SLE. In one study of complement levels in SLE patients, total complement and C3 levels were lowered in 13 patients. Of these, 12 had a low C4 level, indicating activation by the classic pathway.

Fluorescent antibody tests to detect patient antinuclear antibody (ANA) still have a useful place in diagnosing SLE and its closely related diseases. Progress in the purification of nucleic acid complexes—both RNA and DNA, and the proteins associated with them—has created a specificity in the diagnosis of SLE, polymyositis, mixed connective tissue disease, and associated illnesses. This is discussed in the section on SLE in this chapter.

---

dsDNA, SLE patients have a high frequency (up to 90% in some studies) of circulating immune complexes. Removal of these in the kidney accounts for the glomerulonephritis characteristic of the disease (Fig. 19-11). About 75% of SLE patients will develop hypocomplementemia. Levels of both C3 and C4 are decreased indicating activation of the classic complement pathway. Deposits of C3b and C4b can be identified in kidneys. The combined chemotactic and anaphylatoxic properties of the complement system contribute significantly to kidney disease in SLE.

The success of immunosuppressive treatment of SLE with cyclophosphamide, azathioprine, and corticosteroids has underscored the immunologic nature of this disease. Although a viral origin is still possible (with viruses of the dsDNA type), current opinion is shifting to a loss of T_S cells as the basis for this disease. This hypothesis has received strong support from studies of murine SLE. In human SLE,

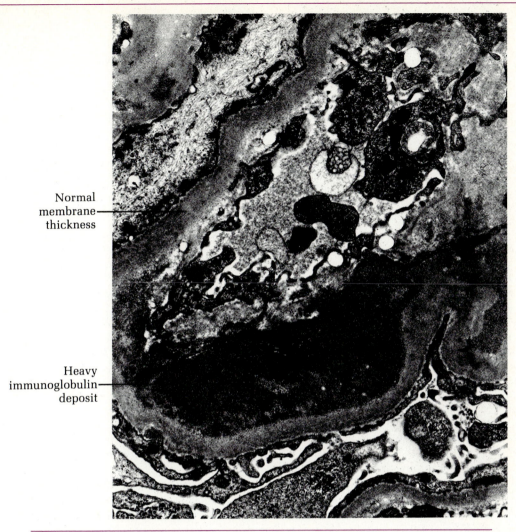

Normal
membrane
thickness

Heavy
immunoglobulin
deposit

FIG. 19-11

An immunoglobulin deposit in the basement membrane of a patient with SLE as seen by the electron microscope. (Courtesy Dr. E. Adelstein.)

a loss of IL-2 producing cells, normally considered as T_H cells, is also noted. A combined loss of T_S cells with other T cell subsets eventually disrupts T cell dependent regulatory events and allows forbidden antibodies to be produced.

The best animal model of SLE is the NZB/NZW progeny that result from mating of New Zealand black (NZB) and New Zealand white (NZW) mice.

These NZB/NZW hybrids develop antibodies versus dsDNA, ssDNA, dsRNA, ssRNA, and other ENA antigens. Virtually 100% of these mice develop and die of immune complex glomerulonephritis. In the first few months of life NZB/NZW mice appear completely normal, but this masks a gradual loss of T_S cell function, which ultimately explodes in the form of undesired B cell activities—the numerous

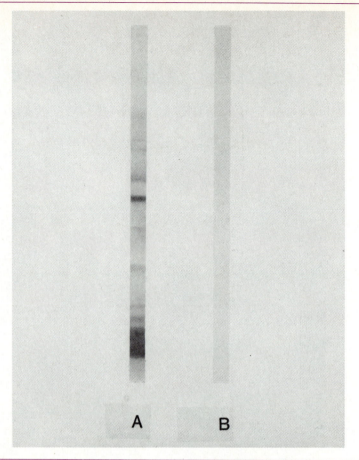

FIG. 19-12

An immunoperoxidase test used to identify the appearance of autoantibodies to RNP. The RNP antigen was separated by electrophoresis on both gels. Sera from an aged (**A**) and young MLR mouse (**B**) were incubated with the antigen on the electrophoretic strips. Then peroxidase-labeled antimouse globulin was used to localize the antibody in the aged mouse serum. The young mouse was negative in this test. (Courtesy Dr. K. Wise.)

autoantibodies (Fig. 19-12), and macroglobulinemia that precede death. These mice will have 4 to 8 times the normal mouse level of 3 to 4 mg of IgG/ml at the time of their death. The more recently described MLR-lpr^{+} mouse is also an excellent model of SLE, showing much the same history as the New Zealand hybrids. Fifty percent of these mice die before they are 6 months of age. The lpr (lymphoproliferating) gene is an autosomal recessive gene that is expressed as a generalized proliferation of lymph node cells. A marked expansion of Lyt1^{+} cells is characteristic of these mice. These mice develop a thymotoxic antibody, an IgM, which reacts with 98% of mouse thymocytes and behaves like an anti-Thy serum. Such antibodies contribute to the loss of T$_S$ cells and allow expression of undesired antibody responses. These mice produce high levels of anti-ds and -ssDNA, as well as anti-IgG. These antibodies plus those directed at a glycoprotein of 70,000 mol wt are the most predictive of murine SLE.

Another excellent model for LE is the canine model, in which characteristics of SLE such as glomerulonephritis, positive LE cells, and antibodies to nuclear antigens and DNA are present. These conditions are accompanied by a host of other physiologic abnormalities, including anemia, thrombocytopenia, polyarteritis, thyroiditis, and a chronic viral infection. A strong possibility exists that many of the symptoms of the autoimmune diseases in these dogs are the direct result of a viral infection or an indirect effect of a virus on lymphoid cells. Aleutian mink disease has a viral cause yet produces many of the immunopathologic aspects typical of SLE.

Drug-induced SLE has been associated with chemotherapy with several compounds, including hydralazine, penicillin, oral contraceptives, and procainamide. Although this form of LE may appear within a few weeks after therapy is initiated, a prodromal period of several months is more common. Anti-dsDNA is less common in drug-induced SLE than in the spontaneous disease.

Other collagen diseases

Rheumatoid arthritis and systemic lupus erythematosus are often described as collagen diseases, diseases exemplified by a combination of immune complex deposition in blood vessels, kidney, joints, and serosal membranes accompanied by complement-mediated tissue damage. Numerous other conditions display similar immunologic phenomena and are classified as collagen diseases. These diseases included mixed connective tissue disease, Sjögren's syndrome, scleroderma, polymyositis-dermatomyositis, and amyloidosis.

Mixed connective tissue disease (MCTD) shares many features with SLE, yet appears to be a distinct illness. The renal disease is often more mild than in SLE, and the response to steroid therapy is more favorable. The FANA test presents a speckled pattern. This staining pattern is associated with anti-RNP and virtually 100% of mixed connective tissue disease have such antibodies, but only rarely have anti-Sm, anti-SS-A, or anti-SS-B.

The presence of antibodies to SS-A and SS-B, both of which are in the ENA fraction of cells, is typical of patients with Sjögren's syndrome, who

TABLE 19-4

Incidence of antibodies to various antigens in connective tissue diseases

Disease	Sm	nRNP	SS-A	PM-1
SLE	24	25	30	Rare
MCTD	Rare	100	0	Rare
Sjögren's syndrome	0	3	70	Rare
Polymyositis	Rare	Rare	Rare	75

virtually never produce antibodies to the Sm antigen. Patients with scleroderma do not have as distinctive an autoimmune response as patients with the diseases already mentioned. Patients with polymyositis have, at a rate of approximately 75%, autoantibodies versus the PM-1 antigen, but almost never versus the aforementioned antigens (Table 19-4).

Of course, a primary goal in studying these antigens is to identify an antigen fraction that is diagnostic for one of these diseases. Already, however, some novel ideas on the evolution of these diseases have arisen from the study of these antigens. A recent publication indicated that some of these antigens were actually enzymes—polymerases and transferases—associated with nucleic acid metabolism. Interference of the function of these critical enzymes by autoantibodies would be expected to have a marked influence on cell health.

Graves' disease

A thyroid disease more common than Hashimoto's disease is Graves' disease, a form of hyperthyroidism. The evidence, accumulated at a rapid pace after 1956, indicates that the hyperthyroidism associated with Graves' disease is caused by a long-acting thyroid stimulator (LATS), an immunoglobulin found in the sera of nearly 85% of all patients. Purified IgG that contains this LATS activity has been further analyzed with the discovery that the Fab and $F(ab')_2$ portions of the molecule contain the LATS activity. The LATS autoantibody is a type of enhancing antibody that operates at the cellular level, much like the thyroid stimulatory hormone, to stimulate thyroid hormone release and thyrotoxicosis.

Autoimmune skin diseases

Three serious diseases of the skin now are recognized to have a strong autoimmune component. These diseases are pemphigus vulgaris, bullous pemphigoid, and dermatitis herpetiformis. The first is characterized by a separation of the epidermis from the underlying intraepithelial cells and bullae (blister) formation. Fluorescent antibody staining for immunoglobulin and complement component C3 has revealed the presence of both in affected areas of the skin. In pemphigus vulgaris it is thought that the autoantibody, an IgG, may be specific for the intercellular cement substance and that fixation of complement results in chemotaxis and a self-destructive attack on the epidermis.

In the case of bullous pemphigoid, autoantibodies directed against the dermal epithelial junction of the skin can be found circulating in the blood and deposited in the skin. C3 also is demonstrable in the skin. Evidence for an activation of the alternate complement pathway is based on the presence of C3 proactivator and properdin in the dermal basement membranes.

The third skin disease, dermatitis herpetiformis, has many features that suggest an autoimmune origin, but these are inconsistent from patient to patient. Deposits of IgA at the dermal-epidermal junction are seen more frequently than are deposits of IgG and IgM. C3 is found frequently, but it is difficult to correlate it with the presence of IgA, which cannot fix complement. Circulating autoantibodies are not detectable in these patients.

Other diseases

Antibodies to tissue antigens have been recognized in a long list of human ailments, including Addison's disease (adrenal disease), Felty's syndrome (a characteristic type of leukopenia), pernicious anemia, gastrointestinal disease, celiac disease, and juvenile onset or insulin-dependent diabetes. In the last of these diseases, a viral infection is nearly always an antecedent to the disease and Coxsackie B-4 virus isolated from a patient will provoke disease in mice. Antibodies versus insulin and islet cells contribute to the disease. This is unlike other diseases, where auto-

antibodies serve as a convenient diagnostic support when present, but this does not reflect any role of the autoantibody in the origin or continuation of the disease. For most of these conditions it simply is not possible to make any conclusions other than stating that autoantibodies often are associated with the disease.

REFERENCES

Alvord, E.C., Jr., Kies, M.K., and Suckling, A.J., editors: Experimental allergic encephalomyelitis. A useful model for multiple sclerosis, New York, 1984, Alan R. Liss, Inc.

Blecher, M.: Receptors, antibodies, and disease, Clin. Chem. **30:**1137, 1984.

Brockes, J., editor: Neuroimmunology, New York, 1982, Plenum Press.

Cohen, A.S., editor: Laboratory diagnostic procedures in the rheumatic diseases, Orlando, 1985, Grune and Stratton, Inc.

Cruse, J.M., and Lewis, R.E., editors: Autoimmunity: basic concepts; systemic and selected organ-specific diseases, New York, 1985, S. Karger Publishers, Inc.

Cruse, J.M., and Lewis, R.E., editors: Organ based autoimmune diseases, New York, 1985, S. Karger Publishers, Inc.

Cummings, N.B., Michael, A.F., and Wilson, C.B., editors: Immune mechanisms in renal disease, New York, 1983, Plenum Medical Book Company.

Eilat, D.: Monoclonal autoantibodies: an approach to studying autoimmune disease, Mol. Immunol. **19:**943, 1982.

Gupta, S., editor: Immunology of clinical and experimental diabetes, New York, 1984, Plenum Publishing Corporation.

Haynes, B.F., and Eisenbarth, G.S., editors: Monoclonal antibodies: probes for the study of autoimmunity and immunodeficiency, Orlando, 1983, Academic Press, Inc.

Lambert, P.H., Perrin, L., and Izui, S., editors: Recent advances in systemic lupus erythematosus, Orlando, 1984, Academic Press, Inc.

Lindstrom, J.: Immunobiology of myasthenia gravis, experimental autoimmune myasthenia gravis, and Lambert-Eaton syndrome, Ann. Rev. Immunol. **3:**109, 1985.

Lubec, G., editor: Renal immunology, Basel, 1983, S. Karger AG.

McCarty, G.A., Valencia, D.W., and Fritzler, M.J.: Antinuclear antibodies, Fairlawn, New Jersey, 1984, Oxford University Press.

Neale, T.J., and Wilson, C.B.: Glomerular antigens in glomerulonephritis, Springer Semin. Immunopathol. **5:**221, 1982.

O'Connor, G.R., and Chandler, J.W.: editors: Advances in immunology and immunopathology of the eye, New York, 1985, Masson Publishing USA, Inc.

Rose, N.R., and Mackay, I.R., editors: The autoimmune diseases, Orlando, 1985, Academic Press, Inc.

Rossini, A.A., Mordes, J.P., and Like, A.A.: Immunology of insulin-dependent diabetes mellitus, Ann. Rev. Immunol. **3:**289, 1985.

Scheinberg, L., and Raine, C.S., editors: Multiple sclerosis: experimental and clinical aspects, Ann. N.Y. Acad. Sci. **436:**1, 1984.

Senitzer, D.: Autoimmune mechanisms in the pathogenesis of rheumatic fever, Rev. Infect. Dis. **6:**832, 1984.

Seybold, M.E., and Lindstrom, J.M.: Immunopathology of acetylcholine receptors in myasthenia gravis, Springer Semin. Immunopathol. **5:**389, 1982.

Shapira, E., and Wilson, G.B., editors: Immunological aspects of cystic fibrosis, Boca Raton, Florida, 1984, CRC Press, Inc.

Smith, H.R., and Steinberg, A.D.: Autoimmunity—a perspective, Ann. Rev. Immunol. **1:**175, 1983.

Steck, A.J., and Lisak, R.P., editors: Immunoneurology, Springer Semin. Immunopathol. **8:**parts I, II and III, 1985.

Stollar, B.D.: Antibodies to DNA, CRC Crit. Rev. Biochem. **20:**1, 1986.

Strakosck, C.R., and others: Immunology of autoimmune thyroid diseases, New Eng. J. Med. **307:**1499, 1982.

Tan, E.M.: Autoantibodies to nuclear antigens (ANA): their immunobiology and medicine, Adv. Immunol. **33:**167, 1982.

Theofilopoulos, A.N., and Dixon, F.J.: Murine models of systemic lupus erythematosus, Adv. Immunol. **37:**269, 1985.

Tsokos, G.C., and Balow, J.E.: Cellular immune responses in systemic lupus erythematosus, Prog. Allergy **35:**93, 1984.

Volpé, R., editor: Autoimmunity and endocrine disease, New York, 1985, Marcel Dekker, Inc.

Walfish, P., Wall, J., and Volpé, R., editors: Autoimmunity and the thyroid, Orlando, 1985, Academic Press, Inc.

Zabriskie, J.B., Fillit, H., Villarreal, H., Jr., and Becker, E.L., editors: Clinical immunology of the kidney, New York, 1982, John Wiley & Sons, Inc.

Immunodeficiency

≡ GLOSSARY

acquired immune deficiency syndrome (AIDS) A loss of immune competence due to the destruction of T_H cells by the HIV virus.

ADA Adenosine deaminase.

agammaglobulinemia A condition in which all the immunoglobulins are absent from the serum.

ataxia telangiectasia A loss of muscle coordination accompanied by blood vessel dilation combined with deficits in IgA production and T lymphocytes.

Bruton's agammaglobulinemia A sex-linked congenital loss of B cells and hence immunoglobulins.

Chédiak-Higashi disease (CDH) A disease based on faulty phagocytic destruction of parasites, related to lysosomal abnormalities.

chronic granulomatous disease (CGD) A sex-linked hereditary disease resulting in faulty phagocytic destruction of ingested parasites.

chronic mucocutaneous candidiasis A T cell deficiency disease resulting in a chronic *Candida* infection.

DiGeorge's syndrome A birth defect in the embryonic development of the thymus, resulting in losses of immune competence related to T lymphocytes.

dysgammaglobulinemia An imbalance from the normal concentration of the immunoglobulins or a malfunction of one or more immunoglobulins.

H chain disease A disease in which incomplete immunoglobulins consisting of H chains, or parts thereof, are synthesized.

hypogammaglobulinemia The opposite of hypergammaglobulinemia, or decreased levels of γ-globulin in plasma.

neonatal hypogammaglobulinemia A transient hypogammaglobulinemia affecting all newborn infants.

nitroblue tetrazolium (NBT) A dye used in a reductase test to measure the oxidative activity of phagocytes.

Nezelof's syndrome A genetic failure of T lymphocyte development and hence cell-mediated hypersensitivity.

PNP Purine nucleoside phosphorylase.

severe combined immunodeficiency disease (SCID) Immunodeficiency of both T and B cells.

Swiss-type agammaglobulinemia A genetic disease resulting in deficiencies in both T and B lymphocyte functions.

Wiskott-Aldrich syndrome A sex-linked genetic disease with combined losses of B and T lymphocytes and especially of IgM production.

■　　　　　　　　■　　　　　　　　■

Resistance to infectious disease is the expression of the body's ability, through its natural and acquired defense forces, to cope with internal and external antigenic threats to its well-being. Just as cuts and scratches of the skin can create a breach in the natural defense system and open the body to infection, so also can fissures in other parts of the defense system—phagocytosis, immunoglobulin synthesis, T cell activities, and the complement system—render the body susceptible to otherwise easily repelled organisms (Fig. 20-1). Immunodeficiencies may arise from a genetic inability to produce a required cell or cell product (primary immunodeficiency), or they may be acquired.

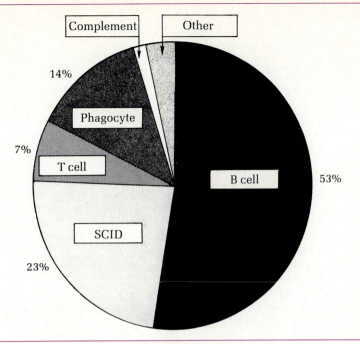

FIG. 20-1

This pie diagram illustrates that pure B cell deficiencies represent 53% of the human immunodeficiencies, T cells only 7%, SCIDs 23%, and phagocytic deficiencies 14%. Complement and undeciphered deficiencies represent less than 3%.

PREDOMINANTLY IMMUNOGLOBULIN DEFICIENCIES

Any interruption in B cell differentiation and maturation from the level of the stem cells in the bone marrow to the mature functioning plasma cells of peripherally situated lymphoid tissues will affect immunoglobulin synthesis. The earlier the rupture in the developmental pathway, the more extensive the loss in antibody-forming capacity. Although breaks in the maturation chain of the B lymphocytes clearly lead to immunoglobulin deficiencies, there is increasing evidence that T cells have a far broader regulatory role on the activities of B cells than previously suspected. Obviously losses of T_H or T_{CS} lymphocytes or a hyperactivity of T_S lymphocytes also could result in impaired immunoglobulin levels.

Although the term *agammaglobulinemia* is well entrenched in the immunologic literature, traces of γ-globulin, perhaps only 5 to 500 μg/ml, can be found in sera of agammaglobulinemic patients. Thus *hypogammaglobulinemia* is a more exact term, but the two are used interchangeably here (Table 20-1).

Diagnosis

Assessment of B lymphocyte functioning is based on the past and present ability of the patient to produce immunoglobulins. Preexisting B cell functions are evaluated on the basis of the current serum immunoglobulin concentration by radial immunodiffusion tests for IgG, IgM, and IgA. Ordinary serum immunoelectrophoresis may be performed first as a screening method, but ultimately the individual globulins must be quantitated. A history of successful immunization against toxoids such as those from tetanus and diphtheria or of bacterial vaccines such as pertussis (but not BCG for tuberculosis) signifies a satisfactory B cell system. Antibody titers should be determined by specific serologic tests. In the absence

TABLE 20-1

Predominantly immunoglobulin deficiencies

Name	Immunoglobulin status	Etiology	Inheritance	Comment
Transient hypogamma-globulinemia of infancy	Low IgG and IgA	Delayed T_H cell maturation	Uncertain	—
Sex-linked agamma-globulinemia (Bruton's disease)	All isotypes markedly decreased	Failure of pre-B cells to differentiate and mature	Sex-linked	B cells absent
Autosomal recessive agammaglobulinemia	All isotypes markedly decreased	Uncertain	Autosomal recessive	—
Common variable immunodeficiency	Various isotype combinations decreased	Defective B cell switch, excess T_S function	Varies	B and T cell numbers often normal
IgA deficiency	IgA1 and IgA2 decreased	Defect in B cell differentiation	Uncertain	Normal B cell numbers, SC produced
Hyper IgM syndrome	Elevated IgM and IgD, other isotypes decreased	Failure in isotype switch mechanism	Varies	—

of an immunization record, past humoral immunity can be judged on the basis of normal levels of the anti-A or anti-B blood group hemagglutinins or antibodies to common bacteria or their products. *Escherichia coli* and streptolysin O are useful antigens in these tests.

The current status of the humoral immune system can be evaluated by the response to antigens not likely to be encountered in ordinary life. For this the rare bacteriophage ΦX174, bacterial flagellin, keyhole-limpet hemocyanin, or other antigens are used. Concurrent B cell evaluation should include an enumeration of circulating B cells, accomplished by identifying Fc receptors on lymphocytes or the presence of surface immunoglobulins by immunofluorescence. B cells also should be purified from the peripheral blood and examined for their capacity to respond to mitogens. PWM is one of the best activators of these cells, but PHA or other lectins can be selected.

Transient hypogammaglobulinemia of infancy

Transient hypogammaglobulinemia of the newborn infant is the culmination of the infant's inability to synthesize significant amounts of immunoglobulin until he or she has been challenged with antigen and the inability of IgA and IgM to pass the placental barrier from mother to fetus. The total amount of γ-globulin in the serum of the newborn infant is 1044 ± 201 mg/dl, or approximately two thirds the normal adult level of 1457 ± 353 mg/dl (Fig. 20-2). Since maternal IgG can pass the placenta, the IgG level in newborn sera (1031 ± 200 mg/dl of serum) compares favorably with the adult level of 1158 ± 305 mg/dl. Neonatal levels of IgM and IgA average 11% and 1%, respectively, of the adult levels of 99 ± 27 mg/dl and 200 ± 61 mg/dl. IgD is difficult to detect in the sera of newborn infants, and IgE is found at approximately 15% of the adult level of 225 μg/ml.

After birth the infant's IgG level falls steadily for approximately 3 months. Between 3 and 6 months of age, when IgG is at its low ebb (300 to 600 mg/dl), the infant displays the greatest sensitivity to infectious disease. After the third month of life the IgG level usually increases steadily so that about 75% of the adult level is achieved by 3 years of age. IgM is synthesized earlier in infancy than IgG and increases in concentration so rapidly after birth that 50% of the adult level is reached within the first 6 months. In

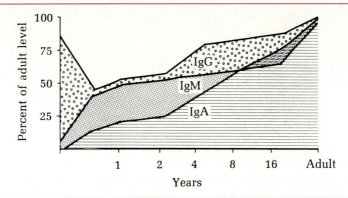

FIG. 20-2

Ontogeny of immunoglobulin formation in the human. IgG acquired by the infant transplacentally from the mother falls quickly in titer during the time that IgA and especially IgM levels are climbing. After 6 months all three immunoglobulins increase gradually toward the adult level.

some infants the IgG and IgA levels remain low for an additional several weeks, possibly due to a delay in T_H cell maturation. IgA does not achieve 50% of the adult level until the child is 1 year of age. At 5 years of age the IgD level is still one third that of adults, and the IgE level reaches approximately two thirds that of adults.

Congenital agammaglobulinemia

Congenital or genetic hypogammaglobulinemia results from a permanent inability to synthesize γ-globulins. The afflicted children suffer from repeated bouts of bacterial disease, often caused by feeble pathogens. If no accompanying disorder of the T cell system is involved, hypogammaglobulinemic children will contract and recover normally from the usual viral and fungal diseases of childhood. In the preantibiotic era these children died of bacterial septicemia before it could be recognized that they were hypogammaglobulinemic. In the 1950s the development and use of broad-spectrum antibiotics kept these children alive long enough for their congenital condition to be diagnosed. Now antibiotics and passive immunization with pooled human γ-globulin allow these individuals to lead a relatively normal life.

Sex-linked agammaglobulinemia (Bruton's disease)

A WHO committee has recommended that "sex-linked agammaglobulinemia" be used as the official

name of the disease commonly known as Bruton's agammaglobulinemia or Bruton's sex-linked agammaglobulinemia. As the new name indicates, this is a disease transmitted by the mother to her male children only. The disease does not become apparent until about 6 months of age, at which time the immunity the child derived from maternal IgG has waned. These young boys then begin what will invariably develop into a series of bacterial infections involving the usual pathogens of childhood, *Hemophilus, Streptococcus, Staphylococcus, Pseudomonas,* and other less pathogenic gram-negative bacilli. These primary bacterial infections do not result in immunity and the synthesis of immunoglobulins; instead they signal that recurrences of otitis media, conjunctivitis, pneumonia, meningitis, pyoderma, and septicemia will follow. The γ-globulin concentration in these children may fall below 25 mg/dl of serum. All classes of immunoglobulins are absent or extremely low. Lymphocyte counts in peripheral blood are within the normal range, but these are T cells, not B cells.

These children respond normally to most viral diseases of childhood (for example, measles, mumps, and chickenpox) and develop a lasting immunity. Their response to chemicals that provoke contact dermatitis is normal, also indicating that their T cell system is functioning suitably. Even after intensive stimulation with antigens, plasma cells rarely are found in lymphoid tissues. All the evidence suggests that infantile sex-linked agammaglobulinemia is a total incapacity to synthesize immunoglobulins concurrent with a normal T cell responsiveness. Since all the immunoglobulin classes are involved in the deficiency, the cellular fault occurs early. Immature B cells are unable to differentiate and thus none of the immunoglobulins can be produced. An autosomally inherited form of this disease has also been recognized (Table 20-1).

A murine analog of human sex-linked agammaglobulinemia was identified in the CBA/N (originally CBA/HN) mouse strain in 1972. Both male and female CBA/N adults are unresponsive or only feebly responsive to TI-2 antigens. F1 males resulting from matings of CBA/N females with mice of responsive strains were immunocompromised, whereas F1 females were not. This characteristic signalled a sex-linked deficiency, termed *xid*. This *xid* character has also been noted in the MLR and BXSB mouse lines.

Common variable hypogammaglobulinemia

Far more common than generalized hypogammaglobulinemia is selective or variable hypogammaglobulinemia, in which only one or a combination of immunoglobulins is missing or present in much lower than normal concentrations (Table 20-1). This condition also is known as dysgammaglobulinemia. Individuals with selective hypogammaglobulinemia cannot always be identified by a decrease in total γ-globulin levels, since a decrease in one class of immunoglobulin may be compensated by a disproportionate hypergammaglobulinemia of another class of immunoglobulin. For example, several patients deficient in IgG and IgA have been described, but they had sufficiently increased IgM levels to have a normal total γ-globulin level. Diagnosis of selective immunoglobulinemia is best made by quantitative radial immunodiffusion analysis for the separate immunoglobulin classes, although a first clue to the diagnosis is often an abnormal immunoelectrophoretic serum profile. An increased incidence of infectious diseases is an unreliable diagnostic criterion, since single deficiencies, except when IgG is the deficient immunoglobulin, do not always lead to an increased incidence of infectious disease. Patients with dys-

gammaglobulinemia often display a malabsorption syndrome with a noninfectious diarrhea of variable severity. When IgG is involved, its level is usually low, often less than 500 mg/dl, but not as low as in sex-linked agammaglobulinemia. IgG levels greater than 250 mg/dl are usually adequate for protection against most bacterial infections.

IgA deficiency

Virtually all mathematically possible forms of dysgammaglobulinemia have been detected, that is, those in which only one of the immunoglobulins is missing and all the possible combinations in which two, three, or more are missing. Of the selective hypogammaglobulinemias, the most frequently recognized is that involving a familial loss of IgA. The incidence of single IgA dysgammaglobulinemia was found to be 1 in 450 in a recent study of 28,000 persons. The criterion for IgA deficiency was less than 1 mg/dl of serum. Both serum and secretory IgA are diminished or absent, although SC is produced. There is frequently a corresponding increase in IgM. Patients with an isolated IgA loss commonly seek medical assistance because of the associated autoimmune disease. The diseases involved include rheumatoid arthritis, LE, and thyroiditis. IgA losses also are associated with sinopulmonary disease, a feature of the deficiency which indicates that secretory IgA is important in protecting mucous membranes. A noninfectious diarrhea is also a common feature of IgA deficiency.

Recent evidence indicates that patients with common variable immunodeficiency have normal or near normal numbers of B lymphocytes, but these cells are unable to mature to plasma cells. The origin of the condition is found in the T cell compartment, in which there is an excessive number of Ts cells or an exaggerated activity of these cells. Cocultivation of B cells from persons who form normal amounts of the immunoglobulins with T cells from the immunodeficient person results in a failure of the normal cells to produce the expected immunoglobulins. This experiment clearly indicates that the immunologic fault resides in the patient's T cell population.

As was expected, a case of genetic inability to form SC eventually was discovered. The conse-

≡ SITUATION 1

SELECTIVE IgA DEFICIENCY

Karen, a 3-year-old girl, was referred to a regional hospital by her local physician in a small farming community because of recurrent respiratory tract infections. On admission she weighed 29 pounds, appeared thin and pale, had a temperature of 37.5° C, had a reddened throat, and had small white foci on her tonsils. The child's history indicated that she had had recurrent tonsillitis since 1½ years of age. Rarely were any significant pathogens isolated, but on one occasion *Streptococcus pyogenes* group A was recovered. Her present white blood cell count was moderately elevated, with a shift to the left. Throat cultures were taken, and blood was drawn for serum electrophoretic analysis.

Questions

1. Why is this child not considered to have agammaglobulinemia?
2. What is the status of secretory IgA in the serum IgA-deficient person?
3. What diseases are associated with IgA dysgammaglobulinemia?
4. Is IgA antigenic for the patient with IgA dysgammaglobulinemia?

Solution

It is the general experience that, even though many IgA-deficient individuals are asymptomatic, recurrent infections are also common. Recognized infectious diseases include tonsillitis, otitis media, febrile disease with cough, nasal discharge, and other upper respiratory tract diseases not further identified. In older children and adults asthmatic episodes are triggered by these infections, which suggests an allergic disposition toward the pathogens. This is not the case in hereditary telangiectasia, where an IgE deficiency accompanies the IgA loss. Since this child had not had a life-threatening illness in the first years of her life, combined immunodeficiency disease was not considered. Because the child was female, Bruton's agammaglobulinemia was discounted.

Individuals deficient in serum IgA are likewise deficient in secretory IgA. Since the patient with IgA dysgammaglobulinemia has never experienced any self-contact with IgA, it is recognized as a foreign antigen. The immune response to external IgA in plasma or blood transfusions could result in anaphylaxis if a prior exposure induced sufficient antibody formation.

---

quence of this is an inability to form secretory IgA (and IgM). Heretofore all examples of IgA insufficiency involved both serum and secretory IgA, since the plasma cell was the absentee. Now, in SC deficiency, a required epithelial cell is missing, and a more restricted loss of only secretory IgA is the result.

Hyper IgM syndrome

Another form of common variable immunodeficiency that has been recognized on enough occasions to give it a special designation is the syndrome in which IgM and IgD serum levels are increased, but the level of other immunoglobulin isotypes is decreased. Since IgM and IgD synthesis are the features of the immature B cell, the hyper IgM syndrome reflects a failure of B cells to effect the isotype switch.

SEVERE COMBINED IMMUNODEFICIENCY DISEASES (SCID)
Diagnosis

The diagnosis of severe combined immunodeficiency diseases (SCID) relies on the recognition of both B and T cell failures. SCIDs are those in which there is a decided loss in both B and T lymphocyte functions. As a consequence of this superimposed loss of humoral and cellular immunity, survival beyond infancy until recently was rare. Persons with combined immunodeficiency diseases have an extraordinarily high incidence of infectious disease and malignancy associated with an abbreviated life expectancy.

It is recognized now that there are many variants of this condition (Table 20-2). In some only a partial loss of T cell functions can be identified; in others the loss appears almost total. Specific enzyme abnor-

TABLE 20-2

Severe combined immunodeficiencies

Name	Immunoglobulin status	T cell status	Etiology	Comment
Severe combined immunodeficiency (SCID)	Decreased	Decreased	Maturation defect of B and T cells	Many variations; some sex-linked, others autosomal, DiGeorge syndrome has embryogenic etiology
Adenosine deaminase (ADA) deficiency	Progressive loss	Decreased	Toxic metabolites due to enzyme deficiency	Passive therapy with whole blood or erythrocyte transfusion
Purine nucleotide phosphorylase (PNP) deficiency	Progressive loss	Decreased	Toxic metabolites due to enzyme deficiency	Passive therapy with whole blood or erythrocyte transfusion
Acquired immunodeficiency syndrome (AIDS)	Progressive loss	Progressive loss	HIV	Incidence higher in homosexual males and drug addicts

malities may or may not be identified. Similar inconsistencies may be observed in the immunoglobulin patterns.

A history of an effective cell-mediated arm of the immune system is judged by conducting skin tests with agents that provoke traditional delayed hypersensitive skin reactions in the majority of normal adults. Mumps vaccine, PPD or OT, trichophytin, candidin, or streptokinase-streptodornase can be used for this purpose. In certain geographic areas histoplasmin and coccidioidin were useful in the past. A history of a normal recovery from viral infections or BCG immunization is also helpful. Since smallpox vaccination is no longer required in the United States, this monitor cannot be used much longer, and a history of successful BCG vaccination is probably most applicable to foreign-born patients.

The contemporary status of T cells can be evaluated on the basis of T cell enumeration by the sheep erythrocyte rosette method and by the in vitro transformation of T cells exposed to Con A or in MLC. The latter is the more important of the two, since it reflects the functional capacity of the cells. The ability of a person to become dermally sensitized by a single exposure to 0.05 ml of 30% dinitrochlorobenzene should be determined. This will evoke a contact dermatitis in greater than 95% of T cell–sufficient

persons. This is determined by the dermal application of 0.05 ml of a 0.1% solution of the chemical 14 days after the sensitizing exposure. Special enzyme studies for adenosine deaminase (ADA) or nucleoside phosphorylase also are useful diagnostic criteria.

Sex-linked agammaglobulinemia

Sex-linked agammaglobulinemia, in which there is a defect in cellular immune mechanisms associated with agammaglobulinemia, must not be confused with infantile sex-linked agammaglobulinemia of the Bruton type, in which no generalized loss of cellular immunity has ever been noted.

Losses in cellular immunity may not be absolute, but the thymus is small, weighing only about 1 g as compared with an expected weight of 4 g for the normal infant. The combination of B cell and T cell losses results in a life expectancy of only 2 years. The condition is seen only in boys and is inherited as a recessive characteristic.

Swiss-type agammaglobulinemia

A second disease embodying losses in both cellular and humoral immunity is Swiss-type agammaglobulinemia. Several dozen cases have been reported since the original description of this disease in 1950 by Glanzmann and Riniker, two Swiss pediatricians. The afflicted children, either boys or girls, since this disease is transmitted as an autosomal recessive disease, are vulnerable to severe diarrhea and severe pyogenic infections caused by the usual bacterial pathogens of childhood. More reflective of their severe immunologic handicap is the inability of these children to resist even feeble pathogens such as *E. coli, Pseudomonas aeruginosa,* and *Pneumocystis carinii.* Childhood viral and fungal diseases—measles, chickenpox, smallpox vaccination, and *Candida* infections—all can be fatal or, contribute to fatality.

Autopsied tissues do not reveal plasma cells or germinal centers, and little, if any, immunoglobulin is present in the blood. The thymus exists as an epithelial structure without lymphoid elements. This is the key to the inability of these patients to resist viral or fungal pathogens or to respond to other T cell stimuli such as the contact sensitizers dinitrochlorobenzene and dinitrofluorobenzene.

Nezelof's syndrome

Infants with Nezelof's syndrome are athymic by virtue of an autosomal recessive trait whose inheritance prevents normal lymphoid development of the gland. Since the connective tissue of the gland is reasonably intact, the defect does not reside in embryogenesis of the thymus gland per se from the third and fourth pharyngeal pouches but in its fulfillment as a lymphoid organ. Consequently the block in cellular development resides in or near the stem cell level and its inability to generate the lymphocytes destined to become T cells. Children with Nezelof's syndrome generate typical germinal centers in the far cortical, or B cell, regions of their lymph nodes, produce plasma cells, and have a reasonably normal immunoglobulin response. However, the lymphoid development of the paracortical and medullary regions of lymph nodes, the T cell regions, is markedly restricted. This is demonstrated early in infancy by the development of infectious diseases that are resisted primarily by a suitable T cell activity: *Candida albicans* infections and those by other yeasts or fungi and severe, even fatal, chickenpox or a fatal outcome from smallpox vaccination. Respira-

tory disease caused by the feebly pathogenic *Pneumocystis carinii* and by bacteria also is prominent. A high incidence of malignancy also is noted in these unfortunate children.

DiGeorge's syndrome

DiGeorge's syndrome is the result of an accidental failure in embryogenesis of the third and fourth branchial pouches and is not a familial, inherited disease like Nezelof's syndrome. In the DiGeorge form of congenital thymic hypoplasia, abnormalities of the aortic arch, the mandible, the ear, and the parathyroid may accompany those of the thymic gland, since all these tissues have a common embryonic origin. Of these accessory deficits, that of the parathyroid gland is the most important from a diagnostic viewpoint. The parathyroid gland is the regulatory organ for blood calcium. During fetal life the level of this mineral in fetal blood is regulated in part by the maternal parathyroid hormone. After birth, when this is no longer possible, the infant progresses toward a condition of hypocalcemia that is soon expressed as an involuntary rigid muscular contraction (tetany). Restoration of the blood calcium level by calcium or parathyroid hormone relieves this condition but of course can do nothing to restore thymic functioning. DiGeorge's syndrome is not a genetic disease; its cause is unknown. It may arise from an intrauterine infection. Presumably this infection would occur before the fourteenth week of gestation, when the development of the involved tissues ordinarily begins.

SCID with abnormal purine enzymes

Until 1983, less than 40 examples of combined immunodeficiency with abnormal purine enzymes had been described. Persons with this condition fall into two major categories, those who are deficient in adenosine deaminase (ADA), or those who are deficient in purine nucleoside phosphorylase (PNP), with the former representing the greatest number of persons (Table 20-2).

Adenosine deaminase irreversibly deaminates adenosine to produce inosine. Purine nucleoside phosphorylase then cleaves inosine to produce hypoxanthine and ribose-1-phosphate (Fig. 20-3). ADA

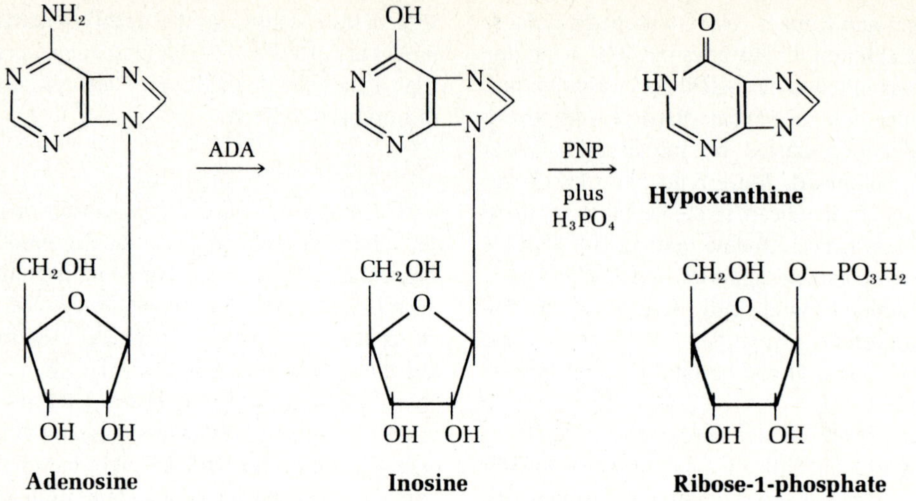

FIG. 20-3
The enzymes ADA and PNP are both present in healthy T cells.

also deaminates 2-deoxyadenosine which is cleaved by PNP to form hypoxanthine and deoxyribose-1-phosphate. Other substrates may be used by these enzymes; for example, PNP will also split quanine nucleotides. Both enzymes are thus part of the salvage pathway of purine metabolism in which preformed purines are recovered as such from nucleosides, rather than being replaced by de novo synthesis.

The immature T cell is normally low in ADA, but this increases 3 to 15 fold as the T cell matures. In SCID with ADA deficiency, this does not occur. SCID patients with ADA deficiency excrete large amounts of adenosine and 2-deoxyadenosine in their urine, plus derivatives of these compounds such as 2-O-methyladenosine. An enormous excess of deoxyadenosine triphosphate (deoxy ATP) is sequestered in lymphocytes.

Among the hypotheses to account for the immunodeficiency in these individuals, the inhibition of ribonucleotide reductase by the excessive deoxyATP is the most favored. Impairment of this enzyme would sharply reduce the availability of deoxynucleotides for normal DNA synthesis. Another possibility is tied to the accompanying increase in S-adenosylhomocystine, one of the adenosine derivatives produced in excess by these patients. Free homocystine normally contributes to methylation reactions, but cannot do so when conjugated with adenosine. These changes would prevent normal T cell maturation.

ADA is plentiful in erythrocytes, and blood transfusion to supply the needed enzyme is a successful therapeutic. Bone marrow transplantation provides a more permanent therapy.

Patients with PNP deficiency have lowered T cell numbers and the cells that are present respond poorly to T cell mitogens and allogenic tissue. The activity and number of B cells, may be normal. *In vivo,* the equilibrium of PNP strongly favors the formation of the free purine bases, and in the absence of this enzyme the nucleosides accumulate. Deoxyguanosine triphosphate is the major component that accumulates, and is thus suspected to be the most toxic to T cells.

Both ADA and PNP deficiency are inherited as autosomal recessive traits.

Acquired immunodeficiency syndrome (AIDS)

In 1981, AIDS was first recognized as a distinct disease in the United States. By January 1986, the Center for Disease Control reported that 16,458 cases had been diagnosed in the intervening 5 years. A WHO report indicated more than 3,000 cases had been diagnosed in Europe. AIDS is a remarkable disease in terms of its etiology and devastation of the immune system.

As early as 1977, a retrovirus was associated with a neoplastic transformation of T cells that resulted in adult T cell leukemia. This discovery made in Japan was confirmed in the U.S. in 1980. In 1982, hairy cell leukemia was associated with a second retrovirus. These agents have since been referred to as HTLV I and HTLV II (human T lymphocyte viruses I and II). In 1984, it was announced that a third retrovirus called HTLV III, and now known as HIV, in the United States and LAV or lymphadenopathy associated virus in France was the etiologic agent of AIDS. In AIDS, the lymphocytes are not transformed to a neoplastic state by the virus; they are destroyed.

HIV attacks $T4^+$ lymphocytes and since anti T4 will prevent virus infection of these cells, it appears that the T4 glycoprotein is the virus receptor. T4 positive cells of the brain also become infected by the AIDS virus, and cells of the monocyte-macrophage system, perhaps infected as the result of phagocytosis, will support HIV growth. Langerhans' and dendritic cells are also susceptible to infection as are some, but not all, EBV infected B cell lines.

Because of the critical role of T_H cells as the source of IL-2 needed for maximal stimulation of the other T cell subsets, loss of T_H cells due to the virus infection initiates a progressive loss in immune capacity. Only 10% of $T4^+$ cells are virus positive by immunofluorescence. This may reflect a low rate of virus production, virus latency or poor transmission of the agent. T cells with IL-2 receptors (the Tac antigen) are also diminished in number.

Homosexual males account for 75% of the AIDS cases, followed by intravenous drug users at 17%. Hatian immigrants to the United States account for 5% of our cases. Comparisons of heterosexual and HIV free homosexual males has not identified any significant difference in their immune status other than a slightly lower level of delayed type hypersensitivity in the latter and this may reflect an inability to detect the virus. Once the disease becomes active,

the T4/T8 ratio diminishes steadily from the 1.8 to 0.7 normal values, to lower values. The prospect of heterosexually acquired AIDS is based on the identification of AIDS antibodies in prostitutes.

Transmission of AIDS via blood transfusion is of major concern. Blood that is positive for AIDS antibody is not used for fear of the simultaneous presence of the virus. ELISA and a radio labeled antigen precipitation test can be used to detect AIDS virus antibodies. These tests are also being used to evaluate genetically engineered virus proteins as potential vaccines.

The relationship of simian retroviruses to HIV is important in our understanding of this virus and AIDS. The high incidence (59% of the prostitutes in Zaire are seropositive) of AIDS in Central Africa is of special interest to those interested in the possible origin and heterosexual transmission of AIDS.

Specific T cell deficiency

There appear to be a few situations in which a clone of T cells with a single antigen specificity are nonfunctional. The first of these to be recognized was cutaneous mucocutaneous candidiasis, a disease of early childhood. Most of the other examples are also associated with infectious diseases, but are more often seen in adults. Leprosy is an example of this group in which it is difficult to determine if the infection itself has rendered the T cells anergic, or whether there is a more complex etiology.

Chronic mucocutaneous candidiasis

Several conditions are known that involve only a partial T cell loss. One of the first infectious diseases recognized to have an attendant defect in the T cell system was chronic mucocutaneous candidiasis. The etiologic agent of this disease, a yeast, is a relatively feeble pathogen and a common part of the normal flora of the birth canal. As a consequence, neonates not infrequently develop mild infections with this yeast. Candidiasis (also known as moniliasis) also can be seen as an extensive and severe disease in persons with a thymus defect. Patients with chronic mucocutaneous candidiasis exhibit extensive destruction of the nail beds and persistent infections of the mucous membranes and the skin. The normal features of the skin may be almost totally obliterated by the serous exudate, crust, and granuloma formation of the affected regions. Patients with this disease do not respond to dermal injections of *Candida* organisms, and in vitro tests of lymphocytes from these patients reveal their inability to produce lymphokines. The cellular defect probably is not identical in all these patients; some may have a generalized T cell defect and others a specific *Candida* organism–related defect. Efforts to treat chronic mucocutaneous candidiasis with TF were at first heralded to give permanent cures but this claim has proven to be exaggerated. Nevertheless, repeated treatments with TF have provided significant improvements in the patient's condition, improvements that could not be accomplished with antibiotic treatment.

Leprosy

The cause of leprosy clearly is established as *Mycobacterium leprae,* and the disease is divided into two easily recognized clinical forms: lepromatous and tuberculoid leprosy. In the former the disease is progressive; the bacterial population is high and increases steadily with an associated increase in the necrotic destruction of tissue, and when untreated, it offers a bleak prognosis. On the other hand, tuberculoid leprosy has a better prognosis; there is less tissue destruction and a lower bacillary load. Diagnostic skin testing of persons with leprosy using lepromin, an extract of human tissue containing *M. leprae,* has revealed that those with the tuberculoid form of the disease give the typical delayed skin reactions, whereas those with lepromatous leprosy are often unreactive to lepromin. Since bacteriologic and histologic evidence can confirm that both types of patients have leprosy, the unresponsiveness of those with the lepromatous disease requires an explanation.

This explanation recently has been discovered. Patients with lepromatous leprosy have depleted paracortical and medullary regions in their lymph nodes; their lymphocytes are unresponsive to mitogens such as PHA or *M. leprae* antigens in vitro and fail to produce lymphokines in culture. The T cell population in the peripheral circulation of persons with lepromatous leprosy (but not those with tuber-

culoid leprosy) is depressed. The degree of this T cell loss is correlated directly with the bacillary load. It is tempting to conclude that the bacteria or products of the leprosy bacillus specifically destroy the T cells which might protect the patient against the disease, but more experimentation is needed before this can be proved. It is interesting that patients with lepromatous leprosy have about twice the B cell population of those with the tuberculoid disease, but since immunoglobulins contribute so little to protection and recovery from leprosy, this is of little benefit to them.

IMMUNODEFICIENCY WITH OTHER DEFECTS

Several immunodeficiency diseases, of which the DiGeorge syndrome has already been mentioned, have other striking symptoms, in addition to an increase in infectious disease, as part of their illness. In ataxia telangiectasia, this has been identified as a loss of DNA repair enzymes and in transcobalamin deficiency, anemia is a significant part of the disease (Table 20-3).

Wiskott-Aldrich syndrome

The Wiskott-Aldrich syndrome is a sex-linked recessive disease whose victims suffer innumerable bacterial, viral, fungal, and protozoan infections as a result of their failure to generate a typical immunoglobulin or T cell response. In terms of the immunoglobulin aspects of their disease it has been noted that the total immunoglobulin level may be normal. This is because of elevated IgA and depressed IgM levels in the presence of an essentially normal or elevated level of IgG. The restriction of the immunoglobulin loss to IgM suggests that the B cell deficit is related primarily to polysaccharide antigens. The true locus of the defect may not be in the lymphocyte cell system at all but in the macrophages that process the polysaccharide antigens for the B cells. Further studies are needed to confirm the site of the metabolic error, but it is well known that patients with Wiskott-Aldrich syndrome respond poorly to *Salmonella* vaccines and have only low levels of hemagglutinins for red blood cells, both of which depend on polysaccharide antigens. The location of the

TABLE 20-3

Immunodeficiencies with other defects

Name	Immunoglobulin status	T cell status	Etiology	Comment
Ataxia telangiectasia	Often decreased IgG, IgA and IgE	Decreased	Defect in T cell maturation and DNA repair enzymes	B cells often normal
Wiskott-Aldrich syndrome	Decreased IgM	Progressive loss	Uncertain	Accompanied by platelet defects
DiGeorge syndrome	Often decreased	Decreased	Embryonic failure to complete 3rd and 4th pharyngeal arch	Hypoparathyroidism
Transcobalamin 2 deficiency	All isotypes decreased	Normal	Vitamin B_{12} transport defect	Anemia

defect in the T cell system is also obscure. The thymus itself is relatively normal; only peripheral lymphoid organs demonstrate losses in T cells. This appears to be a progressive condition associated with thrombocytopenia and eczema.

Ataxia telangiectasia

Ataxia telangiectasia is described as a disorder in which a progressive loss of muscle coordination (ataxia) is associated with a dilation of small blood vessels (telangiectasia), most notable in conjunctivae but also seen in the skin. It is transmitted as an autosomal recessive disease with an estimated incidence of 1.5 in 100,000 persons. There is a deficiency of both humoral and cellular immunity in homozygotes, which also can be demonstrated in heterozygotes. Most patients display an increased susceptibility to sinopulmonary infections and malignancy.

The cellular immune deficit is indicated by the finding that a third of the patients have lymphopenia. Virtually all patients have an aplastic or hypoplastic thymus with an unfulfilled T cell population. Repeated or serious viral infections are not as significant in patients with ataxia telangiectasia as in others with abnormal thymus development. Low-reactive skin tests or an absence of positive skin tests to normal antigens of fungal or mycotic origin is typical. It also has been difficult to sensitize these patients to dinitrochlorobenzene; 10 of 21 resisted sensitization in one study, and 12 of 16 did so in another. The re-

markable sensitivity of patients with ataxia telangiectasia to x-rays, and their 10% incidence of malignancy, prompted a biochemical study that identified a failure of DNA repair enzymes as the major fault in this disease. This is clearly related to T cell growth and differentiation.

In terms of the patient's humoral status the IgG levels are normal or exceed the normal as a result of repeated infections. IgE levels are depressed in 65% of the patients, but this is unrelated to the heightened incidence of upper respiratory tract infection. This is more certainly caused by loss of IgA, which is total or very nearly so in about 90% of the patients, and the presence of the abnormal 7S variety of IgM in about 78% of the patients. The low IgA levels may not reflect a loss of IgA lymphocytes but may be the result of faulty T cell–B cell interaction, since thymectomized laboratory animals also lose their serum IgA.

Transcobalamine deficiency

An inheritable deficiency in the synthesis of transcobalamine II is expressed as a combination of several hematopoietic defects—anemia, thrombocytopenia, and leukopenia. With this disease, there is also a decrease in the concentration of all immunoglobulin isotypes. Since there appears to be no alteration in T cell numbers or function, the immunoglobulin loss must be attributed directly to alterations in B cell activity.

Transcobalamine II is the blood transport protein for vitamin B_{12} (cobalamine). This vitamin-protein complex is endocytosed and degraded by intracellular enzymes to release B_{12}. Methylation of cobalamine allows it to participate in the conversion of homocysteine to methionine. Adenosylation allows the vitamin to contribute to the formation of succinyl coenzyme A. The loss of these activities in B cells due to the lack of transcobalamine has not yet been directly linked biochemically to the failure of these cells to synthesize normal amounts of the immunoglobulins.

DEFICIENCIES OF THE PHAGOCYTIC SYSTEM

Deficiencies of the phagocytic system can result from several causes, among which those of congenital origin are perhaps the best understood (Table 20-4). Idiopathic, acquired conditions also may influence the behavior of phagocytes. Since the half-life of neutrophils in the blood may be as short as 6 hours and that of the monocytes only 1 to 2 days, the susceptibility of this cell population to transient damage is magnified. Many conditions ranging from the use of chemotherapeutic agents, the presence of kidney disease or cancer, autoimmune disease, and even infections themselves may produce a neutropenia. Cyclic neutropenia of all blood elements occurs in some individuals as the result of an inherited autosomal condition.

TABLE 20-4

Deficiencies in the phagocytic system

Condition	Characteristic
Chronic granulomatous disease (CGD)	Failure to form toxic forms of oxygen
G6PD deficiency	Failure of phagocyte to oxidize via shunt
Myeloperoxidase deficiency	Failure to use H_2O_2
Chédiak-Higashi disease (CHD)	Failure to release myeloperoxidase
Actin dysfunction	Granulocytes have reduced locomotion

Diagnosis

The evaluation of phagocytic cell defects is made from the clinical history and by in vitro tests to determine the oxidative and cell-killing capacity of the patient's white blood cells. The nitroblue tetrazolium (NBT) reductase test may be used but is not as popular as it once was. Intraphagocytic killing methods are not available in the usual clinical immunology laboratory. Reliance often must be placed on research scientists for a definite diagnosis of a phagocytic defect.

Chronic granulomatous disease (CGD)

Chronic granulomatous disease (CGD) is a sex-linked disease of male infants that usually is recognized within the first few months of life. A second, less severe form of the disease is found in girls and probably is transmitted as an autosomal recessive trait. Differences in the exact nature of CGD in different patients also are reflected in their biochemistry. An inconsistency in the levels of G6PD from patient to patient is one example of this. Immunologic examination of infants with CGD has confirmed that they have a normal or even elevated immunoglobulin level, that they respond normally to vaccines, and that they have normal B and T lymphocyte functions and complement levels. Nevertheless victims of CGD develop a series of infections early in infancy caused by bacterial pathogens such as *Klebsiella* species, *Proteus vulgaris, Staphylococcus epidermidis, E. coli, Enterobacter aerogenes, Serratia marcescens*, and the more virulent *Staphylococcus aureus*. Feebly virulent yeasts and fungi such as *Candida albicans* and *Aspergillus* species also may be involved in infections that are far more serious in these children than in the usual child. Surprisingly the pathogenic bacteria that cause the most serious diseases of childhood—*Neisseria meningitidis, Hemophilus influenzae, Streptococcus pyogenes,* and *Streptococcus (Diplococcus) pneumoniae*—are combated effectively.

As a result of these repeated infections, CGD patients typically have elevated immunoglobulin levels. Leukocytosis and granulomatous lymphadenitis are also hallmarks of the disease. Tissue biopsies will reveal granuloma formation in virtually every organ. Granulomas typically include tissue macro-

≡ SITUATION 2

LEUKOCYTE FUNCTION—CGD

Mark, a 3-year-old boy, entered the hospital for the sixth time in the past 2½ years. His admission was for a fever of unknown origin. His white blood cell count was 18,500 per mm^3, of which 46% were PMNs. His temperature was 38.8° C, and the liver and spleen were enlarged. Blood cultures were taken and reported to be positive for *E. coli*. On previous hospitalizations for septicemia, boils, cervical lymphadenopathy, and pneumonia, bacterial cultures had been positive for *E. coli* and/or *Klebsiella* organisms and coagulase-positive staphylococci. A diagnosis of CGD was considered, and the following laboratory tests were ordered: total γ-globulin, NBT reductase test, and bactericidal killing test.

Questions

1. What is CGD, and what are the hallmarks of leukocyte function in this disease?
2. What is the importance of the three special laboratory procedures, and what are the normal values of these tests?
3. How is CGD treated?

Solution

CGD is typified by repeated, slow-healing infections caused by ordinarily feeble infectious organisms. The disease is seen only in young boys because of its sex-linked inheritance, although similar diseases are seen in girls. Granulomatous deposits in visceral organs, especially the lungs, facilitate radiologic diagnosis; however, deficits in neutrophil function with normal T and B lymphocyte functions are instrumental in confirming the diagnosis.

Patients with CGD, because of the high incidence of bacterial infections, have higher γ-globulin levels than normal, and this was seen in the case of Mark, who had a total γ-globulin level of 1,400 mg/dl. The presence of such high levels of immunoglobulins promotes phagocytosis of bacteria but does not necessarily accelerate the intraphagocytic death of the ingested bacteria. For this reason a bactericidal killing test is performed. The buffy coat of heparinized blood from the patient is adjusted to a suitable neutrophil cell count rather than to some specific dilution. Cell counts are necessary be-

cause of the fluctuation in granulocyte counts in such patients. Generally 10^6 white blood cells per milliliter and 10^6 bacteria per milliliter are attained in the final mixture, which is contained in a tissue culture fluid supplemented with normal serum to the extent of 10%. After incubation of the mixture at 37° C for 30 minutes and at 30-minute intervals thereafter penicillin and streptomycin are added to kill extracellular bacteria. (Penicillin-sensitive *Staphylococcus aureus* is used in the test.) The centrifuged pellet is subjected to total plate counts for surviving bacteria. The normal control uses white blood cells from a healthy subject.

Normal leukocytes kill staphylococci and most other bacteria rapidly, with a 1% viable remainder being typical after 2 hours of incubation. Patients with CGD may have as much as 95% bacterial survival in the same test, although 70% survival would be more typical. PMNs from Mark reduced the staphylococcal population from 10^6 to only 8 × 10^5. Examination of white blood cell smears revealed that adequate ingestion had occurred.

Because the bactericidal killing test is cumbersome and time consuming, the NBT reductase test may be used to evaluate neutrophil performance instead. The test is based on the knowledge that phagocytosis is accompanied by a burst in respiratory metabolism that can be detected by the ability of white blood cells to transfer hydrogen to the NBT dye. This reduces the dye and causes appearance of dark blue dye granules inside the neutrophils. Neutrophils from patients with CGD are genetically incapable of leaving their glycolytic energy-deriving system for the oxidative pathways associated with intraphagocytic killing. In the NBT reductase test latex spherules are used as the phagocytic subject for white blood cells incubated with NBT. About 50% of the neutrophils will have phagocytosed at least five latex beads and be positive. Patients with CGD have decidedly lower scores, as do some other restricted patient categories and neonates. Mark had a score of 5%, which was definitely below the normal and compatible with the diagnosis.

There is no suitable therapy for CGD other than treatment of the bacterial infections as they occur. For this reason the average life expectancy of such patients is only 10 years.

phages in various stages of digestion of bacterial cells, giant cells containing several nuclei, monocytes, and epithelioid cells. All parameters of the immune defense system function normally in these patients except for their intraphagocytic destruction of certain bacteria. Even the phagocytic cells of patients with CGD have normal chemotactic responses and are as active in engulfment as other phagocytes. Neutrophils of CGD patients kill engulfed bacteria at a reduced rate, and the recovery of 50% to 100% of ingested bacteria at a time when only 1% to 10% of bacteria can be recovered from normal leukocytes is typical (Fig. 20-4).

The biochemical lesion in neutrophils of CGD pa-

tients has been identified as a failure to accumulate H_2O_2 during phagocytosis and is based on an inability of the NADPH oxidase to function normally. Prior to phagocytosis these cells use anaerobic glycolysis as their source of energy. During and after phagocytosis normal neutrophils demonstrate a burst in respiratory activity as they shift to the HMP shunt as their energy source. Use of the HMP pathway typically results in the formation of H_2O_2 as hydrogen is transferred by the nicotinamide-adenine dinucleotide phosphate (NADP) system to oxygen. The resultant hydrogen peroxide functions in cooperation with lysosomal myeloperoxidase to iodinate and kill intracellular bacteria. This may be mediated by sing-

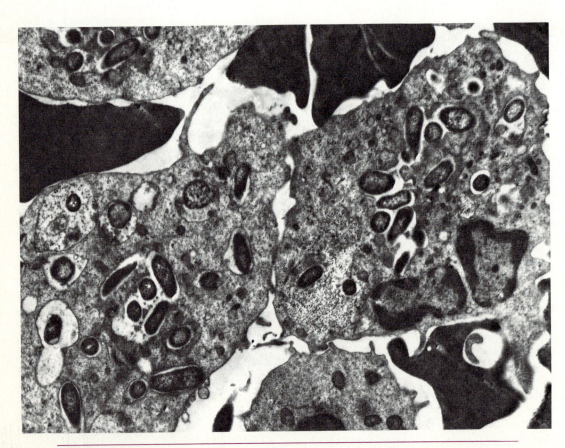

FIG. 20-4
Undigested bacteria are numerous within the phagosomes of these phagocytes taken from a patient with CGD. (Courtesy Dr. E. Adelstein.)

let oxygen, the superoxide radical, the hydroxyl radical, or other forms of oxygen derived from the hydrogen peroxide. Neutrophils of CGD patients do not make the shift to aerobic metabolism and therefore fail to accumulate H_2O_2 and to kill intracellular bacteria.

The role of H_2O_2 clearly is related to the type of pathogen that causes the most trouble for the CGD patient. Organisms such as *Hemophilus, Neisseria,* and *Streptococcus* species produce H_2O_2 but lack a catalase that can destroy it. Consequently these bacteria develop a microenvironment just like that created in normal phagocytes, and this is suicidal. The feebler pathogens that so often are involved in CGD infections have a high level of catalase, an enzyme that converts H_2O_2 to water and oxygen. Neutrophils of the CGD patient simply do not produce enough H_2O_2 to overcome the bacterial catalase. The microorganisms that cause infections in CGD patients are typically those which do produce catalase, whereas bacteria that lack catalase but produce their own H_2O_2 are resisted by these patients.

The metabolic shift of normal phagocytes to oxidative metabolism can be determined easily by the NBT reductase test. In this test neutrophils in the act of phagocytosing latex spherules are incubated in a solution of NBT dye that serves as a hydrogen acceptor instead of oxygen as oxidative metabolism ensues. This reduces the dye to its insoluble formazan, which is seen as distinct blue intracytoplasmic granules. Leukocytes of the CGD patient are not engaged in active oxidative metabolism and thus cannot reduce NBT. Female carriers of CGD have approximately a 50% loss in their ability to reduce NBT.

Chédiak-Higashi disease (CHD)

Chédiak-Higashi disease (CHD) is characterized by a pigmentary dilution of the eyes and skin (oculocutaneous albinism), extreme sensitivity to light (photophobia), rapid involuntary eye movements (nystagmus), and frequent pyogenic infections. Neutropenia, thrombocytopenia, and recurrent fever are also symptoms of the disease. The primary cellular defect noticed in victims of CHD is the presence of abnormally large granules in all phagocytic cells.

Because of the recurrent infections, these persons have fever, lymphadenopathy, and hepatosplenomegaly and a mean survival age of 6 years. In only 13 of 56 cases reported in one study did the patients live beyond 10 years of age.

In patients with CHD giant granules are found in the highly active phagocytic cells of the tissue and blood such as the tissue macrophages, alveolar macrophages and neutrophils, and other cells of the myeloid series. This makes diagnosis of the disease simple through the direct examination of stained blood films. An analysis of host defenses in CHD patients has revealed that immunoglobulin synthesis, CMI, and phagocytic endocytosis are all normal. The central defect is an inability to form normal primary granules in cells of the granulocytic series. Primary granules are the typical lysosomal granules that contain β-glucuronidase, myeloperoxidase, lysozyme, several hydrolases, etc. and can be compared with the secondary granules that contain alkaline phosphatase. Even though the engulfment by granulocytes in CHD patients is normal, bactericidal activity against *Staphylococcus aureus,* streptococci, pneumococci, and lesser pathogenic bacteria has proved to be deficient. Retarded intraphagocyte killing is not the result of depressed H_2O_2 formation, but it is associated with an inability of cells to degranulate normally and to deliver myeloperoxidase to the phagocytic vacuole. In CHD there is also an impaired chemotactic response, which would favor bacterial pathogens.

A striking defect recently observed in CHD patients is a severe loss of NK cell activity. Enriched NK cell preparations from a CHD patient failed to kill any of five NK-sensitive tumor cell lines. NK cell activity was estimated to be 400-fold less in CHD patients than in normal persons despite essentially equal NK cell numbers in the two groups.

The animal model that most resembles human CHD is the beige mouse. The beige mouses originated from a point mutation on chromosome 13 of the black C57BL/6 mouse. Beige mice lack NK cells and are virtually unable to reject allografts or tumors. They are likewise unable to muster NK-dependent ADCC reactions, although their macrophage and T cell dependent cytotoxic activities are normal.

Hyperimmunoglobulinemia E or Job's syndrome

Patients with Job's syndrome, true to the biblical origin of the name for their condition, have repeated skin infections. Group A *Streptococcus pyogenes, Candida albicans,* and *Staphylococcus aureus* are the primary offenders, the last especially producing the deep abscesses, furuncles, and boils that so troubled Job. These lesions are described as cold abscesses because of the scant inflammatory infiltration of phagocytic cells. Phagocytes from patients with Job's syndrome are also chemotactically depressed when examined *in vivo,* but are normally active in endocytosis. Nevertheless, the ingested microbes are highly resistant to intracellular killing. Cytocidal forms of oxygen are not formed and the nitroblue tetrazolium reductase test is negative. The exact location of the chemotactic and oxidative defects is unknown.

Job's syndrome patients also display other important immune abnormalities, the most regularly recognized being a hyperimmunoglobulinemia E and eosinophilia. IgE levels of 50,000 IU/ml are not unknown, although values between 5,000 and 25,000 are more common. This compares to normal values of 25 to 50 units. The source of the hyper IgE condition has been ascribed to a loss of T_S cells, since T_S cells ($T8^+$ cells) from normal individuals, but not autologous T_S cells, will suppress the intense production of IgE seen in cultures of B cells from Job patients. The situation appears to be more complicated than this, however, since allogenic matching of T_S cells from Job patients with B cells of other patients *does* result in IgE suppression.

G6PD deficiency

An inability of neutrophils to destroy engulfed bacteria also has been associated with a deficiency in the enzyme G6PD. This enzyme is the first in the HMP shunt, where it diverts G6P from the glycolytic pathway. Accordingly, individuals who are devoid of this enzyme have a defective ability to generate H_2O_2; in fact it is estimated that their phagocytes produce only 25% of the normal level of hydrogen peroxide. *Staphylococcus, Escherichia,* and *Serratia* organisms survive inside these phagocytes, but H_2O_2-producing microbes do not.

Myeloperoxidase deficiency

Benzidine staining of granulocytes for myeloperoxidase activity has exposed a deficiency of this enzyme in certain patients with severe acute infections. During phagocytosis the shift of phagocytic metabolism to the oxygen-consuming pentose pathway occurs normally in these patients, which suggests that normal amounts of H_2O_2 are formed. Cell studies have revealed that little or no iodination of intracellular microbes occurs and that the killing rate is depressed. The similarity of myeloperoxidase deficiency to CGD is obvious; patients with the latter disease have myeloperoxidase but little H_2O_2, whereas patients with the former disease have H_2O_2 but no myeloperoxidase. Both are required for protection against many pyogenic bacteria. In this syndrome only PMNs are affected. Monocytes and eosinophils remain normal.

Dysfunction of neutrophil actin

At least one example of recurrent skin and intestinal infections with gram-negative and gram-positive bacteria has been attributed to a failure of actin in neutrophils to polymerize. In its rest state actin exists in a monomeric form but is converted to a polymeric or filamentous form during pseudopod formation and locomotion. Neutrophils unable to transform actin into its contractile state cannot respond properly to chemotactic stimuli, and this accounts for the failure of the patient to develop pus at the site of infections. Other metabolic functions of the neutrophils, including oxygen metabolism and degranulation, are normal, and the patient's monocytes function normally.

DEFICIENCIES OF THE COMPLEMENT COMPONENTS

Inadequate amounts of the various components of the complement system, including the inhibitors and inactivators that regulate the activation cascade, may arise from genetic conditions in which the component is not synthesized at all or is produced at subnormal levels. It is also possible that the molecule may be synthesized in the normal amount, but it may be structurally defective and functionally inert. Hypercatabolism also may produce a deficiency of one of the complement proteins, and this may be difficult to distinguish from activation of the molecule, especially if only a late-acting component is involved. Before it is possible to establish that a deficiency of some complement molecule exists, it is necessary to have a reliable method for quantitating the individual component or the whole complement system.

Quantitation of complement
Hemolytic titration

The total complement level of a serum is determined in a hemolytic assay system. In the titration of complement sheep red blood cells that have been preincubated with a slight excess of antisheep hemolysin are added to varying amounts of the complement source. Such erythrocytes are known as sensitized sheep cells because they are susceptible to lysis in the presence of complement. The exact volumes used in the test will vary according to whether it is a macroscopic tube test (final volume 3 to 7.5 ml) or a microtiter test (final volume 0.2 to 0.5 ml). The erythrocyte suspension also is adjusted according to the dimensions of the test, with its final concentration ranging from 1% to 0.25%. After a suitable incubation period at 37° C the tubes or wells containing the several complement dilutions are examined for hemolysis. The amount of complement present in the test material usually is expressed as the dilution of complement necessary to achieve lysis of half the red cells added, that is, the CH50 dilution. This can be determined very accurately by a spectrophotometric determination of the amount of hemoglobin released in different tubes in the complement dilution series compared with a standard containing half the amount of cells used in the titration that have been lysed with distilled water.

Complement components

Quantitation of the individual components of the complement system is possible by serologic means or by hemolytic assays. It should be remembered that the latter method measures the functional capacity of the molecule, whereas the former measures only the antigenic integrity of the molecule. For example, it is known that the activation of C3 removes such a small peptide, C3a, from the parent molecule

that nearly all the serologic activity of the parent molecule is left with C3b. When C3b is acted on by Factor I, another low molecular weight peptide, C3d, is freed. The remainder is hemolytically inactive but serologically identical (with respect to most antisera) to total C3. Thus, if one recovers C3 as an antigen, it could be C3, C3b, or C3c that is being measured, but if C3 is measured by hemolytic assays, only C3 (C3b) is being determined.

Measuring each of the components in sera is a useful way to determine if a classic or alternate pathway of complement activation is in progress. If levels of C1, C4, and C2 are normal in company with low C3 levels and a low hemolytic activity of the serum, then it can be assumed that the complement level of the serum was lowered by activation of the alternate pathway.

Commercially available Mancini plates with the specific antiserum incorporated into agarose are used for the quantitative immunodiffusion determination of C3 and C5. Standards are provided with the test kits. Mancini plates can be prepared for C4, C8, C9, and properdin from commercially available antisera. Other antisera undoubtedly will be available soon.

To measure the biologic activity of human or other sources of the individual complement components, special serum reagents are available that are devoid of the component to be quantitated. A sample containing an unknown quantity of the component to be measured is added to sensitized sheep erythrocytes; this is incubated to allow lysis to take place. The amount of lysis that occurs is relatable to the quantity of the component being measured, since an excess of all the other components is present in the mixture.

Genetic complement deficiency
C1q and C1r

Human deficiency of C1q initially was reported in 1961, and several examples have been added since that time. Most of these cases have been associated with a sex-linked agammaglobulinemia or a combined immuno-deficiency disease. The C1q level is reduced to about half that of normal levels. In 5 patients in one study the average C1q concentration was 6.4 μg/ml, compared with 20.2 for control subjects. Bone marrow grafting was performed to repair the immune deficit and was successful, restoring the C1q levels to normal. The basis for the C1q loss is uncertain. In some persons a hypercatabolism of the molecules has been suggested as the cause, although restoration of C1q blood levels by marrow transplants indicates that the cellular origin of the molecule is lacking in these persons. Since C1q deficiency is regularly associated with a loss of B and T lymphocytes, it is difficult to recognize any single defect associated with the C1q deficiency.

Normal C1q levels were noted in those few persons in whom C1r levels were markedly depressed. It is striking that all patients with the C1r deficiency had an extensive medical history, including multiple episodes of upper respiratory tract disease, chronic kidney disease, or a lupus erythematosus (LE)–like syndrome. Genetic studies indicate that the C1r loss is transmitted as an autosomal recessive trait.

C1s and C$\overline{1s}$ INH

Patients with C1r deficiency may have a loss of nearly 50% of their C1s. Little is known about the relationship of C1s deficiency and human health, although several of the individuals studied had an LE-like syndrome. This is not the case the C$\overline{1s}$ INH deficiency, which is clearly associated with HANE, also known as hereditary giant edema or giant edema. This disease is transmitted as an autosomal dominant deficiency in which the afflicted individuals average but 31 µg/ml of C$\overline{1s}$ INH, compared with 180 µg/ml for normal persons. A second form of C$\overline{1s}$ INH deficiency should be classified as a dysfunction or paraproteinemia, since a protein antigenically identical to the α_2-neuraminoglycoprotein is present in serum but is functionally inert.

The importance of α_2-neuraminoglycoprotein in homeostasis is best represented by its genetic deficiency disease, HANE. Persons with this disease suffer sporadic attacks of subcutaneous edema, which may be more or less localized, often associated with minor trauma of the affected part. In extensive reactions, edema of the face, neck, and joints may develop. The edema usually resolves within 72 hours, is not especially bothersome, and may not be associated with extensive pain, itching, or marked erythema. However, edema in the throat may make breathing difficult, and abdominal pain of considerable intensity is associated with edema of the viscera. The pathogenesis of the disease is not entirely known but may ultimately reside in a kinin released from C2. It is possible that Hageman's factor becomes activated by tissue enzymes released by the local trauma, and this is followed by the formation of plasmin from plasminogen and the activation of C1. In the absence of C$\overline{1s}$ INH, C2 kinin may be released. Patients with HANE have depleted plasma levels of C4 and C2 (and of C$\overline{1s}$ INH) consistent with this hypothesis. Injection of C1s into the skin of these patients produces a local edema. Prevention of this edema or attacks of angioneurotic edema with antihistamines or adrenergic drugs is not successful, suggesting little, if any, contribution of C3a or C5a to the disease. Infusion of plasma that contains the normal level of C$\overline{1s}$ INH and treatment with ϵ-aminocaproic acid, which inhibits plasmin formation from plasminogen, are both therapeutic. Androgen therapy is preferred since it will restore C$\overline{1s}$ INH to normal levels in those previously devoid of the molecule and convert those with a non-functional C$\overline{1s}$ INH to production of a functionally normal protein.

C4

An autosomal recessive deficiency of C4 first was recognized in an inbred strain of guinea pigs. In the homozygous condition absolutely no C4 could be detected, whereas in the heterozygous state up to 30% of normal values were observed. Homozygotes could be successfully immunized with guinea pig C4. The C4-deficient guinea pigs developed feeble immune responses to egg or bovine serum albumin but developed normal Arthus and passive cutaneous anaphylactic reactions. The alternate complement pathway is intact and may be the major source of protection for these animals against bacterial and viral infections.

Eight human examples of C4 deficiency have been reported, and one of the victims had a pronounced skin rash of uncertain cause.

C2

The C4-deficient guinea pigs just mentioned have about 40% of the normal C2 levels, and this has been attributed to a decreased synthetic rate of this protein and is not directly related to the C4 loss as such.

Human C2 deficiencies of both homozygous and heterozygous origin have been described on numerous occasions. Over 60 cases have been recognized, making this the most common of the human complement deficiencies. The heterozygous individuals have 30% to 70% of the normal C2 serum level, whereas the homozygous deficient persons range below 4% of normal values, based on hemolytic assays. Immune adherence assays for C2 are normal for both classes of individuals, probably because only 100 molecules of C3 need to be fixed for immune adherence to occur, whereas many thousand C3 molecules must be bound before hemolysis can occur. The frequency of hypersensitive disease such as LE and dermatomyositis and repeated infectious disease in C2-deficient persons exceeds what would be expected on the basis of random distribution. The basis for these relationships is not known.

C3

Over 20 separate hospital admissions for multiple bouts of middle ear infections, meningitis, pneumonia, etc. are in the medical history of the one known human with total C3 deficiency (2.5 μg/ml of serum, compared with a normal level of 1,250 μg/ml). Five other children in the same family plus the mother had about half-normal C3 levels. The preponderance of infections by the patient emphasizes the critical role of C3 not only in linking the classic and alternate pathways but also in immune adherence, opsonization, and chemotaxis, all of which are important defense functions. Approximately a half dozen C3-deficient persons are recorded in the medical literature.

C5

About 40% of inbred mice lack a functional C5 but produce a unique protein termed MuB1. Because of antigenic similarities between MuB1 and C5, the former is considered an inactive form of the normal complement component. The hemolytic deficiency of C5-deficient mouse serum is totally replaced by fresh whole mouse serum or by pure C5. These mice are apparently as healthy as other mice, although there is provisional evidence that they are more susceptible to infection with *Corynebacterium kutscheri* and *Candida albicans*.

Human dysfunction of C5, unlike that of mice, is more clearly relatable to recurrent infectious disease. Only seven examples are known, and in these the C5 level as determined immunochemically was normal, but hemolytic titrations of complement could detect no C5. Phagocytosis was depressed and could not be restored to normal with C5-deficient mouse sera but could be with human C5. This loss of the expected phagocytic activity accounts for the higher incidence of infectious disease in these patients.

C6 and C7

A strain of rabbits with a genetic deficiency of C6 is known. This is apparently only part of a more generalized fault in the immunologic functions of complement, since serum of the affected individuals is not chemotactic, a property related to C5 but not to C6. These rabbits also develop only a feeble delayed hypersensitivity to tuberculin and retain skin grafts longer than is typical, phenomena that are quite unrelated to complement function and indicate a broad immunodepressed condition in these animals. Sera of these rabbits are devoid of bacteriolytic as well as hemolytic properties, both ascribable to their complement deficit. These latter defects were correctable with addition of purified C6. The deficiency was inherited as a single autosomal recessive characteristic. A C6 deficiency in hamsters also has been recognized.

Human C6 deficiency has been described in 24 individuals who lacked hemolytically or immunochemically active C6. The parents and siblings of the individuals had half-normal serum levels of C6. C6 deficiency appears to be associated with a heightened susceptibility to *Neisseria* infections. Several patients have been described who are deficient in C7, and more than 20 individuals lacking C8 also has been identified. C9 deficiency has been recognized in 5 families.

IMMUNOLOGIC RECONSTITUTION

Restoration of a suitable immune status to persons with uncomplicated agammaglobulinemia presents no novel problems; it is only necessary to provide them passive immunity by periodic injections of pooled human γ-globulin (Table 20-5). Since purification of γ-globulin often creates aggregates that will fix complement and produce anaphylactoid reactions, transfusions with plasma may be used to supplant injections of γ-globulin. When hepatitis-free donors are available, this is a safe and practical procedure.

Selective deficits in T cell responses also are subject to correction by a simple technical procedure (Table 20-5). Nonviable T cell extracts or transfer factor prepared from the T cells of donors with a normal status of CMI can be injected into the T cell–deficient person to convert him or her to the immune condition of the donor. T cell extracts are not injected in their crude form. The lymphocytes of a donor with good T cell responses are subjected to several freeze-thaw cycles. Cell fragments are removed by centrifugation, and high molecular weight molecules are trapped inside a dialysis membrane. The low molecular weight dialysate, the fraction originally described by Lawrence as transfer factor, is used. Human transfer factor is an antigen-specific low molecular weight oligonucleotide or peptide. Its mode of action in the recipient is unknown, but the recipient's lymphocytes are converted to a condition in which they will respond to foreign antigens in the typical way. This generally is determined externally by a skin test of the recipient with PPD, dermatophytin, coccidioidin, or some other preparation known to provoke a delayed skin reaction in the donor.

Transfer factor injections have been applied in the treatment of chronic mucocutaneous candidiasis, coccidioidomycosis, Swiss-type agammaglobulinemia, sex-linked agammaglobulinemia, ataxia telangiectasia, Wiskott-Aldrich syndrome, leprosy, and several forms of cancer. The results have been encouraging. Of seven patients with mucocutaneous candidiasis, four showed definite improvement; of 11 patients with Wiskott-Aldrich syndrome, six responded with a change in skin test results, five no longer have the eczema, and four became free of infection; and some patients with coccidioidomycosis showed improvement after treatment with transfer factor.

Successful reconstitution of the immune status with transfer factor demands that the individual have

---

TABLE 20-5
Immunologic reconstitution of immunodeficiency diseases

Condition	Method
B lymphocyte deficiencies	
Transient agammaglobulinemia	None needed; self-correcting
Bruton's agammaglobulinemia	Pooled human γ-globulin
Common variable hypogammaglobulinemia	Pooled human γ-globulin if IgG missing
T lymphocyte deficiencies	
Nezelof's syndrome	Thymus grafts ± bone marrow
DiGeorge's syndrome	Thymus grafts ± bone marrow
Leprosy, chronic mucocutaneous candidiasis	Transfer factor
Combined B and T lymphocyte deficiencies	
Sex-linked agammaglobulinemia	
Swiss-type agammaglobulinemia	Transfer factor plus pooled human γ-globulin or bone marrow
Wiskott-Aldrich syndrome	and thymus, depending on extent of T and B cell loss
Ataxia telangiectasia	
Phagocytic system deficiencies	Granulocyte transfusions (temporary value only)

a reasonably normal population of lymphocytes. Transfer factor merely triggers existing lymphocytes into activity; it does not generate lymphocytes. When these lymphocytes are not present or are present in extremely low numbers, transfer factor injections can be expected to fail. In these instances (Nezelof's and DiGeorge's syndromes and some cases of combined immunodeficiency disease) transplantation of bone marrow or thymus may be required to provide the needed T lymphocytes. Bone marrow transplants also would provide the B lymphocytes, but this usually is not the primary purpose of bone marrow transplants, since B cell products (immunoglobulins) are readily available. Bone marrow transplantation suffers the innate hazard of creating GVH reactions, since immunoresponsive cells are being transferred to an immunodeficient host. This problem is not met when the transplantation is between identical twins or between a histocompatible donor and recipient.

Since DiGeorge's and Nezelof's syndromes are characterized by the loss of only the cell-mediated arm of the immune response, marrow grafts to supply B cells are unnecessary, and thymus grafting alone is sufficient. Fetal thymus that has not yet reached immunologic maturity is the preferred tissue and has successfully reconstituted patients with Nezelof's or DiGeorge's syndrome. More recently it has been possible to transplant fragments of thymus cultured in vitro to patients with SCID and effect recovery from the condition. The fragments, which lose their lymphocytes during cultivation, are composed almost entirely of epithelium. Lymphocytes or prolymphocytes leaving the bone marrow of the transplant recipient repopulate the thymus fragments and are converted into functional T lymphocytes. This reveals the possibility that the thymic hormones required for T cell maturation are produced by the nonlymphoid portion of the thymus gland. One interesting aspect of this is that the thymus fragments can be successfully transplanted across the HLA barrier.

REFERENCES

Bertazzoni, U., and Bollum, F.J., editors: Terminal transferase in immunobiology and leukemia, New York, 1982, Plenum Press.

Buckley, R.H.: Immunodeficiency, J. Allergy Clin. Immunol. **72:**627, 1983.

Chandra, R.K., editor: Primary and secondary immunodeficiency disorders, Edinburgh, 1984, Churchill Livingstone.

DeVita, V.T., Jr., Hellman, S., and Rosenberg, B.A., editors: AIDS-etiology, diagnosis, treatment, and prevention, Philadelphia, 1985, J.B. Lippincott Company.

Gallin, J.I.: Neutrophil specific granule deficiency, Ann. Rev. Med. **36:**263, 1985.

Gallin, J.I., and Fauci, A.S., editors: Acquired immunodeficiency syndromes, New York, 1985, Raven Press.

Gluckman, J.C., Klatzmann, D., and Montagnier, L.: Lymphadenopathy-associated-virus infection and acquired immunodeficiency syndrome, Ann. Rev. Immunol. **4:**97, 1986.

Klein, E., editor: Acquired immunodeficiency syndrome, Prog. Allergy, **37:**1, 1986.

Lane, H.C., and Fauci, A.S.: Immunologic abnormalities in the acquired immunodeficiency syndrome, Ann. Rev. Immunol. **3:**477, 1985.

Quie, P.G.: Disorders of phagocyte function: biochemical aspects, Prog. Clin. Biol. Res. **13:**157, 1977.

Rosen, F.S.: The primary immunodeficiencies, New Eng. J. Med. **311:**300, 1984.

Selikoff, I.J., Teirstein, A.S., and Hirschman, S.Z., editors: Acquired immune deficiency syndrome, Ann. N. Y. Acad. Sci. **437:**1, 1984.

Tritsch, G.L., editor: Adenosine deaminase in disorders of purine metabolism and in immune deficiency, Ann. N. Y. Acad. Sci. **451:**1, 1985.

Webster, A.D.B.: Metabolic defects in immunodeficiency diseases, Clin. Exp. Immunol. **49:**1, 1982.

Wedgwood, R.J., Rosen, F.S., and Paul, N.W., editors: Primary immunodeficiency diseases, New York, 1983, Alan R. Liss, Inc.

Weiss, A., Hollander, H., and Stobo, J.: Acquired immunodeficiency syndrome: epidemiology, virology and immunology, Ann. Rev. Med. **36:**545, 1985.

READINGS IN IMMUNOLOGY

The inclusion of these readings in immunology is intended to serve at least three instructional purposes. It will be seen immediately that several of the readings have been chosen for their historical significance—the reporting of important firsts in immunology. The articles chosen for this purpose are from the recent rather than the early historical records so that the modern language used and the possibility of current applications of the information reported will give additional appeal to the reading lesson. Even so, the student will note in the earlier papers that briefly written reports based on unsophisticated procedures can be as vital to the development of a science as the longer, more complex reports so common in the present literature. A second purpose of these readings is to support the summary views in the body of the text with specific selections from the scientific literature, with the intent to exemplify the exact procedures and terminology used. It is not possible to present samples corresponding to each chapter in the text; nevertheless those presented do introduce cause and effect relationships and other aspects of the scientific method that are applicable to diverse subtopics in immunology. A third purpose, embodied especially in the recent selections, is to provide an opportunity for students to gain confidence in their mastery of immunology by realizing that, from the base of classroom lectures and text assignments, they in fact have learned enough immunology to comprehend current scientific writings.

No foreign language readings have been included in order that the intended purpose of this volume—instruction of beginning students of immunology— might be achieved.

Readings in immunology

≡READING 1

One of the perplexing questions that recur in biology is, how does the cell that produces a poisonous or toxic substance protect itself against the toxin? How does the tissue producing a proteolytic enzyme protect itself against self-digestion? How does the electric eel keep from shocking itself? How does the phagocyte keep from oxidizing and digesting itself? Insight into the solution of the last problem is presented in this discussion from *Infection and Immunity* **12:**252-256, 1975.

In this report the high intracellular content of ascorbic acid in phagocytes is noted to be divided between ascorbate and dehydroascorbate. Phagocytic studies with ascorbic acid-deficient guinea pigs indicated that dietary vitamin C did not influence the capacity of the cells to kill *Staphylococcus aureus* or to produce H_2O_2. During phagocytosis by human PMNs, dehydroascorbate in the cells increased, with a decrease in reduced ascorbate. This suggests that the PMNs use the ascorbate-dehydroascorbate system as an oxidation reduction balance during phagocytosis.

ASCORBATE AND PHAGOCYTE FUNCTION

Libuse Stankova, Nancy B. Gerhardt, Larry Nagel, and Robert H. Bigley*

Scorbutic guinea pig neutrophils (PMN) were found to produce H_2O_2 and kill Staphylococcus aureus *as well as control PMN, suggesting that ascorbate does not contribute significantly to phagocyte H_2O_2 production or bacterial killing. Total and reduced ascorbate contents of human PMN were observed to fall upon phagocytosis, whereas dehydroascorbate increased to a lesser extent. These observations are consistent with the view that ascorbate constitutes a functional part of the PMN's redox-active components and may thus function to protect cell constituents from denaturation by the oxidants produced during phagocytosis.*

In a previous study,[1] we found that human neutrophil leukocytes have impressive capacity for reducing dehydroascorbate and thus for regenerating their content of reduced ascorbate upon oxidation. This property of neutrophils (PMN), along with their relatively high ascorbate content, suggests that ascorbate may play an important role in PMN function. Phagocyte ascorbate might promote oxidative denaturation of bacterial components and thus potentiate bacterial killing, as proposed by Miller[2] and by Drath and Karnofsky.[3] Ascorbate also might function to preserve cell integrity by inactivating free radicals and oxidants[4-6] produced during phagocytosis.[7-9]

To determine whether physiological concentrations of ascorbate are critical for optimal phagocytosis and bacterial killing, we assayed H_2O_2 production and bactericidal activity in scorbutic guinea pig PMN. To examine the possibility that ascorbate is a redox-active component of oxidant-producing cells, we have measured changes in human PMN ascorbate contents during phagocytosis.

Materials and methods
Ascorbate contents

Ascorbate contents of tissues and cell preparations were measured by the method of Roe et al.[10] This method quantitatively distinguishes reduced ascorbate, dehydroascorbate, and diketogulonate from each other and from other organic compounds. De-

*Department of Medicine and Department of Microbiology and Immunology, University of Oregon Health Sciences Center, Portland, Oregon 97201.

hydroascorbate, the oxidized derivative of ascorbic acid, is reducible to ascorbate in most mammalian tissues. Diketogulonate, the hydrated derivative of dehydroascorbate, is not converted to dehydroascorbate in mammalian tissues.

Guinea pig experiments

Two-month-old guinea pigs weighing 325 to 375 g were divided into two groups. Both groups were fed for 18 days with an ascorbic acid-deficient diet (Nutritional Biochemicals Co., Cleveland, Ohio). Control animals were also fed by gavage 1 mg of ascorbate per g of body weight daily. Single experiments utilized pairs of animals, one scorbutic and one control. The order of harvest of control and scorbutic cells was alternated in successive experiments.

Guinea pig peritoneal PMN were harvested 12 h after intraperitoneal injection of 15 ml of 20% autoclaved sodium caseinate. Cells were suspended in calcium-free Krebs-Ringer phosphate buffer (KRP), pH 7.4. After 2 volumes of 0.87% ammonium chloride was added to lyse contaminating erythrocytes, leukocytes were collected by centrifugation for 10 min at $150 \times g$, washed twice in KRP, counted in a hemocytometer, and diluted with KRP to an approximate concentration of 100×10^6 phagocytes (PMN plus macrophages)/ml. Final suspensions contained 74 to 95% neutrophils, 3 to 25% macrophages, 0 to 8% lymphocytes, and 0 to 2% eosinophils.

H_2O_2 production was measured continuously as the rate of $^{14}CO_2$ production from [1-^{14}C]formate[9,11] (New England Nuclear Corp., Boston, Mass.), using the gas flow-ionization chamber system of Davidson and Tanaka.[12] This technique converts charge accumulated in an ionization chamber to a millivolt signal. Unstimulated reaction mixtures (1 ml) containing 20×10^6 to 40×10^6 leukocytes, 0.7 μmol of sodium formate including 0.86 μCi of [^{14}C]formate, and 5.6 μmol of glucose in KRP were incubated in 20-ml flat-bottomed glass vials in a Dubnoff shaking incubator (Precision Scientific Co., Chicago, Ill.) at 37° C, 80 oscillations/min. Phagocytosing signals were recorded after the addition of approximately 2×10^9 thrice-washed polystyrene latex spheres (0.81 μm in diameter; Bacto-Latex, Difco Laboratories, Detroit, Mich.) in 0.2 ml of KRP. The depth of the reaction mixtures was 2 mm and the surface area

was 5 cm^2. Vials were gassed with 5% CO_2 in air, flowing at 73 ml/min. Nanomoles of formate oxidized were calculated from the millivolt signal, using factors derived from calibrations previously reported.[1]

Bacterial killing by guinea pig peritoneal PMN was measured using a modification of the method of Pincus and Klebanoff,[13] within 2 to 4 h of cell collection. Assay mixtures (1 ml) contained 30×10^6 phagocytes, 5×10^6 colony-forming units of *Staphylococcus aureus* 502A (kindly supplied by G. Mandell), 0.1 ml of serum separated from blood obtained by cardiac puncture at the time of cell harvest, 10 μmol of glucose, and KRP. These were incubated at 37° C in stoppered siliconized glass tubes (12 by 75 mm), which were rotated on a model 150 Multi-Purpose Rotator (Scientific Industries, Inc.) at 24 rpm. At intervals noted in Fig. 1, 0.1-ml aliquants were removed, diluted in distilled water, vortexed heavily to disrupt PMN, and plated in duplicate in Trypti-

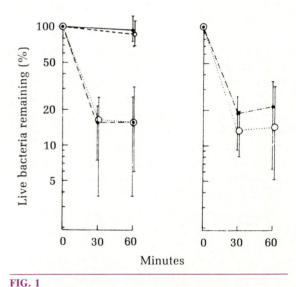

FIG. 1

In vitro killing of *S. aureus* 502A by scorbutic and control guinea pig PMN. n = 3 for scorbutic PMN plus control serum; n = 4 for the other groups; mean values and ranges are indicated. Symbols for left-hand panel: ○ – – – ○, Scorbutic serum; ● – · – ●, control PMN plus serum; ●—●, control serum; ○ · · · · ○, scorbutic PMN plus serum. Symbols for right-hand panel: ●, Control PMN plus scorbutic serum; ○, scorbutic PMN plus control serum.

case soy broth containing 15% agar. Colonies were counted after 44 to 48 h of culture at 37° C.

Human experiments

Human PMN were separated from peripheral blood as previously described.[1] These preparations contained 85% neutrophils, 5 to 15% monocytes, 0 to 8% lymphocytes, and 0 to 5% eosinophils.

Ascorbate contents of resting and phagocytosing PMN were measured by using the entire 1.5-ml reaction mixtures: 0.7×10^8 to 1.2×10^8 phagocytes, with or without approximately 2×10^9 latex particles, suspended in KRP containing 8.25 µmol of glucose. Samples were incubated in the shaking incubator at 80 oscillations/min at 37 C for the times indicated in the tables.

Results

The ascorbate contents of scorbutic guinea pig peritoneal PMN, whole blood, liver, and kidney were about 15% of normal (Table 1). These values agree well with published data for comparably treated animals.[14]

Scorbutic guinea pig leukocytes produced normal amounts of H_2O_2 during phagocytosis (Table 2). Four of thirteen scorbutic peritoneal exudates were grossly bloody. PMN in those samples were packed with ingested erythrocytes and exhibited high resting H_2O_2 production (mean, 1.69 nmol of formate oxidized/10 min per 10^8 PMN), which did not increase upon addition of latex particles. Giemsa-stained smears showed that less than 1% of these cells had ingested latex spheres. These findings were reproduced in PMN from a control guinea pig given isologous whole blood intraperitoneally 12 h before PMN harvest. Such bloody samples were excluded from this study.

Scorbutic PMN killed *S. aureus* as efficiently as did control guinea pig cells (Fig. 1). It can also be inferred from Fig. 1 that normal and scorbutic sera supported opsonization equally well, since phagocytosis-dependent bacterial killing did not vary significantly with serum source.

The total ascorbate content of phagocytosing human peripheral blood PMN decreased during the 60 min after phagocytosis and then remained stable (Table 3). Table 4 shows that total ascorbate decreased by an average of 12% in phagocytosing normal human PMN but did not change during phagocytosis in cells from two patients with chronic granulomatous disease. The decrease in total ascorbate content of phagocytosing normal cells was accompanied by a marked decrease in reduced ascorbate which was not accounted for by a moderate increase in dehydroascorbate. Only trace amounts of diketogulonate were detectable in both resting and phagocytosing samples.

Discussion

The present study shows that PMN obtained from scorbutic guinea pigs produce H_2O_2 and kill *S. aureus* as well as do control cells, at least briefly after phagocytosis. Since these functions depend on phagocytosis, our results argue against the conclusion of Nungester and Ames that phagocytosis is impaired in scorbutic guinea pig phagocytes.[15] The discrepancy

---

TABLE 1

Total ascorbate content of scorbutic and control guinea pig tissues

| Tissue | Total ascorbate | | Ratio (scorbutic/control) |
	Control	Scorbutic	
Peritoneal PMN*	42.4 (34.8-51.0)	4.5 (3.2-5.5)	0.11
Blood†	4.9 ± 0.3	0.6 ± 0.17	0.12
Liver‡	126.7 ± 23.8	18.8 ± 1.7	0.15
Kidney‡	68.8 ± 10.7	10.8 ± 2.8	0.16

*$n = 3$ control, 3 scorbutic; expressed as nmol/10^8 cells; mean (range).

†$n = 6$ control, 6 scorbutic; expressed as nmol/0.1 ml; mean ± standard deviation.

‡$n = 6$ control, 6 scorbutic; nmol/100 mg of tissue; mean ± standard deviation.

TABLE 2

H_2O_2 production by scorbutic and control guinea pig PMN without and with latex particles

| PMN | Formate oxidation* | | Ratio (phagocytosing/unstimulated) |
	Unstimulated	Phagocytosing	
Control†	0.532 ± 0.206	1.480 ± 0.552	2.8 ± 0.3
Scorbutic‡	0.575 ± 0.294	1.401 ± 0.367	2.7 ± 0.7

*Expressed as nmol of formate oxidized/10 min per 10^8 PMN; mean $\pm$ standard deviation.
†$n = 10$.
‡$n = 9$.

TABLE 3

Total ascorbate content of human PMN; effect of time of incubation without and with latex particles*

Incubation time (min)	Unstimulated	Phagocytosing
0	73	73
40	73	68
60	71	65
90	74	66
120	72	66

*Expressed as nmol of ascorbate/10^8 PMN.

is best explained by the fact that the peritoneal exudates in the study of Nungester and Ames were hemorrhagic, as often occurs with advanced ascorbate deficiency. As we have demonstrated, erythrophagocytosis interferes with further particle ingestion and therefore with enhanced H_2O_2 production upon incubation with latex spheres. Experiments using bloody exudates were excluded from the present study.

The observations that H_2O_2 production and bacterial killing are unimpaired in scorbutic PMN imply that these activities are not sensitive to changes in ascorbate concentration over the range studied here. The 15% of normal ascorbate residual in scorbutic cells might suffice to support H_2O_2 production, since neutrophils possess efficient dehydroascorbate reducing activity.[1] However, it would be unusual for a biological reaction to be insensitive to a decrease in substrate concentration to less than one-fifth of the physiological level. Therefore, we doubt that ascor-

bate participates directly in phagocyte H_2O_2 production or bacterial killing.

Upon phagocytosis, human PMN oxygen consumption increased by 100 to 300 nmol/10^8 cells per min:[16,17] Measurements of the H_2O_2 and activated oxygen species produced during phagocytosis account for up to 80% of the increment in oxygen consumption.[16,17,18,19,20] Despite exposure to these potent and largely diffusible denaturants, PMN survive and function at least briefly[21] and do not accumulate lipid peroxides[22] after phagocytosis. Catalase, myeloperoxidase, and glutathione peroxidase catalyze destruction of H_2O_2; glutathione peroxidase also catalyzes lipid peroxide reduction.[24] Ascorbate and other small molecules, including reduced glutathione and α-tocopherol, are effective antioxidants and free radical scavengers.[4,5,6] Human leukocytes (10^8) contain 107 to 205 nmol of reduced glutathione,[25] 3.2 ± 0.2 nmol of oxidized nicotinamide adenine dinucleotide (NAD^+), 2.5 ± 0.2 nmol NADH, 0.8 ± 0.2 nmol of $NADP^+$, and 2.4 ± 0.4 nmol of NADPH.[28] The cell contents of these redox-active molecules are comparable to the ascorbate contents measured in the present study (Table 4). Human PMN can reduce more than 200 nmol of dehydroascorbate/10^8 cells per min.[1] This activity would appear sufficient to maintain ascorbate in reduced form, able to act as a significant part of the PMN's capacity for inactivating free radicals and oxidants and thus for preventing denaturation of cell constituents.

Chronic granulomatous disease neutrophils phagocytose normally,[26] but their ability to produce H_2O_2 and activated oxygen species is markedly impaired.[18,19] In the studies reported here, ascorbate

TABLE 4

Ascorbate contents of human PMN after 60-min incubation without and with latex particles*

PMN	Ascorbate content (nmol/10^8 cells)					
	Total		Reduced		Dehydroascorbate	
Normal*						
Unstimulated	78.1 ± 8.3		54.9 ± 10.3		23.2 ± 8.9	
Phagocytosing	68.6 ± 4.8		40.0 ± 7.4		28.6 ± 7.6	
Difference	(−)9.5 ± 4.6†		(−)14.9 ± 4.4†		(+)5.4 ± 4.6‡	
Chronic granulomatous disease§						
Unstimulated	54.7	52.9	46.8	44.6	7.8	8.3
Phagocytosing	54.7	53.5	41.2	43.4	13.4	10.2
Difference	0.0	(+)0.6	(−)5.6	(−)1.2	(+)5.6	(+)1.9

*$n = 10$; mean ± standard deviation.
†$P < 0.001$ by paired t test.

‡$P < 0.005$ by paired t test.
§$n = 2$; recorded separately.

levels were stable during phagocytosis in chronic granulomatous disease phagocytes but fell significantly in normal phagocytes. The latter observation probably reflects degradation of ascorbate, mediated by oxidants produced during phagocytosis, to compounds other than those assayable as total ascorbate. The degraded ascorbate may be sequestered from the cell's dehydroascorbate reducing activity, perhaps in phagolysosomes.

The ratio of $NADP^+$ to NADPH in PMN was observed to increase from 0.11 to 0.31 during phagocytosis.[27] This has been interpreted to reflect NADPH oxidation in the process of H_2O_2 production[27] or the oxidation of reduced glutathione by H_2O_2.[18] Neutrophil-unsaturated membrane lipid, an easily oxidized cell component, is not detectably oxidized after phagocytosis.[23] This suggests that extensive oxidation of cell constituents is not a general phenomenon in phagocytosing PMN. The present study demonstrates that ascorbate is oxidized during phagocytosis. This observation is consistent with the view that ascorbate is a functional part of the cell's redox-active components.

Acknowledgments

This work was supported by Public Health Service grant no. AM 13173 from the National Institute of Arthritis, Metabolism, and Digestive Diseases and Medical Research Foundation grant no. 7412.

The expert technical assistance of John Niedra, Department of Microbiology and Immunology, is gratefully acknowledged.

REFERENCES

1. Bigley, R.H., and Stankova, L.: Uptake and reduction of oxidized and reduced ascorbate by human leukocytes, J. Exp. Med. **139:**1084-92, 1974.
2. Miller, T.E.: Killing and lysis of gram-negative bacteria through the synergistic effect of hydrogen peroxide, ascorbic acid, and lysozyme, J. Bacteriol. **98:**949-955, 1969.
3. Drath, D.B., and Karnofsky, M.L.: Bactericidal activity of metal-mediated peroxide-ascorbate systems, Infect. Immunol. **10:**1077-1083, 1974.
4. Demopoulos, H.B.: Control of free radicals in biologic systems, Fed. Proc. **32:**1903-1908, 1973.
5. DiLuzio, N.R.: Antioxidants, lipid peroxidation and chemical-induced liver injury, Fed. Prod. **32:**1875-1881, 1973.
6. Tappel, A.L.: Lipid peroxidation damage to cell components, Fed. Proc. **32:**1870-1874, 1973.
7. Allen, R.C., Stjernholm, R.L., and Steele, R.H.: Evidence for the generation of an electronic excitation state(s) in human polymorphonuclear leukocytes and its participation in bacterial activity, Biochem. Biophys. Res. Commun. **47:**679-684, 1972.
8. Babior, B.M., Kipnes, R.S., and Curnutte, J.T.: The production by leukocytes of superoxide, a potential bactericidal agent, J. Clin. Invest. **52:**741-754, 1973.
9. Iyer, G.Y.N., Islam, D.M.F., and Quastel, J.H.: Biochemical aspects of phagocytosis. Nature (London) **192:**535-541, 1961.
10. Roe, J.H., Milles, M.B., Osterling, M.J., and Damron, C.M.: The detection of diketo-l-gulonic acid, dehydro-1-ascorbic acid and 1-ascorbic acid in the same tissue extract

by the 2,4-dinitrophenylhydrazine method, J. Biol. Chem. **174:**201-208, 1948.

11. Aebi, H.: Detection and fixation of radiation-produced peroxide by enzymes. Radiat. Res. **3**(Suppl.):130-152, 1963.

12. Davidson, W.D., and Tanaka, K.R.: Continuous measurement of pentose phosphate pathway activity in erythrocytes. An ionization chamber method, J. Lab. Clin. Med. **73:**173-180, 1969.

13. Pincus, S.H., and Klebanoff, S.J.: Quantitative leukocyte iodination, N. Engl. J. Med. **284:**744-750, 1971.

14. Penney, J.R., and Zilva, S.S.: The fixation and retention of ascorbic acid by the guinea-pig, Biochem. J. **40:**695-706, 1945.

15. Nungester, W.J., and Ames, A.M.: The relationship between ascorbic acid and phagocytic activity, J. Infect. Dis. **83:**50-59, 1948.

16. Homan-Muller, J.W.T., Weening, T.S., and Roos, D.: Production of hydrogen peroxide by phagocytosing human granulocytes, J. Lab. Clin. Med. **85:**198-207, 1975.

17. Klebanoff, S.J., and Hamon, C.B.: Role of myeloperoxidase-mediated antimicrobial systems in intact leukocytes, RES J. Reticuloendothel. Soc. **12:**170-196, 1972.

18. Baehner, R.L., Gilman, N., and Karnofsky, M.L.: Respiration and glucose oxidation in human and guinea pig leukocytes: comparative studies, J. Clin. Invest. **49:**692-699, 1970.

19. Curnutte, J.T., Whitten, D.M., and Babior, B.M.: Defective superoxide production by granulocytes from patients with chronic granulomatous disease, N. Engl. J. Med. **290:**593-597, 1974.

20. Holmes, B., Page, A.R., and Good, R.A.: Studies of the metabolic activity of leukocytes from patients with a genetic abnormality of phagocyte function, J. Clin. Invest. **46:**1422-1432, 1967.

21. Zatti, M., Rossi, F., and Patriarca, P.: The H_2O_2 production by polymorphonuclear leucocytes during phagocytosis, Experientia **24:**669-670, 1968.

22. Rosner, F., Valmont, I., Kozinn, P.J., and Caroline, L.: Leukocyte function in patients with leukemia. Cancer **25:**835-842, 1970.

23. Mason, R.J., Stossel, T.P., and Vaughn, M.: Lipids of alveolar macrophages, polymorphonuclear leukocytes, and their phagocytic vesicles, J. Clin. Invest. **51:**2399-2407, 1972.

24. Little, C., and Obrien, P.J.: An intracellular GSH-peroxidase with a lipid peroxide substrate, Biochem. Biophys. Res. Commun. **31:**145-150, 1968.

25. Hardin, B., Valentine, W.N., Follette, J.H., and Lawrence, J.S.: Studies on the sulfhydryl content of human leukocytes and erythrocytes, Am. J. Med. Sci. **228:**73-82, 1954.

26. Stossel, T.P., Root, R.K., and Vaughan, M.: Phagocytosis in chronic granulomatous disease and the Chediak-Higashi syndrome, N. Engl. J. Med. **286:**120-123, 1972.

27. Zatti, M., and Rossi, F.: Early changes of hexose monophosphate pathway activity and of NADPH oxidation in phago-cytosing leucocytes, Biochim. Biophys. Acta **99:**557-561, 1965.

28. Silber, R., and Gabrio, B.: Studies on normal and leukemic leukocytes. III. Pyridine nucleotides, J. Clin. Invest. **41:**230-234, 1962.

☰ READING 2

This reading, entitled "The Bursa of Fabricius and Antibody Production," is taken from *Poultry Science* **35:**224-225, 1956 (copyright 1956, *Poultry Science*). This succinct report attributed for the first time a dependence of immunoglobulin production by chickens to a cloacal organ known as the bursa of Fabricius. Even though this paper was published in 1956, it is still possible to consider it as a paper of historical interest because of the important first that it describes. The evidence for the conclusion drawn is presented in the form of a single table, which needs no statistical interpretation.

This article inaugurated two major types of investigation: the search for similar immunoglobulin-dependent tissues in higher animals and a search for the basis (either cellular or humoral) for the bursa's contribution to birds. Regrettably only the latter of these has been finally determined; however, this in no way detracts from the keystone position of this paper to the phylogenetic basis of comparative immunology.

THE BURSA OF FABRICIUS AND ANTIBODY PRODUCTION

BRUCE GLICK, TIMOTHY S. CHANG, AND R. GEORGE JAAP*

The bursa of Fabricius is a structure peculiar to *Aves*. It is a blind sac connected by a small duct to the dorsal part of the cloaca. Often nicknamed "cloacal thymus," the function of the bursa is believed to be similar to that of the thymus.[1,2] There is no question that the bursa of Fabricius functions as a lymph gland during the first two to three months after the chicken hatches.[3-5] Like the thymus, the bursa in birds is believed to have some endocrine function in relation to growth and sexual development.[1,6]

---

*The Ohio Agricultural Experiment Station, Columbus, Ohio.

Although reticular cells of lymph glands and lymphocytes may participate in globulin and antibody synthesis,[7] suspicion regarding the importance of the bursa in antibody production arose in the following accidental manner. A source of chicken blood possessing a high titre of antibody for antigen O of *Salmonella typhimurium* was desired for other experiments. Seventeen and one-half milliliters of a 48 hour, heat inactivated, broth culture[8] were injected intravenously during a 20 day period. Surplus 6 month old females from an experiment designed to study the effect of bursectomy were used. To our surprise six females which had been bursectomized at 12 days of age died as a result of the injections. Three survived but produced no antibodies. The non-bursectomized females seemed unaffected and built up normal titres of antibodies in their blood.

To test whether the bursa of Fabricius was involved in antibody production, 85 out of 168 male and female chickens were bursectomized at two weeks of age. Twenty of these White Leghorns received 8.5 ml of *S. typhimurium* antigen per bird in six intramuscular injections at four day intervals between the 3rd and 6th week after hatching. Blood samples taken one week after the last injection were tested by the homologous antigen-antibody reaction test at 1:25 dilution. Out of ten bursectomized birds antibodies to *S. typhimurium* were present in three individuals while eight of the ten normal controls developed antibodies.

The larger group composed of 74 White Leghorns and 74 Rhode Island Reds were each injected with 17.5 ml of the suspension of *S. typhimurium* in six intramuscular injections at four-day intervals from the 13th to the 16th week after hatching. Their reaction to the test for antibodies at 17 weeks of age is given in Table 1.

Antibody titres were demonstrated for 63 out of 73 controls. This is considered to be a normal result with the typhimurium antigen. Only 8 of the 75 bursectomized birds developed antibodies. These results demonstrate that the bursa of Fabricius plays a vital role in the production of antibodies to *S. typhimurium*. No information is available concerning the possible role of the bursa in the production of antibodies for other antigens.

TABLE 1

Number of chickens and antibody production resulting from injections of O antigen *(S. typhimurium)* between the 13th and 17th week after hatching

	Bursectomized		Controls	
	Positive	Negative	Positive	Negative
Rhode Island Red	5	33	35	1
White Leghorn	3	34	28	9
TOTAL	8	67	63	10

The bursa of Fabricius reaches its maximum size as early as 4 to 5 weeks in White Leghorns and as late as 9 to 10 weeks in Rhode Island Reds.[5] This rapid growth period for the bursa coincides with the period when chickens attain the ability to develop many antibodies to foreign proteins.[9] Once the bird has developed the ability to produce antibodies this ability is maintained throughout life.

The bursae of White Leghorns begin to atrophy about seven weeks after hatching. In Rhode Island Reds atrophy of the bursa begins later, about the 13th week.[5] It is unlikely that the atrophic bursae of chickens between the 13th and 17th week after hatching could have a direct influence on antibody production. To determine where and how the bursa is involved in antibody production should prove promising for further research.

The White Leghorn breed has a greater resistance to *S. pullorum* than Rhode Island Reds during the first two weeks after hatching.[10] The more rapid growth rate and larger mature size of the bursa in White Leghorns has been demonstrated. Disease resistance in general may be associated with rate of growth and size of the bursa during the period when the bird first develops the capacity to produce many of its antibodies.

REFERENCES

1. Riddle, O.: Growth of the gonads and bursa of Fabricius in doves and pigeons with data for body growth and age at maturity, Amer. J. Physiol. **86:**243-265, 1928.
2. Taibel, A.M.: Effetto della bursectomia sul timo in *Gallus domesticus,* Riv. Biol. **24:**364-372, 1938.

3. Jolly, J.: La bourse de Fabricius. Et les organes lymphoepithéliauz, Arch. d'Anat. Micr. **16**:316-546, 1914.

4. Calhoun, M.L.: Microscopic anatomy of the digestive tract of *Gallus domesticus,* Iowa State College J. Sci. **7**:261-382, 1933.

5. Glick, B.: Growth and function of the Bursa of Fabricius in the domestic fowl. Ph.D. dissertation, Ohio State University, 1955.

6. Woodward, M.: Studies in bursectomized and thymectomized chicken, M.S. thesis, Kansas State College, 1931.

7. Raffel, S.: Immunity, New York, 1953, Appleton-Century-Crofts, Inc.

8. Kauffmann, F.: The Diagnosis of *Salmonella* types, Illinois, 1950, Charles C Thomas.

9. Wolfe, H.R., and Dilks, E.: Precipitin production in the chicken. III: Variation in antibody response as correlated with age of animal, J. Immunol. **58**:245-250, 1948.

10. Hutt, F.B., and Scholes, J.C.: Genetics of the fowl, 13, Breed differences in susceptibility to *Salmonella pullorum,* Poultry Sci. **20**:342-352, 1941.

≣ READING 3

The article "Thymus-Marrow Immunocompetence. III. The Requirement for Living Thymus Cells" often is quoted as among the first articles to clearly substantiate the importance of the interaction between thymus cells and bone marrow cells in the formation of immunoglobulins. As indicated in the title, this is actually the third of a series of articles from this group of experimenters on essentially the same subject. The importance of this particular article is its proof that the thymus-marrow (currently referred to as the T cell–B cell) interaction is clearly synergistic and depends on living thymus cells. Irradiated or sonic-treated thymus cells improved the response slightly compared with animals that did not receive any type of thymus stimulant, and this type of data often has been presented as evidence of the thymus hormone. Note that the authors emphasize the contribution of living syngeneic thymus tissue, since the response is so much greater than with dead or foreign thymus tissue, which could have low activity merely as a nonspecific adjuvant effect. Note also that the numbers appear more meaningful when expressed as plaque-forming centers rather than as the titer of the antisera.

This article is reprinted from the *Proceedings of the Society of Experimental Biology and Medicine* **127**:462-466, 1968.

THYMUS-MARROW IMMUNOCOMPETENCE. III. THE REQUIREMENT FOR LIVING THYMUS CELLS* (32715)

HENRY N. CLAMAN, EDWARD A. CHAPERON,† AND JOHN C. SELNER‡

The immunocompetence of thymus-marrow cell suspensions has been demonstrated.[1,2] Suspensions containing both thymus and marrow cells produced mcre antibody to sheep erythrocytes (SRBC) when transferred to irradiated syngeneic hosts and stimulated with antigen than could be accounted for by the summation of the activities of thymus or marrow cell suspensions considered singly. Thymus-marrow interaction has also been demonstrated in other systems.[3-6]

The nature of the thymus-marrow interaction is obscure. The purpose of these experiments was to investigate the system using the Jerne plaque assay method and to determine whether isologous living thymus cells could be replaced by irradiated cells, cell sonicates, or heterologous cells. The importance of the recipient thymus was also investigated.

Materials and methods

LAF₁ mice were used and the description of the mice, method of cell suspension preparation and hemolysin assay have already been published.[1,2] Immunization was with 0.2 ml of 10% washed SRBC. Rat thymus cell suspensions were made from freshly sacrificed young adult Sprague-Dawley Rats (Simonson Laboratories). Fetal liver cell suspensions were made by passing fetal LAF₁ livers through a graded series of needles as was done with marrow. "Minced" thymus preparations each consisted of a pair of thymic lobes cut into 8-12 pieces with scissors; these pieces were injected ip through a 20-

*This work was supported by USPHS grants, 5 TI AI 13, AM-10145, AM-07529, AI-04152, and AI-33165.

†Postdoctoral Fellow, USPHS grant AM-33525.

‡Departments of Medicine and Pediatrics, University of Colorado Medical Center, Denver, Colorado 80220.

gauge needle. Chilled thymus cells suspensions were disrupted by sonication for 5 min. Thymectomy was done under secobarbital anesthesia one week before irradiation and cell transfer. The sternum was split, the fascia incised, and the thymus aspirated. Sham thymectomies were done similarly except that aspiration was omitted.

Irradiation was carried out either with a 250 kV$_p$GE Maxitron or a 220 kV$_p$ Westinghouse therapy unit. HVT for both units was 1.57 mm Cu. Radiation was delivered at 26r/min.

In most of the experiments the recipient mice were irradiated on day 0 and cells from normal donors together with SRBC were injected iv several hours later. On day 4 recipients were given an additional ip injection of SRBC. At sacrifice on day 8 the mice were bled and the sera from each group were pooled for hemolysin titrations. The recipient spleens were removed and passed through a stainless steel screen to make a single cell suspension. Plates were made according to the method of Jerne *et al.*[7] as described in detail elsewhere.[8] Plaques were counted with an image amplifier and the geometric mean number of plaque-forming cells (PFC) per

spleen for each group was calculated together with the 95% confidence limits.

Histological examination of tissues was made by fixation in Zenker-formalin, imbedding in methyl methacrylate, sectioning and staining with hematoxylin-eosin-azure.

Results

Tables 1 and 3 show that the enhanced effect of thymus-plus-marrow combinations over the sum of thymus and marrow taken singly may be demonstrated using the Jerne plaque-assay method. The importance of the route of injection of cells is shown by comparing groups A, B, and C in Table 1. If marrow was given iv thymus cells were effective if given either iv (A) or ip (C). If marrow was given ip, however, thymus cells iv were ineffective in augmenting the PFC in host spleens (B). The hemolysin titer of group B, on the other hand, was as great as A or C. We interpret this to indicate that antibody-producing cells were present in the body outside the spleen (see *Discussion*).

Table 2 shows that the sonicated cells of one thymus per day injected ip daily into each mouse for 8

TABLE 1

Immunocompetence of thymus-marrow cell combinations

Group	No. of animals	Cells received on day 0*	Results day 8	
			PFC/spleen (±95% limits)	Log$_2$ hemolysins
A	5	Thymus iv + marrow iv + SRBC iv	892 (276-2233)	4
B	5	Thymus iv + marrow ip + SRBC iv	13 (3-68)	5
C	5	Thymus ip + marrow iv + SRBC iv	468 (86-2570)	4
D	4	Thymus iv + SRBC iv	11 (1-125)	0
E	4	Marrow iv + SRBC iv	110 (19-624)	2
F	4	SRBC iv	2 (1-5)	0

*All recipients were given 855r 250 kV$_p$ X-rays on day 0 prior to injection of cells, and on day 4 were given SRBC ip. Doses of cells were: thymus (5.1×10^7) and marrow (3.6×10^7).

TABLE 2

Effects of suspensions of whole and sonicated mouse thymus cells

Group	No. of animals*	Cells received on day 0	Daily	PFC/spleen (±95% limits)	Log$_2$ hemolysins
				Results day 8	
A	5	Mouse thymus (3×10^7) iv Marrow (9.1×10^6) + SRBC iv		383 (180-812)	3
B	6	Marrow (9.1×10^6) + SRBC iv	Sonicated thymus ip†	90 (33-249)	0
C	5	Marrow (9.1×10^6) + SRBC iv		76 (15-375)	0
D	4	SRBC iv	Sonicated thymus ip†	3 (1-17)	0

*All recipient mice received 855r on day 0.
†Each mouse in Groups B and D received the cells of one thymus, sonicated ip daily.

TABLE 3

Effects of rat thymus cell suspensions

Group	No. of animals*	Cells received on day 0	Daily	PFC/spleen (±95% limits)	Log$_2$ hemolysins
				Results day 8	
A	4	Mouse thymus (5×10^7) iv Marrow (10^7) + SRBC iv		404 (107-962)	4
B	5	Rat thymus (3×10^7) iv Marrow (10^7) + SRBC iv	Rat thymus ip†	42 (14-131)	0
C	3	Mouse thymus (5×10^7) + SRBC iv		12 (3-55)	0
D	5	Mouse (10^7) + SRBC iv		16 (6-38)	0
E	5	Rat thymus (3×10^7) + SRBc iv	Rat thymus ip†	8 (1-45)	0
F	5	SRBC iv		2 (1-3)	0

*All recipients given 855r irradiation and SRBC as in Table 1.
†Each mouse in Groups B and E received 1/12 fresh rat thymus suspension ip daily, days 1-7.

days did not interact with iv marrow, while 3×10^7 iv thymus cells given once only on day 0 with iv marrow did result in production of significant antibody.

Table 3 shows that daily injections of suspensions of rat thymus cells ip were unable to substitute for a single iv injection of mouse thymus cells.

Other workers have shown that the immunocompetence of thymus cells was resistant to 500r *in vitro* and may be associated with the radioresistant thymic epithelial and reticular cells rather than the radiosensitive thymic small lymphocyte.[9] Our previous experiments, on the contrary, showed that the immunocompetence of the thymus component in this thy-

TABLE 4

Effects of minced normal or irradiated mouse thymus preparations

| Group | No. of animals | Cells received on day 0* | Results day 9 | |
			PFC/spleen (±95% limits)	Log$_2$ hemolysins
A	11	1 Normal thymus (minced) ip Marrow + SRBC iv	1006† (550-1756)	4.5†
B	8	1 Irradiated thymus (minced) ip Marrow + SRBC iv	209† (98-448)	1†
C	5	1 Normal thymus (minced) ip SRBC iv	15 (15-45)	0
D	5	Marrow + SRBC iv	69 (17-276)	0
E	3	SRBC iv	10 (2-47)	0

*All recipients were given 742-795r on day 0 prior to injection of cells, and on day 4 were given SRBC ip. Marrow dosage was 7.4-10.0 × 10^6. Group-B recipients received minced thymus from donors which had received 530r 2-3 hours before transfer of cells.
†Groups A and B are pooled from two experiments.

TABLE 5

Effect of thymectomy of hosts

| No. of animals | Treatment | Cells received on day 0* | Results day 8 | |
			PFC/spleen (±95% limits)	Log$_2$ hemolysins
7	Thymectomy	Thymus + marrow + SRBC	1810 (920-3557)	4
6	Sham thymectomy	Thymus + marrow + SRBC	1566 (926-2650)	4
3	None	SRBC	11 (2-48)	0

*Hosts were thymectomized or sham thymectomized on day 7. On day 0 hosts received 742r and then were given 5 × 10^7 thymus cells plus 10^7 marrow cells plus SRBC iv.

mus-marrow system was abolished by 500r *in vivo*.[2] One possible explanation for this discrepancy is that in using screened suspensions of thymus cells prepared after irradiation, a selected population of epithelial and reticular cells adhered to the stroma during preparation and was not passed through the screen nor injected into the recipient. To test this, minced whole thymus preparations, presumably containing all the cells of the thymus, were injected ip. While these minced preparations showed immunocompetence when injected with iv marrow (Table 4, A), similar minced thymus preparations from irradiated donors (530r) showed very little antibody production (B) when injected with iv marrow.

Thymectomy 1 week prior to the injection of cells (Table 5) had no significant effect on the antibody-forming potential of transfused thymus-marrow suspensions. Histological examination of tissue from the anterior mediastinum showed no thymic remnants in the thymectomized group.

Other experiments have shown that fetal liver may substitute for marrow since fetal liver-plus-thymus combinations were more immunogenic than the sum of both cell suspensions alone. Fetal liver suspensions were about half as effective as suspensions containing equal numbers of marrow cells.

Discussion

These data clearly demonstrate that the phenomenon of thymus-marrow "synergism" may be seen using the Jerne plaque assay on recipient spleens. This technique is more readily quantitated than the previously used technique of Playfair et al.[9] A drawback of the Jerne technique, as used here and in other experimental systems, is that it measures antibody production only in the tissue sampled, e.g., spleen in these experiments. Serum-antibody titers probably reflect antibody production in the *whole* animal to a greater degree than do spleen PFC. On the other hand, it is known that the antibody response of mice to iv SRBC is concentrated in the spleen. These factors, together with the known migration of antibody-forming cells between tissues,[8] complicate the interpretation of the numbers of spleen PFC. This is particularly obvious in Group B of Table 1 where the discrepancy between spleen PFC and serum hemolysins is large. We interpret this discrepancy to indicate that antibody is being formed by thymus- or marrow-cell descendants in tissues other than the spleen. Since this discrepancy was seen only with iv thymus and ip marrow, the route of injection of marrow becomes crucial. These data suggest that the marrow cells must be present within the spleen in order to get PFC in that organ while the thymus cells probably do not appear in the spleen in significant numbers. This conclusion is based on the findings that iv marrow is more effective in thymus-marrow interaction than ip marrow, and that dividing cells from iv marrow "home" to the spleen in 8 days.[11] Marrow cells given ip "home" to the spleen in much less efficient manner. Dividing thymus cells given iv do not appear in the recipient spleen in significant numbers,[11] and in our experiments, both ip thymus cells and ip minced thymus were effective in thymus-marrow synergism.

These data show that the thymus component of the "synergistic" combination must consist of living cells. Thymic cell suspensions from irradiated donors and thymic cell sonicates are ineffective.[9] In view of the large amount of sonicated thymic tissue given (Groups B and D in Table 2 received approximately

10 times more thymus tissue than did Group A), it is unlikely that a "humoral factor" is involved. The absence of activity following large daily doses of living rat thymus cells indicates a need for genetically related thymus cells. Recent experiments in our laboratory have shown that allogeneic (parental) thymus cells are less effective than are syngeneic cells.[12]

The failure of recipient thymectomy to alter the thymus-marrow synergism indicates that this synergism does not depend on the presence of recipient's thymus during the period following irradiation and cell transfer. The mechanism of the phenomenon of thymus-marrow interaction remains obscure.

Summary

The enhanced immunocompetence of transferred thymus-marrow cell combinations was demonstrated using the Jerne plaque assay method. Suspensions containing both thymus and marrow cells produced more antibody to sheep erythrocytes when transferred to irradiated syngeneic hosts and stimulated with antigen than could be accounted for by the summation of thymus- or marrow-cell activities considered singly. Living homologous thymus cells were required, since the following materials were incapable of interacting with isologous marrow cells: sonicated or irradiated (530r) mouse thymus cells or living rat thymus cells. The thymus of the host was not necessary for demonstrating thymus-marrow immunocompetence.

We are grateful to Jean Baughman for excellent technical assistance and to the Department of Radiology for aid in irradiating the mice.

REFERENCES

1. Claman, H.N., Chaperon, E.A., and Triplett, R.F.: Proc. Soc. Exptl. Biol. Med. **122:**1167 1966.
2. Claman, H.N., Chaperon, E.A., and Triplett, R.F.: J. Immunol. **97:**828, 1966.
3. Miller, J.F.A.P., Leuchars, E., Cross, A.M., and Dukor, P.: Ann. N.Y. Acad. Sci. **120:**205, 1964.
4. Globerson, W., and Auerbach, R.: J. Exptl. Med. **126:**223, 1967.
5. Cheng, V., and Trentin, J.J.: Federation Proc. **26:**641, 1967.
6. Davies, A.J.S., Leuchars, E., Wallis, V., Marchant, R., and Elliott, E.V.: Transplantation **5:**222, 1967.
7. Jerne, N.K., and Nordin, A.A.: Science **140:**405, 1955.
8. Chaperon, E.A., Selner, J.C., and Claman, H.N.: Immunol. **14:**553, 1968.

9. Miller, J.F.A.P., DeBurgh, P.M., Dukor, P., Grant, G., Allman, V., and House, W.: Clin. Exptl. Immunol. **1**:61, 1966.
10. Playfair, J.H.L., Papermaster, B.W., and Cole, L.J.: Science **149**:998, 1965.
11. Micklem, H.S., Ford, C.E., Evans, E.P., and Gray, J.: Proc. Royal Soc. Ser. B. **165**:78, 1966.
12. Chaperon, E.A., and Claman, H.N.: Federation Proc. **26**: 640, 1967.

≡ READING 4

This reading (from *Science* **102**:400-401, 1945) by Ray D. Owen, entitled "Immunogenetic Consequences of Vascular Anastomoses Between Bovine Twins," has been selected, as was the second reading, for its historical import. In this brief communication Professor Owen combines information that he retrieved from the scientific literature of the previous 30 years with the then unexplainable observations about blood group patterns in twin calves. The scientific harvest from this article was not simply the solution of this blood grouping problem but also the opening of new vistas in immunotolerance and immunogenetics. Today immunologists are actively involved in research on the subjects of skin and tissue grafting, histocompatibility testing, fetal immune tolerance, and the ontogeny of the immune response, any one of which would be an adequate reason for the inclusion of this article here.

IMMUNOGENETIC CONSEQUENCES OF VASCULAR ANASTOMOSES BETWEEN BOVINE TWINS*

Ray D. Owen

Almost thirty years have passed since Lillie[1] used the demonstrated union of the circulatory systems of twin bovine embryos of opposite sex to explain, on an endocrine basis, the frequent reproductive abnormalities of the female twin. Since the appearance of Lillie's paper, the freemartin, as the modified female is called, has become an important example of the effects of hormones on sex-differentiation and sexual development in mammals.[2] Consequences other than endocrinological of nature's experiment in parabiosis have, however, received little attention.

Estimates of the frequency of identical as compared with fraternal twinning indicate that the former is relatively rare in cattle.[3] Tests for inherited cellular antigens in the blood of more than eighty pairs of bovine twins show, however, that in the majority of these pairs the twins have identical blood types. Identity of blood types between full sibs not twins is infrequent, as might be expected from the large number of different, genetically controlled antigens[4,5] (now approximately 40) identified in the tests. If, therefore, the frequent identity of blood types in twin pairs can be explained neither as the result of monozygotic twinning nor as chance identity between fraternal twins, nor as the sum of these two factors, it is evident that some mechanism is operating to produce frequent phenotypic identity of blood types in genetically dissimilar twins. The vascular anastomosis between bovine twins, known to be a common occurrence,[1] provides an explanation.

Three additional, independent sources of evidence help to define the action of this mechanism. (1) One twin sire failed to transmit to any of his twenty progeny certain of the antigens found in his blood. In other words, the genotype of this bull as determined from his progeny appeared to lack factors responsible for some of the antigens found in his phenotype. Tests showed that cells containing these antigens could have been derived from his twin, whose genotype did contain the necessary factors. (2) In a case of superfecundation in cattle, involving twins of opposite sex and by different sires,[6] the twins had identical blood types, each possessing two antigens the genetic factors for which could not have come from his own sire or from the dam. Cells containing those critical antigens could in each case have been derived from the co-twin. (3) It has been demonstrated, by a simple immunological technique developed for this purpose, that there is a mixture of two distinct types of erythrocytes in certain twins.

*From the Departments of Genetics (No. 346) and Veterinary Science, University of Wisconsin, in cooperation with the Bureau of Animal Industry, U.S. Department of Agriculture. This is part of a program aided by grants from the American Guernsey Cattle Club, the Holstein-Friesian Association of America, the Rockefeller Foundation and the Wisconsin Alumni Research Foundation. Appreciated contributions to various phases of the investigation have been made by Professor M.R. Irwin, C.J. Stormont and Mary W. Ycas. This study has been possible only through the generous cooperation of workers at many state experiment stations and of numerous private breeders of cattle.

These facts are consistent with the conclusion that an interchange of cells between bovine twin embryos occurred as a result of vascular anastomoses. Since many of the twins in this study were adults when they were tested, and since the interchange of formed erythrocytes alone between embryos occurs as a result of vascular anastomosient modification of the variety of circulating cells, it is further indicated that the critical interchange is of embryonal cells ancestral to the erythrocytes of the adult animal.[7] These cells are apparently capable of becoming established in the hemapoietic tissues of their co-twin hosts and continuing to provide a source of blood cells distinct from those of the host, presumably throughout his life.

Several interesting problems in the fields of genetics, immunology and development are suggested by these observations. Most of them are still largely speculative and will not be considered here. An application that may be mentioned is the tool now provided by the blood tests for selecting, with a high degree of reliability, those heifers, born twin with bulls, that are potentially not freemartins but normal, fertile individuals. A heifer whose blood type is the same as her twin brother's will very probably be a freemartin, while a difference in even a single antigen between twins of opposite sex may indicate that vascular anastomosis did not occur, and therefore that the heifer will be normal. Thus clinical observations on the heifer alone, probably not always reliable when the heifer is young, can be supplemented by an objective laboratory test applicable as soon as the twins are born. Possible limitations of this application, as well as a more complete presentation of the data and further discussion of the implications of the present study, will be included in another paper.

REFERENCES

1. Lillie, F.R.: Science, **43:**611-613, 1916.
2. See "Sex and Internal Secretions," edited by Edgar Allen (Baltimore, 1939, Williams and Wilkins) for general discussions of and references to the literature on the freemartin.
3. Sanders, D.: Zeit. fur Zuchtung B, **32:**223-268, 1935.
4. Ferguson, L.C.: J. Immunol., **40:**213-242, 1940.
5. Ferguson, L.C., Stormont, C., and Irwin, M.R.: J. Immunol., **44:**147-164, 1942.
6. A description and discussion of this case will be published elsewhere by Mr. B.H. Roche, who called it to our attention and provided us with blood samples from the animals involved.
7. Cf. Jordan, H.E.: Physiol. Rev., **22:**375-384, 1942.

≣ READING 5

The importance of complement in nonhemolytic reactions, in company with the unraveling of its structural complexities, has been the center of research with complement over the past decade. During this same period considerable debate has existed as to how lymphoid cells and monocytes participated with antibody and complement in ADCC reactions. In this report from *Science* **192:**563-565, 1976 (copyright 1976, the American Association for the Advancement of Science), a system of ADCC attack on sheep red blood cells, which could be blocked by normal IgG, is released from this block by coating the target cells with complement and antibody. Thus the complement receptor of the ADCC effector cells, in an as yet unidentified fashion, generates with C3b a lytic attack that can overcome the normal antibody blockade. This may be important in the interpretation of some aspects of transplantation and tumor immunity as well as the area of autoimmune disease.

COMPLEMENT-DEPENDENT IMMUNOGLOBULIN G RECEPTOR FUNCTION IN LYMPHOID CELLS

JUAN CARLOS SCORNICK*

Abstract. *Lymphoid cells are unable to lyse antibody-coated target cells in the presence of normal immunoglobulin G (IgG), presumably because their surface receptors for IgG are blocked. However, when target cells are sensitized with antibodies and complement, IgG receptors are unblocked and cytotoxicity occurs even in the presence of normal IgG. Thus, IgG receptors may function in vivo despite the relatively high concentrations of IgG in serum and interstitial fluid.*

Cell-mediated cytotoxity induced by immunoglobulin G (IgG) antibodies to target cell (antibody-dependent cell-mediated cytotoxicity, ADCC) has been

*Hematology Section, Department of Clinical Chemistry and Laboratory Medicine, University of Texas System Cancer Center, M.D. Anderson Hospital and Tumor Institute, Houston, Texas 77025. Present address: Department of Pathology, University of Florida College of Medicine, Gainesville, Fla. 32610.

advocated as a possible mechanism involved in allograft rejection,[1] viral infections,[2] tumor immunity,[3] and autoimmune diseases.[4] However, no direct evidence of its participation in vivo has been obtained. Furthermore, ADCC is inhibited by normal IgG[5] at concentrations below those in normal serum or interstitial fluid.[6] I now report an in vitro model in which ADCC is induced even in the presence of inhibitory concentrations of IgG, providing an experimental basis for a possible in vivo function of the IgG receptors.

Effector cells were obtained from spleens surgically removed from patients undergoing staging laparotomies.[7] A cell suspension was prepared and mononuclear cells were concentrated by Ficoll-Hypaque centrifugation.[8] Sheep red blood cells (SRBC), used as target cells, were labeled with 100 μc of ^{51}Cr ($Na_2{}^{51}CrO_4$, New England Nuclear)[9] and treated with different antibody preparations. The following groups of sensitized target cells were prepared: EA-G, SRBC coated with IgG antibodies;[10] EA-M, SRBC sensitized with IgM antibodies; EAC-M and EAC-G, SRBC sensitized with IgM or IgG antibodies and complement (C); EA-M-G, SRBC sensitized with IgM first and subsequently with IgG; EAC-M-G, SRBC sensitized with IgM and C and subsequently with IgG.

Effector cells (30×10^6) and target cells (2×10^6) were placed in plastic petri dishes (35 by 10 mm; Falcon Plastics) in 1 ml of Ham's F-10 medium (Grand Island) supplemented with 20 percent fetal calf serum and 50 μg of gentamicin (Schering) per milliliter. Inhibitors were added prior to the addition of the target cells. The cell mixtures were incubated (on a rocking platform) in an atmosphere of 5 percent CO_2 at 37 ° C for 18 hours and the percentage of cytotoxicity was determined.[11] Values were expressed as specific cytotoxicity after subtraction of nonspecific lysis obtained in the absence of spleen cells. Nonspecific lysis was determined for each type of target cell (EA-G, EAC-G, EAC-M, and others).

Lymphoid cells carry on their surface receptors for the third component of complement (C3), which enable them to bind SRBC coated with C.[12] However, such a binding does not induce lysis of the target cell, an observation that has led to the suggestion that the C3 receptor does not have a major role in

ADCC.[13] The following results indicate that the C3 receptor does have a major role since it allows the induction of ADCC in the presence of inhibitory concentrations of serum IgG. Lysis of EA-G is inhibited by human serum at dilutions of 10^{-2} and 10^{-1}. However, lysis of EAC-G is inhibited to a much lesser extent, and a significant degree of cytotoxicity is still observed at the higher concentrations of serum (Fig. 1). The same effect is observed when C is bound to the erythrocyte by IgM antibody, and IgG antibody is added later (EAC-M-G); the lysis of EA-G is not affected by the simultaneous presence of IgM (EA-M-G). Similar results were obtained in four independent experiments.[14]

An excess of free molecules of serum IgG may block the IgG receptors but not the C3 receptors. However, since the binding through C3 receptors does not trigger lysis of the target cells, an explanation must be offered for the cytotoxicity of EAC-G (but not of EA-G) obtained in the presence of serum IgG. Taking into account that the IgG antibody must be present on the target cell for the induction of cy-

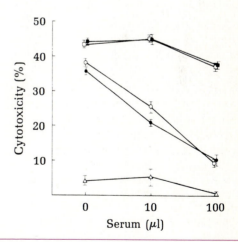

FIG. 1

Inhibition of cytotoxicity by human serum. Human serum, obtained from normal donors, was pooled, inactivated by heat, and absorbed with SRBC. Cytotoxicity was induced by human spleen lymphoid cells against SRBC sensitized in different ways. △, EAC-M; ●, EA-G; ○, EA-M-G; ■, EAC-G; □, EAC-M-G. The total volume of the cell mixture was 1 ml. The bars correspond to the range of duplicate determinations.

totoxicity and that the binding of free monomeric IgG molecules to the IgG receptors is weak,[15] then it can be postulated that the intimate contact between effector and target cell, brought about through the C3 receptor, promotes the displacement of the free IgG from the lymphocyte receptor by the IgG antibody bound to the target cell, making possible the occurrence of ADCC. If this hypothesis is correct, blocking of the IgG receptors with soluble antigen-antibody complexes, whose binding with the IgG receptor is stronger than that of free IgG (and more difficult to displace), should lead to a pronounced inhibition of the lysis of EAC-G.

The following experiments support this possibility. Serum from a rabbit immunized against *Candida albicans* antigens[16] produced significant inhibition of cytotoxicity of EA-G, but little effect on the lysis of EAC-G (Fig. 2, *A*). However, when the antigen was also added to the cell mixture, cytotoxicity for both EA-G and EAC-G was inhibited (Fig. 2, *B*). Antigen

alone did not inhibit cytotoxicity. In other experiments, antigen-antibody complexes did not inhibit binding of EAC-G.[17]

The foregoing results suggest that the antigen-antibody complexes do not block the C3 receptors, and hence binding of EAC-G ensues unaffected. Antigen-antibody complexes do not block IgG receptors, in a reaction not easily reversible; and lysis of target cells does not occur in their presence. Thus, the lysis of EAC-G obtained in the presence of monomeric serum IgG represents an induction of the classical ADCC, generated through the IgG receptors.

Most cells that carry IgG receptors (B lymphocytes, granulocytes, monocytes, macrophages), which are efficient effector cells for ADCC,[11,18] also carry C receptors.[12] This may be a structural arrangement designed for a cooperative function of C and IgG receptors.[19]

In conclusion, the classical mechanism of ADCC

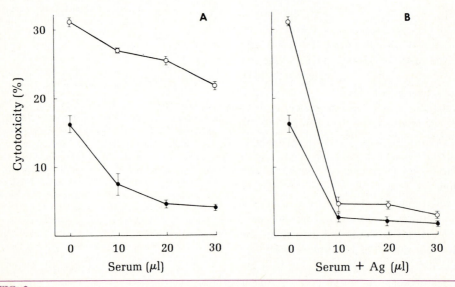

FIG. 2

Inhibition of cytotoxicity by rabbit serum and antigen-antibody complexes. Cytotoxicity was induced by human spleen lymphoid cells in a total volume of 1 ml. The target cells used were as follows: ●, EA-G; ○, EAC-G. Lysis of EAC-M was 2.2 percent. **A,** Effect of increasing concentrations of rabbit antiserum to *Candida albicans* antigens. **B,** Effect of the rabbit antiserum plus equal volume of *Candida albicans* antigen. No inhibition of cytoxicity was observed with 10, 20, or 30 μl of the antigen preparation in the absence of the rabbit antiserum. The bars correspond to the range of duplicate determinations.

may operate in the presence of normal IgG, provided that both IgG antibody and C are present on the target cell. The function of the C3 receptor is to promote the binding of effector and target cells, generating favorable conditions for the interaction of the IgG antibody and the lymphocyte receptor, and overcoming the inhibitory effect of normal IgG.

The occurrence of IgG antibodies and the presence of C on target cells or tissues are features frequently found in some autoimmune diseases[4] and in allograft reactions.[20] Consequently, the above results suggest that the participation of ADCC in those situations is not only possible but is also likely to occur.

REFERENCES AND NOTES

1. Strom, T.B., Tilney, N.L., Carpenter, C.B., and Busch, G.J.: N. Engl. J. Med. **292:**1257, 1975; Ting, A., and Terasaki, P.I.: Transplantation **18:**371, 1974.
2. Shore, S.L., Nahmias, A.J., Starr, S.E., Wood, P.A., and McFarlin, D.E.: Nature (London) **251:**350, 1974.
3. Landazuri, M.O., Kedar, E., Fahey, J.L.: J. Natl. Cancer Inst. **52:**147, 1974.
4. Steblay, R.W., and Rudofsky, U.: Science **180:**966, 1973; Rudofsky, U.H., Steblay, R.W., and Pollara, B.: Clin. Immunol. Immunopathol. **3:**396, 1975.
5. MacLennan, I.C.M.: Clin. Exp. Immunol. **10:**275, 1972; Holm, G., Engwall, E., Hammarström, S., and Natvig, J.B.: Scand. J. Immunol. **3:**173, 1974; Scornik, J.C., Cosenza, H., Lee, W., Köhler, H., and Rowley, D.A.: J. Immunol. **113:**1510, 1974; Scornik, J.C., Salinas, M.C., and Drewinko, B.: ibid. **115:**901, 1975.
6. Poulsen, H.L.: Scand. J. Clin. Lab. Invest. **34:**119, 1974. Poulsen reported an IgG concentration of approximately 10 mg/ml in serum and 6 mg/ml in interstitial fluid.
7. Nine spleens were used in this study, all from patients with Hodgkin's disease of the nodular sclerosing or mixed cellularity type. Six spleens were macroscopically and microscopically normal. In three cases the spleen was involved, and areas without macroscopic nodules were used to prepare the cell suspensions. Two patients received radiotherapy 1 month before splenectomy; the remaining patients were untreated at the time of the study. Experiments were also done with mouse spleen cells as effector cells; the results were similar to those obtained with human cells.
8. Böyum, A.: Scand. J. Clin. Lab. Invest. **21:** (Suppl. 97), 1, 1968. The cells collected at the interphase were washed three times with Hanks solution before use. Viability was 85 to 90 percent, and the cell population comprised more than 90 percent lymphoid cells, the rest being mainly monocytes and granulocytes.
9. Perlmann, P., and Perlmann, H.: Cell Immunol. **1:**300, 1970.
10. Packed SRBC (50 μl) were incubated with 0.5 ml of the appropriate dilution of antibodies for 15 minutes at 37° C and then washed three times. The IgG (7S) fraction of a rabbit antibody to SRBC was used at 1:400 dilution, whereas a rabbit antibody to SRBC stromata [the immunoglobulin M (IgM) fraction] was used at a 1:120 dilution. Both preparations were obtained from Cordis, (Miami, Florida). A 1:5 dilution of mouse serum in Hanks solution, which was the source of complement, was added for 30 minutes at 37° C to the sensitized RBC for the preparation of EAC.
11. Scornik, J.C., and Cosenza, H.: J. Immunol. **113:**1527, 1974. The content (1 ml total volume) of each petri dish was placed in a tube (tube A), and the saline (1 ml) used to rinse the petri dish was added. The tube was centrifuged, and the supernatant was placed in another tube (tube B). The cells remaining in the petri dishes were removed with 2 ml of distilled water and placed in tube A. The radioactivity in both tubes was counted in a well-type gamma counter and the percentage of cytotoxicity was calculated by dividing the radioactivity of tube B by the total radioactivity (tube A + tube B) and multiplying by 100.
12. Nussenzweig, V.: Adv. Immunol. **19:**217, 1974.
13. Van Boxel, J.A., Paul, W.E., Green, I., and Frank, M.M.: J. Immunol. **112:**398, 1974; Perlmann, P., Perlmann, H., and Müller-Eberhard, H.J.: J. Exp. Med. **141:**287, 1975.
14. Experiments where the human serum concentrations were more than 50 percent are not reported because they produced agglutination of SRBC (despite repeated absorptions). However, purified human IgG at 4 mg/ml produced complete inhibition of lysis of EA-G but not of EAC-G.
15. Cerottini, J.C., and Brunner, K.T.: Adv. Immunol. **18:**67, 1974.
16. Antigen and antiserum were provided by Dr. Roy Hopfer. Soluble *Candida albicans* antigens were prepared by mechanically disrupting the organisms and discarding insoluble particles by centrifugation and filtration through a 0.22-μm Millipore filter. Rabbit antiserum was obtained after repeated immunizations with the antigen preparation in complete Freund's adjuvant. The rabbit antiserum was inactivated by heat and absorbed with SRBC before use. The antigen preparation was used at a 1:20 dilution, which was optimal for obtaining precipitation lines in counterelectrophoresis.
17. Spleen cells attached to plastic petri dishes treated with poly-L-lysine [Kennedy, J.C., and Axelrod, M.A.: Immunol. **20:**253, 1971] were incubated with ^{51}Cr-labeled target cells (E, EA-G, EA-M, EAC-M, EAC-G) for 1 hour at 37° C in a rocking platform. Each petri dish was then washed three times with saline and immersed three more times in a beaker with saline. The target cells that remained attached to the spleen cells were lysed with distilled water, and radioactivity was measured in a well-type gamma counter [Scornik, J.C., and Drewinko, B.: J. Immunol. **115:**1223, 1975].
18. Van Boxel, J.A., Paul, W.E., Frank, M.M., and Green, I.: J. Immunol. **110:**1027, 1973; Gale, R.R., and Zighelboim, J.: ibid. **113:**1793, 1974; Holm, G., Engwall, E., Hammar-

ström, W., and Natvig, J.B.: Scand. J. Immunol. **3**:173, 1974.

19. A similar cooperative effect has been described in the phagocytosis of erythrocytes by human monocytes [Huber, H., Polley, M.J., Linscott, W.D., Fudenberg, H.H., and Müller-Eberhard, H.J.: Science **162**:1281, 1968] and mouse polymorphonuclear leukocytes [Mantovani, B.: J. Immunol. **115**:15, 1975.]

20. D'Apice, A.J., and Morris, P.J.: Transplantation **18**:20, 1974; Porter, K.A.: Transpl. Proc. **6** (Suppl. 1):79, 1974.

21. I thank B. Drewinko for his support for this work and A. Gage for technical assistance. Supported by NIH grant CA 17072-01.

22. August 1975; revised 16 January 1976.

≣ READING 6

"Barbiturates: Radioimmunoassay" by Sydney Spector and Edward J. Flynn is an article that reveals the simplicity by which immunoassays of great sensitivity can be developed for low molecular weight compounds of biologic importance. This article illustrates by chemical formulas how modification of the barbituric acid compound was necessary before it could be coupled to a carrier protein by carbodiimide conjugation and used as a hapten-antigen conjugate for the production of antisera. Fig. 2 presents the data for the determinations that were necessary preludes to the development of the radioassay itself, that is, the titrations of antiserum and of hapten against varying concentrations of hapten and antiserum, respectively. The data precisely fit the theoretic curves. In the complete test some variance from a straight line was observed in determining the concentration of barbiturates in biologic fluids, but this is not greater than observed by other methods or in other RIAs. The results reveal that the test is 20 to 200 times more sensitive than other procedures.

This article is reprinted from *Science* **174**:1036-1038, 1971 (copyright 1971, the American Association for the Advancement of Science).

BARBITURATES: RADIOIMMUNOASSAY

SYDNEY SPECTOR AND EDWARD J. FLYNN*

Abstract. *The development of a radioimmunoassay for barbiturate is described. The barbiturate is made antigenic by coupling it to a protein, bovine gamma globulin. The radioimmunoassay can measure as little as 5 nanograms of barbiturate.*

For the study of the metabolism of barbiturates, quantitative assays that are rapid, sensitive, specific, and reliable even for small amounts of barbiturates would be most advantageous. Methods now available are suited for qualitative and quantitative analysis only if an adequate sample of biological tissue, 1 to 5 ml, is available.[1] In addition, these methods require solvent extraction[1] and, in some instances, filtration and evaporation.[2] Gas chromatography and spectrophotometry are sensitive to 10 μg/ml but require solvent extraction.[3] Immunologic methods for assaying polypeptides, hormones, and drugs have been reported.[4] We have conjugated a barbiturate to bovine gamma globulin (BGG), produced antibodies against the barbiturate hapten, and developed a radioimmunoassay capable of measuring nanogram levels of barbiturates.

Antibodies were induced by immunization of rabbits with a barbiturate-protein conjugate. The barbiturate, 5-allyl-5-(1-carboxyisopropyl) barbituric acid, was converted to 5-allyl-5-(1-*p*-nitro-phenyloxycarbonylisopropyl) barbituric acid by reacting the free base (10 mg) with *p*-nitrophenol (12 mg) in *N,-N*-dimethylformamide for 24 hours at 4° C. The 5-allyl-5-(1-*p*-nitrophenyloxycarbonylisopropyl) barbituric acid was coupled to BGG (10 mg) in a glycerin-water solution (1:1, by volume) in the presence of dicyclohexylcarbodiimide (5 mg).[5] The mixture was incubated overnight at 4° C, and the protein-hapten complex was dialyzed against distilled water. Conjugation of the barbiturate to the protein carrier was confirmed by the increase in absorbance at 202 nm of the barbiturate-BGG conjugate as compared to control BGG solutions. From the molar extinction coefficient of the barbiturate (E_m = 19,500), the degree of substitution was estimated to be 2 to 3 moles of barbiturate per mole of protein. New Zealand albino rabbits were immunized with 1 mg of barbiturate-BGG (Fig. 1). The immunogen (100 μg) in phosphate-buffered saline, *p*H 7.2, was emulsified with an equal volume of complete Freund's adjuvant. The initial dose was 1.6 ml, 0.4 ml injected into each footpad. A booster injection of 100 μg of antigen in adjuvant was given every 6 to 8 weeks,

*Department of Physiological Chemistry, Pharmacology Section, Roche Institute of Molecular Biology, Nutley, New Jersey 07110.

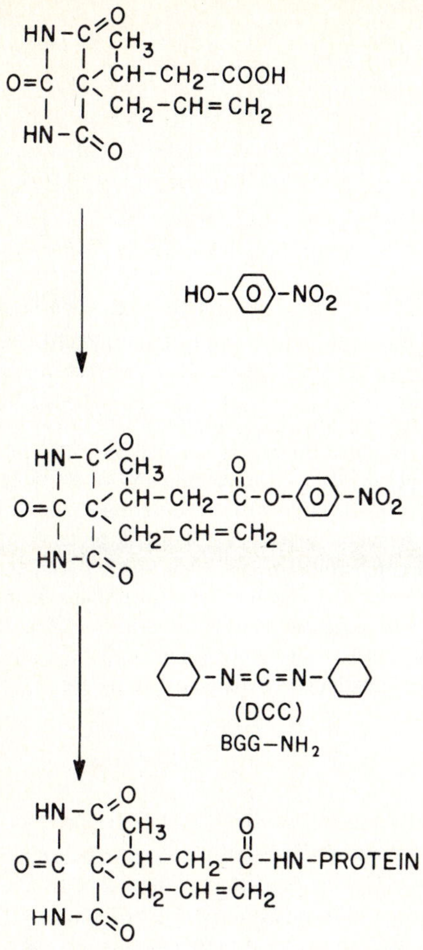

FIG. 1

Synthesis of the barbiturate antigen. *DCC,* Dicyclohexyl-carbodiimide; *BGG,* bovine gamma globulin.

25 µg in each of the footpads. Blood was collected 5 to 7 days after booster injections and the serum was examined for antibodies to barbiturates.

Various dilutions of antiserums were incubated with 8×10^{-4} µc of [^{14}C]pentobarbital sodium (New England Nuclear, 4.13 mc/mmole), approximately 1000 count/min, at 4° C overnight. After incubation, a neutral saturated ammonium sulfate solution (volume equal to incubation medium) was added to all tubes. The precipitate, containing pentobarbital bound to antibody, was washed two times with an equal volume of 50 percent saturated ammonium sul-

fate and then dissolved in 0.5 ml of Nuclear-Chicago Solubilizer,[6] and the radioactivity was counted in a liquid scintillation spectrometer (Packard Tri-Carb). While normal rabbit serum failed to bind labeled pentobarbital, the serum from immunized rabbits bound 75 to 80 percent of the added labeled pentobarbital, and there was a linear relationship between bound [^{14}C]pentobarbital and the concentration of added antibody (Fig. 2, *A*). When variable amounts of [^{14}C]pentobarbital were added to a constant amount of antibody, there was a linear relationship between added and bound [^{14}C]pentobarbital (Fig. 2, *B*).

The radioimmunoassay depends on competition between unlabeled pentobarbital and a standard of [^{14}C]pentobarbital for combination with barbiturate antibodies in rabbit antisera. A tube that contained radioactive pentobarbital and antiserum, but no unlabeled pentobarbital, measured maximum radioactivity bound to antibody. The addition of increasing amounts of unlabeled pentobarbital to fixed amounts of [^{14}C]pentobarbital and antiserum resulted in competitive inhibition of binding of labeled pentobarbital by antibody (Fig. 3). The similarity of the standard curves obtained when pentobarbital was added in plasma, urine, or buffered saline indicates that there are no interfering substances in the two body fluids. In addition, the data demonstrate the sensitivity of the method. Pentobarbital (5 ng) in a sample volume of 10 µl caused a 20 percent inhibition of binding of the labeled compound. The same amount of pentobarbital can be assayed in a larger sample volume (200 µl), which increases the sensitivity 20-fold.

The antibody bound barbital, pentobarbital and phenobarbital equally well. These three compounds differ only by the substituents on the C-5 position. Since BGG was conjugated to the barbituric acid moiety at C-5 it is understandable that the antibody fails to differentiate between these barbituric acids. In contrast, at equimolar concentration of hexobarbital or thiopental the antibody bound these compounds to a lesser degree. These compounds have different substituents at either position 2 or 3 in the barbituric acid ring. Thus, the urea portion of the ring may be critical in determining antibody specificity.

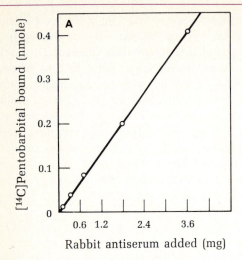

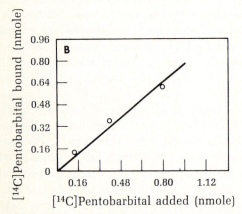

FIG. 2

Binding of [^{14}C]pentobarbital by rabbit antiserum. In **A**, varying amounts of antiserum (milligrams of protein per reaction tube) were added to a constant amount of [^{14}C]pentobarbital (0.8 nmole). In **B**, varying amounts of [^{14}C]pentobarbital were added to a constant amount of rabbit antiserum (3.5 mg of protein per reaction tube).

The barbiturate-BGG antigen was effective in eliciting antibodies against barbituric acid derivatives. We believe that this is the first report of the experimental production of antibodies capable of recognizing barbiturates. The radioimmunoassay technique reported here is rapid and extremely sensitive, and should be useful for the determination of barbiturate concentrations in biological tissues and

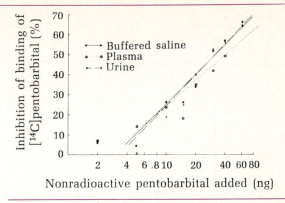

FIG. 3

Inhibition of binding of [^{14}C]pentobarbital to rabbit antiserum by nonradioactive pentobarbital in buffered saline (●—●), plasma (○ · · · ○), or urine (X——X). Incubation medium consisted of 0.10 ml of normal rabbit serum, 0.10 ml of rabbit antiserum (0.4 mg of protein), 0.01 ml of [^{14}C]pentobarbital (0.1 nmole), and 0.01 ml of either standard unlabeled pentobarbital (1 to 100 ng) or unknown sample and sufficient phosphate-buffered saline (0.01M phosphate, pH 7.4) to make a final volume of 0.50 ml. Lines of regression were calculated by the method of least squares.

fluids. Theoretically, since metabolic products with changes at the C-5 position may also be detected by the antibody, our procedure, coupled with a solvent extraction, could measure both total concentration of barbiturate and its hydroxylated metabolites. Antibodies directed against steroid haptens[7] and digitalis[8] have been reported to modify the physiological actions of these agents, and it would be interesting to determine whether antibodies against barbiturates interfere with the pharmacological effects of barbiturates.

REFERENCES

1. Koppanyi, T., Dille, J.M., Murphy, W.S., and Krop, S.: J. Amer. Pharm. Ass. **23**:1074, 1934; Jailer, J.W., and Goldbaum, L.R.: J. Lab. Clin. Med. **31**:1344 1946; Deininger, R.: Arzneim. Forsch. **5**:472, 1955.
2. Parker, K.D., and Kirk, P.L.: Anal. Chem. **33**:1378, 1961; Martin, H.F., and Driscoll, J.L.: ibid. **38**:345, 1966.
3. Anders, M.W.: ibid. **38**:1945, 1966; Walker, J.T., Fisher, R.S., and McHugh, J.J.: Amer. J. Clin. Pathol. **18**:451, 1948; Hellman, L.B., Shettles, L.B., and Strau, H.: J. Biol. Chem.

148:293, 1943; Goldbaum, L.R.: J. Pharmacol. Exp. Ther. **94:**68, 1948.

4. Yalow, R.S., Glick, S.M., Roth, J., and Berson, S.A.: J. Clin. Endocrinol. Metab. **24:**1219, 1964; Utiger, R.D.: J. Clin. Invest. **44:**1277, 1965; Berson, S.A., and Yalow, R.S.: ibid. **38:**1966, 1959; Vallotton, M.B., Page, L.B., and Haber, E.: Nature **215:**714, 1967; Spector, S., and Parker, C.W.: Science **168:**1347, 1970.

5. Ott Chemical Company, Muskegan, Michigan.

6. Amersham/Searle.

7. Goodfriend, L., and Sehon, A.H.: Can. J. Biochem. Physiol. **39:**941, 1961; Neri, R.O., Tolksdorf, S., Belser, S.M., Erlanger, F., Agate, J., and Lieberman, S.: Endocrinology **74:**593, 1964.

8. Butler, V.P.: N. Engl. J. Med. **283:**1150, 1970.

9. Supported by a postdoctoral fellowship (E.J.F.) from Hoffmann-La Roche Inc.

☰ READING 7

This reading indicates some of the known facts and future possibilities about interferon. Drs. Norris and Loh in their article "Coxsackievirus Myocarditis: Prophylaxis and Therapy with an Interferon Stimulator," from *Proceedings of the Society of Experimental Biology and Medicine* **142:**133-136, 1973, utilized double-stranded polyinosinic acid–polycytidylic acid (poly I · C) as an interferon inducer in mice. This complex is one of the most commonly used inducers, and the prevention of cytopathic effects of vesicular stomatitis virus in tissue culture, which these authors also used, is a common indicator for interferon. After establishing that the degree of pathology resulting from Coxsackie virus injection in young mice was related to the virus dose (except for large doses of virus), the authors present data to illustrate the protective effect of a single dose of poly I · C given prior to and as late as 1 day after virus injection but not if given later. Interferon levels were determined at various intervals after injection of the inducer. The results indicate high levels of interferon were present in blood within 4 hours and began to wane by 48 hours, as expected. Application of this type of information to domestic animals prior to exposure to certain disease agents, as in shipping fever in cattle, is a real possibility, although poly I · C is perhaps too toxic a compound for human use.

COXSACKIEVIRUS MYOCARDITIS: PROPHYLAXIS AND THERAPY WITH AN INTERFERON STIMULATOR* (36975)

DAVID NORRIS AND PHILIP C. LOH†

It is becoming increasingly evident that viral infections play a significant role in the etiology of heart diseases.[1-3] Coxsackie B viruses, which have been implicated as responsible agents in fatal myocarditis in the newborn[4-6] as well as adult myocarditis and pericarditis,[3,7-9] are currently thought to be the commonest cause of virus-induced heart illness in man.[3,9] The susceptibility of weanling mice to myocarditis in a nonlethal, experimental coxsackievirus B-3 infection[10] has provided us with a host-virus model which imitates the coxsackievirus-human relationship.

Numerous studies have demonstrated that interferon (IF) and interferon inducers are highly effective when used prophylactically in a variety of experimental viral infections.[11-14] The present investigation was conducted to determine the effect of treatment with an IF inducer polyinosinic · polycytidylic acid (poly I · poly C) on myocarditis produced during an experimental coxsackievirus B-3 infection of mice.

Materials and methods

Mice

Thirteen-day-old general purpose Swiss mice obtained from the Animal Colony, University of Hawaii, were used in all experiments.

Virus

Coxsackievirus B-3 was obtained from the Department of Health, State of Hawaii, and was passed three times in suckling mice (<72 hr) by the intraperitoneal route (ip). A stock 20% carcass suspension was prepared after the final passage and yielded a LD_{50} of $10^{-5 \cdot 3}$/ml in 1-day-old mice inoculated ip.

*Supported in part by a Biomedical Sciences Grant from the University Research Council.
†Virus Laboratory, Department of Microbiology, University of Hawaii, Honolulu, Hawaii 96822.

Histological examination and scoring of lesions

The hearts were removed and examined microscopically. They were then fresh frozen and cut into 8 μm sections. Each 30th section was mounted and stained with haematoxylin and eosin. The severity of microscopic lesions was scored as described by Grodums and Dempster[15] with 1+ = lesions involving <25% of the myocardium, 2+ = lesions involving 50% of the myocardium, 3+ = lesions involving 75% of the myocardium, and 4+ = most of the myocardium has undergone pathological change. Susceptibility of each experimental group was graded on a percentile basis using "cumulative lesion score," divided by "maximum possible score" as described by Rytel and Kilbourne.[16]

Interferon inducer

A commercial sterile preparation of double-stranded poly I · poly C obtained from Microbiology Associates, Bethesda, MD, was used for interferon induction.

Interferon assay

Serum IF concentrations were determined by the viral plaque reduction method[17] employing vesicular stomatitis virus (VSV) and mouse L cells.

Results and discussion

Testing host-virus system and determination of virus dose

To establish the degree of myocarditis to be expected, and to determine the appropriate virus challenge dose to be used in interferon studies, groups of 4-6 mice were inoculated ip with 0.5 ml of varying dilutions of the stock virus suspension. After 7 days, the mice were sacrificed and the hearts were examined. The affected hearts with gross damage exhibited yellow-white streaks or patches on the ventricular surface. Microscopic examination revealed focal areas of necrosis and degeneration of the myocardium with a mononuclear cell infiltrate. The results of histological examination of a representative experiment are shown in Table 1.

All of the mice challenged with virus dilutions to 10^{-3} developed myocarditis with the most severe damage occurring when the 10^{-2} dilution was used. However, animals inoculated with the higher concentration of virus (10^{-1} or undiluted) showed less damage. The reason for the decreased severity of damage with the lower dilutions is unknown. It can be speculated that at these dilutions the virus suspension contains a factor(s) which either passively inhibited the viral infection or induced a host response which interfered with the infectious process. This "factor(s)," which could be either IF in the inoculum or IF-induction by the large virus inoculum, is no longer effective at the higher dilutions. Also, it is possible that inoculation of high concentrations of virus may induce early antibody formation which may play a role here.[18]

Effect of poly I · C on virus induced myocarditis

To determine the prophylactic and therapeutic effect of poly I · C on coxsackievirus B-3–induced myocarditis, groups of 4-6 mice were given a single 150 μg dose of the interferon inducer ip at intervals from 48 hr prior to, to 96 hr after virus challenge. The challenge dose consisted of 0.5 ml of a 10^{-2} dilution of the stock virus suspension administered by the ip route. Seven days after challenge the mice were sacrificed and the frequency and severity of histological lesions of the hearts were examined.

The results of a representative experiment shown

TABLE 1

Degree of myocarditis in mice inoculated intraperitoneally with (0.5 ml) varying dilutions of virus

Dilution of stock virus suspension	Frequency and severity* of histological lesions					
	−	1+	2+	3+	4+	Score %†
Undiluted	0	0	4	2	0	58
10^{-1}	0	0	1	0	3	87
10^{-2}	0	0	0	1	3	94
10^{-3}	0	0	2	3	0	65
10^{-4}	2	2	0	1	0	25

*Severity is graded as follows: 1+ = lesions involving <25% of the myocardium, 2+ = lesions involving 50% of the myocardium, 3+ = lesions involving 75% of the myocardium, 4+ = most of the myocardium involved.
†The score percentage was calculated according to the method of Rytel and Kilbourne.[16]

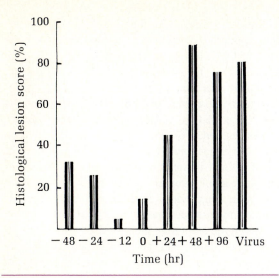

FIG. 1

Comparison of lesion severity in mice inoculated ip with 150 μg of poly I · C at intervals from 48 hr prior to, to 96 hr after challenge with 0.5 ml of 10^{-2} dilution of the stock coxsackievirus B-3 (ip). Histological lesions were graded as described in the text. Score percentage for each experimental group was calculated according to the method of Rytel and Kilbourne.[16]

TABLE 2

Serum interferon response in mice at different times after poly I · C inoculation*

Poly I · C time (hr)	Log_{10} IF/ml
None	<1.0
4	3.6
12	4.3
24	3.6
48	3.3

*A single dose of 150 μg of poly I · C/animal was injected intraperitoneally in mice. The animals were sacrificed at different times after inoculation and their serum interferon levels were determined by the 50% VSV plaque reduction technique.[17]

in Fig. 1 indicate that significant protection was provided when the poly I · C was given between 48 hr prior to, and 24 hr after challenge. Protection was almost complete when poly I · C was given 12 hr prior to challenge. In contrast no protection was observed when the inducer was given on the second or fourth day after challenge.

When serum IF concentrations were determined at different times after poly I · C inoculation, maximal production was obtained 12 hr after induction (Table 2). This time period coincided with the period when the animals exhibited maximal protection to challenge with coxsackievirus. The protection decreased with increasing intervals between induction and challenge.

Previous studies have shown that poly I · C induces high levels of serum IF in mice within a few hours of inoculation.[13,19] Numerous studies have also demonstrated that IF provides resistance to a variety of experimental viral infections.[12-14] The inhibition of myocarditis by poly I · C in the present study can therefore also be attributed to be due to the induction of IF. The fact that the inducer no longer provides protection when administered 48 hr after challenge indicated that by this time the infectious process may have either progressed to the point that IF was ineffective in preventing damage, or the protective effect of the single induction of IF may have waned. Rytel and Kilbourne[16] have shown that in experimental infection of mice with coxsackievirus B-3, the severity of cardiac lesions begins to increase rapidly after 24 hr postchallenge attaining almost maximum severity by 72 hr. Furthermore, the present results show that the protective effect induced by poly I · C decreases as a function of time when it is given 24 hr or more before the challenge. This is in agreement with the reported kinetics of IF induction and duration.[16,20,21]

Since a single dose of poly I · C in the present experiment provided a significant degree of therapeutic effect, it would be interesting to examine the effect of a multiple dose schedule on coxsackievirus-induced myocarditis. Daily treatments of Semliki Forest virus–infected mice with 100 μg of poly I · C (ip) have been reported to be most effective in reducing mortality compared to other dose schedules tested.[22]

Summary

A single dose of the synthetic double-stranded polynucleotide poly I · C inoculated intraperitoneally into mice 12 to 48 hr before challenge with coxsackievirus B-3 resulted in almost complete protection from virus-induced myocarditis. Protection was related to the presence of high titers of circulating IF in the serum. Significant protection was also obtained even when poly I · C was given 24 hr after challenge with coxsackievirus.

REFERENCES

1. Woodward, T.E., Togo, Y., Lee, Y., and Hornick, R.B.: Arch. Intern. Med. **120**:279, 1967.
2. Smith, W.G.: Amer. Heart J. **73**:439, 1967.
3. Smith, W.G.: Amer. Heart J. **80**:34, 1970.
4. Javett, S.N., Heymann, S., Mundel, B., Pepler, W.J., Lurie, H.I., Gear, J., Measroch, V., and Kirsch, Z.: J. Pediat. **48**:1, 1956.
5. Sussman, K.L., Strauss, L., and Hodes, H.L.: AMA J. Dis. Child. **97**:483, 1959.
6. Burch G.E., Sun, S-C., Chu, K-C., Sohal, R.S., and Colcolough, H.L.: J. Amer. Med. Ass. **203**:1, 1968.
7. Fletcher, E., and Brennan, C.F.: Lancet **1**:913, 1957.
8. Burch, G.E., and Colcolough, H.L.: Ann. Intern. Med. **71**:(5), 963, 1969.
9. Grist, N.R., and Bell, E.J.: Amer. Heart J. **77**:295, 1969.
10. Grodums, E.I., and Dempster, G.: Can. J. Microbiol. **5**:605, 1959.
11. Field, A.K., Tyrell, A.A., Lampson, G.P., and Hilleman, M.R.: Proc. Nat. Acad. Sci. USA **58**:1004, 1967.
12. Gresser, L., Bourali, C., Thouas, M.T., and Falcoff, E.: Proc. Soc. Exp. Biol. Med. **127**:491, 1968.
13. Catalano, L.W., and Baron, S.: Proc. Soc. Exp. Biol. Med. **133**:684, 1970.
14. Richmond, J.Y., and Hamilton, L.D.: Proc. Nat. Acad. Sci. USA **64**:81, 1969.
15. Grodums, E.I., and Dempster, G.: Can. J. Microbiol. **5**:595, 1959.
16. Rytel, M.W., and Kilbourne, E.D.: Proc. Soc. Exp. Biol. Med. **137**:443, 1971.
17. Wagner, R.R.: Virology **13**:323, 1961.
18. Murphy, E.R., and Glasgow, L.A.: J. Exp. Med. **127**:1035, 1968.
19. Youngner, J.S., and Hallum, J.V.: Virology **35**:177, 1968.
20. DuBuy, H.G., Johnson, M.O., Buckler, C.E., and Baron, S.: Proc. Soc. Exp. Biol. Med. **135**:349, 1970.
21. Buckler, C.E., DuBuy, H.G., Johnson, M.L., and Baron, S.: Proc. Soc. Exp. Biol. Med. **136**:394, 1971.
22. Worthington, M., and Baron, S.: Proc. Soc. Exp. Biol. Med. **136**:323, 1971.

≡ READING 8

The opinion that sensitized T lymphocytes exert their major cytotoxic effects only by cell-cell contact with the target cell is an idea which has by now totally collapsed, despite its long history as a basic tenet of CMI. In this article, reprinted from *Science* **172**:729-731, 1972 (copyright 1972, the American Association for the Advancement of Science), the investigators have exposed PPD-sensitive lymphocytes to PPD, to medium lacking antigen, and to a heterologous antigen. This latter type of control with an unrelated antigen now is becoming standard in studies of cellular immunity, although it has been a traditional part of serologic studies for years. Only recently, in comparison, have cellular immunologists guarded themselves against nonspecific stimulatory effects by incorporating additional controls. Purified supernatant fluids, with potent MIF activity, and fluids from the control systems were tested in vivo for their ability to impair tumor growth, and only the experimental MIF material was active. This material was inactive on distantly placed tumors (thereby possibly limiting its potential therapeutic use). Nonetheless an anti-tumor product is released by cells that are not specifically sensitized to the tumor, and this material can be purified easily. The article reveals the type of experiments and data being accumulated and published currently in the area of tumor immunology.

TUMOR IMMUNITY: TUMOR SUPPRESSION IN VIVO INITIATED BY SOLUBLE PRODUCTS OF SPECIFICALLY STIMULATED LYMPHYOCYTES

Irwin D. Bernstein, Daniel E. Thor, Berton Zbar, and Herbert J. Rapp*

Abstract. Supernatant fluids of specifically stimulated lymphocyte cultures were purified. Fractions containing migration inhibition factor when injected intradermally into strain-2 guinea pigs produced a reaction similar in appearance to delayed cutaneous hypersensitivity. There was an accumulation of mononuclear cells at the injection sites and the growth of syngenetic tumor grafts at the sites was suppressed.

The immunologic rejection of tumors in syngeneic animals is mediated by specifically sensitized lymphoid cells.[1] Delayed hypersensitivity has been

*Biology Branch, National Cancer Institute and Laboratory of Virology and Rickettsiology, Division of Biologics Standards, Bethesda, Maryland 20014.

associated with the rejection of some syngeneic hepatomas induced by diethylnitrosamine.[2] However, hepatomas that do not provoke a delayed hypersensitivity reaction can be inhibited at the site of a delayed hypersensitivity reaction initiated by an unrelated antigen. Delayed hypersensitivity reactions consist of the specific recognition of an antigen by a relatively small number of sensitized lymphocytes followed by the accumulation of a relatively large number of mononuclear cells.[3] We have found that macrophages from unimmunized animals, but not neutrophils or lymphocytes, can inhibit the growth of one of these tumors in vivo and in vitro.[4] Cell-mediated tumor immunity, therefore, requires at least two distinct reactions: (i) specific interaction of sensitized lymphocytes and tumor cell antigen, and (ii) the local accumulation of mononuclear cells that prevent the growth of tumor cells at that site.

Lymphocytes incubated in vitro with the specific antigen to which they were sensitized produce substances that (i) inhibit the migration of macrophages from capillary tubes,[5] (ii) are cytotoxic in vitro,[6] (iii) are leukotactic,[7] and (iv) can give skin reactions similar to delayed hypersensitivity.[8] Tumor cell antigens have been shown to cause the release of macrophage migration inhibition factor (MIF).[9] We have been able to obtain inhibition of tumor growth at sites of inflammatory reactions produced by the intradermal injections of crude supernatants of specifically stimulated lymphocyte cultures.[10] In this report we show that intradermal injection of tissue culture fluids containing MIF is followed by the accumulation of mononuclear cells and an inflammatory response at the site of injection. The growth of tumors at these sites is inhibited.

Age-matched, adult, Sewall-Wright NIH inbred strain-2 guinea pigs were used. Induction of primary hepatomas by the administration of diethylnitrosamine in the drinking water and the formation of an ascites variant have been described.[11] Ascites cells from the sixth generation of a transplantable hepatoma (line 10) were prepared.[12] In all experiments 10^6 tumor cells mixed with the appropriate reagent were injected intradermally in a volume of 0.1 ml. Each result given is the mean for three animals.

Inbred strain-2 guinea pigs were immunized by the injection of heat-killed *Mycobacterium tuberculosis* (0.1 ml, H37Rv strain 2 mg/ml in a 1:1 mixture of 0.15M NaCl and 15 percent Arlacel A in Bayol F) into each footpad and posterior nuchal area (five injections). Fourteen to 18 days later the animals were killed, the lymph nodes collected, and cell suspensions made as previously described.[13] The cells were washed with Hanks balanced salt solution and resuspended in RPMI-1640 tissue culture medium to contain 3 to 4×10^6 viable cells per milliliter (1.2 to 1.6×10^7 per 4-ml of culture). The medium contained fresh frozen glutamine (15 mg/liter) and Ampicillin (100 µg/ml at 288 milliosmoles, pH 7.4). Cultures for MIF production contained PPD-S antigen (10 µg/ml) without preservation. Two control cultures were included: one without antigen (control A) and one with coccidioidin, an antigen unrelated to tubercle bacilli (control D). The supernatants, after 36 hours, were harvested, dialyzed against distilled water, lyophilized, and kept frozen at $-70°$ C. Lyophilized samples were reconstituted with distilled water, and fractionated by gel filtration on Sephadex columns; the peak of biologic activity was located by testing the fractions for capillary migration inhibition.[13] Sephadex G-75 was eluted with 0.01M borate buffer, pH 8, and the fraction having a molecular weight of 30,000 to 40,000 was collected and found to contain the MIF activity by the indirect assay. Pooled fractions of this peak were lyophilized and redissolved in 0.01M tris buffer, pH 8.7, and fractionated further by electrophoresis on polyacrylamide gel. With a 10 percent gel, separation pH 10.2, concentration pH 9.65, on a 1 by 20 cm column, electrophoresis was performed at $4°$ C (200 volts, 5 to 10 ma). The active MIF fraction migrated ahead of albumin. In the stained gel there was no visible band in the area containing active MIF. Active MIF could be eluted from the gel either by extraction of minced sections of gel in distilled water or by continued electrophoresis from individual sections into dialysis bags. The purified MIF fraction was dissolved in a volume of medium equal to the volume of the original supernatant fluid obtained from the lymphocyte cultures. MIF activity was present at this final concentration. Corresponding fractions of control A from Sephadex and polyacrylamide gels were used. An additional control consisting of supernatant fluid from unstimulated lymphocyte cultures and an amount of PPD-S equivalent to the maximal possible amount in the purified material had shown neither inflammatory nor tumor-inhibiting activity.

Fluids containing MIF and control fluids were injected intradermally. Skin reactions to fluids contain-

ing MIF were present at 3 to 4 hours and reached maximal size between 12 and 24 hours; there was no reaction to the intradermal injection of control fluids. Histologic sections of reaction sites taken at 24 hours revealed a typical picture of tuberculin hypersensitivity reaction. There was a preponderance (70 to 80 percent) of mononuclear cells. Supernatants incu-

---

TABLE 1

Inhibition of tumor growth in vivo by tissue culture fluids containing MIF

Supernatant injected*	Delayed hypersensitivity skin reactions at 24 hours† (mm²)	Size of intradermal tumor papule on day 14† (mm²)
Control A	0	15 ± 1.0
Supernatant containing MIF	15.6 ± 2.5	0
Control D	0	9.3 ± 0.7
Medium 199	0	6.0 ± 1.0

*10^7 Tumor cells per milliliter of supernatant were incubated at 37° C for 10 minutes; 0.1 ml of the mixture was injected intradermally at each site.
†Results are expressed as means of the average radius squared (mm²) ± standard error of the mean.

TABLE 2

Tumor growth in vivo at a site adjacent to MIF-mediated rejection of tumor cells

Supernatant injected*	Growth of tumor cells inoculated in medium 199: size of papule on day 14†	Growth of tumor cells inoculated in MIF or control supernatants: size of papule on day 14†
Control A	19.9 ± 1.0	20 ± 2.3
Supernatant containing MIF	17.7 ± 3.0	0
Control D	16.2 ± 2.3	18.1 ± 1.2

*10^7 Tumor cells per milliliter of supernatant or medium 199 were incubated at 37° C for 10 minutes; 0.1 ml of the mixture was injected intradermally at each site. The distance between sites of tumor rejection and adjacent tumor sites was 1.5 to 2.0 cm.
†Results are expressed as mean of the average radius squared (mm²) ± standard error of the mean.

TABLE 3

Inhibition of tumor growth at sites of skin reactions to MIF

Supernatant injected*	Size of skin reaction at 24 hours† (mm²)	Size of tumor papule at 14 days† (mm²)
Control A	0	7.1 ± 2.6
Supernatant containing MIF	16.4 ± 1.2	0.2 ± 0.2
Control D	0	5.9 ± 3.2

*0.1 ml of each supernatant was injected intradermally 24 hours prior to the injection of 10^6 tumor cells in a volume of 0.1 ml into each site.
†Results are expressed as mean of the average radius squared (mm²) ± standard error of the mean.

bated with tumor cells were injected intradermally. The results of this experiment are shown in Table 1. It can be seen that fluids containing MIF inhibit tumor growth and control fluids do not.

We next tested whether tumor rejection initiated by MIF at one intradermal site would affect tumor growth at another intradermal site. The design and results of this experiment are given in Table 2. It can be seen that a tumor adjacent to a rejected tumor was unaffected. This observation opposes the view that tumor rejection initiated by MIF was due to a systemic adjuvant effect.

It is possible that supernatants containing MIF exert a direct cytotoxic effect on tumor cells. In order to test this possibility, tumor cells were inoculated into skin sites where MIF or control supernatants had been injected 24 hours earlier. Tumor cell growth was inhibited (see Table 3) at sites where an inflammatory reaction was present before tumor cells were injected. This observation favors the view that tumor rejection was due to host cells rather than to a direct effect by MIF.

These experiments support the concept that animals immunized to a given tumor contain lymphocytes capable of specific immunologic interaction with that tumor and that following this interaction, the lymphocytes elaborate substances that cause the accumulation of mononuclear cells; these mononuclear cells are then responsible for the rejection of tumor grafts. Present evidence indicates that this activity of the mononuclear cells is immunologically nonspecific, and, therefore, tumor rejection by these cells does not require their specific recognition of tumor antigen.

REFERENCES

1. Old, L.J., Boyse, E.A., Clarke, D.A., and Carswell, E.A.: Ann. N.Y. Acad. Sci. **101**:80, 1962-63; Klein, G., Sjögren, H.O., Klein, E., and Hellström, K.E.: Cancer Res. **20**:1561, 1960.

2. Zbar, B., Wepsic, H.T., Rapp, H.J., Borsos, T., Kronman, B.S., and Churchill, W.H., Jr.: J. Nat. Cancer Inst. **43**:833, 1969; Zbar, B., Wepsic, H.T., Borsos, T., and Rapp, H.J.: ibid. **44**:473, 1970.

3. McCluskey, R.T., Benacerraf, B., and McCluskey, J.W.: J. Immunol. **90**:466, 1963.

4. Zbar, B., Bernstein, I.D., Wepsic, H.T., Stewart, L., Borsos, T., and Rapp, H.J.: in preparation: Oppenheim, J., Zbar, B., and Rapp, H.J.: Proc. Nat. Acad. Sci. U.S. **66**:119, 1970.

5. Bloom, B.R., and Bennett, B.: Science **153**:80, 1966; Bennett, B., and Bloom, B.R.: Proc. Nat. Acad. Sci. U.S. **59**:759, 1968; Bloom, B.R., and Bennett, B.: Ann. N.Y. Acad. Sci. **169**:258, 1970; David, J.R., in Landy, M., and Lawrence, H.S., editors: Mediators of Cellular Immunity, New York, 1969, Academic Press; David, J.R.: Proc. Nat. Acad. Sci. U.S. **56**:72, 1966; Thor, D., Jureziz, R.E., Veach, S.R., Miller, E., and Dray, S.: Nature **219**:5155, 1968; Thor, D., in Landy, M., and Lawrence, H.S., Editors: Mediators of Cellular Immunity, New York, 1969, Academic Press.

6. Ruddle, N.H., and Waksman, B.H.: Science **157**:1060, 1967; J. Exp. Med. **128**:1267, 1968; Granger, G.A., and Kolb, W.P.: J. Immunol. **101**:111, 1968; Granger, G.A., in Landy, M., and Lawrence, H.S., Editors: Mediators of Cellular Immunity, New York, 1969, Academic Press.

7. Ward, P.A., Remold, H.G., and David, J.R.: Science **163**:1081, 1969.

8. Bennett, B., and Bloom, B.R.: Proc. Nat. Acad. Sci. U.S. **59**:756, 1968; Pick, E., Krevci, J., Coch, K., and Turk, J.L.: Immunology **17**:741, 1969; Turk, J.L., in Landy, M., and Lawrence, H.S., Editors: Mediators of Cellular Immunity, New York, 1969, Academic Press.

9. Kronman, B.S., Wepsic, H.T., Churchill, W.H., Jr., Zbar, B., Borsos, T., and Rapp, H.J.: Science **165**:296, 1969; Bloom, B.R., Bennett, B., Oettgen, H.F., McLean, E.P, and Old, L.J.: Proc. Nat. Acad. Sci. U.S. **64**:1176, 1969.

10. Bernstein, I.D., Thor, D.E., Zbar, B., and Rapp, H.J.: unpublished observations.

11. Rapp, H.J., Churchill, W.H., Jr., Kronman, B.S., Rolley, R.T., Hammond, W.G., and Borsos, T.: J. Nat. Cancer Inst. **41**:1, 1968.

12. Churchill, W.H., Jr., Rapp, H.J., Kronman, B.S., and Borsos, T.: ibid., p. 13.

13. Thor, D.E., and Dray, S.: J. Immunol. **101**:51, 1968; Thor, D.E., in Bloom, B., and Glade, P., Editors: In vitro Methods of Cellular Immunity, New York, 1971, Academic Press.

INDEX

Index

A

Abequose, structure of, 247
ABO(H) blood group system, 232-236
Acidic radicals and serologic specificity, 42
Acquired immune deficiency syndrome, 394-395
  definition of, 386
Actin, neutrophil, dysfunction of, 402
Actinomycin D, 162
ADA; *see* Adenosine deaminase
ADCC; *see* Antibody-dependent cell cytotoxicity
Adenosine deaminase, 393-394
Adherence, immune, 180
  definition of, 165
Adjuvant therapy, 296-297
  definition of, 272
Adjuvants, 43-46
  definition of, 25
Adrenaline, 331
Adsorption, agglutinin, definition of, 232
AFP; *see* α-Fetoprotein
Agammaglobulinemia, 387
  Bruton's, 389-390
    definition of, 386
  congenital, 389
  definition of, 386
  sex-linked, 392
  Swiss-type, 392-393
    definition of, 386
Agar plaque technique, 150
Age and immunity, 253
Agglutination, 232-247
  bacterial, 11, 242, 244-247
    H, 242, 244
    O, 242, 244
  cross, 245-246
  definition of, 232
  passive, 240-242
    for human chorionic gonadotropin, 242
Agglutinins
  adsorption of, 245-246
  cold, definition of, 357

Agglutinins—cont'd
  definition of, 232
  warm, definition of, 357
AHP; *see* α₂-Hepatic protein
AIDS; *see* Acquired immune deficiency syndrome
Alexin, 12
ALG; *see* Antilymphocyte globulin
Alkaline phosphatase, 212
  isozymes of, 291
Alkylating agents, 159-161
  definition of, 146
Allelic exclusion, 72-73
Allergen, definition of, 301
Allergy
  anaphylactic, definition of, 301
  cytotoxic, definition of, 301
  definition of, 301
  immune complex, 213
  of infection, 350-352
    definition of, 337
  ingestant, 334
  inhalant, 333-334
  injectant, 334-335
  introduction to, 301-306
  precipitin, 338
  T cell–mediated, definition of, 301
Alloantibody, definition of, 25
Alloantigen, definition of, 25
Allogenic, definition of, 272
Allograft, definition of, 272
Alloimmunization, 35
  definition of, 25
ALS; *see* Antilymphocyte serum
Am marker, definition of, 47
Amethopterin, 159, 160
Amine, vasoactive, definition of, 308
p-Aminobenzylcellulose, 74-75
Aminopterin, 159, 160
Ana INH, 181
  definition of, 165
Anamnestic response, definition of, 146